PRINCIPLES AND PRACTICE OF AVIATION MEDICINE

PRINCIPLES AND PRACTICE OF AVIATION MEDICINE

editors

Claus Curdt-Christiansen

International Civil Aviation Organization, Montreal

Jörg Draeger

University of Hamburg, Germany

Jürgen Kriebel

Aero Medical Center, Lufthansa AG, Frankfurt, Germany

World Scientific

NEW JERSEY • LONDON • SINGAPORE • BEIJING • SHANGHAI • HONG KONG • TAIPEI • CHENNAI

Published by

World Scientific Publishing Co. Pte. Ltd.
5 Toh Tuck Link, Singapore 596224
USA office: 27 Warren Street, Suite 401-402, Hackensack, NJ 07601
UK office: 57 Shelton Street, Covent Garden, London WC2H 9HE

Library of Congress Cataloging-in-Publication Data
Principles and practice of aviation medicine / editors, Claus Curdt-Christiansen, Jörg Draeger, Jürgen Kriebel.
p. ; cm.
Includes bibliographical references and index.
ISBN-13: 978-981-238-861-2 (hardcover : alk. paper)
ISBN-10: 981-238-861-3 (hardcover : alk. paper)
1. Aviation medicine. I. Curdt-Christiansen, Claus. II. Draeger, Jörg, Prof. Dr. III. Kriebel, Jürgen.
[DNLM: 1. Aerospace Medicine--methods. 2. Aerospace Medicine--standards. WD 700 P952 2009]
RC1062.P75 2009
616.9'80213--dc22

2009013320

British Library Cataloguing-in-Publication Data
A catalogue record for this book is available from the British Library.

Typeset by Stallion Press
Email: enquiries@stallionpress.com

Printed by FuIsland Offset Printing (S) Pte Ltd. Singapore

Prologue

Aviation is at the heart of world development. Man, with all his physical and mental shortcomings, is at the heart of aviation. But just as modern life is inconceivable without aviation, aviation cannot exist without its weakest link, the human being. The aviation environment, however, is hostile to humans. Soon after the first balloon flights more than 200 years ago, it became clear that man was unable to function and survive at altitude without special protection and support. With the advent of powered flight more than 100 years ago, the need for physiological and medical support became obvious. Doctors supporting the military flight operations of World War I realized that selection criteria had to be developed to reduce the high number of losses of both aircraft and pilots. Following the Peace Conference in Paris in 1919, the first international medical requirements for licensing of aviators were agreed upon, and over the ensuing years these international standards have been further developed. Since then powered flight has evolved considerably and so has the specialty of aviation medicine. The medical standards for licensing of pilots, i.e. the medical requirements an applicant must meet to be accepted for initial training and which all trained and licensed pilots must meet at their regulatory renewal examinations, have always been restrictive and conservative. This is an obvious necessity. The purpose of the requirements is to maintain and secure the high level of safety that characterizes modern aviation — a goal that leaves little room for experimenting with or relaxing the requirements. However, many medical conditions that were considered permanently disqualifying in the past are now allowed as a result of continuous improvement in our understanding of the physiology of flight, the evolution of evidence-based medicine, and the vast technical advances of recent years in diagnosis and treatment.

All medical standards have three different aspects that always must be considered together. The first is the requirement *per se*, e.g., epilepsy entails unfitness for all classes of medical certification, or blood pressure shall be within normal limits. The second aspect is the method or methods traditionally employed or sometimes prescribed by the Licensing Authority for carrying out the examination. The third aspect is the definitions applied to the requirements. For example, how is epilepsy defined or what are the normal limits for arterial tension? Although most countries have accepted the international standards and recommended practices developed and continually updated by the International Civil Aviation Organization (ICAO), there are still significant differences from one country to another pertaining to the methods of examination. Examining the visual fields of a pilot by confrontational testing with finger movements compared to examining by automated, computerized perimetry provides results on very different levels of reliability. The use of different methods of examination vary from country to country is hardly a surprise; different countries have different cultures, different socio-economical conditions, different prevalences of many diseases, different medical traditions, and different attitudes to the relevance of safety precautions.

Modern civil aviation, however, is international. A modern airliner has the same needs and demands for ground support wherever it happens to be in the world. Almost 200 countries are currently connected with each other by regular commercial flights and none can afford to reject the international community and refuse to provide the infrastructure necessary to ensure the safety of aviation. All signatories to the Convention on International Civil Aviation ("Chicago Convention") of 1944, currently totaling 191 countries, have undertaken to collaborate in securing the highest practicable degree of uniformity in relation to aircraft, aviation personnel, licensing procedures, etc., including medical certification of pilots and air traffic controllers. Even so, there are still significant differences regarding national approaches to aeromedical certification. To some extent, these differences are related to the influence that military aviation medicine has had upon civil aviation medicine. Also relevant is the comparative level of development that aviation medicine (as a medical specialty) has reached in different countries. While in some countries aviation medicine was a highly-developed medical specialty even before World War II, in other countries aviation medicine is only beginning to establish itself as a recognized specialty.

Most countries have agreed on the need to implement medical requirements for aviation personnel and have adopted the ICAO International Medical Standards and Recommended Practices or developed their own medical standards in accordance with the ICAO provisions. The next step towards uniformity in medical certification must be to help medical examiners and medical assessors worldwide adopt similar methods of examination and similar definitions of diseases and disorders. In particular, agreement on definitions and similar interpretation of the signs and symptoms of diseases and disorders are required if global harmonization in aeromedical certification is to be achieved.

This book contains detailed, experience-based, practical knowledge written to assist aviation medical examiners (AMEs) and other clinicians, as well as medical assessors of the Licensing Authorities, in the often confusing world of medical treatment and aeromedical evaluation of safety-critical aviation personnel such as pilots, cabin crew members, and air traffic controllers. In addition, it provides medical guidelines for physicians who have patients with medical conditions who wish to travel by air. This book is written by AMEs and clinicians from a wide range of medical specialties that are important to the field of aviation medicine. It initially began as a reference book for German physicians who may or may not be AMEs, yet who are involved in the health care of pilots. It has expanded to this current English version to address an international audience in order to provide guidance and advice to colleagues in the practice of clinical aviation medicine. Considering the European background of the authors, this book represents European points of view and international or European criteria regarding the determination of fitness for duty among civil aviation personnel. It is, nonetheless, an excellent and detailed international guide for medical practitioners in all parts of the world who deal with aircrew members and airline passengers.

Aviation medicine is a scientific discipline that involves the study of the physiological, psychological, operational, and environmental factors that determine the adaptive responses of a human being during flight. With regard to flight crews, the focus is different from that of the "conventional" clinical specialties which primarily deal with abnormal physiology within a normal environment, as it is concerned with normal physiology within an abnormal environment. With regard to passengers, however, conventional and aviation medicine intersect because at times abnormal physiology may be placed within an abnormal environment. This is also the case when it comes to determining exactly to what degree, i.e., with what limitations or restrictions or under what conditions, a pilot with a medical disorder may be able to perform his duties without endangering flight safety. It is to this highly specialized field of clinical aviation medicine that most chapters of the book are dedicated.

Flying represents a hostile environment that imposes a variety of physical, physiological, and psychological demands on human beings who are not genetically adapted to function in such an environment. Promoting the health and well being of aviation personnel worldwide is essential for the safety of all flight operations in civil aviation. It is also very important to recognize the potential consequences that the flight environment can have on those individuals who have pre-existing medical conditions and wish to travel by air or are required to be transported or medically evacuated by aircraft. Therefore, medical practitioners must possess basic knowledge of aviation physiology and medicine in order to make appropriate decisions concerning medical certification of pilots and other flight personnel. Such knowledge is also essential in making the correct decisions concerning the safe medical transport of diseased passengers aboard commercial aircraft or the medical transport (elective or emergency) of patients by air ambulance.

Most university programs that train medical professionals do not include instruction in the basic principles of aviation physiology or medicine. Some countries offer basic and advanced post-graduate training in aviation medicine, but very few offer formal residency programs (specialty) in aviation medicine. Therefore, this book will benefit medical practitioners in many countries that do not have national access to post-graduate training in aviation medicine. It will also be a good source of clinical, aeromedical knowledge for those who are enrolled in post-graduate training programs in aviation medicine.

Any professional publication that contributes to our existing body of knowledge in aviation medicine is very welcome since there are not many up-to-date publications that specifically address the clinical aspects of aviation medicine. Therefore, this book represents an important addition to the international literature on aviation medicine in general, and to its clinical aspects in particular.

The contributing authors' knowledge of aviation medicine, significant clinical experiences, and international professional recognition among colleagues make this book an excellent addition to any aviation medicine practitioner's personal library.

Dr. Melchor Joaquín Antuñano
Director, Civil Aerospace Medical Institute —
Federal Aviation Administration

Past-President and Fellow,
Aerospace Medical Association

Past-President, Space Medicine Society

Past-President, Iberoamerican
Association of Aerospace Medicine

Member and Chancellor of the International
Academy of Aviation and Space Medicine

Member of the International Academy of Astronautics

Honorary Member of the Colombian, Greek,
Brazilian, Mexican, Slovenian and Turkish
Aerospace Medicine Societies

Preface and Acknowledgement

Aviation medicine is a medical specialty which combines aspects of preventive, occupational, environmental and clinical medicine with the physiology and psychology of man in flight. It is concerned with the health and safety of those who fly, both crew and passengers, as well as the selection and performance of those who hold aviation licences.

This book provides practice-oriented information on evaluation of fitness to fly and medical certification of those who want to acquire or maintain an aviation licence. The focus is on uniform methods of examination and assessment of pilots, both professional and private, cabin crew members, and air traffic controllers. In order to increase the book's clarity and usefulness for practical application, common diseases and disorders are discussed; those rarely encountered in aviation medicine practice are excluded.

A symbolic summary of this book is depicted on the cover by the "aeromedical homunculus." As the area of anatomical representation increases with the complexity of the sensory-motor function, the sensory-motor homunculus represents the connection between different body parts and the corresponding areas in the hemispheres of the brain. The body on the left side is the *motor homunculus,* lying in front of the central sulcus (CS) of the brain. The bigger the body parts in this picture are, the more brainpower is required to control them. The body half on the right is the *sensory homunculus,* lying behind the CS. It is similar to the motor homunculus except that it depicts how much brain power is dedicated to receiving sensory input from the different body parts. By analogy, the "aeromedical homunculus" in the middle has organs whose relative size symbolizes their aeromedical significance. The dominance of the heart (and therefore of aviation cardiology) makes an extracorporeal depiction necessary. The importance of the eyes and ears (and therefore of aviation ophthalmology and otology) leaves hardly any room for the brain, which — being the most important of all organs — has been moved to the front and given its own, separate space. The gap where the liver should have been alludes to the easily overlooked exogenous and toxic risks.

The different sizes of the organs of the "aeromedical homunculus" are also correlated to the selection of medical topics and the degree of detail and comprehensiveness with which they are treated in the various chapters of the book.

Regarding the significance of clinical aviation medicine, one should not overlook the fact that aviation incidents and accidents have remained relatively constant in recent decades, with human factors causing or contributing to about 80 percent. This gives emphasis to the importance of aviation psychology. The criteria for mental fitness and psychological testing as well as the significance of crew coordination and cockpit resource management are described. A separate chapter deals with the less understood and often underestimated influence of psycho-social stressors. Through disruption of the man-machine interface, the problems of daily life may become a threat to aviation safety. Consequences of head injuries or diseases affecting the brain are sometimes overlooked as licence holders construct facades to hide their loss of flying skills. This is discussed in depth in a chapter on the relevant neuro-psychological conditions and disorders.

An aeromedical book intended for an international readership constantly collides with transcultural issues. In order to minimize the risk inherent in all aviation activities, international regulations (ICAO International Standards and Recommended Practices, SARPs) have been developed and agreed to by virtually all countries in the world. In this context, it is surprising that aviation medicine still exhibits a large degree of international variation. Each country issues its own aeromedical requirements in accordance with, but not necessarily identical with, the international SARPs of ICAO, but each country has it own aeromedical traditions and a national understanding of the medical problems involved in flying. Even the nomenclature of medical certification is not uniform, e.g. FAA Class 3 medical certification corresponds to JAA Class 2. In addition, there are still national differences with regard to the retirement age for commercial pilots, although the international age limit of 65 years is gaining global acceptance.

The editors are proud to have succeeded in acquiring the co-operation and contributions of several of the leading experts from the various fields of operational aviation medicine. The majority of these experts have for years been engaged in both the clinical and the regulatory aspects of aviation medicine in their capacity as members of the Aviation Medicine Committee of the Federal Minister of Transportation.

The physiological basis for aviation medicine, outlined by two eminent experts, provides the basic theoretical foundation for the following clinical sections.

A chapter on the history of aviation medicine gives the interested reader a stimulating insight into the methodological development of a very specialized field of medicine which, in the words of Dr. Silvio Finkelstein, former Chief of Aviation Medicine Section of ICAO is "invisible but essential."

In addition to the International Standards and Recommended Practices of ICAO, the JAR-FCL 3 medical requirements as well as the FAA rules for licensing are described.

Finally, a chapter on passenger health, written by Dr. Petra Illig, has been added. It deals with several aspects of aviation medicine of importance not only for those who practise aviation medicine but for all medical practitioners who in their daily practice meet people who fly.

Claus Curdt-Christiansen
Jörg Dräger
Jürgen Kriebel

Contents

List of Abbreviations, Acronyms and Units

ACC	American College of Cardiology
ACE	angiotensin converting enzyme
AED	automated external defibrillator
AeMC	aeromedical centre
AF	atrial fibrillation
AHA	American Heart Association
AI	aortic insufficiency
AIDS	acquired immuno-deficiency syndrome
AMC	aeromedical center; acceptable means of compliance
AME	authorized medical examiner
AMS	aeromedical section (of the Licensing Authority) ~ CMO's office
ANC	active noise compensation
AP	angina pectoris
AS	aortic stenosis
ASA	acetyl salicylic acid (Aspirin®); atrial septal aneurysm
ASD	atrial septal defect
AsMA	Aerospace Medical Association
AT_1	angiotensin type 1
ATP	adenosine triphosphate
ATPL	airline transport pilot licence
BPPV	benign positional paroxysmal vertigo
BMI	body mass index

BP	blood pressure
CAA	civil aviation authority
CAB	civil aeronautics board
CABG	coronary artery by-pass graft
CACS	coronary artery calcium score
CAD	coronary artery disease
CAMI	Civil Aerospace Medical Institute (in Oklahoma City)
CCS	Canadian Cardiovascular Society
CCT	cranial CT
CDC	Centers for Disease Control & Prevention (in Atlanta)
CDT	carbohydrate-deficient transferrin
CHD	coronary heart disease
CHF	congestive heart failure
CMO	chief medical officer
CMRI	cardiac MRI
CNS	central nervous system
COPD	chronic obstructive pulmonary disease
CPL	commercial pilot licence
CRM	crew resource management
CRP	C-reactive protein
CT	computerized tomography
CVA	cerebrovascular attack
D	dioptre
DCS	decompression sickness
DES	drug eluting stent
DIWS	document, imaging and workflow system
DNA	deoxyribonucleic acid
DSM-IV	Diagnostic and Statistic Manual of Mental Disorders, 4th Edition (American Psychiatric Association)
DVT	deep vein thrombosis
EASA	European Aviation Safety Agency
EBCT	electron beam computed tomography
EC	European Commission
ECG	electrocardiogram

EEC	electroencephalogram
EEMK	enhanced emergency medical kits
EF	ejection fraction
ENT	ear, nose and throat
ESC	European Society of Cardiology
EU	European Union
EURATOM	European Atomic Energy Community
FAA	Federal Aviation Administration
FCL	flight crew licensing
FFA	free fatty acids
FO	first officer
g	gravity, i.e. the gravitational attraction of the Earth
G	accelerative force (in multiples of g).
γ-GT	gamma-glutamyl-transferase
GND	ground
Gy	gray
HDL	high density lipoprotein
HEPA	high efficiency particulate air filter
hs-CRP	high-sensitivity CRP
Hz	hertz
IATA	International Air Transport Association
ICAO	International Civil Aviation Organization (a specialized agency of the United Nations with HQ in Montreal, Canada)
ICD	implantable cardioverter defibrillator
ICD-10	International Statistical Classification of Diseases and Related Health Problems, 10th revision (WHO).
ICRP	International Commission on Radiological Protection
IFR	instrument flight rules
IMA	internal mammary artery
INR	international normalized ratio
IPPPSH	International Prospective Primary Prevention Study in Hypertension
IR	implementing rule

ISA	international standard atmosphere
JAA	Joint Aviation Authorities
JAR	Joint Aviation Regulations
K	Kelvin
KeV	kilo electron volt
LA	left atrium
LAD	left anterior descending coronary artery
LBBB	left bundle branch block
LDL	low density lipoprotein
Lp(a)	lipoprotein a
LV	left ventricle
MAR	minimum angle of resolution
MCV	mean corpuscular volume
MEDIF	medical information sheet (IATA)
MET	metabolic equivalent
MeV	mega electron volt
MIDCAB	minimally invasive direct coronary artery by-pass
MRA	magnetic resonance angiogram
MRI	magnetic resonance imaging
MS	mitral stenosis
MSCT	multi-slice CT
MSL	mean sea level
mSv	milli sievert
MVP	mitral valve prolapse
N	newton; north
NOTAM	notification for airmen
NSAID	non-steroidal anti-inflammatory drug
NYHA	New York Heart Association
OML	operational multicrew limitation
OSL	operational single pilot limitation
P	pressure
Pa	pascal
PAC	premature atrial contraction
PBW	phonetically balanced words
PCI	percutaneous coronary intervention
PE	pulmonary emboli

PET	positron emission tomography
PFO	patent foramen ovale
PPL	private pilot licence
PS	pulmonary stenosis
PTCA	percutaneous transluminal coronary angioplasty
PTS	permanent threshold shift
PVC	premature ventricular contraction
R	specific gas constant
RBBB	right bundle branch block
RCA	right coronary artery
RQ	respiratory quotient
RV	right ventricle
SARP	Standards and Recommended Practices (ICAO)
SARS	severe acute respiratory syndrome
SHBG	sex hormone-binding globulin
SJM	St. Jude medical prosthesis
SODA	statement of demonstrated ability
SMR	standard mortality rate
SPECT	single photon emission computed tomography
SSRI	selective serotonin re-uptake inhibitor
SST	super sonic transport
STPD	standard temperature, pressure and air density
T	temperature
TEE	transesophageal echocardiography
TIA	transitory ischemic attack
TTS	temporary treshold shift
TUC	time of useful consciousness
URI	upper respiratory infection
V	volume
VAT	visceral adipose tissue
VF	ventricular fibrillation
VFR	visual flight rules
VOC	volatile organic compounds
VPN	virtual private network
VSD	ventricular septal defect
VLDL	very low density lipoprotein

VT	ventricular tachycardia
WHO	World Health Organization (a specialized agency of the United Nations with HQ in Geneva, Switzerland)
WHR	waist-to-hip ration
WOSCOPS	West of Scotland Coronary Prevention Study
WPW	Wolff-Parkinson-White syndrome
WRIGHT	WHO Research Into Global Hazards of Travel

Part 1

INTRODUCTION

Chapter 1

The History and Development of Aviation Medicine

Viktor Harsch*

The development of aviation medicine can only be understood in the context of the scientific advances and technical innovations that made flying possible, with balloons in the 18th century, with gliders in the 19th century, and with powered aircraft in the 20th century. The forerunner of aviation medicine was the study of high mountain physiology. The Jesuit priest J. A. de Acosta described the hypoxia symptoms he experienced during his stay in the Andes in the 16th century and thereby coined the term "mountain sickness." Chinese tradesmen also suffered from the symptoms of mountain sickness on their journeys through the Hindukush and the Karokorum mountains and reported these 1600 years before de Acosta did so in 1590.[1–3] Evangelista Torricelli (1608–1647) made an important contribution to altitude physiology with the development of the mercury barometer in 1643. Additionally, he coined the term "air-pressure" and was the first to perform animal experiments under negative pressure conditions.

Otto von Guericke (1602–1686) developed the air pump in 1650 and was thereby the first person to create a "vacuum" (1654). Only a few years later, in 1659, Robert Boyle (1627–1691) constructed an air pump. With the help of his colleague Robert Hooke (1635–1703), he operated the prototype of a vacuum chamber in 1677 (Fig. 1). By

[a] Paul Bert, 1878, includes 264 references about mountain sickness.[10]

* Joseph-Haydn-Weg 5, Neubrandenburg, Germany.

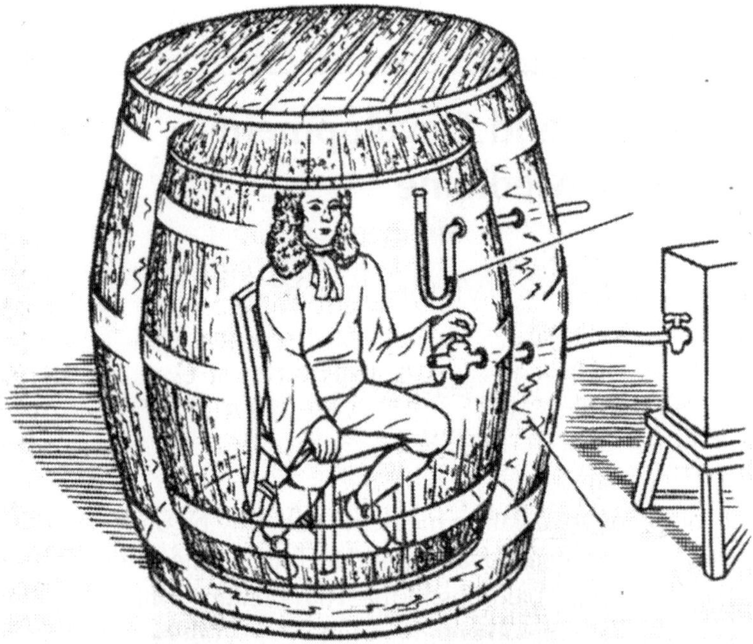

Figure 1. First altitude chamber used by Robert Hooke in 1677. In: Gazenko, 1987.

means of a self-experiment, he was able to form the first conclusions about altitude physiology after spending 15 minutes in the vacuum chamber at an equivalent altitude of about 2400 m (7875 ft). Another significant contribution was presented by Joseph Priestley (1733–1804), who discovered oxygen in 1774. Antoine Lavoisier (1743–1794) shortly afterwards recognized its meaning for oxidation.[2,4–6] By now, the fundamental knowledge for the understanding of altitude physiology had been established.

On November 1, 1783 the first manned flight took place when the French physicist Jean Francois Pilâtre de Rozier (1756–1785) and the officer François Laurent, Marquis d´Arlandes (1742–1809) undertook an ascent with a balloon, built by the Montgolfier brothers, reaching an altitude of 2700 feet (900 m). This date is known as the day aviation was born. de Rozier entered the annals again only two years after his first flight, but this time as the first victim of an aviation accident. In

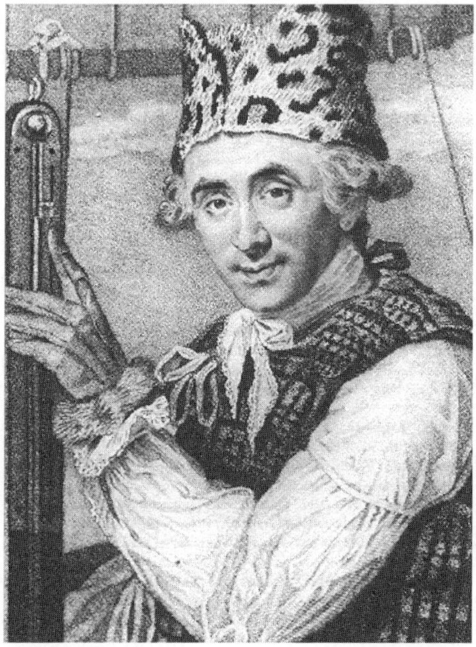

Figure 2. First flight-surgeon John Jeffries (1745–1819). In: Crough, 1983.

1785 the Frenchman Jean Pierre François Blanchard (1753–1809) and the American physician John Jeffries (1745–1819) crossed the British Channel in a balloon (Fig. 2), carrying out meteorological experiments. The development of the hydrogen balloon by the French physicist Jacques Alexandre César Charles (1746–1823) allowed greater heights to be reached, which raised serious medical problems: during his first ascent on December 1, 1783 Charles reached a height of over 8200 feet (2700 m) and in doing so experienced ear pain caused by the pressure change, hypothermia and the symptoms of mild hypoxia.[3,6,7]

In 1803, close to Hamburg in Germany, the French physicist, magician and balloonist Etienne-Gaspar Robert, better known as "Robertson," together with M. Lhoest reached a height of over 21 000 feet (7000 m) and reported a general apathy and an acceleration of the pulse[8]: "Our chest seemed expanded and lacked resilience, my pulse was hurried; that of M. Lhoest was less so; like mine, his lips were swollen, his eyes bloodshot; all the veins were rounded out and stood up in relief on my hands. The blood had rushed to my head so much that I noticed that my hat seemed too small."[b]

During the ascent by the Italians Andreoli, Brasette and Zambeccary in 1804 up to an altitude of more than 18 000 feet (6000 m), the limit of endurance for further altitude ascents became evident: the aeronauts suffered from frostbites in the upper and lower extremities, nausea and dizziness. However, all of them survived this adventure into the heights. Just over half a century hereafter, on September 5, 1862, the ascent of "Zenith" took the English scientists James Glaisher (1809–1903) and Henry Tracey Coxwell (1819–1900) within just under an hour to a height of over 26 800 feet (8800 m). They, too, fainted. Already at a height of 17 200 feet (5640 m) they noticed tachycardia, difficulties in breathing, and palpitation. Their lips and hands became cyanotic and they experienced difficulties in reading their instruments. 3000 feet (1000 m) higher, Glaisher felt clearly "seasick," and at 26 500 feet (8700 m) they were overpowered by exhaustion and slackness.[1–3,8,9] A scientific dealing with the most urgent high altitude physiological questions was therefore a condition sine qua non.

In his laboratory, the French physiologist Paul Bert (1830–1886) undertook a comprehensive investigation of the physiological effects of air-pressure, often using himself as a subject. His experiments laid the foundation for modern altitude physiology and explained the causes of altitude and decompression sickness: His publication "*La pression barométrique; recherches de physiologie expérimentale*" (1878) was a milestone, not just in the area of altitude physiology but also of experimental medicine in a broad sense. Bert used the altitude chamber in order to establish the physiological effect of pressure change and collected experimental results up to an altitude of 8800 m. This chamber was also used by the balloonists Joseph E. Crocé-Spinelli (1843–1875) and H. Theodore Sivel (1834–1875) for preparation of their altitude ascents (Fig. 3). In this connection they recognized

[b] Citation after P. Bert, 1878: 175.

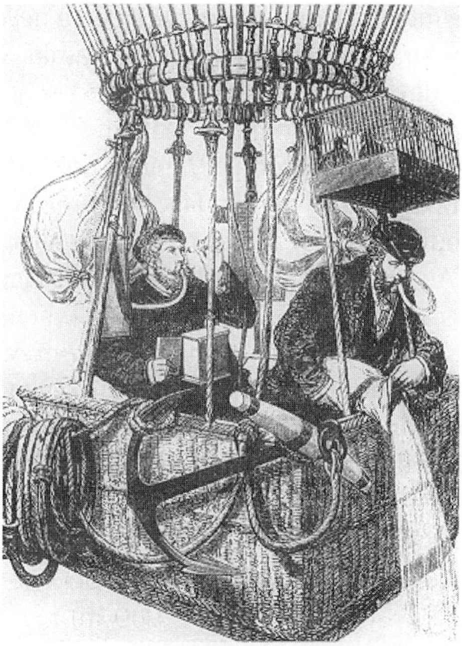

Figure 3. Ascent of H. T. Sivel and J. E. Crocé Spinelli on March 22, 1874. In: Paris, Bibl. des Arts décoratifs.

the advantage of extra oxygen at high altitude; nevertheless, on April 15, 1875, a tragic incident occurred: despite Bert's warning that they were carrying an insufficient supply of oxygen, together with the meteorologist Gaston Tissandier (1843–1899) they conducted a balloon ascent from Paris up to over 8000 m (26 250 ft); only Tissandier survived.[11]

On July 31, 1901, in Berlin, the meteorologists Arthur Berson (1859–1943) and Reinhard Süring reached a height of 32 000 feet (10 500 m) with their balloon "Preussen." While Süring lost consciousness at this altitude, Berson was able to start the lifesaving descent. After the landing both scientists reported that after using extra oxygen, the difficulties in breathing and the feeling of fear ceased; however, a leaden fatigue, exhaustion, a weakness to the stomach and, to a lesser degree, a headache continued. In fact, oxygen was provided through glass-tube mouthpieces instead of the recommended face-fitting oxygen masks.[10,11]

This advance into the stratosphere heralded a new chapter in altitude physiology: stratosphere ascents. The results were especially valuable for the development of aviation and space medicine. As early as 1905, aviation physiologists Nathan Zuntz (Berlin) and his colleague Hermann von Schrötter (Vienna) not only suggested the use of face-fitting breathing masks (Fig. 4) to reach greater heights, but also the employment of a hermetically sealed cabin.[12,13] The Swiss physicist Auguste Piccard (1884–1962) successfully applied this principle in cooperation with Paul Kipfer when they reached a height of 48 132 feet (15 781 m) at an ascent from Augsburg on May 27, 1931 (employing liquid and pressurized oxygen, as well as carbonic acid absorption). In 1933, Russian aeronauts reached a height of about 58 000 feet (19 000 m) in a sealed cabin. The Explorer II

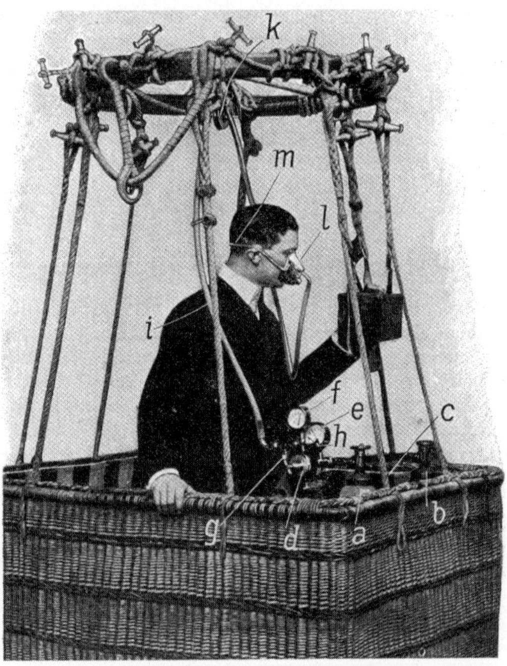

Sauerstoffausrüstung für Hochfahrten.

a Sauerstofflasche, b Reserve-Sauerstofflasche, c Verbindungsrohr, d Reduzier-Ventil, e Inhaltsmesser, f Durchlaßanzeiger, g Regulierschraube, h Abstellschraube, i Schlauch, k Schlauchführung, l Maske, m Maskenhalter (Spirale).

Figure 4. Aeronaut with respirator in 1908. In: Flemming, 1909.

ascended up to over 67 000 feet (22 000 m) in the 1930's in the USA.[7,8] US aviation physician David G. Simons set another milestone in 1957, when he reached a height of about 94 500 feet (31 000 m) as part of the US Man-High-II program in preparation for space travel.[7,11,14]

Technical progress demanded, as demonstrated in the example of the stratosphere ascent, a solution of the medical problems it created. Physiological research at high mountain camps and expeditions provided the necessary preparatory work for aviation medicine (Kronecker, Zuntz, Loewy, Barcroft, Schneider, Haldane, Douglas, Grollmann, Hartmann and others). Berlin physiologist Nathan Zuntz (1847–1920) had been occupied for years with altitude physiological questions in his "pneumatic cabinet," a therapeutically used altitude chamber in a Berlin hospital. His laboratory supported work was complemented by high mountain expeditions as well as practical flight experience. In 1910 he undertook an expedition to Tenerife together with Durig, von Schrötter, Barcroft (Cambridge) and Douglas (Oxford).[15] Zuntz´ fundamental treatise *"Zur Physiologie und Hygiene der Luftfahrt"* (About Aviation Physiology and Hygiene) was published in 1912. In the same year von Schrötter published his treatise *"Hygiene in Aeronautik und Aviatik"* (Hygiene in Aeronautics and Aviation). With their treatises both of them created an awareness of aviation medical tasks.[1,12,13,16]

Scientific and technical advances have always been put to use by the military. For example, the foundation in 1881 of the "German Association for the Promotion of Airship Travel" (Deutscher Verein zur Förderung der Luftschiffahrt) — the first of its kind worldwide — was followed by the opening of the first Prussian airship battalion in 1884. Of special medical interest is the account by medical officer Dr. Flemming, who reported on several sudden deaths caused by arsenic oxygen (composed of sulphuric acid and iron swarfs) in personnel working in the balloon shed or operating the hydrogen generators in the open: (12:173): "In many cases the nausea and the headache were slight so that some of the critically poisoned remained on duty for several hours before reporting sick. Only later did they experience a slight difficulty in breathing, they felt dizzy and noticed a tingling feeling in the skin or the sensation that their extremities had gone to sleep. Under the moderate appearance of fever the body became sensitive to pressure and soon followed a nearly unappeasable vomiting of a yellow-green-black substance which only stopped with the increase of exhaustion shortly before death." Nathan Zuntz dedicated an entire treatise to the influence of balloon gases on the state of health of the aeronaut, paying special attention to carbon monoxide poisoning. For the resuscitation of the poisoned persons, Zuntz propagated the methods of artificial respiration after Hall and Silvester, if necessary with the aid of inhalation masks and the use of oxygen (Fig. 5).[13]

The development of aircraft "heavier than air" is inseparably connected with the name of the German engineer and air pioneer Otto Lilienthal (1848–1896).[c] His extensive experimental foundations

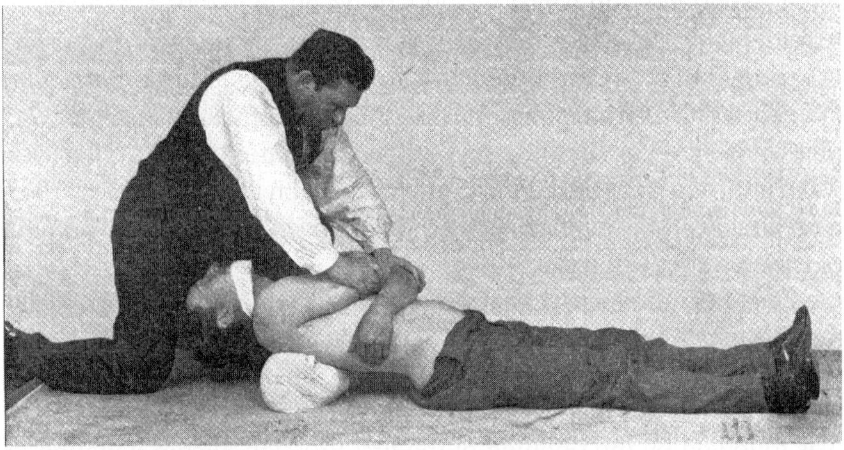

Figure 5. Pulmonary resuscitation after the method of Silvester (picture shows expiration). In: Zuntz, 1912.

[c] To mention all those who have been concerned with the development of aviation would go far beyond the scope of this chapter. Albrecht Ludwig Berblinger (1770–1829) could be mentioned as a representative. Known as the "Tailor of Ulm," he planned to cross the Danube River with a flight apparatus, designed by the Vienna watchmaker Jacob Degen; however, because of an unexpected fast descent into the water, he demonstrated little more than the limits of the technological capabilities of his time.

were followed by the first glider flights in Drewitz in 1891. In 1896 Lilienthal became the victim of a flight accident in one of his own self-built glider-aircraft. He paved the way for the first motorized flight by the American brothers Wilbur and Orville Wright in December 1903. By the means of serial production of their aircraft, they made aviation available for a greater circle of people. Worldwide, the military also became more and more interested in aviation development: war catalysed the development, which furthered the work in aviation medicine. The employment of aircraft at high altitudes, like zeppelins and Gotha-bombers at the beginning of World War I, exposed the crews to hypoxia, hypothermia and fatigue, and demanded efforts from the medical-psychological, the technical and the military tactical side to protect the aviators. Besides altitude physiological questions, to which it became more and more urgent to find answers with the increasing altitude of the aircraft, also the acceleration and sensory physiology became important fields of aeromedical research. Other areas of increasing importance were the assessment of fitness of the aviators, the practical applications of aviation hygiene and occupational health and, last but not least, how best to use the knowledge gained from aviation accidents.[11]

During the record ascent of G. Linnekogel on December 27th, 1913 a continuous-flow regulator was used. During exhalation the incoming oxygen was collected into a breathing bag and could therefore be fed in higher concentration during the inhalation phase. The required additional breathing volume, however, was taken from the ambient air,

Table 1. Evolution of Flight Altitudes of Airplanes

Year	Country	Name of Pilot	Altitude in meters	Use of Oxygen
1909	France	Latham	410	no
1910	USA	Drexel	2.050	no
1911	France	Garros	3.910	no
1913	Germany	Linnekogel	6.120	yes
1920	Germany	Schroeder	10.000	yes
1929	Germany	von Neuenhofen	12.700	yes
1938	Italy	Pezzi	17.000	yes (pressure)

which was the major disadvantage of this method. The continuous-flow procedure has an altitude limit, but is still used for emergency oxygen supply in commercial aeroplanes in case of rapid decompression. In Germany, demand regulators came into use in the mid 1930's, allowing greater heights to be reached. At lower altitudes, the outside air could be mixed with oxygen, resulting in better economy with the oxygen supplies carried along. Higher up, pure oxygen was supplied but only during the inhalation phase. This way, the oxygen requirements were reduced, while the aeronaut was supplied with oxygen according to his needs at various altitudes. With the use of a demand regulator, W. von Neuenhofen reached a height of 12 739 m (41 795 ft) on May 26th, 1929 in a Junkers W 34. For ascents above this limit, either pressure devices with close-fitting breathing masks or pressurized cabins and pressure suits are necessary. Later on portable breathing devices were built, which operated on demand or with continuous flow; they were employed for high altitude gliders and parachute jumpers.[11,17]

With the growth of aviation at the beginning of the 20th century, the rapid increase of aviation accidents was unavoidable. In Germany alone, 42 fatal accidents occurred between 1908 and 1912. Every 13th aeronaut in France died within a period of six months in 1911. The frequency of accidents was mainly attributed to the insufficient medical selection and care of the pilots. However, opinions varied[18]: "One of our most successful pilots expressed the opinion that 80% of all accidents happened because of mechanical failures. Another blamed solely the panic of the pilots (!) for all of the accidents. A third aeronaut perceived the danger to be gliding and demanded the descent to be as vertical as possible. A fourth person blamed the innate clumsiness of the pilots for a third of all accidents. The majority confessed that the feeling of loneliness described by me attacked them as often as a suddenly appearing somnolence." This example demonstrates how differently the importance of the "human factor" has been judged in connection with the occurrence of aviation accidents. Technical improvements and minimum requirements for the medical fitness of the pilots should counteract this development. Ernst Koschel from the Medical Committee of the Scientific Society for Aviation Technology (Medizinischer Ausschuss der Wissens-chaftlichen Gesellschaft für Flugtechnik (WGF)) presented extensive guidelines for pilot selection in Germany on June 5, 1913, whose introduction into practical aviation, however, was prevented by the war. On the other hand, the military requirements for pilots were raised during the course of the war[19–21]:

> "The enemy's planes were equipped with guns so quickly that our pilots, unable to do the same, could no longer defend themselves. The enemy's defensive weapons were improved, their number of pilots grew more and more, just like the number of tasks for our observers. First he had to operate the heavy aerial camera in the growing headwind, to suffer more and more from the cold in the faster aeroplanes and at increasing altitude, then he had to drop the heavy air-raid bombs with his bare hands, and then he had to operate the machine gun, turn the heavy rotating assembly, remove jams in strong headwind and install the new drum, and finally he had to operate the RT device. During all this he had the responsibility for navigation and the success of the mission."

This rapidly advancing technological development with more and more strenuous demands on the aviation personnel had a negative influence on the accident rate. The high number of pilots who were lost during the first years of the war was considered a consequence of insufficient selection. Losses due to technical failure or enemy action played a relatively subordinate role. When the number of pilots who became unfit for flying because of medical conditions grew more and more, strict examination guidelines were developed for the German air force troops in October 1915; it contained the following demands (26:12)[d]:

1. Heart, kidneys and lungs absolutely healthy.
2. Eyes and ears fine. Pilot students who constantly wear glasses will not be taken on any more; those already taken on will remain.

---

[d] In the USA, the U.S. War Department released as early as in 1912 guidelines for the selection of pilots candidates. Beside vision and hearing, the cardiovascular and breathing systems were examined.[1]

Apart from this: at least 5/7 of normal eyesight; when on the right only 1/2 eyesight, then on the left 1/1, or reverse. With glasses in all cases full eyesight and only corrected with regular glasses.

3. Tight, elastic muscular system.
4. Healthy nervous system, no persons who have suffered a nervous breakdown or brain symptoms; no alcoholics and syphilists.
5. In general not under 19 and not over 35 years of age. However, decisive are firstly flexibility and moral qualities.

In 1916, the Chief of the German Army Field Flight Corps (Chef des Feldflugwesens) created a department of aviation medicine, of which he put Koschel in charge, and introduced a multistaged medical examination of the applicants before the training began. By means of a thorough examination of the sense organs, the central nervous system, and the respiratory and circulation systems by a body of medical specialists as well as employing aviation psychological principles, he planned not only to assess the fitness to fly, but also to lower the number of pilots dismissed during training, which lay at about a third of all trainees.[11,21] A parallel development could be observed in other aviation nations. In 1916, a Special Royal Flying Corps Medical Board was founded, which mainly dealt with the medical requirements for pilots. The focus of the examination was on the assessment of the cardiovascular capacity and the capacity to endure at altitude with the "rebreather-bag." In addition, examination of the eyes, the sense of balance and the respiratory tract were included.

The following year, an Air Board Research Committee (Medical) was established to coordinate aviation medical work and research.[22,23] In France, the main focus of the psychophysical test was on the excitability of the test subjects, while in Italy it was on their time of reaction.[9,22] In the USA, the Medical Research Board of the US Air Force was established in 1917 in Hazelhurst Field, Mineola, Long Island (New York). It was among other things entrusted with the compilation of suitability guidelines, besides with the following[24]:

— Research of all those factors which influence the capacity of the pilot

— Examination of the psychophysical capacity of pilots at altitude
— Oxygen supply for the pilots at altitude
— Creation of a database concerning all questions in connection with the bodily fitness of pilots

The research laboratory with training facilities for flight surgeons (Medical Research Laboratory and School for Flight Surgeons of the Air Service, Signal Corps of US Army (ASMRL)), which was founded in Hazelhurst, New York in 1918, was already equipped with an altitude chamber. From this facility sprang the School of Aviation Medicine (SAM) in 1922. The school was moved to Brooks Field near San Antonio, Texas four years later. Looking back on a long tradition as the most renowned facility in this field worldwide, it is now known as the USAF School of Aerospace Medicine. From the beginning this school trained the new generation of flight surgeons, and it was here aviation personnel and pilot candidates were assessed and attended to by aeromedical specialists. The aim was that the flight surgeon should practice his profession directly within the environment of the aviators and that he also should possess flying experience himself. The first flight surgeon graduated from this institution in May 1918. The following were conveyed during a training period of four months (Ref. 24)[e]:

— The organization and administration of the Medical Department as related to the special requirements of the Air Corps
— The principles and technique of physical examination of candidates for flying, training, and testing of fliers, including the use of special equipment required in conducting such examinations
— The application of tests for physical efficiency
— The physical care of fliers

---

[e] In continuation of this course, a connection to the training institution was maintained for two years in the form of a correspondence course, followed by a six week period of practical training at the SAM. Apart from this basic course, further education was offered at the school. In the 1950's a three year residency training was founded, which is a specialist physician training program.

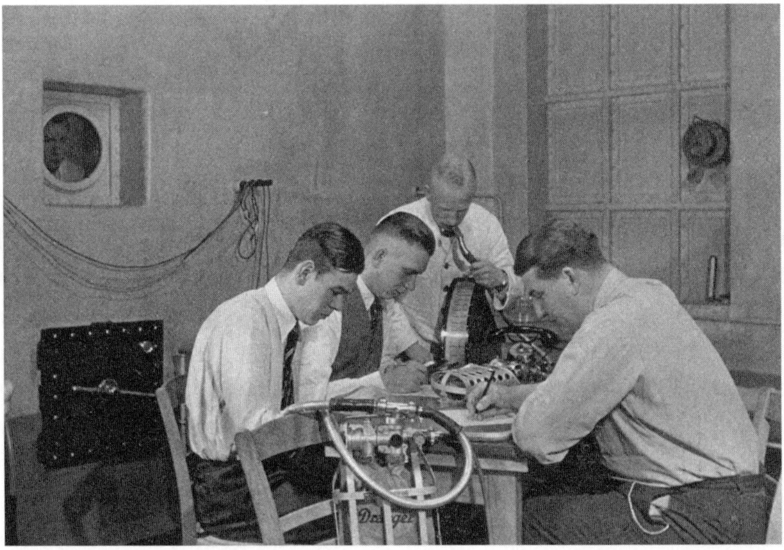

Figure 6. Examination of performance of airmen at high altitudes at the Institute for Medical Research in the Field of Aviation in Hamburg-Eppendorf. In: Harsch, 2003.

— Medical specialties as related to aviation, including neuropsychiatry, physiology, ophthalmology, otology, psychology and cardiology.

The civilian side as well was occupied more and more with selection criteria for pilots. The flight surgeon Louis Hopewell Bauer (1888–1964), the first head of the School of Aviation Medicine, released the first civil medical selection criteria in the USA in December 1926; these are, in their fundamentals, still valid. In 1929, the Aeromedical Association was founded in the USA; it is today the most renowned aviation medical society worldwide. Bauer was elected its first president.[17,19,25]

Practical aspects of aviation medicine were also being pursued in Europe. In 1928, at the Würzburg university, the physiologist Hubertus Strughold (1898–1986) held the first aviation medical lecture, which was complemented by experimental flights with interested students. At this university, Heinz von Diringshofen (1900–1967) started his application orientated acceleration physiological experiments.

Inspired by the transatlantic flight by Charles Lindbergh in 1927, Ludolph Brauer[26] (1865–1951) founded an institute for medical research in the field of aviation (Institut für medizinische Forschung auf dem Gebiet der Luftfahrt) in Hamburg. Here both aviation medical research and the processing of application related questions of altitude physiology were conducted. Students were trained in aviation medicine, pilots and pilot candidates were examined for their fitness to fly, and "physiological training" was offered for aviators and extreme-mountaineers.[26]

In 1928 the Berlin flight physician Ernst Gillert executed a simulated ascent in the altitude-chamber of DVL in Berlin-Adlershof, up to a height of 14 300 m (46 915 ft), in which he fainted[27] (Fig. 7). The need for a pressurized cabin — as that first installed in the Junkers Ju 49 in 1929 — or a pressure-suit was realized for flights within the stratosphere. Nonetheless, the first operational jet and rocket-plane, the Messerschmitt Me-262 "Schwalbe" and the Me 163 "Komet" were not equipped with a pressurized cabin; furthermore, operational pressure suits were not available for their pilots. However, hypoxia-symptoms were not reported, as the time of ascent, at altitude and descent at critical altitudes were shorter than the "Zeitreserve" (time reserve, i.e., time of useful consciousness — TUC).[11] While the development of protective suits, in spite of the promising work of Klanke and Tietze, did not produce operational usable pressure suits, the US pilot Wiley Post (1898–1935) did achieve a breakthrough of pressurized suits when using the first functional one in 1934. Among his other achievements are several aviation records in the 1930's and, moreover, this monocular aviation pioneer is known as the discoverer of the jetstream.[11,28]

Due to the increasing altitudes reached by modern aircraft, altitude physiology remained the focal point of aviation medicine up to the 1940's. Of special interest in this connection was the effect of acclimatisation and whether the airman was 'altitude proof.' Altitude physiologist Hans Hartmann was in charge of an expedition into the Himalayas in 1931, where significant observations were made. In altitude physiological research facilities, like the Mosso-Institute, situated at a height of 3000 m on the Monte Rosa, and at the facility on

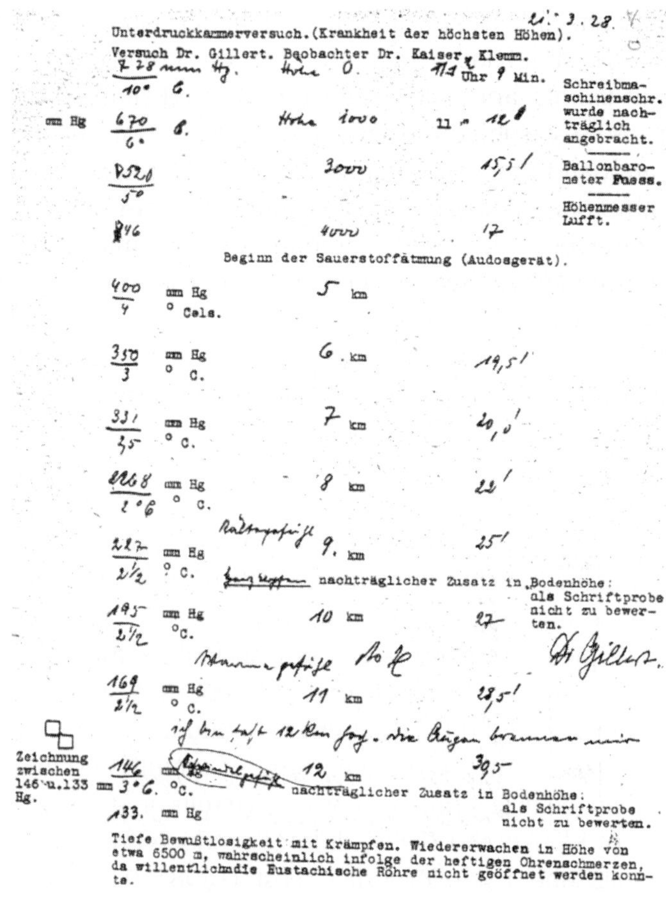

21. 3. 28.

Unterdruckkammerversuch. (Krankheit der höchsten Höhen).
Versuch Dr. Gillert. Beobachter Dr. Kaiser, Klemm.

728 mm Hg. Höhe 0. 11 Uhr 9 Min.
10° C.

mm Hg 670 / 6° C. Höhe 1000 11 " 12
520 / 5° 3000 15,5'
446 4000 17

Schreibmaschinenschr. wurde nachträglich angebracht.

Ballonbarometer Fuess.

Höhenmesser Lufft.

Beginn der Sauerstoffatmung (Audosgerät).

400 mm Hg / 4 ° Cels. 5 km
350 mm Hg / 3 ° C. 6 km 19,5'
331 mm Hg / 3,5 ° C. 7 km 20,0'
268 mm Hg / 2 ° C. 8 km 22'
227 mm Hg / 2½ ° C. 9 km 25'
nachträglicher Zusatz in Bodenhöhe: als Schriftprobe nicht zu bewerten.
195 mm Hg / 2½ °C. 10 km 27
Dr Gillert.
169 mm Hg / 2½ ° C. 11 km 28,5'
Zeichnung zwischen 146 u.133 mm Hg.
146 mm Hg / 3° C. 12 km 30,5
nachträglicher Zusatz in Bodenhöhe: als Schriftprobe nicht zu bewerten.
133. mm Hg

Tiefe Bewußtlosigkeit mit Krämpfen. Wiedererwachen in Höhe von etwa 6500 m, wahrscheinlich infolge der heftigen Ohrenschmerzen, da willentlich die Eustachische Röhre nicht geöffnet werden konnte.

Figure 7. Self-experiment by Dr. E. Gillert in the DVL-altitude chamber up to 14 300 m in 1928. In: Harsch, 2002.

the Jungfraujoch, at a height of 3400 m, lengthy studies were conducted, which methodically were not possible in this form in an altitude chamber. In England, for example, J. Barcroft conducted altitude physiological studies on the effect of hypoxia and acclimatisation during high-mountain expeditions to Mt. Everest and into the Andes. Furthermore, in training examinations on the German side near the front in the 1940's, transportable examination devices for altitude effects after Bruno Müller (1912–1997) were put to use. A mixture of oxygen and nitrogen was employed, which, with an oxygen concentration of 7%, simulated a height of 7500 m (24 600 ft) through a technically simple and safe procedure. The aim was primarily to acquaint the test subjects with the subjective warning signals of hypoxia in order to prevent aviation accidents — this is also today an important part of the physiological training worldwide. Furthermore, the time reserves (TUC) were determined for the assessment of the altitude threshold; this was mainly done by use of the writing test after Lottig[29] (Fig. 8).

In civilian as in military aviation, and here especially in amateur flying, the role of altitude physiology was becoming more and more

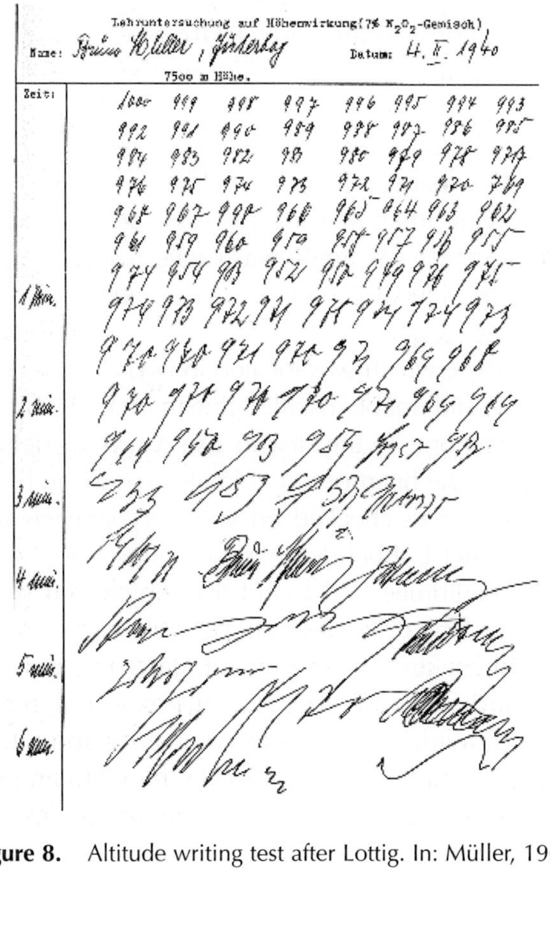

Figure 8. Altitude writing test after Lottig. In: Müller, 1967.

important. The first glide without loss of height succeeded in the landscape of the Rhön in 1916. It was also here the first gliding competition took place in 1920. With the Olympic motto "citius, altius, fortius" (faster, higher, stronger), more and more records were established, which took the glider pilots to their psycho-physical limits: in 1940 the stratosphere was reached for the first time with a "Kranich" soaring plane (11 400 m ~ 37 400 ft). The admission of gliding into the Olympic Games in Helsinki was planned for the same year, however the war prevented this from happening. Since then, with ultra-light flying, hang gliding, paragliding and parachute jumps, many people have found new, although sometimes also dangerous, kinds of sport activities in the third dimension.[11,30]

Beside altitude physiology, acceleration research was another topic of major interest. In the early 1930's, the effects of prolonged in-flight acceleration were first studied by the flight surgeon Heinz von Diringshofen. He suggested selecting small, but strong flight students with a high G-tolerance (due to a resistant circulatory system) for high-performance aircraft. In addition, body positioning as a means of improving tolerance to G-stress was recognized, and the supine positioning at a 45° angle was suggested.

To obtain more standardized conditions than are possible in flight, examinations were supplemented with a centrifuge (16 ft., 45 G max., first 4 G within 40 s), which was located in Berlin. At the time, a larger 66 ft. centrifuge could not be installed due to air-raids. The physiologist Otto F. Ranke was one of the first to use X-rays to demonstrate the decreased filling of the heart of test-animals exposed to high G_z-forces. These results were cross-checked on voluntary subjects in flight. The medical officer cadet L. Buehrlen exposed himself to 17 G_x over two minutes on the centrifuge and found the supine and prone position effective to sustain high G_z-forces in flight.

In dive-bombers such as the Junkers Ju 87 "Stuka," pilots used to crouch forward and contract their muscles through the pullouts. In addition, these widely accepted manoeuvres were accompanied by increasing the intrathoracic pressure by grunting an e-sound (M-1 manoeuvre) (Fig. 9). Only one aircraft loss due to G-LOC was reported in Germany during WWII. Most likely, no attempts were

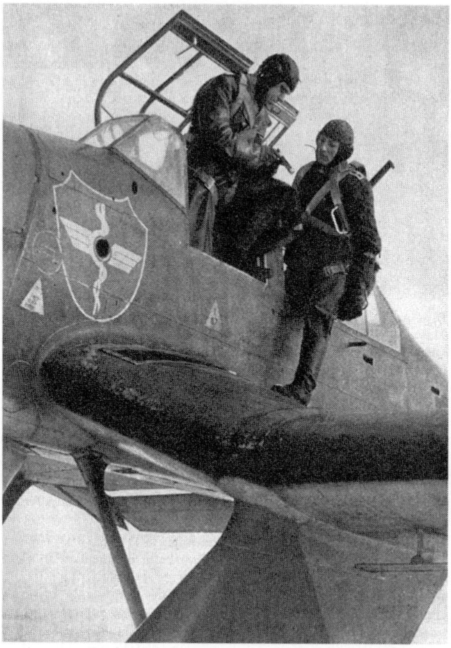

Figure 9. Flight surgeon (and test-pilot, front) and volunteer (back) preparing for aero-medical high-G flight at GAF Testflight-Center in Jüterbog (south of Berlin) in the 1940s. In: Müller, 1967.

made to develop and introduce anti-G suits in Germany because the use of such suits seemed to cause more trouble than it was worth.[11,29,31,32] Since then the use of anti-G suits has gained general acceptance and has made the use of high-performance aircraft more tolerable for pilots. New developments are being made within the field of liquid-filled anti-G suits (e.g. "Libelle"/"Dragon Fly"), as was originally proposed by Otto Gauer in the 1930's.

Beside prolonged acceleration, as described above, the effects of short-term acceleration, caused by vibrations or on impact, ejections etc., were also of physiological and patho-physiological interest. The American officer A. Berry succeeded as early as in 1912 with the first parachute jump from a biplane. However, the parachute was first employed as a life-saving device by the Germans at the end of World War I; one of the rescued was flying ace Ernst Udet who jumped from

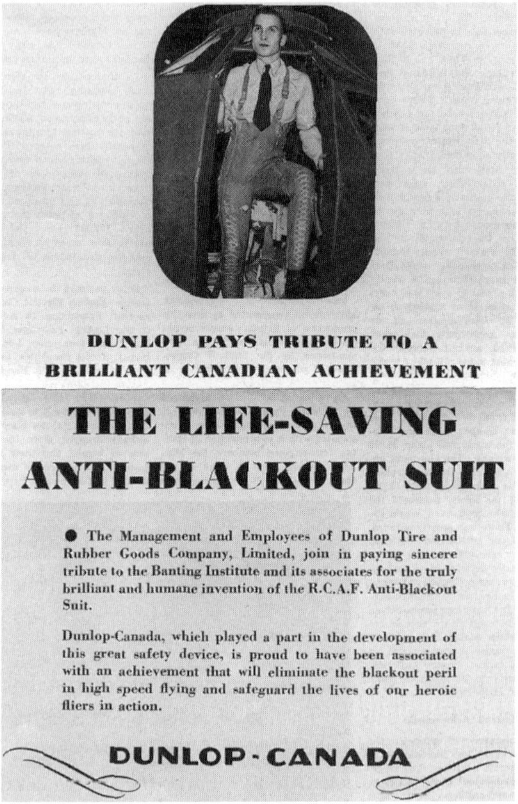

Figure 10. Canadian anti-G suit. In: Canadian Aviation, Mai 1945.

his Fokker D VII on June 29, 1918 and survived with a sprained ankle.[16] With the increasing flying altitudes in World War II, the issue of rescue possibilities from life-threatening heights was evaluated. After parachuting, the development of catapult and ejection seats was taken up. The first ejection seat ever was installed in the Junkers Ju 88 in 1938. The number of accidents increased in which the pilot managed to disembark the plane only to receive fatal injuries afterwards by being struck by the plane's tail. In 1940, the company Heinkel developed catapult seats, of which more than a thousand were built before the end of the war, saving the lives of many pilots. The acceleration sustained was a controllable element, parachute

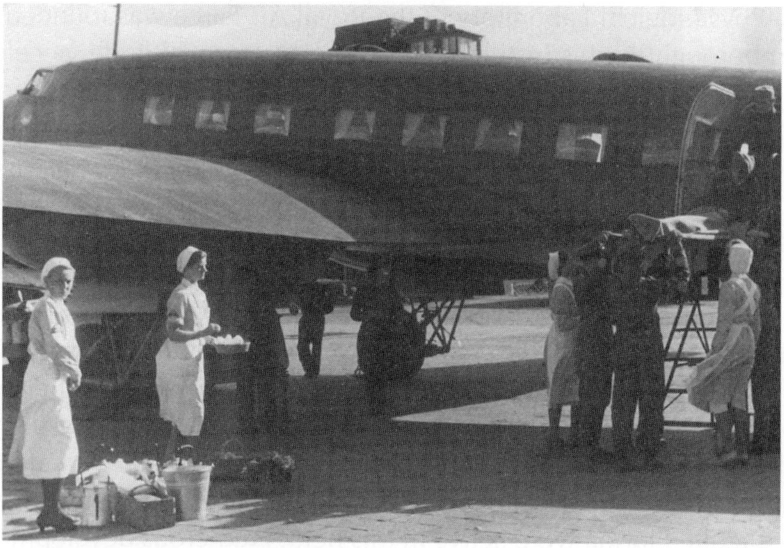

Figure 11. Strategic aeromedical evacuation during WWII: Patients are deployed from Focke-Wulf FW 200 "Condor". Picture Archive of Dr. Harsch.

deployment at great heights and thermal factors on the other hand demanded a technical solution.[11,31,34] Modern ejection-seats have to function under extreme conditions (under "zero-zero" conditions and during high speed and high G). After the Columbia tragedy in 2003, a retrofit of the remaining shuttle fleet for the rescue from high altitudes with ejection seats, as had been the case during the flight test phase, is being discussed again.[f]

Next to the development of aviation medicine, ambulance service by air (AirMedEvac) gained practical relevance: by 1943 more than one million patients had been transported by air on the German side of the front. On the opposing side, especially the Americans reported similar numbers and experiences.[11,35]

Also in other countries, WWII catalyzed further development of special fields within aviation medicine. In England, for example,

[f] In the 1950's, Captain Kittinger managed a successful free-fall jump from over 31 000 m, before he opened the stabilizing chute at about 27 000 m and approached the earth with extremely high speed.[7]

the Physiological Laboratory of the Royal Air Force was founded in Farnborough. In this institute, as in others before, altitude, acceleration and physiology were the main targets for investigation. During the course of the war, the number of staff grew, and the institute also dealt with questions of pilot selection, noise, survival, the influence of heat and cold, decompression sickness, physiological training of the pilots, the development of aircrew equipment, and operational medical support. A part of the experiments were performed through experimental flights by the scientists themselves.[22] In the USA, the Aeromedical Laboratory in Wright Field, Ohio, was the leading force of the development in the field of applied aviation medicine, headed by Harry G. Armstrong. Additionally, the AAF School of Aviation Medicine in Randolph Field, Texas, and the Navy's School of Aviation Medicine in Pensacola, Florida were active in this field. Numerous development projects were carried out as well in the civilian section, especially in the Mayo Clinic in Rochester, Minnesota.

After WW II, the advanced state of aviation medicine was continued at the AAF Aeromedical Center in Heidelberg where the physiologist Otto Gauer and the astrophysicist Heinz Haber reported further development in the field of extraterrestrial physiology. In 1948, a meeting of specialists focussing on the visionary topic *"Aeromedical Problems of Space Travel"* took place in San Antonio, Texas. Aviation physiologist Hubertus Strughold was made first director of the department for space travel medicine at the USAF SAM and was joined by German colleagues K. Büttner, K. Haber and H. Haber in the following year. The biomedical preparatory work for the American manned space programme was initiated under their decisive participation.[11,32,35–37] In 1951 H. Oberth's student Wernher von Braun stated (5:A63): "I believe that the time has arrived for medical investigation of the problems of manned rocket flight, for it will not be the engineering problems but rather the limits of the human frame that will make the final decision as to whether manned space flight will eventually become a reality." We need to remember that the aviation preparatory work contributed decisively to the rapid success of manned space travel.

Charles Lindbergh's flight of 1927 had heralded another new chapter in the history of aviation, namely that of mass air traffic. Strughold stated at the annual scientific conference of the Aeromedical Association in New York City 1937[11]: "The airplane is changing the world. The distance between countries is shrinking. (...) We all can fervently hope that this is leading to a better understanding among the nations." In the following year the four-engine powered Focke-Wulf Fw 200 "Condor" of German Lufthansa flew from Berlin to New York non-stop and back again the following day and paved the way for the upcoming postwar trans-oceanic air travel.

Today the advancing globalization of medicine is a challenge as well as an opportunity. Aviation medicine has evolved from the stage of high-performance physiology and is now a multidisciplinary science concerned with the well-being of humans under aerospace conditions. While Strughold, at the Olympics of 1936, still defined aviation medicine as 'the sports medicine most connected with technique,' nowadays a broader definition of the interdisciplinary field of aviation medicine is preferable: one which subsumes aviation and space medicine, work and travel medicine, as well as further border sciences into one. Its aim is to protect man in his unity of mind, body and soul in the four dimensions of aerospace and, furthermore, gaining knowledge for the earth-bound technical fields of medicine and the biosciences. In essence, aviation medicine is an applied science with the aim of protecting the most vulnerable link in the man-machine complex, the human being. This encompasses the assessment of the fitness to fly for aviators and passengers, even for space travel, as well as assessment of injured and sick persons for air transport. The aerospace physician follows, in this context, the traditional bioethical rules.

The manifold employment possibilities of telemedicine were catalyzed and brought to functioning maturity through the demands of space travel medicine. However, globalization was not solely achieved through the progress in information technology but also through the substantial contribution of mass air traffic. Connected with this, travel medical aspects have gained more and more importance, as highlighted during the outbreak of infectious diseases of international public health concern such as SARS. A further focal point of practical aviation medicine remains in the training of pilots and pilot candidates in the field of human performance limitations (HPL), which as the factors most frequently causing aviation accidents still require intensive attention, always with our common goal in sight: *"Keep 'm flying!"*

REFERENCES

1. Ward MP, Milledge JS, West JB. (1995) High Altitude Medicine and Physiology. Chapman & Hall Medical, London-Glasgow-Weinheim-New York-Tokyo-Melbourne-Madras.
2. West JB. (1998) High Life. A History of High-Altitude Physiology and Medicine. Oxford University Press, New York, Oxford.
3. De Hart RL. (ed.) (1985) Fundamentals of Aerospace Medicine. Lea & Febiger, Philadelphia.
4. Gazenko OG. (1987) Physiology of Men under the Conditions of High Mountains (in Russian). Nauka, Moscow.
5. Hoff EC, Fulton JF. (1942) A Bibliography of Aviation Medicine. Publication No. 5, Yale Medical Library. Charles C. Thomas, Springfield — Baltimore.
6. Schmidt I. (1938) Bibliography of Aviation Medicine (Bibliographie der Luftfahrtmedizin. Eine Zusammenstellung von Arbeiten über Luftfahrtmedizin und Grenzgebiete bis Ende 1936). Springer, Berlin.
7. Crough TD. (1983) The Eagle Aloft. Two centuries of the Balloon in America. Smithsonian Institution Press, Washington D.C.
8. Robinson DH. (1973) The Dangerous Sky. A History of Aviation Medicine. G. T. Foulis & Co. Ltd., Oxfordshire.
9. Dille JR. (2002) In the Beginnings. In De Hart RL, Davis JR (eds.), *Fundamentals of Aerospace Medicine*, pp. 1–18. Williams & Wilkins, Philadelphia.
10. Flemming. (1909) The Physician in the Balloon (Der Arzt im Ballon). In: Broeckelmann (ed.), *Wir Luftschiffer (We the Aviators)*, pp. 127–138. Verlag von Ullstein & Co., Berlin-Wien.
11. Harsch V. (2000) Aerospace medicine in Germany: From the very beginnings. *Aviat Space Environ Med* **71**: 447–450.

12. Schroetter Hv. (1912) Hygiene of Aviation (Hygiene der Aeronautik und Aviatik). Braumüller, Wien-Leipzig (1912).
13. Zuntz N. (1912) Physiology and Hygiene of Aviation (Zur Physiologie und Hygiene der Luftfahrt). Springer, Berlin.
14. Berry CA. (1986) The beginnings of space medicine. *Aviat Space Environ Med* **57**: A58–A63.
15. Gunga HC, Kirsch KA. (1995) Nathan Zuntz (1847–1920) — A German pioneer in high altitude physiology and aviation medicine. *Aviat Space Environ Med* **66**: 168–176.
16. Bauer LH. (1926) Aviation Medicine. The Williams & Wilkins Company, Baltimore.
17. Ruck M, Ruff S, Sedlmayr G. (1989) Safety and Rescue in Aviation (Sicherheit und Rettung in der Luftfahrt). Bernard & Graefe Verlag, Koblenz.
18. Friedlaender. (1912) Physiology and Pathology of Aviation (Zur Physiologie und Pathologie der Luftfahrt). Jahrb WGF 1: 70–83.
19. Engle E, Lott AS. (1973) Man in Flight. Biomedical Achievements in Aerospace. Leeward Publications Inc., Annapolis, Maryland.
20. Koschel E. (1913/14) Requirements for Airmen's Health (Welche Anforderungen müssen an die Gesundheit der Führer von Luftfahrzeugen gestellt werden)? *Jahrb WGF* **2**: 143–156.
21. Koschel E. (1922) Hygiene of the Air Forces (Hygiene des Einsatzes bei den Luftstreitkräften. In: O von Schjerning (ed.), *Medical Experiences in WWI (Handbuch der Ärztlichen Erfahrungen im Weltkriege 1914/1918),* Vol. VII (Hygiene) pp. 10–33. Johann Ambrosius Barth, Leipzig.
22. Gibson TM, Harrison MH. (1984) Into thin Air. A History of Aviation Medicine in the RAF. Robert Hale, London.
23. Harrison MH, Gibson TM. (1999) British Aviation Medicine Research up to 1939. *Aviat Space Environ Med* **70**: 360.
24. Kirby DJ. (2001) A brief overview of the development of aerospace medicine in the United States. *Aviat Space Environ Med* **67**: 96.
25. Benford RJ, Thomas CC. Doctors in the Sky. The Story of the Aeromedical Association. Charles C. Thomas, Springfield.
26. Brauer L. (1933/34) The Institute for Aviation Medicine and Climate Research at the Hamburg Eppendorf Hospital (Das Institut für Luftfahrtmedizin und Klimaforschung am Eppendorfer Krankenhaus zu Hamburg). *Acta Aerophysiologica*: 5–13.

27. Harsch V. (2003) The Institute for Aviation Medicine in Hamburg-Eppendorf (Das Institut für Luftfahrtmedizin in Hamburg-Eppendorf (1927–1945)). Rethra-Verlag, Neubrandenburg.
28. Mohler SR. (1998) The world´s first practical flight pressure suit. *Aviat Space Environ Med* **69**: 802–805.
29. Müller B. (1967) Aviation and Space Medicine (Die gesamte Luftfahrt- und Raumflugmedizin). Droste Verlag, Düsseldorf.
30. Behringer W, Ott-Kopschalijski C. (1991) The Dream of Flight (Der Traum vom Fliegen). S. Fischer, Frankfurt a. M.
31. Harsch V. (2000) German acceleration research from the very beginnings. *Aviat Space Environ Med* **71**: 854–856.
32. Strughold H. (1950) Development, Organization and Experiences of Aviation Medicine in Germany during World War II. In: USAF (ed.). *German Aviation Medicine World War II,* pp. 12–51. US Govt Print Office, Washington D.C.
33. Harsch V. (2002) History of Aviation Medicine (Flugmedizingeschichte: Ein kurzgefasster Abriss zur Entwicklung der praktischen Flugmedizin in Deutschland). In Draeger J, Kriebel J (eds.), *Practical Aspects of Aviation Medicine (Praktische Flugmedizin),* pp. 25–32. Ecomed, Landsberg/L.
34. Armstrong HG. (1939) Principles and Practise of Aviation Medicine. The Williams & Wilkins Company, Baltimore.
35. Gauer O, Haber H. (1950) Man under gravity-free conditions. In: The Surgeon General (ed.), *German Aviation Medicine World War II,* pp. 641–4. Washington, DC: US Department of the Air Force; US Govt Print Off, Vol. 1.
36. Lauschner EA. (1984) The beginnings of aviation medicine in Germany. *Aviat Space Environ Med* **55**: 355–357.
37. Marbarger JP (ed.). (1951) *Space Medicine.* The University Press, Urbana.

Part 2

INTERNATIONAL STANDARDS AND REQUIREMENTS

Chapter 2

ICAO International Medical Standards and Recommended Practices

Claus Curdt-Christiansen*

INTRODUCTION

Following World War I (1914–1918), a convention providing for the creation of a permanent International Commission for Air Navigation (ICAN) under the direction of the League of Nations was presented to the Supreme Council of the Paris Peace Conference and signed in Paris on October 13, 1919. The "Convention relating to the regulation of aerial navigation" came into force in 14 of the signatory States on July 11, 1922.[a] ICAN was set up to establish the regulation of aerial navigation by developing standards and rules for universal application in order to prevent controversy and encourage the peaceful intercourse of nations, and because such regulations "will be to the interest of all." In the ensuing decades, the Convention was ratified by several more States, and at the 27th and last meeting of ICAN in Copenhagen in June 1939, it was in force in 33 States around the world.

---

* Former Chief of Aviation Medicine Section at ICAO, Montreal.

[a] In 1922, ICAN had 28 members: The United States of America, Belgium, Bolivia, Brazil, The British Empire, China, Cuba, Ecuador, France, Greece, Guatemala, Haiti, The Hedjaz, Honduras, Italy, Japan, Liberia, Nicaragua, Panama, Persia, Peru, Poland, Portugal, Romania, The Kingdom of the Serbs, Croats and Slovenes, Siam, Czechoslovakia, and Uruguay.

DEVELOPMENTS OVER THE YEARS

A Medical Sub-Commission of the ICAN formulated the international minimum standard of medical requirements and outlined the methods of medical examination. This first set of international medical standards for civil aviation, published as Annex E to the Paris Convention, was remarkably complete and detailed and to the surprise of many modern readers, neither very demanding nor very rigid. The following excerpt from paragraph 8 of Section IV of Annex E, Medical Examination, Medical requirements for licences for pilots of private aerodynes (mechanically driven), may serve as an example:

> Eye examination — The candidate must not be completely deprived of the use of one eye. He must possess, with correction by glasses if necessary, a visual acuity equal to at least 70% of the normal visual acuity for each eye taken separately. When this first measurement has been effected with correction by glasses, the medical examiner shall in addition see that the visual acuity of the candidate, measured without correction by glasses, after such candidate has had time to adapt himself to these new requirements, is equal to at least 10% of the normal visual acuity, for each eye taken separately.
>
> (Excerpt taken from the latest edition, February 1940)

The Medical Sub-Commission of ICAN met several times in the 1920s and 1930s, further developing and polishing the regulations. The following excerpt shows both the degree of detail and the style of the regulations:

> ... with regard to the maintenance of efficiency of the pilot, pulmonary emphysema will entail rejection only when the pulmonary capacity falls below three and a half liters at rest after a full exhalation and inhalation and when the duration of the breath holding falls at rest below 50 seconds, or only 40 seconds if the candidate

is less than one meter and 65 centimeters in height or is of the female sex.

(Excerpt from paragraph 9, Medical requirements for licences for pilots of public transport or aerial work aerodynes (mechanically driven))

THE BIRTH OF ICAO

The outbreak of World War II put an end to further developments in the work of ICAN. But towards the end of the war, in November–December 1944, a meeting was held in Chicago, where delegates from 52 States convened, deliberated for five weeks, and conceived the *Convention on International Civil Aviation* ("Chicago Convention"), which led to the establishment of the International Civil Aviation Organization (ICAO). The Canadian government offered to host this new organization, and ever since ICAO has had its headquarters in Montreal, Quebec. As a specialized agency of the United Nations, ICAO carried on the work of ICAN, and in May 1946 "Recommendations for Standards, Practices and Procedures — Personnel Licensing (PEL)" was published in which the medical provisions for licensing were spelled out.

DEVELOPMENTS OVER THE YEARS

In 1948, the first edition of Annex 1 to the *Convention on International Civil Aviation* was published. It contained the Standards and Recommended Practices (SARPs) for Personnel Licensing. The Standards were then, as they are today, rules that ICAO's Contracting States have an obligation to adhere to, whereas the Recommended Practices are rules that States should endeavor to follow if possible. Notes that do not alter the meaning of the Standards or Recommended Practices were included whenever it was necessary to clarify an intention, to stress a particular point or to draw the attention of the reader to related provisions elsewhere in the Annex. Pursuant to Article 38 of the Chicago Convention, States are obligated to inform

ICAO of differences between national regulations and practices and the international Standards and Recommended Practices. A decision by the ICAO Council a few years later modified this article so that only differences to Standards had to be reported, and moreover, this obligation was limited to national regulations that were less demanding than the international Standards.

In the second edition of Annex 1, published in 1951, the entire text of the medical requirements was phrased as Recommended Practices, where "should" was the operative verb:

> *Color perception requirement No. 1. The candidate should be required to have normal color perception.*
>
> *Color perception requirement No. 2. The candidate should be required to demonstrate his ability to identify readily colored lights of signal red, signal green, and white.*

Beginning with the third edition of Annex 1, published in 1953, and in all later editions, the provisions were phrased as Standards and Recommended Practices. In the text of a Standard, the operative verb is "shall," and in the text of a Recommended Practice, the operative verb is "should." In order to indicate at a glance the status of each statement, the Standards were now printed in regular typeface, and the Recommended Practices and the Notes in italics.

In the following decades, amendments to Annex 1, which included additional Standards and Recommended Practices as well as modifications to existing Standards, were primarily based on recommendations from the Personnel Licensing Division sessions, large meetings with participation from the majority of the Contracting States. A Special Meeting on Hearing and Visual Requirements for Personnel Licensing was held in 1955, with participation of doctors from around the world, and a Personnel/Medical Divisional meeting was held in 1970. In 1980, an International Medical Study Group was established to review the medical provisions in Annex 1. In its final report, the group wrote that the ICAO medical provisions had stood the test of time, and that no further amendments were required. In 1997, an international Vision and Color

Perception Study Group reviewed and updated the visual requirements, and in 2003/2004, a Medical Provisions Study Group, with participation of aeromedical experts from Canada, Egypt, France, New Zealand, Singapore, Russian Federation, United Kingdom, United States, IFALPA, IATA, IAASM and AsMA overhauled and modernized the entire body of medical provisions in Chapters 1 and 6 of Annex 1. These new medical provisions were adopted by the ICAO Council on February 21, 2005 and became applicable in all 188 Contracting States on November 24, 2005. During the approval process, the Council requested that further study of certain areas of the medical provisions should be carried out in the near future. Consequently, the Medical Provisions Study Group reconvened the following year, and on 5 February 2009 the Council adopted additional amendments with regard to the content and nature of the certificatory examination, increasing the emphasis on health education and prevention of ill health, especially in applicants under 40 years of age. Also, the requirements for female applicants and for applicants infected with HIV underwent some changes, and the possibility of treatment with antidepressant medicines was introduced in a Recommendation. These changes represent a modest shift towards a performance-based approach to medical assessment and give further support to evidence-based aeromedical decision-making. They emphasize that the incidence of medical conditions varies with age, that health education and prevention of ill health can be beneficial to flight safety, that the routine periodic medical examination is not very effective at detecting or predicting medical conditions of flight safety relevance, especially in the younger pilot, and that stringent medical standards may not necessarily improve flight safety if they result in licence holders withholding relevant medical information from the Licensing Authority. These additional amendments to the medical provisions in Annex 1 will come into force in all Contracting States on the 19 November 2009 (see Appendix 1).

THE MEDICAL PROVISIONS TODAY

The International Standards and Recommended Practices (SARPs), in force worldwide since November 2005, contain regulations (in

Chapter 1 of Annex 1) that govern the administration of the aeromedical certification system. Contracting States shall designate medical examiners to conduct the regulatory medical examinations, the medical examiners shall have adequate knowledge of aviation medicine, and they shall be familiar with the aviation environment; their competence shall be tested before designation, and they shall undergo refresher training at regular intervals. The national civil aviation authority shall appoint a medical assessor, a specialist in aviation medicine, to oversee the work and conduct of the medical examiners, and to review the medical reports they submit to the licensing authority. Medical confidentiality shall be safeguarded at all times, although the medical assessor may discuss a particular case with other officials of the licensing authority when required by operational concerns. The SARPs in Chapter 1 also regulate the intervals between health examinations, set a limit of 45 days for the "grace period" (i.e. the number of days before the expiry date of a medical assessment, where renewed examination can be performed without changing the annual or semi-annual renewal dates), and permit States to mandate shorter intervals when needed on clinical grounds. The SARPs further contain regulations (in Chapter 6 of Annex 1), which define the medical (mental and physical) requirements for professional pilots (Class 1), private pilots (Class 2), and air traffic controllers (Class 3). The so-called flexibility clause (paragraph 1.2.4.8) is, however, part of Chapter 1. It states that an applicant who does not fully meet the requirements of the medical provisions in Chapter 6 may still be assessed as fit if an accredited medical conclusion[b] can be reached that he or she is unlikely to jeopardize flight safety.

> 1.2.4.8 If the Medical Standards prescribed in Chapter 6 for a particular licence are not met, the appropriate Medical

[b] Accredited Medical Conclusion (AMC): A conclusion reached by one or more medical experts acceptable to the Licensing Authority for the purposes of the case concerned, in consultation with flight operations or other experts as necessary.

Assessment shall not be issued or renewed unless the following conditions are fulfilled:

a) accredited medical conclusion indicates that in special circumstances the applicant's failure to meet any requirement, whether numerical or otherwise, is such that exercise of the privileges of the licence applied for is not likely to jeopardize flight safety;
b) relevant ability, skill and experience of the applicant and operational conditions have been given due consideration; and
c) the licence is endorsed with any special limitation or limitations when the safe performance of the licence holder's duties is dependent on compliance with such limitation or limitations.

A consequence of this clause, which is a Standard, is that a licence holder, who is deemed to meet the requirements of 1.2.4.8, is considered to meet the Standard even when not meeting a specific medical requirement in Chapter 6. The term "waiver," frequently used about the application of flexibility, is a misnomer. The licensing authority does not waive any requirement but applies a Standard (1.2.4.8) which, under certain specified circumstances and in unusual cases only, allows a licence holder to be assessed as fit. It is important not to apply 1.2.4.8 routinely for a certain condition as this may lead to widely differing practices in different States. Frequent use of 1.2.4.8 may indicate that certain medical requirements in Chapter 6 do not reflect the demands of contemporary aviation. In such cases, ICAO should be approached with a request to review the SARPs concerned.

The medical provisions in Chapter 6 contain both physiological performance requirements and health requirements. In addition to the former, specific testing requirements are given. In many, the Standards containing the health requirements are divided in two parts: an initial medical requirement (using the verb "shall") and a subsidiary requirement (using the verb "may" or "need not"):

> 6.3.2.12 Applicants with active pulmonary tuberculosis shall be assessed as unfit.
>
> 6.3.2.12.1 Applicants with quiescent or healed lesions which are known to be tuberculous, or are presumably tuberculous in origin, may be assessed as fit.
>
> —
>
> 6.3.2.26 There shall be:
>
> —
>
> c) no unhealed perforation of the tympanic membranes.
>
> 6.3.2.26.1 A single dry perforation of the tympanic membrane need not render the applicant unfit.

This structure has been chosen for two reasons: (1) to facilitate the administration of the provisions by allowing the authority to ground licence holders who need to have their medical condition further investigated before a final aeromedical disposition can be made; and (2) to allow applicants with certain medical conditions, which are usually but not always, incompatible with flight duties, to pursue an aviation career.

In other cases, the phrasing of the requirement contains a second part, beginning with the word "unless":

> 6.3.2.20 Applicants who are seropositive for human immunodeficiency virus (HIV) shall be assessed as unfit unless the applicant's condition has been investigated and evaluated in accordance with best medical practice and is assessed as not likely to interfere with the safe exercise of the applicant's licence or rating privileges.

This structure has been chosen to allow licence holders who are willing to undergo certain additional examinations or accept certain treatments to obtain a fit assessment.

The medical provisions in Annex 1 are supported by "guidance material" — the *Manual of Civil Aviation Medicine* (Doc 8984; this document can be accessed on-line at www.icao.int). This manual gives background information, explains the requirements in detail, gives guidance on how to examine applicants and how to investigate various medical conditions, and gives advice on how to interpret pathological findings in the context of an aeromedical disposition.

Chapter 3

Federal Aviation Administration — Aviation Medicine[1]

Warren S. Silberman*

HISTORICAL INFORMATION

Civil aviation medicine had its beginnings in the USA on May 20, 1926 when President Calvin Coolidge signed the Air Commerce Act. This act gave the responsibility of civil aviation to the Department of Commerce. Herbert Hoover, who was the secretary of commerce, created the Aeronautics Branch to manage these responsibilities. This Aeronautics Branch was divided into the Air Regulations Division and the Air Information Division. Aviation Medicine was placed in the Air Regulations Division.

The initial draft of the aeronautical regulations, drawn up in August 1926, did not stipulate what the physical standards would be, just that a physical examination would be required for licencure and that the cost of this examination would not be more than five dollars.

When the physical standards finally became effective on December 31, 1926, they were contained in Section 66 of the Air Commerce Regulations. Physically disqualifying conditions for any of the classes of medicals were *"certain diseases and conditions ... medical experts had concluded could cause sudden incapacitation or death while at aircraft controls, or could otherwise compromise a pilot's ability to operate an*

* Civil Aerospace Medical Institute, Mike Monroney Aeronautical Center, 6700 South MacArthur Blvd, Oklahoma City, OK 73125.

aircraft in a manner compatible with an acceptable level of safety."[2] (pp. 2–3). Three levels of physical qualifications were established, one for each of the pilot classes that were created:

> *"Private Pilots: Absence of organic disease or defect which would interfere with safe handling of an airplane under the conditions for private flying: visual acuity of at least 20/40 in each eye; less than 20/40 may be accepted if a pilot wears correction in his goggles and has normal judgment of distance without correction, good judgment of distance; no diplopia in any position; normal visual fields and color vision; no organic disease of eye or ear.*
>
> *Industrial pilots: Absence of any organic disease or defect which would interfere with the safe handling of an airplane; visual acuity of not less than 20/30 in each eye, although in certain instances less than 20/30 may be accepted if the applicant wears correction to 20/20 in his goggles and has good judgment of distance without correction; good judgment of distance; no diplopia in any field; normal visual fields and color vision; absence of organic disease of the eye, ear, nose or throat.*
>
> *Transportation pilots: Good past history; sound pulmonary, cardiovascular, gastrointestinal, central nervous and genito-urinary systems; freedom from material structural defects or limitations; freedom from disease of the ductless glands; normal central, peripheral and color vision, normal judgment of distance; only slight defects of ocular muscle balance; freedom from ocular disease; absence of obstruction or diseased conditions of the ear, nose and throat, no abnormalities of the equilibrium that would interfere with flying"*[3] (p. 3).
>
> Waivers were granted provided the "*experience of the pilot will compensate for the defect.*" The waiver would continue provided the "*defect for which it was granted has not increased or unless canceled by the Secretary of Commerce*"[4] (p. 3).

Louis Hopewell Bauer, who was the first medical director of aeronautics, designed his system around a group of specially designated physicians known as aviation medicine examiners or AMEs. They would be knowledgeable or trained in the factors of flight as they relate to medicine. These physicians would be appointed or specially designated by the Department of Commerce and would be delegated authority to conduct physical examinations of pilot applicants and pilots. They could issue medical certificates to those who met the physical standards and deny issuance to those who did not.

On July 1, 1934, the Aeronautics Branch became the Bureau of Aeronautics. This organization was still under the Department of Commerce.

In 1938, President Roosevelt and Congress created the Civil Aeronautics Authority. They consolidated all aviation functions into this independent agency. The Civil Aeronautics Act of 1938 gave the economic and safety regulation of the air transportation industry and all civil aviation operations to a five-member Civil Aeronautics Authority. The quasi-legislative responsibility for looking into the cause of aircraft accidents was given to a three-member Air Safety Board. The Act also created an Administrator who was given the power of executive functions, which were at that time the fostering of civil aeronautics and commerce, operation of the civil airways, maintaining the air navigation facilities, and regulation of air traffic.

On August 22, 1940, the President and Congress placed into operation a plan for the reorganization of federal aviation. This reorganization disbanded the five-member Civil Aeronautics Authority and created the Civil Aeronautics Board (the CAB) and placed the CAB back into the Department of Commerce. The organization retained its independence for aviation rulemaking, adjudication, and accident investigation. It reported to the President and Congress through the secretary of commerce. The Air Safety Board was disbanded and its functions were assigned to the CAB, which formed the Aviation Safety Bureau. The Administrator's functions were assigned to the secretary of commerce who created the Civil Aeronautics Administration (the CAA), which was to be run by a new Administrator of Aeronautics.

The CAB passed an amendment to the Civil Air Regulations on August 20, 1940 that reinstituted a former practice of licencing the physically handicapped. This amendment would allow them to fly under appropriately "restricted" conditions (p. 120). The amendment No. 67 read:

> *"Exceptions to the Physical Requirements: An applicant may receive a certificate in spite of failure to comply with the above physical requirements [in Section 20] if his physical deficiency is such as to not interfere with his safe piloting of aircraft. Any applicant receiving a certificate under these conditions may be restricted to particular types of operations or types of aircraft"*[5] (p. 120).

In early 1942, the CAB changed the time intervals between examinations from every 24 months to 12 months for student and private pilots and lengthened them from six months to 12 months for commercial pilots. This regulation became effective on April 1, 1942. Also effective on this date was the separation of the pilot licence and the medical certificate.

On May 1, 1945, the CAA announced that it was going to decentralize its operations from its Washington headquarters to regional offices. The Washington officials would continue to set "... overall plans, general policies and standardization procedures"[6] (p. 147), while operational responsibility for programs would fall to regional managers. These managers were then called "Regional Administrators."

The Federal Aviation Act was passed by Congress and signed by the President on August 23, 1958. The Federal Aviation Agency began its operations under retired Lieutenant General Elwood R. Quesada on December 3l, 1958. The act continued the Civil Aviation Board, which was assigned the economic regulation of the airlines and investigation of aircraft accidents. Safety regulation was removed from the Board's responsibilities and became the responsibility of the FAA Administrator. The CAB retained the responsibility of adjudicating appeals in cases where an appellant believed that the FAA had improperly applied a federal aviation regulation. The regulation of pilot medical standards became the responsibility of the FAA administrator.

Administrator Quesada created the "Office of the Civil Air Surgeon", which was to be independent of the Bureau of Flight Standards.

One of the first acts of the acting Civil Air Surgeon Dr. John E. Smith was to transfer back to medical control the pilot medical certification and physical examination records, which had been removed from medical custody in September 1957.

THE SITUATION TODAY

The current physical standards for medical certification are contained in part 67 of Title 14 Code of Federal Regulations. These regulations are further divided into sections 67.100, 67.200 and 67.300 series corresponding to respectively, a first-, second- and third-class airman medical certificate.

The requirements for the different classes and time limitations for medical certificates are based on part 61.23, which states that to perform piloting duties, an airline transport pilot must hold a first-class medical, a commercial pilot must hold a second-class medical, while private, student, and recreational pilots are to hold a third-class medical certificate. The duration of medical certificates is also contained in the same regulation. First-class medical certificates for airmen under 40 are good for the remainder of the month that the examination was performed and for an additional 12 months; over age 40, the examination is good for the remainder of the month that it was performed and for an additional six months. A second-class examination is good for the rest of the month in which it was performed and for an additional 12 months. A third-class examination for under age 40 is good for the remainder of the month in which it was performed and an additional 60 months (5 years), and for over age 40, is good for the remainder of the month that it was performed and an additional 24 months. A first-class medical certificate lapses to a second-class medical after the last day of the six-month period in which it was taken and to a third-class after the last day of the twelfth month in which it was taken. The same applies for the second-class medical certificate, which lapses to a third-class medical after the last day of the twelfth month after it was taken.

In the US, a medical certificate is not required for operations that include glider operations, balloon operations, student pilot in glider or balloon, flight instructor in gliders, nor in regular aircraft when not acting as pilot-in-command or required flight crewmember.

The authority of the FAA Administrator to issue or deny a medical certificate is delegated to the Federal Air Surgeon. The Federal Air Surgeon further delegates the responsibility for medical certification to the Manager of the Aerospace Medical Certification Division (AAM-300) and to the Regional Flight Surgeons in the nine regions.

All Aviation Medicine Examiners (AMEs) are permitted to perform second- and third-class airman examinations, but only Senior AMEs may perform first-class examinations. An AME may request a designation as a senior AME after he demonstrates competency for three years or sooner if he has specialty training in aerospace medicine.

A medical certificate, issued by an aviation medical examiner, is affirmed issued unless the Federal Air Surgeon or one of the other designated agency officials as mentioned above reverses the issuance. Should these officials find a need to reverse the issuance of the medical certificate, they must accomplish this within 60 days after the date of issuance of the certificate. Otherwise, the certificate becomes legally valid and must therefore be revoked. Should the FAA request the certificate holder to submit to more medical testing, the authorizing official has 60 days after receipt of this material to reverse the issuance of the medical certificate.

Some peculiarities that separate the medical standards of the FAA from those of other certifying authorities will be discussed in the next several paragraphs. The FAA medical standards do not have any requirements for uncorrected vision. A first-class airman must be correctable to 20/20 Snellen vision in each eye distant, and 20/40 in each eye near. A second-class airman must be correctable to the same standards as the first-class. A third-class airman must be correctable to 20/40 distant and 20/40 near in each eye. There is also a 20/40 requirement for intermediate visual acuity over age 50 for first- and second-class airmen. There are no refractive limitations in the FAA standards. For color vision in all classes, the airman must be able to distinguish aviation colors. A variety of color vision screening tests are acceptable, such as pseudoisochromatic plates, Dvorine plates, Farnsworth Lantern, Titmus tester, and OPTEC 900.

An airman can pass either of three tests to demonstrate hearing capability. These are the conversational voice test at six feet, standard audiometer with a better ear/worse ear requirement, or a speech discrimination test. Hearing amplification is permitted should the airman require this to pass any of these tests. The airman would then receive a restriction on the medical certificate that he must use hearing amplification. Deaf airmen have also been granted medical certification with stipulation on their medical certificates that they cannot serve as a required pilot in radio-controlled airspace.

67.401 is the section in the medical regulations that deals with discretionary issuance of a certificate to a person who does not meet the medical provisions, i.e. gives the FAA the ability to authorize a special issuance of a medical certificate or grant a "waiver" for disqualifying medical conditions. A "waiver" is granted by the FAA if *"the person shows to the satisfaction of the Federal Air Surgeon that the duties authorized by the class of medical applied for can be performed without endangering public safety during the period the Authorization would be in force."*[7] The Federal Air Surgeon or any of his appointees may request a special medical flight test, practical test or medical evaluation for the purpose of issuing this "waiver." There are two types of "waivers" issued by the FAA: a Statement of Demonstrated Ability or SODA for a medical condition that does not usually change over time, and an Authorization for Special Issuance for a medical condition that may change. An example of a condition for which a SODA would be appropriate is a pilot who has monocular vision. SODAs generally require a special medical flight test. Airmen with treated coronary artery disease require an Authorization for Special Issuance.

Medical certificates issued to airmen under an Authorization are usually time-limited because the airman must regularly demonstrate to the Federal Air Surgeon that there is no adverse change in his underlying medical condition. In general, the duration of these time-limited medical certificates is six, 12, or 24 months, depending on the existing pathology. The airman is still required to obtain a medical examination for the class of medical he is required to hold based on the requirements as set forth in Part 61.23.

In the United States, a third-class licence holder, i.e. a private pilot, is permitted to accept reasonable risks to his person and property that are not acceptable for the conduct of airline transport or commercial pilot operations. Often, the FAA grants medical certification to private pilots flying single crew operations for medical conditions and treatments that by many other aviation authorities around the world are seen as disqualifying. Limitations such as "without passengers only" or "with safety pilot only" are not used in the United States. These are some of the more significant differences between the medical certification philosophy of the United States and that of many other countries.

In the United States, airmen must only demonstrate to the FAA that they are safe to pilot an aircraft during the time period that the medical certificate is valid. The examination is not intended to serve as a warranty of a normal full aviation career. It is done to assess whether the airman is likely during the validity period to develop a condition that could compromise safety or lead to sudden incapacitation. The only routine medical testing required for all classes of medical certificates is a urinalysis to detect the presence of sugar and protein, and for first-class certification, an electrocardiogram at ages 35 and 40, and then annually after age 40.

There are 15 medical conditions set forth in the regulation that are disqualifying on the basis of an established medical history or clinical diagnosis. If an airman of any class demonstrates or is suspected of having one of these medical conditions, the AME is required to defer or deny the issuance of the medical certificate. These 15 medical conditions are:

1. A personality disorder severe enough to have repeatedly manifested itself by overt acts
2. A psychosis
3. A bipolar disorder
4. Substance dependence
5. Substance abuse
6. Epilepsy

7. A disturbance of consciousness without satisfactory medical explanation of the cause
8. A transient loss of nervous system function(s) without satisfactory medical explanation of the cause
9. Myocardial infarction
10. Angina Pectoris
11. Coronary heart disease that requires treatment, or if untreated, that has been symptomatic or requires treatment
12. Cardiac valve replacement
13. Permanent cardiac pacemaker implantation
14. Heart replacement, and
15. Diabetes mellitus that requires insulin or any other hypoglycemic for control.[8]

As in most airman medical certification regulations, there are provisions that allow the Federal Air Surgeon or his representatives to deny certification if there is *"other organic, functional, or structural disease, defect, or limitation that the Federal Air Surgeon, based on the case history and appropriate qualified medical judgment relating to the condition involved, finds* — makes the individual unable to safely perform or exercise the privileges of the medical certificate or may *reasonably be expected* to do so for the duration of the medical applied for or held."[9]

Part 61.53 is another regulation that can be found in the US physical standards as well as in the regulations of other countries. To paraphrase, it states that should an airman develop a medical condition that is disqualifying or should he be given a disqualifying medical treatment or therapy, he is to cease flying.

The federal regulations also require that the airman sign a statement on his medical application that authorizes the FAA Administrator to request the National Driver Register to transmit information contained in the Register about that person to the Administrator. The Register contains information concerning convictions for driving while intoxicated.

The right of airmen to appeal, should they disagree with a denial of their medical certificate, is first to the Federal Air Surgeon, then to an administrative law judge of the National Transportation Safety Board, and then to the full National Transportation Safety Board. A decision by the Board may be appealed to a US Court of Appeals, and finally, the Supreme Court of the United States may be asked for consideration.

In 2007, the number of airmen granted medical certificates by class were: 219 481 first-class, 84 207 second-class, and 125 993 third-class. In 2007, there were a total of 590 349 pilots.

The actual process of reviewing cases for medical certification is described in the following paragraphs. A study done by the Human Resources Research Division of the Civil Aerospace Medical Institute (CAMI) several years ago revealed that 95% of airmen receive their medical certificates at or within a few days of the date of the medical examination. The other 5% are deferred to the Regional Medical Offices or the Aerospace Medical Certification Division. The examinations are required to be transmitted over the Internet. The "hard copy" of the FAA medical examination report (Form 8500-8) must still be completed by the airman and signed. The airman's signature on the form establishes a legal basis for revocation of the certificate issued if there is a falsification of the airman's medical history. When the examination findings are transmitted via the Internet, they immediately reside in a server located at the CAMI in Oklahoma City. All of the nine regional medical offices have the capability to review and work on cases in the Document, Imaging, and Workflow System (DIWS). In this way FAA has a virtual office where a medical case can be viewed and electronically worked on by an approved individual in any place at which there is access to the computer system.

At the present time, all paper documents that relate to the medical certification, including Form 8500-8, are optically scanned into the airman's case file upon arrival at CAMI. Each airman in the FAA system has an electronic file. When the electronically transmitted medical examination results are joined with the hard copy of Form 8500-8 and any associated documents, they are electronically transferred to legal instrument examiners, who are the employees who perform the initial review of the cases. The cases are sorted out for review using electronic messages stored in the system. These legal instrument examiners are non-medical professionals that perform the major portion of the review. It takes a minimum of six months and sometimes up to two years to adequately train these examiners. Should a legal instrument examiner have a medical question concerning a case under examination, the case is forwarded for review by one of the physicians. If the physician is confronted by a medical issue that is beyond his or her expertise, the case is referred to a consultant. All first- and second-class airmen with myocardial infarction, angina pectoris, treated or untreated coronary disease, valve replacement and permanent pacemaker insertion have their cases reviewed by the Federal Air Surgeon's Cardiology Consulting Panel. These consultants make recommendations to the FAA as to whether the airman should be issued a medical certificate.

"Waivers" are processed in much the same way. Letters to airmen, medical certificates, SODAs, and Letters of Authorization for special issuances are produced electronically as well. Approximately 130 legal instrument examiners, physicians, and support personnel make up the Aerospace Medical Certification Division (AMCD).

The DIWS system of processing cases has come a long way since its inception. Currently as I mentioned above the processing of cases is essentially a virtual one with physicians able to work on medical case files anywhere in the world as long as they have Internet capability with connection to the VPN. Recently, the last process of working on hard copy cases was converted to electronic capability so the entire processing is now paperless. The time it takes to process a priority case was significantly reduced by changing the business process. Currently this is less than 30 days! Airmen can go online, as long as they have a personal email address, obtain a username and password and complete the medical history portion of the FAA Medical Examination online. The Aviation Medical Examiner can view the entire medical history that the FAA has on an airman.

The capabilities of the DIWS system are extensive. In the future airmen will be able to have the hospital or physician submit medical records electronically. Their records will be inserted directly into their electronic medical file. Radiographic images could be digitally scanned into an airman file so the FAA medical officers could view the original image. Perhaps even the medical examination will be performed via telemedicine!

Some relevant websites with good information about various medical standards issues are www.AOPA.org, www.aviationmedicine.com, www.EAA.org, www.faa.gov/about/office_org/headquarters_offices/avs/offices/aam/,www.leftseat.com.

REFERENCES

1–5. Holbrook, HA. (1974) *Civil Aviation Medicine in the Bureaucracy.* Banner Publishing Co, Inc, Bethesda, MD.

6–9. Federal Aviation Administration. (1999) *Guide for Aviation Medical Examiners.*

Chapter 4

Joint Aviation Authorities (JAA) and European Aviation Safety Agency (EASA) — Medical Requirements for Pilots in Europe

Joerg Siedenburg*,† and Annetje Roodenburg

INTRODUCTION

In the second half of the 20th century, the idea of Europe as an area with a common cultural, political and economic background was borne. After the European "common market" was established in 1957, European cooperation had evolved in all fields, and in 1993 the European Union was formed, guaranteeing free movements of citizens and exchange of goods throughout the member states. European cooperation had achieved a common political body and peaceful understanding among the nations of a continent that had been plagued by war for centuries at the turn of the millennium. In view of the tremendous growth of aviation, harmonization within the area of aviation safety was considered a priority. The Joint Aviation Authorities (JAA) was established and the transformation of JAA into the European Aviation Safety Agency (EASA) is now well under way and will soon be completed.

* Corresponding author.

† Aero Medical Center, Deutsche Lufthansa AG, Lufthansa Basis, Torzi, D-60546 Frankfurt, Germany.

JAA

Primarily as an answer to the needs of the industry, harmonization in European aviation began in the 1970s. The work began with the Joint Airworthiness Authorities, a cooperative body whose first task was to develop common certification codes for large aircraft and engines. In 1987, the scope was extended to include maintenance, later flight operations, and licensing of aircraft. In 1990, the Directors General of 12 European states signed the Cyprus Arrangements, committing the member states to develop and implement common European safety standards and procedures.

The Joint Aviation Authorities (JAA) was an executive and cooperative body that was created under the auspices of the Cyprus Arrangement. The objectives were to harmonize the safety standards and procedures for civil aviation within Europe, to reach a common high level of aviation safety in the JAA member states, and to create "a level playing field" for aviation in Europe. According to the principles of the European Union, freedom of movement of goods and people had to be guaranteed. Technically, this was achieved in the field of aviation safety by developing and adopting Joint Aviation Requirements (JARs), as well as procedures for their implementation.

Provisions for licensing are covered by JAR-FCL (Flight Crew Licensing). A prerequisite to exercise a pilot's privileges is a private or professional licence, including a class or type rating, and a medical certificate — Class 1 for professional or Class 2 for private pilots. The requirements for a medical certificate are promulgated in JAR-FCL 3 (Medical).

DRAFTING OF THE JAA MEDICAL REQUIREMENTS

The requirements of JAR-FCL 3 had been drafted by the FCL Medical Sub-Committee (in 2001 renamed the Licensing Sub-Sectorial Team (Medical)) consisting of the chief medical officers of the licensing authorities of the JAA member states[a] and representatives of interested parties. The work to harmonize the medical requirements for pilots' licences began in 1991 and was based on the ICAO medical provisions in Annex 1 and existing national standards. However, the ICAO medical provisions are designed to ensure a minimum standard and ICAO's contracting states are free to develop more stringent requirements. In most European states at least some medical requirements for pilots were more demanding than those of ICAO.

The new JAA requirements were to be the "sole code," leading to equal and uniform medical assessments in all JAA member states. Consequently, the Medical Sub-Committee concluded that very detailed requirements would be needed to avoid different interpretations. The price to pay for having these detailed and precise requirements was that there would be very little room for flexibility.

One of the difficulties of drafting harmonized requirements was the fact that the European states had different approaches to determine medical fitness to fly, which had led to different approaches to the aviation medical examination and assessment.

In several European states, the requirements for civilian pilots had been derived from the requirements for military pilots and included occupational health aspects. In some states all professional pilots, military as well as civilian, and sometimes even private pilots, were examined by aeromedical specialists at specialized centers, staffed with highly trained personnel, and given immediate access to the relevant special equipment. The result was a high entry level, close monitoring during the entire career, and an early detection of relevant pathology. The benefits for the pilot were clear: a comprehensive

---

[a] In 1990, the JAA countries participating in the work of the JAA FCL Medical Sub-Committee were Belgium, Denmark, Finland, Ireland, Italy, Netherlands, Sweden, Switzerland, and the United Kingdom. Over the years, JAA membership has grown, and in 2007, more than 30 European countries, eight interested parties, ICAO, FAA, and Transport Canada have nominated members to the Licensing SubSectorial Team (LSST(M)).

medical examination at the beginning of the aviation career that included occupational health aspects and minimized the risk of a pathology later during the career, with the aim to keep the pilots in the best possible physical state during their whole professional life. Examinations included screening with various routine medical tests, like stress ECG, biochemistry, etc.

In other states, strict military standards and occupational or preventive health concerns were not of immediate importance. Pilots were examined by designated medical examiners, usually by family practitioners who had an interest in flying but a varying degree of aeromedical training. In this system, a pilot would normally be examined by an individual doctor and never pass through a specialized center. Laboratory tests were required only on clinical indication, with the exception of a urine test for glucose and, for Class 1 applicants, a blood test for hemoglobin. The scope of the aeromedical examinations was limited to establish clinical normality at a given moment and to ensure flight safety for a determined period of time. A pilot was required to have a certain level of mental and physical health and be likely to maintain this level for the duration of validity of his medical certificate, usually between six months and two years. Furthermore, there were other contrasts such as centralized versus decentralized systems, and different legal philosophies: Anglo-Saxon ("If the rule does not say you can't, then you can.") versus Roman philosophy ("If the rule does not say you can, then you can't.").

The JAA Medical Sub-Committee adopted the philosophy that the primary goal of aviation medical requirements is to assure a high level of flight safety, and combined the aeromedical cultures outlined above. This resulted in a compromise with clear characteristics concerning the chosen parameters and threshold values as well as detailed provisions for the practical completion of the medical examination.

With the implementation of JAR-FCL medical requirements in 1999, not only the national requirements starting from 1999 had to change but also the examination and assessment systems. When compared to previous national standards, the JAA requirements and corresponding aeromedical examinations were less demanding for pilots in several JAA member states, but for others, they were more demanding.

As could be expected, it was not easy for licence holders and regulators in some JAA member states to accept medical requirements and health examinations that were more stringent than those they were used to and which had been considered safe before. But it was probably even more difficult in other JAA member states to accept the relaxation of the requirements while still considering the former more stringent ones necessary to ensure flight safety and to comply with the duty of care for maintaining the health of the pilots.

Like aviation itself, medical and aeromedical knowledge develops at a quick pace. Therefore, the medical provisions had to develop as well. Furthermore, lessons learned after the implementation of the new rules had to be considered, editorial errors discovered during application of the rules had to be corrected, and further improvements had to be incorporated. A change mechanism for the evolution of the requirements was necessary. The Licensing Sub-Sectorial Team (Medical) was the working group tasked with adjusting the medical provisions in a procedure called Notice of Proposed Amendment. All those affected were invited to participate in the development of the proposal and subsequent consultation on drafts concerning new JARs or amendment of existing ones before the final adoption process ('consensus through participation').

OUTLINE OF JAR-FCL 3 (MEDICAL)

JAR-FCL 3 provides for a system of Authorized Medical Examiners (AME), who are entitled to perform initial and revalidation/renewal aeromedical examinations for private pilots, and revalidation/renewal examinations for commercial pilots. Aeromedical Centers (AMCs) have the privilege to also examine initial applicants for commercial licences and to carry out more extended examinations. AMEs and AMCs are supervised by the Aeromedical Section (AMS), which is normally part of the National Aviation Authority of the respective JAA member state and consists of aviation medicine specialists. This institution ensures the high level of medical confidentiality required under EU law. Medical data are only circulated between medical personnel and medical files are accessible to specially authorized medical personnel only.

The responsibilities of AMEs, AMCs, and AMS, the period of validity of medical certificates, the extent of medical assessments, examination methods, and physical and psychological standards are laid down in JAR-FCL 3. This document is divided into two sections. Section 1 contains the administrative and medical requirements in three subparts (Subpart A for general requirements, Subpart B for Class 1 and Subpart C for Class 2 medical requirements) and the pertaining appendices to those subparts. Section 2 contains guidance material such as information for national authorities regarding the training course syllabi for AMEs, and guidelines for AMCs and AMEs on how examinations have to be carried out, forms to be used, etc. Furthermore, a Manual of Civil Aviation Medicine contains guidelines for examining and assessing applicants together with the aeromedical background for the requirements. This text book is available by free access to the JAA website (see below). In some countries it is the only reference available for AMS, AMC, and AME, and has proved to be of immense value for all those involved in aviation medicine and the medical assessment of pilots.

MEDICAL STANDARDS OF JAR-FCL 3

Aviation safety is the principal objective of JAA (Joint Aviation Authorities) and JARs (Joint Aviation Regulations). This encompasses the safety of pilots, passengers, and third parties, i.e., the general public, people, and their property on the ground. Therefore, any policy permitting a decrease in medical fitness of pilots or any relaxation of the medical requirements must be accompanied by proof that aviation safety is not jeopardized.

For safe operation in the aviation environment, particular standards of visual acuity, color vision, hearing, cardiovascular, and physical capability are required. Sex and age are no reasons for denying a certificate. However, pilots above age 60 shall not engage in commercial air transport except when acting as a pilot in multi-crew operations and only when the other pilot is younger than 60 years. No commercial air transport is possible above age 65. However, since ICAO Annex 1 kept the historical "age 60 rule" until November 2006, some countries in compliance with this provision had imposed an age limit of 60 years for commercial air transport until their national codes were changed.

Wounds, injuries, sequelae from operations, abnormalities, disabilities, whether congenital or acquired, acute, latent, or chronic might bear a certain potential for functional incapacity. Diseases or disabilities, use of prescription or non-prescription drugs, or other treatments might interfere with aviation safety and result in a decrease in medical fitness. Pilots shall not fly if they are aware of such a condition or if they are not absolutely sure that any drug or treatment will not have any adverse effect. If certain conditions prevail, or if the pilot is in doubt, AMS, AMC, or AME have to be asked for advice (this applies in case of hospital admission of more than 12 hours, operations or other invasive procedures, regular medication, need for regular use of glasses), or be informed in writing and the medical certificate to be deemed suspended until otherwise decided by the authority (in case of significant personal injury, unfitness for more than 21 days, and pregnancy).

During or after certain diseases or operations (e.g., during cardiovascular disease, after refractive surgery), the medical certificate may be suspended for a certain time or permanently withdrawn (e.g., after a diagnosis of insulin dependent diabetes).

REVIEW PROCEDURES

An AME or AMC may assess pilots as fit to fly if the examination results are within the standards laid down in Subparts B or C of JAR-FCL 3. If the results are outside these limits, a fit assessment cannot be made by an AME or AMC. However, if they are in line with the Appendices to Subparts B and C, the AMS may perform a review procedure of the individual case and can assess the applicant as fit, taking into account experience, operational environment, etc.

If doubts about whether a fit assessment could be granted still prevail or if a rejected applicant appeals, a secondary review and a final decision by accredited medical conclusion is possible. A board of experts in aviation medicine, medical specialties, representatives of airline industry, and aircrew associations may be put together to give their opinion to the AMS. The latest Amendment 5 of JAR-FCL 3 allowed the authorities to delegate review procedures to AMCs or AME, and states like Germany do so. The latter has proven to be safe, as well as strengthened the role of aeromedical expertise, led to a quicker processing of reviews, and reduced administrative burden on pilots, the industry and administration.

Subsequent to review procedures, medical certificates are sometimes issued with a limitation. This may be a reduced validity of the medical certificate, mandatory additional tests, etc.

The provisions of JAR-FCL 3 do not allow as much flexibility as the Flexibility Standard of ICAO Annex 1, 1.2.4.8, and the review procedure is standardized. However, should an applicant be outside the requirements of JAR-FCL 3, an exemption may be granted by the Authority (JAR-FCL 3.045) following the prescribed procedures.

MUTUAL RECOGNITION OF MEDICAL CERTIFICATES

One of the aims of the Joint Aviation Requirements is to achieve mutual recognition of products, organizations, and licences among the JAA member states without further formalities. This applies to mutual recognition of medical certificates as well. Preconditions are implementation of the common codes and standardization of their application. The latter is achieved by an auditing system focussing on compliance with the JAR provisions. After many years of drafting JAR-FCL 3, auditing began after 1999, when the first JAA member states invited standardization teams to monitor their implementation of and compliance with JAR-FCL. By 2008, 28 JAA member states have been recommended by Central JAA for mutual recognition of licences and medical certificates.

EASA — THE EUROPEAN AVIATION SAFETY AGENCY

The limitation of the JAA was always that it was not a legal body but merely a cooperation of the JAA member states in the field of civil aviation. JARs had to be adopted by the individual member states and incorporated into national law to become binding, thus sometimes leading to different levels of implementation. It was concluded that a uniform level of implementation could only be achieved by acting on a European community level and creating an agency with a legal executive and enforcement power. The corresponding proposal was made by the European Commission (EC) in 1996.

The legislative process led to the creation of the European Aviation Safety Agency (EASA) and the common rules in the field of civil aviation were laid down in the "EASA Regulation" or "Basic Regulation" (Regulation 1592/2002 of the European Parliament). EASA was established in September 2003. The agency, first located in Brussels (Belgium), was relocated to Cologne (Germany) in September 2004. The agency forms part of the European Community System and is controlled by the European Commission. It has legislative power, taken over from the National Aviation Authorities (NAAs). The agency assists the European Commission in drafting regulations; it will cover all areas of civil aviation and neighboring areas such as air traffic control and, in the future, also management of airports.

In a multinational context, decisions in the field of aviation safety have to be made by a neutral and independent agency with the necessary authority and responsibility. The independence of EASA is ensured by its executive director, who is appointed by an executive board, consisting of representatives of the EU member states and the European Commission. He reports to an independent chamber of appeals and is controlled by a management board.

A basic idea of EASA is mandatory standardization, and the agency is the certifying entity and acts as authority in the field of airworthiness and continuing airworthiness. After extension of the scope to flight operations, flight crew licensing and medical certification, it will be the body determining the policy and setting the standards in this field as well. The National Aviation Authorities will still be responsible for the legal findings (examination and assessment, issue of licences and medical certificates), based on binding codes — the so-called technical findings. In contrast to the JAA system, mutual recognition is mandatory. This means that licences and authorizations issued by one member state must be accepted by all other member states.

NEW EASA REQUIREMENTS

The process to extend the competencies of EASA to flight operations and flight crew licensing began already in 2003. The development of the relevant amendment of the "EASA regulation" and of Essential Requirements (ERs) for personnel licensing — outlining the legal scope — also began in 2003. Articles 7 to 10 of the amended Regulation 1592/2002 related to pilot licensing. However, the legislative process slowed down and was delayed several times. After final approval by the European Parliament, the Council of Ministers and the European Commission at the end of 2007 and beginning of 2008, EASA achieved legal competence *inter alia* in the field of licensing and medical certification from March 2008 on, with the publication of a new Basic Regulation 216/2008 repealing the old one.

The medical provisions were included in the Draft Essential Requirements for Pilot Proficiency, containing the common rules for issuing and maintaining licences and certificates. The draft ERs were based on the concept of hazard-risk-mitigation, compliance with ICAO Standards and Recommended Practices (SARPs), and the use of existing JAR-FCL as Implementing Rules (IR). The requirements are designed to mitigate unavoidable risks; consequently, hazards and risks associated with aviation have been identified and analyzed. Pilot competence (qualifications), quality of training, medical fitness (physical and mental), and age related degradation were identified as hazard areas. With respect to age, education, physical and mental maturity as well as experience had to be balanced against age-related degradation of the cognitive functions and motor skills required for the safe performance of aviation tasks. The mitigating criteria were based on ICAO Annex 1 — *Personnel Licensing* and JAR-FCL. The underlying philosophy is that regulations have to mitigate the risks as much as reasonably achievable, but on the other hand, they should not go beyond that goal, creating undue restrictions not justified by their objectives. With respect to age, anti-discrimination principles had to be taken into account throughout the requirements.

All flight crewmembers have to demonstrate medical and physical fitness. They must not suffer from any disease or disability that might interfere with their ability to operate an aircraft safely and perform their duties correctly. Flexibility is necessary because the demands vary with the type of aircraft flown and activities performed. Deviations may be acceptable if it is ensured that the level of safety is maintained by appropriate mitigation measures. Pursuant to ICAO Annex 1 (Standard 1.2.4.8), certification of applicants with medical conditions or disabilities compensated by operational or technical measures is possible.

Full compliance with the established requirements is an essential safety element. Only appropriately qualified medical examiners should perform the assessment, and certain criteria for the authorization as Aeromedical Examiner (AME) have to be met. In more complicated cases, the medical assessment has to be performed by a well-structured and adequately equipped organization — an Aeromedical Center (AeMC).

Implementing Rules (IR) specify the details for pilot licensing and medical assessment. In contrast with the JAA principle of achieving consensus of all those affected by a regulation by a constitutional right of participation in the relevant regulation drafting groups (consensus by participation), EASA chose the approach of having small working groups, consisting of technical experts, proposed by advisory groups and selected by EASA to develop the drafts. Consensus building will be by public consultation only. The medical IRs are based on existing JAR-FCL 3. Acceptable Means of Compliance (AMC) and Guidance Material (GM) will provide further guidance for implementation of the future system and have to satisfy the requirements of ERs and IRs. However, stakeholders may choose a different AMC, provided that the same level of safety can be achieved (EASA "soft law"). The IRs on licensing, including medical certification, will be promulgated as a separate commission regulation. The drafts for the Implementing Rules have been completed once EASA had achieved legal competency in those areas (March 2008). The new IRs will be implemented at the beginning of 2009 at the earliest, and there will be a transition period of four years at the most. Once the legal framework is operative, it has to be implemented by the National Aviation Authorities of the EU member states. The public consultation started in June 2008. The original consultation period of three months was extended for some months, because the drafts for the pertaining Authority Requirements was not published until end October 2008 to allow for a clear picture of the administrative architecture.

As the new requirements no longer include the institution of an AMS, and as medical assessments are in the remit of the "licensing authority," a problem with medical confidentiality may arise due to conflicting requirements. Those who examine applicants for a medical certificate are responsible for safeguarding medical confidentiality. On the other hand — as required by ICAO Annex 1 and JAR-FCL 3 — these persons are obliged to submit reports and — in the case of applicants exceeding certain physiological and medical limits — detailed records of their examinations and findings to the "licensing authority." The requirements do not state that only medical personnel shall deal with the information submitted to the "licensing authority." A senior representative of EASA announced that adopting the system implemented in Germany in 2007 might solve the conflict. There, the complete files with records of examinations and assessments are kept by the AeMC or AME. After aeromedical assessment or review procedures, the German AMS only receives the information whether an applicant is unfit or fit and whether limitations are imposed. Information about limitations or whether a review procedure has been conducted is included in the medical certificate to make the next examiner aware in case of "doctor hopping." Detailed information about the review and subsequent obligations for the applicant is included in a document handed over to the applicant, which has to be presented to the next AME or AeMC. Thus, the authority can concentrate on its intrinsic and most important job to control and audit the system, without being distracted by a large amount of routine technical work, better to be done by those having direct access to the applicant, and without jeopardizing medical confidentiality.

A change mechanism to allow for adaptation and improvement of the requirements (as that described for JAR-FCL 3 above) is not stipulated; a team or working group tasked with the medical requirements or a focal point for aviation medicine within the agency does not exist anymore. Amending the IRs or even the ERs involves a complex legal mechanism. To enable an adaptation of standards and limits, these particular rules are included in Acceptable Means of Compliance (AMC) and Guidance Material (GM) — which can be more easily changed; in addition, numerical standards have been omitted wherever possible.

A totally new concept was introduced with the new requirements. In particular, less demanding requirements for airworthiness, continuing airworthiness, operations and licensing, tailored around the concept of a European light aircraft for general aviation, were introduced as JAR requirements were felt to be excessive. The concept encompassed another class of medical certificate for the new Light Aircraft Pilot Licence (LAPL), for which the requirements are included in the AMC of the new commission regulation. The medical requirements are much less stringent than those for JAR-FCL 3 Class 2 medical certificates and below those of ICAO Annex 1. The assessment for the LAPL medical certificate will include a comprehensive questionnaire to be answered by the applicant, a basic mandatory examination (including distant visual acuity, testing of the visual field, urine glucose, and systolic blood pressure) and — in case of doubt — some additional tests (BMI, whispered voice, mobility and strength of upper and lower limbs). Besides Aeromedical Centres (AeMCs) and Aeromedical Examiners (AMEs), general practitioners (GPs) with some training and experience in aviation medicine or a pilot licence may conduct aeromedical assessments for the LPL.

Even though being a transposition of JAR-FCL 3, the new medical requirements are published in a different format and show a different structure than JAR-FCL 3. They contain some items not mentioned in JAR-FCL 3 and are promulgated as Annex II of the new Commission Regulation on Personnel Licensing. Subpart A resembles Subpart A in JAR-FCL 3 and contains general requirements in three sections. Subpart B contains the general and specific requirements for Class 1 and Class 2 medical certificates — both merged together — arranged in paragraphs for the different organ systems. Subpart C contains the requirements for AMEs, Subpart D those for general practitioners involved in aeromedical assessments for the LPL. The specific standards and limits are published as AMC (Acceptable Means of Compliance)/GM (Guidance Material), which follow the structure of the subparts and refer to the appropriate paragraphs. However, the medical requirements for the LPL as well as the questionnaire to be used (Subpart A, Section 1) are listed as AMC. The AMC/GM are divided into subparts like the requirements they refer to. Consequently, Subpart A, which consists of one section, contains general material and the questionnaire for the LPL (Subpart A, Section 1). Subpart B is further divided into three sections. Section 1 General consists of the specific guidelines for the medical certificates for the LPL, Section 2 of the specific requirements for Class 1 and Class 2 medical certificates, with Chapter A relating to Class 1 and Chapter B relating to Class 2. Subparts C and D relate to the authorization of AMEs and general medical practitioners respectively.

The JAA is actively participating in the transition from the JAA system to EASA, which was outlined in a "roadmap" promulgated in the so-called FUJA (Future of JAA) Report. However, as normally only EU member states will be members of EASA, those JAA member states that were not or not yet members of EU, were not directly covered by EASA. The problem was that the JARs were part of their national aviation legislation. For this reason, these countries will still apply the JARs in the future and JAA acted as a liaison between those states and EASA during a transition period. JAA continued as JAAT (JAA in transition) with two different scopes: as liaison office (JAA-LO) for non-EU

JAA members (existing most probably until 2009), and as training office (JAA-TO). Furthermore, JAA coordinated the continued JAA rulemaking procedures as long as EASA had not yet achieved legal competency in rulemaking in the field of flight operations and licensing. Further amendments of the JARs will be in parallel to the development of EASA provisions, which means that EASA's legislative procedures has to be transposed into JARs. With EASA having gained momentum and competency in licensing and operations, a new FUJA Report II was launched in 2008 to determine the end of JAA by end June 2009. However, the JAA-TO will continue to offer training in aviation safety, including courses in aviation medicine. All JAA member states had to withdraw from the Cyprus Arrangement. A successful story with great achievements in aviation safety will be completed and an important chapter in aviation history be closed.

REFERENCES

1. JAR-FCL 3 — Flight Crew Licensing (Medical). Amendment 5, 01 December 2006, Joint Aviation Authorities (see: www.jaa.nl → Publications and NPAs → JARs → Section 1 → JAR-FCL 3).
2. JAA Manual of Civil Aviation Medicine. Amendment 5, 01 November 2006, Joint Aviation Authorities (see: www.jaa.nl → Liaison Office → Licensing → JAA Manual of Civil Aviation Medicine).

Part 3

PHYSIOLOGY AND RADIATION

Chapter 5

Fundamentals of Aviation Physiology

Dietrich Wirth† and Ekkehart Rumberger*,‡

INTRODUCTION

Many types of demands are placed upon the pilot. These can be demonstrated by analyzing different occupational requirements of various aircraft, by determining the physical loads placed on pilots during flight, and by analyzing the skills required during various flight activities.

The relationship between the pilot and the aircraft, in the sense of a man-machine-system, requires close attention and careful management. An ergonomically adequate design of the cockpit and proper working conditions during flight are necessary to assure flight safety.

HIGH ALTITUDE PERFORMANCE

Physical Fundamentals

Gas laws of the atmosphere

The gas laws apply to ideal gases only. They are, however, generally applicable to real gases at low pressures and high temperatures. The properties of the gaseous components of atmospheric air correspond, within a large temperature and pressure range, to the properties of

* Corresponding author.

† Böhmerstraße 7, D-01099 Dresden, Germany.

‡ Willistrasse 5, 22299 Hamburg, Germany.

an ideal gas. Thus the equation of state for an ideal gas is valid also for air:

$$P \times V = n \times R \times T$$

P = pressure
V = volume
n = number of moles of gas
R = specific gas constant
(for dry air: 8.3144 joules per mole Kelvin)
T = temperature in °K.

or

$$P \times \frac{V}{T} = n \times R = \text{constant}$$

Gas law according to Boyle
At constant temperature, the volume of a gas increases when the pressure decreases:

$$P \times V = \text{constant}$$

or

$$P_1 \times V_1 = P_2 \times V_2$$

P_1 = initial pressure at altitude 1
V_1 = initial volume at altitude 1
P_2 = final pressure at altitude 2
V_2 = final volume at altitude 2

Consequently, a volume of gas at 18 000 ft (5486 m) is twice as large as it was at sea level, and at 39 000 ft (11 887 m) it is five-fold larger.

Gas law according to Dalton

The total pressure (P_t) of a mixture of gases is the sum of the partial pressures (p_x) of all the separate gases in the mixture:

$$P_t = p_1 + p_2 + p_3 + \cdots + p_n$$

The partial pressure of each gas in a gas mixture corresponds to its fractional concentration (percentage by volume):

$$p_x = P_t \times \text{fractional concentration of gas} \times \text{(vol\%) in the mixture}$$

The partial pressure of oxygen at mean sea level is thus

$$pO_2 = 20.95 \times 760 \text{ mmHg} = 159.2 \text{ mmHg}$$

Gas law according to Henry

The amount of a gas (c) absorbed in a liquid is proportional to the partial pressure of the gas above the liquid. Thus when the ambient pressure falls, the partial pressure falls correspondingly (according to Dalton's law) and the amount of gas absorbed in the solution decreases — "goes out" of the liquid. This is the basis of decompression sickness.

The formula for Henry's law is most commonly given as $p = k \times c$, where k is the constant of Henry's law. k is also called the solubility coefficient and varies with the gas and the temperature.

It should be noted that both oxygen and carbon dioxide are also chemically combined with the blood.

International standard atmosphere

Air pressure results from the weight of the air in the atmosphere. A 1 m^2 column of air weighs approximately 100 kN (equivalent to about 10.2 tonnes as sea level). The column of air becomes shorter with increasing altitude, and the pressure correspondingly becomes less.

Due to the compressibility of air, this decrease of pressure occurs exponentially, but is also affected by the differential heating of the atmosphere from exposure to the sun.

In 1964, the International Civil Aviation Organization (ICAO) standardized the measurements of air pressure and temperature variations in the atmosphere up to an altitude of 100 000 ft. This standard atmosphere consists of clean, dry air and is presumed to behave as an ideal gas. The computations are based on a set of standardized values for the atmosphere at mean sea level.

Physiological Fundamentals

Respiration

Oxygen transport in the blood

— Mechanisms of transport

1. Physically absorbed

The transport of oxygen in the plasma follows Henry's law about the partial pressure of a gas, $c = k \times p$. k is the solubility coefficient (α) and depends on the temperature and the characteristics of the liquid. At 37°C, the blood carries about 0.3 mL O_2 per 100 mL blood.

2. Carried in the erythrocytes

Here oxygen transport takes place chemically, bound to hemoglobin. Hemoglobin is a chromoproteid, consisting of a globin and four heme molecules. The globin of the adult consists of four subunits, two α- and two β-chains, each of which carries a heme molecule. The heme molecule is constructed from a protoporphyrine ring, consisting of four pyrrol rings, connected by methyl groups, and carrying characteristic side groups. The heme molecule is anchored to a histidine segment of the globin via at the Fe^{++}-atom. The reversible attachment of O_2 (oxygenation) takes place at the bivalent iron atom in the center of the heme molecule. The S-shaped oxyhemoglobin dissociation curve, which is also known as the

Table 1. International Standard Atmosphere (ISA)[a]

Altitude		Air Pressure			O_2 Partial Pressure				
					Air		Alveolar		O_2 Saturation of
(ft)	(km)	(mmHg)	(kPa)	Temperature	mmHg	kPa	mmHg	KPa	Hemoglobin (%)
0	0	760	101.3	+15.0	160	21.6	103	13.7	97
3.000	0.914	681	90.8	+9.1	143	19.1	89	11.9	
5.000	1.524	632	84.2	+5.1	132	17.6	81	10.8	95
7.000	2.134	586	78.1	+1.1	123	16.4	79	10.5	93
8.000	2.438	565	75.3	−0.9	118	15.7	69	9.2	
10.000	3.048	523	69.7	−4.8	110	14.7	61	8.1	90
12.000	3.658	483	64.3	−8.8	101	13.5	54	7.2	86
15.000	4.572	429	57.1	−14.7	90	12.0	45	6.0	80
18.000	5.486	380	50.7	−20.7	80	10.7	38	5.1	72
20.000	6.096	349	46.5	−24.6	73	9.7	34	4.5	67
22.000	6.706	321	42.8	−28.6	67	8.9	33	4.4	65
25.000	7.620	282	37.6	−34.5	59	7.9	30	4.0	60

(*Continued*)

Table 1. *(Continued)*

Altitude		Air Pressure			O_2 Partial Pressure				
					Air		Alveolar		O_2 Saturation of Hemoglobin (%)
(ft)	(km)	(mmHg)	(kPa)	Temperature	mmHg	kPa	mmHg	KPa	
30.000	9.144	228	30.3	−44.4					
40.000	12.192	141	18.8	−56.5					
50.000	15.240	87	11.6	−56.5					
65.000	19.812	42	5.6	−56.5					

[a] Defined by ICAO (in reference to pressure, altitude and temperature, as well as partial pressure of O_2, and O_2-saturation of hemoglobin (R. Amendt, 1993)

Notes:
- the standard atmosphere presumes dry, clean air behaving as an ideal gas;
- the computations are based on fixed default values for the terrestrial atmosphere at sea level (air pressure P_0 = 101,325 Pa; Temperature $T_0 = 288.15$ K = 15°C; Density $\rho = 1.2250$ kg/m^{-3}; acceleration due to the gravity constant of 980.665 cm/s^2);
- composition of air (volume %): N_2 78.08; O_2 20.95; argon 0.93; carbon dioxide 0.03; noble gases 0.01;
- the aforementioned pressure and temperature levels represent approximate values at 40°N.

oxygen saturation curve, corresponds to the O_2-saturation, expressed as percentage, as a function of O_2 partial pressure.

— O_2 transport capacity

This capacity is primarily given by (1) the actual affinity of oxygen to hemoglobin, i.e. the volume of oxygen that is bound by fully saturated hemoglobin (values of 1.34 to 1.36 mL O_2/g Hb — Hüfner's number — are normal), and (2) the concentration of hemoglobin in the blood (145–155 g L^{-1}). Sex specific differences exist (men: 210 mL O_2 L^{-1}, women: 195 mL O_2 L^{-1}).

— Variation of O_2 affinity of hemoglobin

Functional changes that affect O_2 affinity of hemoglobin are reflected by a right–left shift of the oxyhemoglobin dissociation curve, as well as situations that create reversible or irreversible changes which block O_2 transportability. Brief functional changes in O_2 affinity occur. A decrease in O_2 affinity, resulting in a right shift of the oxyhemoglobin dissociation curve, may be caused by an increase in H^+ ion concentration, increase in CO_2 concentration, increase in body core temperature, and/or an increase in the concentration of 2,3-diphosphoglycerate (DPG). An increase of O_2 affinity, resulting in a left shift of the oxyhemoglobin dissociation curve, occurs when the aforementioned factors change in the opposite direction. These effects of H^+ ions and CO_2 concentration are called the Bohr-effect, and are caused by the allosteric reciprocal changes between H^+ and O_2 bonds.

— Inactive forms of hemoglobin

Carboxyhemoglobin (HbCO) is a strong reversible bond of carbon monoxide and bivalent iron. Since the affinity of CO to hemoglobin is about 300 times larger than that of O_2, CO displaces O_2, creating a strong leftward shift of the oxyhemoglobin dissociation curve.

Methemoglobin (metHb) results from oxidizing bivalent iron (Fe^{++}) in the hem molecule to trivalent (Fe^{+++}), either spontaneously or from oxidizing agents (e.g. nitrates, nitrites, aniline containing materials) making it impossible for O_2 to bond reversibly. The reduction of trivalent Fe^{+++} takes place physiologically via methemoglobinreductase.

CO_2 transport in the blood

— Mechanisms of transport

1. Physically dissolved in the plasma
The solubility of carbon dioxide is over 20 times greater than that of oxygen. The solubility coefficient α_X depends on the characteristics of the molecules X and of the liquid as well as the temperature. At 37°C, $5.06\ ml_{STPD}\ CO_2 \times L^{-1} \times kPa^{-1}$ is physically dissolved in the plasma.

2. As bicarbonate in the erythrocyte and in the plasma
$CO_2 + H_2O \leftrightarrow HCO_3^- + H^+$ (for the most part, a reversible bond).

3. As carbamino compounds at the free amino acid portions of blood proteins, particularly hemoglobin
$CO_2 + R - NH_2 \leftrightarrow R - NH - COO^- + H^+$. Buffering of H^+ ions occurs primarily by hemoglobin; as O_2 saturates hemoglobin, the affinity for carbamino formation decreases.

— CO_2 affinity curve

This curve results from the relationship between the concentrations of all three forms of CO_2 and the CO_2 partial pressure in the blood. There is no "saturation" and no "CO_2 capacity" of blood. At the same p_{CO_2}, deoxygenated hemoglobin binds substantially more CO_2 than oxygenated hemoglobin; this is called the Haldane effect. This process is due to the allosteric reciprocal effects of H^+ and O_2 bonds at the level of the hemoglobin molecule.

— Exchange procedures in the blood

The buffering capacity of the non-bicarbonate buffers in the erythrocytes (hemoglobin) is 7–8 times greater than that of plasma (plasma proteins). The normally slow process of the equilibrium $CO_2 + H_2O \leftrightarrow HCO_3^- + H^+$ is substantially accelerated by the enzyme carbonic anhydrase.

These exchange procedures are also promoted by other mechanisms. Since the concentration of HCO_3^- rises faster in the erythrocytes than in the plasma, a chemical gradient is established, resulting in an exchange of bicarbonate for Cl^- from the erythrocytes into the plasma (Hamburger-shift). In addition, an opposing cycle has been discovered recently, the endothelium of the capillaries mediates, by use of carbonic anhydrase, a back-transport of HCO_3^- into the erythrocytes, leading to a reaction forming CO_2 (Jacob–Stewart cycle.)

Control of ventilation

— Autonomous ventilation rhythm

Rhythmic breathing is governed from the ventral medulla oblongata and is coupled with other neuronal networks to regulate the tone of the bronchial muscles as well as to influence the sympathetic and parasympathetic nervous systems. A spontaneously active formatio reticularis sends impulses to the respiratory neurons. Following this primary network are the inspiratory, post-inspiratory and expiratory "exit neurons" which rhythmically activate the spinal motor neurons of the respiratory musculature. The rhythmicity of breathing results from the oscillating activity exchanges between these groups of neurons on the basis of inhibitory and excitatory synaptic interactions.

— Chemical control of ventilation

The autonomy of ventilation rhythm adjusts itself to cellular metabolic needs by way of chemical controls. The etiology of ventilatory changes can be differentiated by determining the changes in p_{CO_2}, p_{O_2} and pH. An increase in p_{CO_2} (hypercapnia) causes a substantial increase of respiratory drive by way of increased respiratory rate and tidal volume. A drop in arterial pH below normal values causes a drive in ventilation rate and respiratory volume, while a rise in arterial pH above normal values leads only to a low-grade reduction of ventilation. Declines in arterial O_2 partial pressure do not begin to affect the ventilatory system until it falls below the values of 6.7–8.0 kPa (50–60 mmHg), at which level substantial hypoxia exists. This apparent insensitivity of oxygen deficiency during hypoxic conditions is a result of a reduced CO_2 drive: hypoxia-generated tachypnoea is counteracted by a reduction in respiratory drive due to a corresponding fall in p_{CO_2}.

— Effects of central and reflexive factors in ventilation

In addition to the aforementioned control systems, respiration has "collateral" innervation along with the cardiovascular regulatory systems and is networked with nearly all sensorimotor activity. An arbitrary or psychopathological increase in ventilation occurs through co-innervation of the respiratory networks via cortical and limbic structures. Respiratory alkalosis develops quickly with maximal respirations, potentiating cerebral vasoconstriction. This causes a reduction in blood flow in the brain leading to changes in consciousness. Of the multiple mechanical and chemical reflexes existing in the upper airways and lungs, only the lung extension reflex (Hering–Breuer), which prevents a hyperextension of the lung will be mentioned here. On the other hand, significant hypothermia causes an inhibitory effect on ventilatory drive.

Abnormal ventilation

— Hyperventilation in norm and hypoxia

A special case may be considered: Alveolar ventilation is increased by increasing tidal volume beyond the requirement of metabolism. Breathing frequency is diminished, so that the respiratory volume per minute is unchanged. Alveolar and arterial p_{CO_2} falls beneath 5.3 kPa (40 mmHg, hypocapnia). Because the slopes of the affinity curves of O_2 and CO_2 are different, the difference in partial pressures between arterial and mixed-venous blood is smaller for CO_2 (0.8 kPa) than for O_2 (6.6 kPa). Thus the rise in partial pressure of CO_2 in mixed venous blood is less than the drop in O_2. Consequently the sum of all partial pressures in mixed venous blood is subatmospheric. This is the basis for resorption of gases from body cavities into the blood. In the case of hyperventilation, the small increase of p_{O_2} does not considerably increase the O_2 absorption into the blood at normal p_{O_2}. However, the CO_2 concentration in the blood and that of all CO_2 reservoirs of the body are considerably diminished. The CO_2 is exhaled, and the respiratory quotient (RQ) rises above 1, which is the limit of normal metabolic processes. A new level of CO_2 concentration depends on the balance between the degree of hyperventilation and metabolic intensity. The reduction of p_{CO_2} due to hyperventilation produces a cerebral vasoconstriction with decreasing cerebral blood flow, bringing on a unique feeling of disorientation.

Under hypoxic conditions at high altitudes the arterial p_{O_2} can drop below a value of 8 kPa (60 mmHg), thereby inducing a state of hyperventilation via peripheral and arterial chemoreceptors. This is followed by respiratory alkalosis. Both the decreased p_{CO_2} and the increased pH further reduce ventilatory drive, so that ventilation at high altitude conditions creates a situation where the competing drives of hypoxia and hypocapnea co-exist.

— Hypoventilation

A reduction of alveolar ventilation below metabolic requirements induces a rise of alveolar and arterial p_{CO_2} greater than 5.3 kPa (40 mmHg). This hypoventilation causes arterial hypoxemia and hypercapnia, with similar absolute changes in p_{O_2} and p_{CO_2}. Since an increased arterial p_{CO_2} induces ventilatory drive, hypoventilation will continue only if a disturbance of the central respiratory center, weakness of respiratory muscles, or a mechanical interference of the respiratory system is present.

Hypoventilation leads to substantial changes in cerebral circulation and function. CO_2 retention causes respiratory acidosis and dilates the cerebral vessels, adding to the same effect of arterial hypoxia. Beyond that, acute respiratory acidosis has a stronger acidifying effect on cerebrospinal fluid than metabolic acidosis of the same degree, because CO_2 can freely diffuse through the blood brain barrier. The consequences are a rise of pressure in the brain ventricles, a reduction in brain metabolism, a degradation of brain function, and, finally, neurological symptoms. Hypoventilation further affects the pulmonary circulation and the work load of the heart, as it creates a hypoxic vasoconstriction of the blood vessels in the lungs, resulting in pulmonary hypertension and increased loading of the right heart, eventually leading to right heart insufficiency.

Cardiovascular system

Cerebral circulation and metabolism

— Under normoxic conditions the cerebral circulation amounts to approx. 50 mL/100 g of brain tissue per minute, while the O_2 consumption per minute amounts to approx. 3 mL/100 g or approx. 15% of the total requirement of the body. Energy is gained almost entirely from glucose metabolism, and cellular uptake and utilization is insulin independent. Ketone bodies are metabolized only when present in very high plasma concentrations (e.g. during fasting or from diabetic ketoacidosis).

— Mechanisms involved in the regulation of brain circulation

An increase of blood pressure in the brain is followed by only a negligible increase of blood flow as the myogenic tone of the arterioles prevents a significant increase of flow. The range of this pressure auto-regulation lies between 80 and 120 mmHg (10.5 to 16.0 kPa). When the upper range of auto-regulation pressure is approached, sympathetic noradrenalin-mediated fibers send signals to activate cerebral vasculature to constrict, thus preventing a pressure-related cerebral circulatory overload.

Local control is mediated through a release of functionally and metabolically dependent factors (K^+, H^+, adenosine) from cells into the interstitial space of the brain, causing a dilatation of the constricted blood vessels. K^+ ions work quickly but weakly, while fine adjustments are mediated via H^+ ions and adenosine. Further changes of arterial p_{CO_2} resulting from either hyper- or hypoventilation lead to respective changes in pH in the cerebrospinal fluid and in the interstitial fluid, causing further vascular changes: decreased arterial p_{CO_2} → interstitial alkalosis → vasoconstriction, and increased arterial p_{CO_2} → interstitial acidosis → vasodilatation.

Hypoxic conditions with an arterial p_{O_2} below approximately 75 mmHg (10 kPa) have been shown to increase cerebral blood flow, at least partly in response to a release of adenosine from brain tissue.

Coronary blood circulation

At rest, the coronary circulation amounts to 80–90 mL per 100 g of muscle tissue per minute, corresponding to about 5% of cardiac output. An increase in the heart's metabolic demand is followed primarily by an increase in circulation rather than by an increased oxygen extraction capability, which, even at rest, is already greater than in most other organs of the body.

One of the strongest stimuli for coronary artery dilatation is the confluence of various hypoxemia signals. A reduction of only 5% in oxygen saturation leads to coronary artery dilatation, probably primarily due to the accumulation of adenosine in the myocardium from the breakdown products of phosphate compounds. Additionally a rise in extracelluar H^+- and K^+-concentration occurs. One of the most important other critical endothelial factors is nitrogen monoxide (NO).

Important physical factors are aortic pressure as the driving force and the compression of the coronary arteries, which influence coronary flow in every systole.

Neurohormonal factors involved in coronary circulation include the chemical transmitters of the autonomic nervous system, reaching the heart either via neural or circulatory pathways. Noradrenalin operates via the α-receptors as a vasoconstrictor, and via the β-receptors as a positive inotrope. This creates a metabolically more active state which overcomes noradrenalin's vasoconstrictive effect. Other mechanisms will not be described here.

Effects of Hypoxia

Energy metabolism and hypoxia sensitivity

Energy metabolism

Immediate energy is obtained by splitting a phosphate bond from the high energy state of available ATP. New ATP formation is created through a reaction catalyzed by creatinine phosphate (CP), which is especially important within the first 3–10 seconds after muscle activity begins. In case of strenuous work, the circulatory and respiratory systems need 2 to 3 minutes to adapt. The metabolic stimulus for adaptation is acidosis, which is caused by anaerobic energy supply in glycolysis. This ATP production is 2–3 times faster than oxidative phosphorylation, but the extent is limited because some enzymes are inhibited by increasing concentration of H^+-ions.

After 2 to 3 minutes, energy has to be supplied by oxidative phosphorylation, otherwise the muscle becomes rigid and the work must be broken off. If oxygen supply is sufficient for the metabolic requirement, fat and carbohydrates are completely changed to CO_2 and H_2O. The process is only limited by exhaustion of glycogen and fat reservoirs. The most essential fuel is glucose, as the brain can utilize only glucose for its metabolism. Additionally, glucose provides the only anaerobic power production; it also provides the largest amount of energy (21.2 kJ/L O_2.).

The importance of glucose in aviation is the considerable need the brain has for this critical power source. The uptake and utilization of glucose in the brain is insulin independent. Normal plasma glucose level is about 5 mmol, i.e. 90 mg/dL. Pronounced hypoglycemic symptoms appear at a blood sugar level of 2.2 mmol. Symptoms include voracious appetite, perspiration, trembling, agitation, loss of concentration, psychological disinhibition. With further decline in blood levels, somnolence, clouding of the consciousness, and loss of consciousness (hypoglycemic shock) will appear. Even small drops in blood sugar can lead to a reduction in mental and physical capacity by interfering with concentration and judgment. Glucose is subject to strict hormonal control. The β-cells of the islets of Langerhans in the pancreas deliver insulin as soon as glucose concentrations rise in the intestines and plasma. In a healthy person, the administration of 100 g glucose produces a transient rise with a return to the prior blood glucose level after approximately three hours. In some sensitive humans, glucose levels swing after the initial peak to subnormal levels, causing symptoms of hypoglycemia. One should advise such individuals not to ingest large quantities of glucose or other easily-digested carbohydrates rapidly. They are either afflicted with an excessive production of insulin or a lack of somatostatin. This hormone is manufactured in the δ-cells of the islets of Langerhans and in the intestinal epithelium. It diminishes intestinal activity and therefore glucose absorption in response to a rising glucose concentration, thereby dampening the oscillations in blood sugar levels. With declining glucose levels, glucagon in the α-cells of the islets of Langerhans releases glucose from glycogen. The hypothalamic-hypophyseal-adrenaline axis has an important role in glucose metabolism, releasing adrenal cortisol and catecholamines during particularly stressful situations. They also increase gluconeogenesis from proteins, thereby increasing performance capacity.

Oxygen reservoirs are of utmost importance for aerobic metabolism, all combined amounting to approximately 1.5 L: 400 mL in the air in the lungs, 50 mL dissolved in the tissues, 800 mL bound to hemoglobin, and 250 mL bound to myoglobin.

Hypoxia sensitivity of tissues

— General principles

Central nervous system structures exhibit a high degree of hypoxia sensitivity, as they possess only a small reserve capacity for glycolytic metabolic processes. Individual brain structures are differentiated in importance by their phylogenetic age, in that the phylogenetically most recent brain structures have the least tolerance to hypoxia. Furthermore, the more complex the cognitive and motor functions are, the greater the effects of hypoxia. The symptomatology is unique to every individual, but rather constant to an individual throughout the course of his life.

— Anoxia and body tissues

The cerebral cortex exhibits the following functional changes after sudden tissue anoxia: first a 4-second symptom-free interval; then, after 4–6 seconds, malfunctions begin; after 10–20 seconds, complete paralysis and loss of consciousness (period of paralysis defined as survival period of organ function); after 20–30 seconds, loss of spontaneous activity (zero line EEG); after 3–5 minutes, irreversible damage; after 8–10 minutes resuscitation may still possible.

The latent recovery time of the cerebrum after a short anoxic phase is approximately one minute; after about 4 seconds of complete cerebral ischemia, it is about 10 minutes. The recovery time of brain function after one minute of cerebral ischemia is about 15 minutes.

A comparison of the times after which resuscitation is still possible for different brain areas and organs underscores the statement at the beginning of this section: 3–5 minutes for the telencephalon (cortex and basal ganglia), 3–4 minutes for the working heart (e.g. in case of atrial fibrillation), as well as for the diencephalon; 7 minutes for the brain stem (medulla oblongata, pons and mesencephalon), 3–4 hours for kidney and liver, several hours more for skeletal musculature.

Changes in organ functions

Ventilatory parameters

Ventilation increases relatively little, as long as the arterial p_{O_2} does not fall below 8.0 kPa, corresponding to an altitude of approximately 10 000 feet (3050 m). At an altitude of approximately 20 000 feet

Table 2. Oxygen Saturation (%) of Hemoglobin ($\bar{x} \pm s$) as a Function of the Ambient Altitude (I. Schmitz, 1997)

Ambient Altitude (in meters)	Peripheral Oxygen Saturation of Hemoglobin (%), Indirectly Measured			
	Time Spent at the Respective Altitude (min)			
	1	3	5	Average Values
180	98 ± 0.8	98 ± 0.5	98 ± 0.7	98 ± 0.7
2000	97 ± 1.2	97 ± 0.8	96 ± 0.8	96.9 ± 0.9
2500	96 ± 1.3	95 ± 1.5	94 ± 1.4	94.9 ± 1.1
3000	94 ± 2.0	93 ± 1.5	92 ± 2.1	92.4 ± 1.9
3500	91 ± 1.9	89 ± 1.9	88 ± 3.7	89.2 ± 3.7
4000	88 ± 3.1	86 ± 4.0	84 ± 4.0	85.1 ± 4.9

(6100 m), ventilatory rate doubles from the initial value with an arterial p_{O_2} of 5.0 kPa. Furthermore, increase in breath volume ensues, but because of the opposing effects of the ventilatory drive (hyperventilation reduces p_{CO_2}!) this occurs to a lesser extent than could be expected proportionally. At an altitude above 25 000 feet (7600 m), breathing becomes dysrhythmic and flat, so that ventilation is reduced quickly and loss of consciousness is imminent.

Cardiovascular parameters

At rest, the normal heart beats 60–80 times per minute and achieves rates between 90–120 beats per minute at altitudes of 20 000 feet **(6100 m)**. Thereafter, it increases at a lower rate with increasing altitude. With physical loads, this increase is greater. The speed of ascent also affects the heart rate. The stroke volume changes only slightly and without a preferential direction.

The mean arterial blood pressure rises only slightly with increasing altitude. When exposed to longer effects of hypobaric hypoxic hypoxia, the pulmonary vasculature can develop vasoconstriction (Euler–Liljestrand mechanism), resulting in pulmonary edema.

Altogether, these cardiac changes (resulting from an increase in heart rate and vasoconstriction, caused by arterial chemoreceptors) are superimposed upon those mediated by local hypoxic vasodilatator reactions. Within the brain, the net effect of vasodilatation due to hypoxia and the vasoconstriction due to hypocapnia is a small increase in cerebral circulation.

In the myocardium, coronary vasodilatation and circulation rise when hemoglobin oxygen saturation falls by only 5% and, depending on the degree of hypoxia, can double or triple.

Pulmonary hypertension secondary to hypoxia

As a result of an alteration of the redox potential due to hypoxia (60–70 mmHg), a K-channel in the smooth muscle of small pulmonary arterial vessels (diameter: 200 to 400 μm) is inhibited. The membrane is depolarized, causing an increasing permeability of a voltage-dependent calcium channel. The rising intracellular calcium concentration results in vasoconstriction, with increasing pulmonary resistance. This mechanism is influenced by histamine, serotonine, angiotensine II, prostaglandine and nitrogenmonoxid.

Therefore, a prolonged stay in altitude produces a hypertrophy of the smooth muscles of the pulmonary vessels and promote the Euler–Liljestrand-effect in its efficacy in the embryonal circulation and in the adaption of the regional perfusion of the lung.

Subjective altitude effects

General symptomatology of hypobaric hypoxic hypoxia

— Subjective signs: fatigue, sleepiness, stupor, feelings of warmth or cold; dizziness and anxiety; pins and needles in fingers and/or toes; visual disturbances (flickering, decreased visual acuity); euphoria or apathy.

— Objectives symptoms: hyperventilation, cyanosis, impaired color and night vision; disturbed cognitive function, diminished judgment and impaired critical thought processes.

Table 3. Measured Values of Heart Rate as a Function Ambient Altitude (D. Wirth *et al.*, 1999)

Ambient Altitude (m)	Heart Rate (min^{-1}): Time Spent at the Respective Altitude (min)			Heart Rate (min^{-1}): Heart Rate Difference to Sea Level	Arterial Blood Pressure (mmHg)		
	1	3	5		Systolic	Diastolic	Differential
180	78 ± 18	74 ± 17	73 ± 17	Not applicable	135 ± 15	82 ± 10	53 ± 10
2000	79 ± 18	80 ± 15	79 ± 15	6.2 ± 6.2	133 ± 12	83 ± 10	50 ± 7
2500	83 ± 15	84 ± 16	82 ± 16	7.2 ± 5.1	133 ± 12	82 ± 9	51 ± 7
3000	83 ± 15	84 ± 14	82 ± 14	8.9 ± 5.3	133 ± 14	81 ± 8	52 ± 8
3500	86 ± 15	83 ± 16	84 ± 13	10.9 ± 6.5	135 ± 15	82 ± 8	53 ± 8
4000	89 ± 14	89 ± 12	87 ± 13	11.9 ± 11.3	131 ± 13	81 ± 8	51 ± 8

Table 4. Normal Values of Heart Rate during a Stay at an Altitude of 5000 m, Sitting and Standing Position (B. Kasprzak, D. Wirth, 1975)

Experimental Conditions			Age of Participants (years)				
Altitude	Position	Time of Measurement (min)	16–20 (N = 61)	21–25 (N = 40)	26–30 (N = 59)	31–35 (N = 59)	36–40 (N = 39)
0 m GND	sit	1	85 ± 14	74 ± 8	78 ± 12	83 ± 11	83 ± 10
5000 m	sit	1	101 ± 15	89 ± 8	94 ± 11	95 ± 12	94 ± 11
		5	103 ± 14	92 ± 9	97 ± 12	96 ± 13	96 ± 10
		10	102 ± 14	90 ± 9	95 ± 11	94 ± 12	93 ± 11
		15	101 ± 15	89 ± 9	93 ± 12	94 ± 12	93 ± 11
		20	100 ± 14	88 ± 9	92 ± 12	92 ± 12	92 ± 11
		25	97 ± 19	88 ± 11	91 ± 11	91 ± 12	93 ± 11
	stand	1	110 ± 15	95 ± 9	100 ± 12	98 ± 13	99 ± 12
		3	112 ± 16	95 ± 9	99 ± 12	98 ± 13	99 ± 13
		5	111 ± 17	93 ± 9	100 ± 12	99 ± 13	98 ± 12
	sit	1	101 ± 15	88 ± 8	92 ± 11	92 ± 13	95 ± 12
		5	96 ± 14	85 ± 8	89 ± 10	88 ± 11	90 ± 10
0 m GND	sit	1	77 ± 12	67 ± 7	71 ± 10	72 ± 10	72 ± 9

— Symptomatology with progressive hypoxia: continued decrease in concentration and critical thinking; memory lapses, restriction of peripheral vision, diminished speech and verbal reactivity, muscle tremor and cramps, circulatory failure, respiratory arrest, unconsciousness.

Hypoxia symptoms experienced by pilots (as indicated by R.O. Reinhart in Ref. 5)

These are: restriction of peripheral vision, such as "tunnel vision"; decreased visual acuity (blurring, difficulty in focusing); difficulties in visual accommodation, particularly in transitioning from near to distant vision; difficulty in changing seat position; fatigue and exhaustion, sleepiness without a recognizable cause (such as boredom); diminished sensitivity to light touch; feeling of not being in control; reduction in pain sensation (even pain of a sprained ankle); headache, especially after 2 hours of hypoxia exposure; light head tremors and dizziness; poor reaction when turning in a tight radius; pins and needles in fingers and toes; impaired muscular coordination; diminished control of movement; stuttering (correct words cannot be found during radio transmissions); cyanosis (blue lips and fingernails); diminished critical thinking (making silly mistakes, slow mentation); loss of self-assessment abilities; overly confident self-assurance ("no problem!"); overly aggressive, reproachful; provocative on radio calls; depression (small irritations become large problems); changed respiration (faster and flatter); prolonged response time (loss of sense of taction); severely impaired night vision (beginning at 1500 m altitude); euphoria (decreased attention to safety issues).

Hypoxia symptomatology at various altitudes

Table 5 shows the symptomatology of hypoxia at increasing altitudes. Corresponding to the altitude, hypoxia is graduated. The steps from one zone to the next are called thresholds.

Table 5. Symptoms of the Central Nervous System at Different Altitudes (R.O. Reinhart, 1992)

Ambient Altitude				
(ft)	(m)	Degree of Hypoxia	O_2-saturation of Hemoglobin (%)	Symptoms
0–5000	0–1823	minimal	90–98	— decreased night vision acuity
5000–10000	1823–3647	compensatory	80–90	— sleepiness — diminished judgment — deteriorating coordination — reduced performance/efficiency
10000–15000	3647–5470			
15000–20000	5470–7293	not fully compensatory	70–80	— deteriorating flight control — deteriorating handwriting — deteriorating speech ability — decreased coordination
20000–25000	7293–9117	critical	60–70	— circulatory break down — failure of the CNS — muscle cramps — cardiovascular collapse — death

Classification of hypoxia

Tissue hypoxia

Definition: Tissue hypoxia is defined as O_2 deficiency in individual tissue regions, caused by a disturbance in oxygen delivery. Such disturbances can be the result of a reduction in available O_2 from arterial hypoxia, anemia or circulatory disturbances or can be caused by interference with O_2 utilization (e.g. poisoning of the oxidative enzymes). In such cases, energy can be made available only for a short period of time, either by release of energy stores or from anaerobic metabolism.

Possible causes of tissue hypoxia:

1. Hypoxemia (respiratory and hypoxic hypoxia): decreased O_2 saturation of hemoglobin due to lung malfunctions (e.g. hypoventilation or disturbance of the ventilation-perfusion system) or inspiratory hypoxia (e.g. high altitude).
2. Anemic hypoxemia: diminished O_2 carrying capacity caused by organic conditions (e.g. blood loss, circulatory disturbances) or functional conditions (CO poisoning or methemoglobinopathy).
3. Ischemia (circulatory hypoxia): decreased organ perfusion with simultaneously increased arterio-venous difference in O_2-concentration in individual organs (e.g. thrombosis, embolism, arteriosclerosis).
4. Tissue diffusion disturbance: caused by tissue edema, poor vascularization, or rapidly-growing tumors.
5. Histotoxic hypoxia: disturbances of O_2 utilization during oxidative phosphorylation by cellular poisons such as cyanide and its potassium salt.

Classification of various altitudes in relation to hypobaric hypoxic hypoxia

There is a high degree of variability of symptoms in response to reduced partial pressure of oxygen at altitude. The following summary may be useful for orientation:

1. Altitude zones

The generally accepted terms for altitude ranges or zones as characterized by physiological changes are efficient, completely compensated,

Table 6. Causes and Types of Hypoxia (RL. De Hart, 1985)

Respiratory Process	Functional Conditions	Specific Causes	Type of Hypoxia
Ventilation	Reduction of the alveolar P_{O_2}	Reduced P_{O_2} of inhaled air due to strangulation, respiratory arrest, laryngospasm, different types of asthma, breath holding, hypoventilation due to high external pressure of the thorax (snorkeling and diving), inhaled gas mixture with an insufficient PO_2. malfunctioning oxygen devices at altitude	Hypoxic hypoxia
	Reduction of gas exchange surface area	Pneumonia, drowning, atelectasis, emphysema, pneumothorax, pulmonary embolism, inborn cardiac anomalies, physiological shunts	
Diffusion	Diffusion barriers	Hyaline membrane disease of the lung (neonatal), pneumonia, drowning	
Transport	Reduction of the oxygen transportation capacity	Anemia, blood loss, hemoglobinopathies (hypochromic anemia, sickle cell disease) medications (sulfanilamide, nitrites); chemical toxins (cyanide, CO)	Hypemic hypoxia
	Reduction of cardiac stroke volume	Cardiac insufficiency, shock, continuous positive pressure, artificial respiration, acceleration (g-forces), pulmonary embolism	Stagnating hypoxia
	Reduction of regional or local blood flow	External ambient temperatures, position changes (continuous sitting, bed-ridden or weightlessness), constrictions (restricting clothing, belts etc.), hyperventilation, gas embolism, cerebrovascular accidents	

(*Continued*)

Table 6. *(Continued)*

Respiratory Process	Functional Conditions	Specific Causes	Type of Hypoxia
Utilization	Metabolic poisoning or dysfunction of enzymes of respiration	Poisoning or reduction of the respiratory enzymes, carbon monoxide, cyanide, alcohol	Histotoxic hypoxia

incompletely compensated and critical. Generally the following distinctions apply:

— Physiologically efficient zone: spans the altitude range from MSL to 3000 m. Physiological changes cannot be observed or are only minimal. Full capacity exists with normal activity, only minimal decrease in capacity occurs with high physical activity lasting more than 2 minutes.
— Zone of complete compensation: from 3000 m to a level of approximately 4500 m, the O_2-saturation of hemoglobin drops to 80–87%, causing a rise in heart rate and ventilation at rest; efficiency is reduced by approximately 25%.
— Zone of incomplete compensation: from 4500 m to a level of approximately 7000 m, oxygen saturation of hemoglobin drops to values around 65–70%. Even at rest, substantial vegetative, psychological and motor symptoms arise.
— Critical zone: begins at an altitude of 7000 m and above 8000 m, all physical capacity is lost rather quickly.
— Dead man's zone: above 14000 m, sufficient partial pressure of oxygen can only be provided to the alveoli by use of a positive pressure breathing apparatus.

2. Threshold levels

Threshold levels are the levels between the altitude zones described above: the reaction threshold is the level between the efficient zone and the zone of complete compensation, the disturbance threshold is the level between the latter and the zone of incomplete compensation, the critical threshold level lies between this and the critical zone, and, finally, the fatal threshold level lies above the critical zone.

Hypoxia tolerance and self rescue time

Hypoxia tolerance

A variety of factors influence individual hypoxia tolerances, which can be constitutional, dependent on conditioning, current state of health, and topical stressors. Tolerance, therefore, is variable and can be increased with high altitude physiological training.

Self- and assisted rescue times

— Synonymous with self rescue time are the terms time reserve (Ruff/Strughold, 1957), reserve time (Papenfuss *et al.*, 1990; Schulze *et al.*, 1990), Time of Useful Consciousness (TUC) (MOS he/franc, 1988; Amendt, 1993) and effective performance time (CEPT) (Reinhart, 1992).

— The self rescue time is defined as the time from the moment the oxygen supply is interrupted to the onset of incapacitation, i.e. loss of the ability to appropriately carry out required actions. During this period, personal warning symptoms may be noticed. The length of this period depends on the cabin altitude; at high altitudes it amounts to only 9 to 12 seconds.

— The self rescue time is affected by the following factors: 1. The cabin altitude at which the oxygen deficiency begins, 2. The pilot's experience in handling hypoxia, 3. Work load and stress load, and 4. General physical fitness. Fatal outcomes can often be avoided by providing assisted rescue, which significantly enhances survival.

— Necessary course of action for the pilot upon recognizing an oxygen deficiency.

Table 7. Relationship of Altitude to Self Rescue Times (R.O. Reinhart, 1992)

Ambient Altitude		Time of Useful Consciousness (TUC)
(ft)	(m)	
18 000	5486	20–30 min
22 000	6706	10 min
25 000	7620	3–5 min
28 000	8534	2.5–3 min
30 000	9144	1–2 min
35 000	10 668	30–60 s
40 000	12 192	15–20 s
43 000	13 106	9–12 s
50 000	15 240	9–12 s

In unpressurized aircraft equipped with oxygen supply: switch the automatic controller to emergency supply, examine the masks and hose connector, pull the green lever (O_2 reserve activated) and carry out a rapid descent to an altitude below 10 000 ft (3048 m).

In passenger aircraft with pressurized cabin: while keeping the oxygen mask on and descend to a safe altitude of less than 18 000 feet (~6 km) as well as donning the oxygen mask.

Additional oxygen supply

Computation of oxygen partial pressure

Formulas for the computation of oxygen partial pressure:

Air as inhaled gas: 1. $p_T\text{-}O_2 = (P - 47)$ H 0.21

2. $p_A\text{-}O_2 = p_T\text{-}O_2 - p_A\text{-}CO_2/RQ$

With 100% O_2: 3. $p_A\text{-}O_2 = p_T\text{-}O_2 - p_A\text{-}CO_2$

Legend: P = total air pressure

$p_T\text{-}O_2$ = tracheal O_2-partial pressure

$pP_A\text{-}O_2$ = alveolar O_2-partial pressure

$p_A\text{-}CO_2$ = alveolar CO_2-partial pressure

The first formula serves for the computation of p-O_2 in the trachea. The second formula serves for the computation of p-O_2 in the lung alveoli. Alveolar p-O_2 is therefore dependent on the carbon dioxide portion and thus on the respiratory quotient (RQ). Higher altitudes are possible with supplemental oxygen. Because of the danger of hypoxia-induced unconsciousness, breathing air only is inadequate above 10 000 ft (3048 m); supplemental oxygen in an air/oxygen mixture is fully sufficient only up to an altitude of 25 000 ft (7620 m), while 100% supplemental oxygen is commonly used above 30 000 feet (9144 m) and becomes necessary above 33 000 feet (10 057 m).

Positive pressure breathing

Because of the needs of military flying at high altitudes with unpressurized or only partially pressurized cabins, several designs for provision of supplemental pressurized oxygen at various barometric pressures have been created. Active exhalation is necessary against the positive pressure of the inhaled air and gives rise to physiological disturbances such as change of respiratory rate, increase in pulmonary vascular resistance, and decrease in cardiac stroke volume

Table 8. Percentage of Supplemental Oxygen Required as a Minimum at Various Altitudes.

Altitude		Barometric Pressure (kPa)		Proportionate O_2-mixing	
(ft)	(m)	Total	pO_2	(kPa)	(%)
0	0	101.3	21.3	0	0
5000	1524	84.2	17.7	3.6	4
10000	3048	69.7	14.6	6.7	10
15000	4572	57.1	12.0	9.0	19
20000	6096	46.5	9.8	11.2	28
25000	7620	37.6	7.9	13.4	41
30000	9144	30.6	6.4	14.9	60
35000	10668	23.9	5.0	16.3	79

and arterial blood pressure. Compensatory sympathetic mechanisms are activated, causing vasoconstriction, elevation of stroke volume and respiratory rate, and utilization of accessory respiratory muscles.

Altitude protective clothing

High-altitude pressurized suits and well-fitting masks serve as mechanical protection against the increased intrapulmonary pressure created by positive pressure breathing devices. The combination of high altitude pressurized suit and pressure helmet makes it possible to attain a positive oxygen pressure of 19.33 kPa in relation to ambient pressure, enabling flights up to 40–50 km.

Toxic effects of oxygen

Hyperoxia

— General data

Increasing the inspiratory oxygen partial pressure above 22 kPa has a very marginal effect on hemoglobin which is already normally saturated at 97%. At 100 kPa, only 24 ml O_2 per L are physically dissolved (according to the Bunsen's absorption coefficient at 37°C).

— Applications of supplemental oxygen

a) Pre-breathing of O_2 prior to high altitude exposure.
b) Use of increased O_2 partial pressure (>50 kPa) in military night flights.
c) Treating ischemic or anemic hypoxia under isobaric pressure conditions. This necessitates therapeutic mechanical ventilation with high O_2 percentages and increased oxygen partial pressure. For chronic therapy of adults, the inspiratory p-O_2 should not exceed 60 kPa, in newborns not over 40 kPa. Under hyperbaric conditions (hyperbaric chambers) medically pure oxygen should only be given for short periods of time, due to its toxic effects as a cellular poison.
d) Diving with compressed gas.

— Benchmarks for the toxic effects of oxygen (dose-effect relationships)

a) With p-O_2 > 100 kPa (755 mmHg): initial pulmonary symptoms.
b) With p-O_2 > 200 kPa (1510 mmHg): preponderance of CNS symptoms.
c) With p-O_2 = 250 kPa (1885 mmHg): under resting conditions a tolerance of 1–2 hours.
d) With p-O_2 > 600 kPa (4530 mmHg): abrupt onset of tonic-clonic spasms and unconsciousness.

— Effects and risks

a) Inhibition of metabolic tissue enzymes (e.g. inhibition of glucose, fructose oxidation and pyruvic acid.
b) CNS disturbances: nausea, headache, paresthesias (particularly at the fingertips), dizziness, confusion, cramps (e.g. twitching lips), and unconsciousness.
c) Pulmonary disturbances: inflammation of the mucous membranes of the upper respiratory system with cough and retrosternal pain upon deep inspiration; decrease of lung elasticity, atelectasis formation, rise of the alveolar-arterial p-O_2 gradients; in severe cases interstitial pneumonia and pulmonary edema with bloody transudate (increased capillary permeability).
d) Cardiovascular disturbances: diminished cardiac output with increased vagal tone, decreased brain and kidney perfusion.

Normoxic Hypoxemia from CO

CO has about 300 times greater affinity to hemoglobin than oxygen. Carboxyhemoglobin (HbCO) is an inactive form of hemoglobin, in which carbon monoxide (CO) has displaced oxygen and is reversibly bound to the bivalent iron-atom of heme. The additional leftward shift of the oxygen hemoglobin dissociation curve reduces O_2 delivery to the tissues. Normally 1% of hemoglobin is present as HbCO. Differential diagnosis of CO poisoning in pilots includes inhaled engine exhaust, smoldering fire in the cockpit, and tobacco smoking.

The effect of smoking is considerable. Tobacco smoke contains 1.5–4.5 of vol% CO; each cigarette increases the percentage of

Table 9. Symptoms of Carbon Monoxide Poisoning as a Function of HbCO-Concentration (W. Forth, D Henschler, W. Rummel, 1987).

HbCO (%)	Symptoms, Effects
2–3	Impairment of mental functions
5–10	Feeling of tightness in the forehead, mild headache, mild decrease of vision (flicker fusion frequency decreases)
10–20	Severe headache, fatigue, malaise, shortness of breath (with moderate effort), palpitations; changed visual evoked potentials
20–30	Pulsating headache, nausea, dizziness, diminished consciousness, impairment of manual talents, limb flaccidity and paralysis
30–40	Decreased consciousness, flattened respiration, circulatory collapse, skin pink
40–60	Deep unconsciousness, paralysis, Cheyne–Stoke respiration, reduction in body temperature
50–60	Death within 10 minutes to one hour
70	Death within few minutes

carboxyhemoglobin by over 2%. Smokers generally have 2–14% HbCO; smoking 20 cigarettes can lead to the formation of 20% HbCO.

The CO bond cannot be neutralized, but the amount of HbCO can be reduced by O_2-breathing; a complete CO elimination takes hours.

Effects of diminished barometric pressure

Pressure equalization in the nasal cavities

Increasing or decreasing pressure in the sinus cavities is equalized passively by means of the ostia into the main nasal cavity. In the frontal sinus, there is not one simple ostium, but a 3 cm long channel. This is why frontal sinus pressure disturbances occur 3–5 times more frequently here than in the remaining sinus cavities. The barofunction is more complicated in the tympanic cavity because of the special opening mechanism of the Eustachian tubes. At rest, the pharyngeal part of the tube is closed and requires an action to open, such as yawning, swallowing, sneezing, or pulling the jaw forward.

In the event that the tympanic membrane is stretched by 20–27 kPa (150–202 mmHg) above the pressure in the nasopharyngeal cavity, the tube opens passively, due to the pressure differential. Therefore, no problems arise while the aircraft climbs. During descent to land, an increase in ambient pressure gives a rising pressure feeling in the ear (over the tympanic membrane), which should initiate equalization procedures. The pressure differential between the middle ear and the environment cannot be alleviated otherwise.

Gastrointestinal features

According to Boyle's gas law, water-saturated gas doubles in volume at an elevation of 16 500 ft, triples at 25 000 ft, expands five-fold at 34 000 ft, and seven-fold at 39 000 ft. This gas expansion has practical application for aviation personnel and passengers during flight. In order to prevent decompression sickness caused by a rapid drop in pressure, cabin pressure is maintained corresponding to an altitude of 2200–2400 m (approximately 7200–7900 ft) or lower. This is accomplished by active pressurization and hermetic sealing of the cabin. Under these conditions intraabdominal gas expands to nearly 40%. Because the cabin lay-out offers few possibilities for passengers to move around, painful intestinal distension and spasms often result, especially during long-haul flights. It is recommended to avoid gas-producing foods and carbonated beverages before flight. Another preventive measure is simethicon which can reduce the surface tension of intraabdominal gas bubbles, thereby facilitating their elimination.

Decompression sickness (DSC)

Decompression sickness due to disturbances of the flight profile

— Origin

The bubbling effects of dissolved inert gases (nitrogen and the noble gases) develop particularly in bradytroph tissues, as well as in fat and nerve tissues. Gas germinates preferentially in structural and biochemical niches, such as in transition areas from hydrophilic to hydrophobic substances that have large abrupt changes in surface tension. Bubbles occur at pressure drops of at least 50%. Obesity, advanced age, prior injuries, cicatrices and physical activities (after pressure drop) accelerate the generation of bubbles.

— Decompression symptomatology

The frequency of symptoms in different tissues and organ structures vary: in 65% of DCS cases joint pain arises, 17% experience "the bends," paresthesias occur in 7%, pseudoparalysis in 5%, scintillating scotomas in 4%, delayed headaches occur, as well as pulmonary symptoms and collapse, in 2%, and acute paralysis in 1% of cases. The temporal course of symptomatology is characterized initially by a rapid rise in symptoms, reaching a maximum in about 30 minutes, with a slow decline over the next two hours.

Symptoms are differentiated according to their localization and the type of the complaint:

a) Bends: exhibited by pain in the joints and muscles, beginning with a numb feeling and, within hours, changing into a dull, sometimes pounding pain. It arises particularly in joints that are utilized the most (shoulder, elbow, hand, foot and hips). Approximately 54% are joint complaints, 26% deep muscle complaints, and 20% deep bone pain.
b) Chokes (N_2 embolism in pulmonary vessels): presents with substernal pain, frequently also dry cough and episodes of asphyxiation.
c) Circulatory failure: characterized by symptoms of shock (cold sweat, pallor, dizziness), delayed shock (after symptom-free interval of 2–12 hours).
d) Paresthesias: a mild form of DCS due to subcutaneous bubble formation, which is characterized by local or diffuse pruritis, a reddish-blue skin coloration, and punctuate hemorrhages.
e) Neurological disturbances: visual disturbances, headache, hearing impairments, tinnitus (inner ear), disturbances of the muscle coordination (muscle tremor, unilateral or bilateral weakness, or paralysis), cross-sectional paralysis including bladder and bowel incontinence.

— Prevention

Barometric injury and hypobaric hypoxia are generally prevented by use of pressurized cabins and/or supplemental oxygen equipment. At cabin altitudes over 10 000 ft (3000 m) continuous oxygen delivery is required.

— Principles of treatment

The amount of time to be spent in a pressure chamber (which equates with submerged depths) and the amount of O_2 supplementation are determined by the severity of the symptoms. As a minimum, a one-day observation period is necessary. Air transport of patients to a pressure chamber requires a cabin altitude of no more than 3000 ft. By breathing 100% oxygen, 30% of nitrogen can be released from the body within 30 minutes. The speed of N_2 elimination from individual tissues is in the following order: blood and lung tissues, internal organs, skin and muscle tissue, fatty tissue and bone.

Flying after diving

— Applicable principles

a) No flying at a cabin altitude of more than 2000 ft (approximately 600 m) within a period of 12 hours after diving with compressed air, or after a stay in a pressure chamber. Also participation in high altitude chamber operations should be avoided.

b) If symptoms of decompression sickness arise during or after diving, the advice of an aeromedical practitioner should be sought before returning to flying. This is an increasing problem as the number of divers and the frequency of flights after diving courses are rising. The problem is furthermore worsened by the frequent concealment of signs of DCS, primarily by male divers (both civilian and military), as DCS is considered a badge of honor.

c) DCS that occurs after diving can cause functional and an anatomical intrapulmonary right-to-left shunts: The functional intrapulmonary right-to-left (type II) can be induced by the so-called yoyo dive profiles,whereby a series of many flat and short dives take place, with episodes of surfacing separated by only a few minutes. Microscopic bubbles and larger bubbles are formed in the pulmonary capillaries and cause an asymptomatic embolism. These vesicles are partially absorbed and then enlarge with new pressure exposures and by further inhalation of nitrogen. A second mechanism is when dive levels oscillate, such as when deep levels are repeatedly, abruptly and rapidly discontinued, even without surfacing.

The anatomical intrapulmonary right-to-left shunt (Type I) is caused by a small asymptomatic atrial septal defect or by a functionally open foramen oval.

— DCS in divers can also be caused by

a) panic ascent because of unusual or irritating events or particularly stressful conditions such as loss of visual contact with the dive partner, increased resistance of the regulator, etc. Unfavorable personality characteristics often play a role in this context;
b) not observing absolute medical and especially psychiatric contraindications to diving. These are particularly common causes of fatal diving accidents;
c) incomplete consideration of all factors involved in DCS when using the dive computer, e.g. computing basis for the "exponential reduction of saturation" is unrealistically optimistic and does not take into consideration the significant individual differences in dispersion of inert gas, the individual predisposition toward bubble formation (bubblers and non-bubblers), and the biochemical reaction to bubble formation.

EFFECTS OF ACCELERATION

Terminology Pertaining to Accelerations

When evaluating the effects of acceleration, a principle to note is that the physiological effects are caused by inertial forces that operate opposite to the direction of the acceleration. Another term found in the literature for the inertial direction is reaction forces.

In general, the following acceleration features are physiologically and pathophysiologically operative:

— magnitude of acceleration in multiples of earth's gravity ($g = 9.81\ m/s^2$);
— duration of acceleration:

a) sudden accelerations: 1/1000–1/100 s (injuries above 50 G)
b) transient accelerations: 0.5–1 s (no hemodynamic changes)
c) sustained accelerations: (>15 s to several min);

— acceleration gradient (G/s): in aeronautical practice often 0.1–3.0 G/s; briefly to 5–7 G/s; when ejecting up to 300 G/s;
— effective direction: in reference to the body axis and the transverse axis of the body (horizontal, sagittal and frontal planes through the body's center of gravity);
— effective area: body shape — seat design;
— effective range: particularly significant in critical overloading situations, e.g. ejections and forced landings;
— frequency response: particularly significant at the limits of tolerance;
— temporal sequence: pertaining to the acceleration-free intervals (recovery) which are important for acceleration training.

Physiological performance with $+G_z$ accelerations

Physiological fundamentals

Orthostatic load and short-term blood pressure regulation

Circulatory control while standing, i.e. during an orthostatic load, results from the summation of the blood pressures attained by the work of the heart and the hydrostatic pressure due to the force of gravity. Thus, the mean pressure in the arteries of the foot while standing amounts to approx. 190 mmHg, in contrast to 100 mmHg while supine. The pressure drops to approx. 70 mmHg in the arteries of the head. With these pressure changes, thin-walled veins in the legs will stretch and can pool a volume of blood of about 400–600 mL. Under these conditions, the mechanisms that promote return of

Table 10. Terminology of Acceleration and Reaction Forces (Biodynamics Committee of the Aerospace Medical Panel)

Direction of Acceleration with Reference to the Body of the Pilot	Physiological Description of Acceleration G	Physiological Symbol	Reaction Direction (Direction of the Force of Inertia)	Deviating Direction of Motion of the Eyeballs and/or the Axes of Vision
Forwards (back to chest)	Transverse anterior to posterior G, straining backward, chest to back G	$+G_x$	Chest to back (the pilot presses into the seat-back)	Inward
Backwards (chest to back)	Transverse posterior to anterior G, straining forward, back to chest G	$-G_x$	Back to chest (the pilot presses into the lap straps one)	Outward
Headwards (pelvis to head)	Positive G (cephalad)	$+G_z$	Head to pelvis (the pilot presses into the seat)	Downward
Footwards (head to basin)	Negative G (caudal)	$-G_z$	Pelvis to head (the pilot is lifted from the seat)	Upward
To the right	Left-lateral G	$+G_y$	Right to left laterally (the pilot is pressed to the left)	To the left
To the left	Right-lateral G	$-G_y$	Left to right laterally (the pilot is pressed to the right)	To the right

venous blood to the heart become especially important. Particularly notable is the so-called muscle pump, which in principle exists because the veins are squeezed together by virtue of the surrounding skeletal muscle contractions. This causes blood to be pushed toward the heart with the assistance of one-way valves. Thus, the pressure also decreases in the foot veins from approx. 90 mmHg to 20–30 mmHg and capillary filtration pressure becomes even smaller, which resists edema formation. Frequent activation of the muscle pump by walking or by conscious leg contractions helps reduce the negative consequences. This elevated venous pressure is exacerbated by activities which require long periods of standing (e.g. sales personnel) or which create venous occlusion (e.g. sitting). Furthermore, the "suction pressure pump" effect of ventilation comes into play, as this occurs due to the effect of negative chest pressure during inhalation, along with associated stretch of the thoracic blood vessels. Intra-abdominal pressure is increased by virtue of lowering the diaphragm, further promoting the flow of blood into the heart. During exhalation, the opposite occurs and the venous return to the heart is reduced.

Control mechanisms during $+G_z$ accelerations

Manifold hydrostatic loads cause substantial disturbances of the hemodynamic system, manifold gravitational loads cause deformations and misalignments of body parts and organs.

Increased hydrostatic pressure changes the pressure circumstances in the venous and arterial system, the blood distribution in the circulation, venous flow reversal and regional perfusion. In hydrostatic equilibrium, pressure in arteries and veins falls above the heart, and rises below this level, and is dependent on the height of the hydrostatic column. Consequentially, circulation is reduced in the head, while the hydrostatic pressure increases in the legs.

Among the reflex counter-regulations of the organism, the pressure sensors play the most important role. They promote vasoconstrictive reactions of the capacitance and resistance vasculature, a rise of the heart rate, and increase catecholamine release from the adrenal glands. During sustained acceleration, blood pressure control can be activated via the renin-angiotensin mechanism. After 10–15 seconds of vasoconstriction of capacitance vessels, venous return begins to increase, and thus the stroke volume of the heart increases. However, initial values cannot be reached, and complete cardiovascular compensation is possible only with low rise gradients (0.1 g s^{-1}) and mild accelerations between +2 G_z and +3 G_z.

Disturbances in the retinal and cerebral perfusion are very important, especially with acceleration values of +4 G_z or more. Peripheral and central vision disturbances are caused by the peripheral reduction of retinal perfusion. Initially, only peripheral vision is affected; central vision is lost later. These visual disturbances precede reduced brain perfusion, and are followed by loss of consciousness.

Respiratory rate and alveolar ventilation rise even during minor accelerations, and ventilation-perfusion defects become increasingly more significant with increasing acceleration.

The objective and subjective symptoms and the decreased ability of the pilot to act during +G_z accelerations depend not only on the types of acceleration involved, but also on the constitutional, conditional and current health status of the pilot, as well as the behavior of the pilot. A compilation of these situational changes are described in the following table.

Symptomatology of +G_z acceleration

Table 11 gives a synopsis of the effect of G_z-acceleration on the human body and several functions.

Physiological and physical factors which affect +G_z acceleration tolerance

Factors which lower +G_z acceleration tolerance

Unfavorable personal characteristics are: tall stature, large heart-to-eye distance, small body mass, high vagal reactivity (particularly a low heart rate), above average vegetative reactions, low emotional stability, as well as a low or absent achievement motivation.

Tolerance is also reduced by the following health issues: low blood pressure, decreased oxygen content in the blood, varicose

Table 11. Symptoms Caused by the Effects of $+G_z$ Acceleration

Magnitude of $+G_z$ Acceleration	Objective Symptoms	Subjective Sensations	Capacity to Act
2	Increased pressure of the body onto the seat, drooping of the soft parts of the face	Feeling of heaviness of the hands and feet, tension in the face	Difficulty with purposeful movements (temporal and spatial), larger amplitudes of motion
3		Intensified feeling of heaviness	Increased heaviness of arms and legs making movement more difficult; normal seating position more difficult to maintain; exiting the airplane not possible without auxiliary systems
4	Initial visual disturbances, usually a restricting of visual field ("tunnel vision") and blurring of the instrument panel ("foggy vision" or grey curtain = grey-out)		Difficulty of movement of the extremities without support esp. over head movements of the hand; substantially lengthened action times
4 to 5	Visual disturbances in 70% of the pilots, essentially peripheral vision; after 5–6 seconds also disturbances of central vision (black curtain = blackout); aural reception intact	Increasing feel of heaviness in the whole body	

(*Continued*)

Table 11. (*Continued*)

Magnitude of $+G_z$ Acceleration	Objective Symptoms	Subjective Sensations	Capacity to Act
	as well as temporal and spatial orientation and ability to cooperate; during a plateau phase of acceleration, shortly after 8–12 seconds, the intensity of the visual symptoms decreases		
5 to 6			The flexed head with protective helmet can be lifted only with difficulty
to 8			With good support of arms and hands, small movements of the thumb (keyboard!) and the hand (control lever!) are possible
to 12			Sitting position still ensured

veins, hemorrhoids, inguinal and umbilical hernias, stomach and intestine illnesses, infections, cataracts, severe myopia, degenerative changes in the spinal column, and disturbances of the heart and circulatory system.

Tolerance is further impaired by problems in the workplace or in the pilot's personal life. Nutritional problems are also important. Other negative factors are: a lowered oxygen partial pressure in the arterial blood, hyperthermia, dehydration, a full stomach, gas-producing and heavy meals, decreased blood sugar values, consumption of alcohol, heavy nicotine use, tachypnea, fatigue, uncontrolled medicine use, poor physical conditioning, unsatisfactory aeronautical training, frequent exposures to acceleration, and motivational issues. Particularly unfavorable is a combination of the above factors.

Methods and means to increase $+G_z$ acceleration tolerance

— Physical (mechanical) methods

Pneumatic anti-g-suits and/or anti-g-trousers: such special flight clothing can be used as a solitary unit or integrated into high-altitude pressurized suits. Control is via inertia-dependent automatic controllers (usually from $+2\ G_z$) or single solenoid valves or electronically steered valves, and results in tolerance increased by $+0.8\ G_z$ to $+2.5\ G_z$. The physiological effects of this acceleration protection equipment is on the internal organs, resulting in an improvement of the venous return flow, an increase of the arterial (especially systolic) blood pressure, and a high riding diaphragm (minimizing downward heart displacement).

Changes of body position can also increase acceleration tolerance to a substantial extent: a forward inclination of the trunk of around 10–25°, or a rearward inclination up to 30°, can result in an increase of tolerance by approx. $+1\ G_z$. The physiological effect of these countermeasures results from a reduction in hydrostatic pressure. Positive pressure respiration: increasing atmospheric air pressure by around 6 kPa (45 mmHg) can improve acceleration tolerance by approx. $+2\ G_z$ increase. The physiological effects occur because of an increase in intrapulmonary pressure, due to active exhalation; unfortunately, it also causes fatigue rather quickly.

— Physiological methods

The primary physiological methods utilized are the "muscle pump" (the leg musculature), to facilitate venous return, and Valsalva maneuver, to increase intrapulmonary pressure and intracranial circulation. The appropriate muscle straining and/or breathing maneuvers are practiced by jet pilots during aeronautical training. In addition, the inhalation of pure oxygen or O_2-CO_2 mixture (with 7% CO_2) increases the tolerance by approximately $+1\ G_z$.

Physical training is directed toward enhancement of maximum force tolerance, high-speed strength training, and force perseverance, rather than long-term perseverance.

— Training on human centrifuge

Principles of training are based on: gradual increase of acceleration exposures, repetition of exposures, and inclusion of maximal and submaximal acceleration values. The physiological effects develop by adjustments to small acceleration increments, as well as improvement in the use of the techniques of muscular strains and breathing maneuvers.

— Aeronautical training

Standards for maximum acceleration and number of daily flights take into consideration the climate, the air temperatures and the flight control features of the aircraft type.

— Use of pharmacologic means

Use of psychotropic substances and sympathomimetic substances can increase tolerance by over $+3\ G_z$ for a duration of up to three minutes. Due to stimulation of the central nervous system, physiological effects occur, such as faster vegetative responses and decreased reaction times.

— Combined utilization of different means and methods.

Performance with $+G_x$ Acceleration Effects

The $+G_x$ accelerations occur constantly in normal civil flight operations, but due to the low ($+0.5$ to $+2.0\ G_x$) accelerations involved during take off and horizontal flight, they play a small role. Taking off with auxiliary jets and on aircraft carriers may increase the values to +4 G_x.

The hemodynamic effects are small: central venous pressure, cardiac stroke volume and mean aortic pressure rise little, however, cardiac arrhythmias arise frequently, due to the stretching of the right atrium. Because of deformations of the eyeballs, visual disturbances can also occur.

The reserve volume and vital capacity of the lungs are reduced due to the increased pressure of the abdominal organs on the diaphragm (by slight rearward pressure).

The subjective symptomatology and the possible reductions in the capacity to act can be summarized as follows:

+3 to +5 G_x: a pressure feeling in the thorax and a noticeable slightly labored breathing;
+5 to +10 G_x: an acute and vague pain develops in the lower third of the sternum and epigastrium that often radiates to the lateral side of the chest, and is worsened with inspiration;
+6 to +10 G_x: tolerance is still relatively good, with effective times of several minutes (space travel!);
+8 G_x: raising the arms and legs becomes impossible;
+10 to +15 G_x: substantial difficulties arise, breathing becomes difficult; finger movements and small amplitude movements of the wrist are still possible;
+20 G_x: clouding of consciousness and unconsciousness, which can continue up to 24 hours, proved by rapid head movements; after termination of exposure, residual feeling of dizziness, nausea, trembling of the eyes, and a degree of disorientation.

Performance with –G_x Acceleration Effects

Negative accelerations (decelerations) of –0.5 to –1.0 G_x, which occur during normal flight operations, play a small role, and arise only from brake applications during horizontal flight and landing. Higher values of –2 to –4 G_x can be achieved by strong and brief brake applications, such as on aircraft carriers. During aircraft accidents, values of –5 to –8 G_x can be attained, for approximately two seconds. Reserve volumes and vital capacity of the lungs are reduced in the inverted position.

The subjective symptomatology and the possible restrictions of the capacity to act can be summarized as follows:

to –4 G_x:	hardly noticeable disturbances;
–4 to –7 G_x:	small impediment to respiration;
from –7 G_x:	extension of the legs;
–8 G_x:	head and trunk are moved forward rapidly;
–15 G_x:	shoulder belt holds the body, but head is hurled onto front chest wall.

During continuous acceleration, blood is displaced from the trunk up to the head, pain develops in the arms and legs, punctiform bruises (petechiae) develop, and respiration is affected.

Flying in the prone position produces breathing difficulties, nasal secretions, increased salivary output and lacrimal flow, and tugging effects on the lower eyelid.

PERFORMANCE AND TOLERANCE OF SENSORY SYSTEMS

Vision Problems in General Aviation as an Ordinary Referral

As a general principle, it can be said that the continuation of a VFR flight (Visual Flight Rules) from VMC (Visual Meteorological Conditions) into IMC (Instrument Meteorological Conditions) is responsible for approximately 25% of all fatal general aviation accidents. Visual flight rules are established on the basis of the cloud base (average height of the lower surface of the cloud layer above ground) and by visibility.

During flights over open water, groundswells are possible even with zero wind. Local winds can produce an additional secondary wave system, which overlays the groundswell on the water surface. The groundswell (primary wave system) is identifiable at best from a flight altitude of approximately 2000 feet, and the locally-developed second wave system from a flight altitude of 1000 feet. During flights over deserts, the change in diurnal atmospheric pressures can become problematic. The visibility in the morning can be quite good at low temperatures, whereas by noon, flickering temperature layers develop in the radiating heat. This can cause many optical illusions (fata Morgana features, e.g., illusion of a lake with islands, or distant mountains appearing much closer than they are). These optical deceptions are further strengthened by a lack of natural points of reference. The illusions can be so realistic that they can even be photographed. Furthermore, reflections from sand, glaring light and violent wind currents can cause a temporary reduction in visibility, especially during twilight and at night. Eye protection is therefore essential. If possible, polarizing sun glasses should be worn during flight.

Other visibility problems can arise from various kinds of fog, which can develop within a few minutes, and may reduce visibility at ground level to below 5 km. Fog arises primarily in coastal regions, but can also arise in industrial areas, due to the presence of condensation nuclei (exhaust gases and other air pollutions). The formation of fog takes place when the air temperature is reduced to the dew point or by admission of additional humidity in close proximity to the ground. Other kinds of fog are radiation fog, advection fog, upslope fog, fog from precipitation, and ice fog. Vapor, smoke and fog can occur together.

Further obstructions of vision can arise as a result of dust and sand. In stable air, dust can be carried up to a height of 5000 ft and distribute itself over large distances, thereby reducing visibility both at ground and at altitude. Flying sand is rarely carried higher than 50 ft, yet visibility in a sandstorm is near zero.

Finally, direct precipitation (rain) needs to be mentioned, although visibility is rarely reduced below 1.5 km. Drizzling rain and snow reduce visibility and may interfere with the determination of the boundary of cloud layers.

The Visual System

Vision is the most important sensory system for flying, as more than 90 % of all information relevant to flight operation reaches the pilot by means of the eye. The pilot must see the instrument panels in the cockpit and must be able to observe and analyze the area around the moving airplane. Therefore, the pilot must be able to resolve signals in form and in situation, i.e., have appropriate visual acuity. He must discriminate different colors, be able to detect signals arising in the periphery, be able to judge signals while in motion, and to discern the horizon.

Visual acuity

In order to quantify the capacity for signal resolution, thresholds must be defined, which can then serve as useful units of measurement. Several such thresholds are appropriate for the concept of visual acuity.

Point visual acuity

Point visual acuity is defined as the ability to recognize an individual point against an otherwise uniform background. It may be quite important in daily life. One can imagine a situation where another airplane is flying at a great distance, and the pilot's eyes "squeeze" this image together into a point. With the involved airspeeds, the perception of this point and the determination of the associated distance are of great interest. In everyday clinical life, however, the point visual acuity is not examined.

Visual acuity of separation

Visual acuity of separation, or resolution visual acuity, is defined as the ability to discriminate two closely neighboring points as separate. This is one of the most important criteria for signal identification. The unit of measurement is the angle subtended by the two points, still just barely visible as two, at the fovea of the eye. It is referred to as the Minimum Angle of Resolution (MAR). It usually has a value of about 1 minute of arc. The reciprocal value of the measured threshold angle is called the visus. Many people, particularly the young, have a visus > 1, i.e., the MAR is smaller than 1 minute. The retina cannot resolve equally well along its entire surface. The maximum discrimination occurs in only one area of approximately 1° in diameter, the fovea centralis. This represents the intersection of the fixation line with the retina. If the image moves away from the fovea to the retinal periphery, the resolution becomes increasingly poor. At a distance of 20 cm from the eye, the clearly visualized area has a diameter of approximately 3.5 mm, while at a distance of a meter, it is about 1.7 cm. This means that reading cannot be accomplished without eye movements, nor can the cockpit instruments be easily discerned at this distance. The eyes move very fast and are precisely directed. Certainty necessitates a structured area, so that specific features can provide orientation. An array composed of perfectly identical units will lead to greater search image errors than one that is composed of units that are dissimilar. This is very important for rapid reading of check lists and maps.

The retinal periphery, composed primarily of rods, has a horizontal field of approximately 150° and a vertical one of 120°, presumably functioning as a detector of important stimuli. It reacts to slow changes of retinal image position. By rapid and accurate sensory interconnections, the eye is guided in such a way that the image falls on the fovea centralis and can, therefore, be analyzed. The period of fixation can last between 0.2 and 2 seconds and can be extended, if necessary. Vision is therefore coupled to continuous eye movements. Every day experience demonstrates that these eye movements are not burdensome and therefore do not lead to asthenopia, the consequences of which are visual symptoms, such as blurred vision, headache, lack of concentration, lacrimation, and, in severe cases, migraine and photophobia. These symptoms develop when, during the course of normal feedback of operational sequences of eye movements, arbitrary or compensatory intervention occurs. When a signal cannot be recognized and interpreted clearly, the normally short period of fixation can be extended, which can impair flight safety. In order to avoid such situations, symbols must be large enough to be above threshold for clear visualization, but not too large to extend beyond the fovea centralis and, therefore, exceed the area of sharpest visual acuity.

Contour visualization

Discrimination is impaired if the distance between symbols becomes too small. People with a normal visus of 1 need 4′ distance for the optimal discrimination. This critical distance becomes greater with diminishing visual acuity.

Localization visual acuity

Localization visual acuity is defined as the smallest recognizable change of the spatial relationship of two objects to one another. Nonius visual acuity is defined as the ability to distinguish two lines, one exactly above the other. Accuracy up to 10 seconds of arc is possible.

Dynamic visual acuity

To maintain permanently sharp images, the eye must follow moving objects in order to keep the image in the fovea centralis. Rates of motion greater than 20–30°/s result in slippage of the image. Fast saccadian movements restore the image briefly onto the fovea centralis, but at the expense of reduced discrimination. This reduction of visual acuity with rapid eye movements is variable among individuals. It is possible that experience plays a role.

Depth perception

Direct depth perception

Direct depth perception is based on binocular stereoscopic vision. In this manner, the objects, which are momentarily outside the

Table 12. Performance of Depth Perception with Distant Accommodation

	Perceptive Spatial Difference	
Observation distance (m)	Absolute (m)	% of the Observation Distance
5	0.05	1
40	1.2	3
100	7.6	7.6
600	275.2	45.8

accommodation zone, are projected incongruently onto the retina. Horizontal disparity corresponding to about 10 seconds of arc produces distance perception and corresponds to a "double image" coverage on the retina of $< 1\ \mu$m.

The augmentation of the parallax (angle between the connecting lines of object perception areas) can be achieved beyond the pupillary distance with a stereotelescope (approx. 6.5 cm).

Horopter is defined as the totality of all points in the environment that, at a given eye position, are projected on corresponding points of the two retinae.

Objects positioned further away are projected onto the retina as uncrossed double images (from the retinal center inward nasally), while closer objects project as crossed double images (from the retinal center outward nasally).

4.2.2.2 *Indirect depth perception*

Indirect depth perception mechanisms are called into play when monocular vision indirectly assesses spatial depth based on experience and judged by specific optical impressions. Effective mechanisms are: geometrical perspectives, motions of individual objects in relation to each other, the reduction of outline clarity and color intensity with increasing distance, as well as the shadows cast by the direction of object illumination. Distant objects appear blurred and bluish due to dust and atmospheric humidity. Distances can be underestimated in clean dry atmosphere due to the lack of such dimming.

Contrast vision

Simultaneous contrast

The perception of a surface is affected by its environment because of lateral inhibition in the retina. Lateral inhibition between the retinal center and the periphery involves the horizontal cells. Because of lateral inhibitory mechanisms, the retina produces concentric and antagonistic receptive fields which result in contrast enhancement.

In ophthalmologic medical practice, visual acuity is measured by utilizing high contrast (85%) optotypes. Diminished contrast reduces visual acuity. For that reason, characters displayed on a monitor are more difficult to recognize than those of equal size in a well-printed book.

Successive contrast (after-images)

When aborting a fixation of approximately 30 seconds, an after-image appears, which is of opposite brightness or of contrasting color due to a local photochemical and neural adaptation.

Gradual movement contrast is defined by the observation that, following lengthy viewing of a moving pattern, there is an illusion that a stationary object moves in the opposite direction.

Refraction and accommodation

Accommodation

Whether the image of an object really projects on the retina, depends on the distance of the object and on the refraction of the eye. The formula: $1/f = 1/g + 1/b$ applies, where by f = focal length; g = object distance, b = image distance. From this, it follows that for any given focal length, an object can be projected onto the retina only if it is at a certain distance from the eye. Emmetropia is achieved when an image of an infinitely distant object falls exactly onto the retina, and when there is a rear focal length of 22.7 mm. This infinite object distance is relatively small because the short focal length of the eye produces a wide-angle camera effect with great depth of focus at greater distances. If the object approaches the eye, the image distance becomes longer, and the image is projected behind the retina. A sharp image therefore requires a shortening of the focal length. A blurred image is the initiating stimulation for the contraction of the ciliary muscle to induce accommodation. From an extreme near point to infinite viewing, a time interval of 0.4 to 0.5 s is required.

This accommodation ability is age-dependent and decreases with increasing age. In children it amounts to 12 diopters. Presbyopia is a completely normal process. Fifty-year old people have a residual accommodation of 1–2 diopters, which indicates that an object must be held at 50 cm to one meter from the eye in order to be seen clearly. Therefore the commonly heard joke that the eyes do not change with age, but the arms become too short, should lead to the following consideration:

a) The closer the object is to the eye, the larger is the visual angle and the higher the demand on the refractive power of the lens. The older person just cannot relax his lens enough to focus a near object clearly onto his retina.
b) Vanity makes it difficult for many people to accept presbyopia and utilize near vision glasses. This becomes relevant not only after the age of 50, but already in the early 40's, especially in those with a degree of hypermetropia. Near vision glasses reduce the near point distance, but do not enlarge the area of visual acuity or the accommodation depth. Therefore, eyeglasses with graduated refraction may be necessary.

Accommodation-convergence coupling

For clear near vision, a convergence of the eye axis is necessary. Convergence and accommodation are not controlled independently, but each accommodation process is coupled with a vergence motion: accommodation-controlled convergence as each vergence motion is connected with accommodation. If accommodation is prolonged because of blurriness of the image, the extraocular muscles can fatigue, thus leading to eyestrain.

Visualization in an aircraft cockpit is characterized by visual distances of 60–80 cm to the instruments. The additional high density of informational displays makes this a comparable situation to a PC workstation. Accommodation is particularly stressed because of the continuous changes in visual distances required when viewing inside and outside of the cockpit, as well as by the requirements of instrument flight.

Refractive errors

A main point distance of 1.4 mm to the apex of the cornea, plus the 22.7 mm rear focal length of the eye, determines a bulbar length of 24.1 mm for clear vision. Many people's eyes do not have this relationship between the bulbar length and the focal length. This results in decreased visual acuity, as clear projections are possible only under certain circumstances. In general, such refractive errors are the most common cause of reduced visual acuity.

In myopics, the bulbar length is too long in relation to the focal length. Images of distant objects are projected in front of the retina. The object can be brought very near to the eye without accommodation. The far point lies in finiteness near the eye. With dispersion (concave) lenses, this "relatively too-short" focal length will be lengthened. Because of accommodations-convergence coupling, these glasses should also be used for reading.

Hypermetropia (hyperopia) exists if the bulbar length is too short in relation to the focal length. The eye compensates with the help of accommodation, even in distant vision. However, eyestrain can occur because of this accommodation-convergence coupling. In other words, hypermetropia should be corrected.

Astigmatism is another anomaly of refraction. The refractive power of the cornea is distributed unequally throughout the cornea.

Physiologically, this applies to the horizontal and vertical layers. Vertically, the cornea is somewhat more strongly curved and, thereby, has a somewhat larger refraction than horizontally. Therefore, symbols with more vertical information, such as the letter E, have a higher threshold value than symbols that have horizontal orientation, such as the letter H. This can lead to difficulties at threshold boundaries. When symbols are recognized, the gaps are filled in with experience, knowledge, and imagination. The 40-year-old pilot with an accommodation of 4–5 diopters can get by just fine in every day life, but is particularly at risk, because of focusing difficulties in borderline situations.

Light and dark adaptation

Flight often involves drastic changes in brightness. While the adaptation to brightness occurs relatively fast, taking not more than 8 minutes or so — complete dark adaptation can take substantially more time (30–45 minutes). Generally, though, sufficient dark adaptation occurs within approximately 5 minutes.

Several mechanisms for adjustment to surrounding luminosity are at the eye's disposal: 1. the pupil diameter, 2. adjustment of sensitivity of individual sensors, 3. rod-cone dualism.

The amount of light entering the pupil can be changed by a factor of 16. Both extremes of pupillary diameter reduces visual acuity: 1. The larger the pupil, the more apparent the physical aberrations of the spherical lens become. Light rays at the edge of the lens are more strongly bent than in the center, and images therefore become blurred. The eye does not compensate for this lens aberration any differently than an expensive camera lens. In addition, visual acuity is reduced with a large pupil. 2. Small pupils from strong light exposure decrease image quality due to diffraction rings. Constriction of the pupil in light adaptation following maximum dark adaptation can take several seconds to minutes, although 90–95% of pupillary reaction can be achieved within 0.5 seconds. Complete pupillary dilatation from dark exposure can take up to approximately 17 minutes.

The sensitivity of the cones produces relatively rapid adaptive responses. If the light intensity falls to below 10 lx, the cones are subthreshold. At this point, the rods become responsible for vision. In dark conditions, their threshold drops to 0.01 lx within 40–50 minutes. Their peak response is at a wavelength of 510 nm, and that of the cones is at 560 nm. This results in an achromatic transition interval from the scotopic to the photopic adaptation: red light excites the rods only slightly and results in marginal color distinction, while green and blue hues can only be seen in gray tones and require greater illumination for more distinct color definition.

Myopia as a result of altitude

Pilots flying at high altitudes lack terrestrial orientation references and are constantly looking at their instruments in the cockpit. This leads to a permanent close accommodation of the eyes, resulting in the so-called myopia of altitude. Consequently the pilot does not see objects at great distances as well, and notices approaching flying objects substantially later, than when flying at lower altitudes.

Sensory latencies

The so-called "blind zone" is due to the sensory latency of the retina, resulting from the time involved in the photochemical process in the retina, to the conduction of action potentials into the cerebral visual cortex. In humans, this amounts to approximately 0.3 seconds and has no negative effects upon the processing of visual information under normal terrestrial conditions. During flight, this can lead to a temporal disparity between actual situations and conscious optical perceptions. The consequence is that the pilot has a "blind zone" in front of him of some 20 m, which he does not see until after having flown over or through it.

If objects are noticed by the retinal periphery and, therefore, additional fixation movements and accommodation procedures are utilized, the times for signal perception and transmission increase steeply, approaching values of 1.0–1.5 s (so-called sensory latency of low order). At an airspeed of Mach 1, this would correspond to a blind zone of 300–500 m.

Furthermore, it should be taken into consideration that the pilot must attach a flight-specific meaning to these perceptions, as at an airspeed of Mach 1 a distance of over 1 km can be overflown ("sensory latency of higher order") before it is seen.

As the time until flight-dynamic activities increase becomes longer, safety margins of approximately 2 km to objects in the proximity of the flight path should be maintained.

Night vision

Night myopia and presbyopia

With low visual field illumination, the phenomena of night myopia and night presbyopia arise when the pilot looks outside the cockpit, or even onto a dimly lit panel. The far point moves closer to the eye, the near point moves further away from the eye. This phenomenon is particularly unpleasant and becomes apparent in pilots with early presbyopia and in insufficient lighting. This phenomenon is caused by the absence of incentive for accommodation in a structureless area. Accommodation is in effect in a resting position, as it is adjusted not in the infinite, but rather in the range of 2–5 m. More time and a greater innervation effort is required to go from this resting position to an accommodation activity than would be necessary for changes of accommodation within a structured area.

Achromatic interval

In order to be able to perceive colored objects, illumination must exceed the threshold of the cones. The degree of the light intensity, which increases the perception from gray tones (via the rods) to colors (via the cones) produces different brightness intervals (achromatic intervals), and varies subjectively for different colors. Because of the relative insensitivity of the rods for red and red-orange, these colors can excite only the cones and are therefore suitable as unambiguous signal or warning lights in conditions of twilight and darkness. However, this achromatic interval is relatively large for green, blue and intermediate colors.

Vision after light flash (glare)

Light adaptation takes place within a few seconds, during which time the pupils reflexively constrict and rhodopsin disintegrates. Glare is caused by sudden light of high intensity occurring during existing dark adaptation. As glare occurs separately for each eye, closing one eye can be protective.

As a consequence, it is recommended that for flight during thunderstorms, viewing should be restricted to the inside of the cockpit, and ambient lighting should be increased. If viewing outside the cockpit is necessary, one eye should be kept closed.

Glare represents the most frequent cause of asthenopia complaints, particularly at the computer screen. Generally the cause is a disproportion of the light densities in the visual field.

The source of greatest glare is the sun. Three main forms can be differentiated: absolute glare, relative glare and reflected glare.

Absolute glare is directly related to the source of the light, either by an unfavorable placement of the light source, or by its overall intensity. Fluorescent lamps have a lower intensity than light bulbs, as the flux radiates out evenly over a large surface, creating minimal glare. Glare is further reduced by arranging the lights parallel to the line of sight, by utilizing a diffusing cover, and by arrangement of the lamps to be out of the line of sight.

Relative glare develops when there is a large brightness differential within the field of vision or if multiple demands for adaptation are placed upon the eye. Light intensity between the work object and the immediate environment should not be greater than 3:1, nor greater than 10:1 between the work object and the distant environment.

Reflected glare is caused by reflection from smooth surfaces, when the beam of light and the viewing angle are equal. This disturbance can be alleviated by a change in the direction of the beam of light, by use of matt surfaces (e.g., matt working documents), by wide lights with low brilliance, by reducing reflective light angles or by indirect lighting.

Color vision

Signals which convey information by color are every day occurrences, but they also play a significant role in air traffic. The high density arrangement of the cones within the fovea centralis is responsible for color vision. This density decreases in the periphery, so that accurate color discrimination is not possible if the image falls onto the retinal periphery. The sensation of green is particularly limited, while red can still be recognized. The visual field is greatest for blue and yellow.

The various color impressions are produced by stimulation of different patterns of cone types, which can be depicted by color equations, such as Grassmann:

$$a\ (\text{red}) + b\ (\text{green}) + c\ (\text{blue}) = \text{color}.$$

a, b and c are the weighted factors for the individual addendum, the sum of which is 1. According to international agreement, red is defined as wavelength of 700 nm; green as 546 nm and blue as 435 nm; white requires equal proportions of the components. In other words each is a third (0.33) of the whole.

The eye can discriminate between individual colors very well. Within the range between 580 and 610 nm, a 1 nm change in wavelength is sufficient to produce another color impression. The perception of a color assigned to a particular wavelength changes with adaptation. By removing brightness, the yellow and blue spectral ranges become more narrow, while the ranges for red, green and violet become more broad (Bezold–Brücke phenomenon).

Chromatic aberrations are not corrected in the eye. This amounts to nearly two diopters within the visible spectrum range. An eye which is emmetropic for the wavelength of 600 nm has a myopic diopter of about 1.5 for 450 nm, because the short-wave light is more strongly bent. Colored symbols on a screen always require some degree of accommodation. Short-wave lights, particularly violet, cannot be resolved sharply while, on the other hand, the visual acuity for monochromatic light is somewhat greater than for white light of mixed wavelengths.

Eye movement

Eye movements are critical for the perception of the environment, and for this purpose they serve to project and analyze objects of interest onto the fovea centralis. There are three different eye movements: the version, the vergence and the rotation. The axes of the eyes run in the same direction in version, counter to each other in vergence, and rotate in the axis of vision in the rotational motion. Optical orientation in space requires horizontal position of the retinal horizon. With a lateral inclination of the head, the vestibular organs compensate by initiating a rolling of the eyes in order to keep the horizon in place. Movements can be controlled by optical and proprioceptive afferent activity. If such optical cues are absent, as when flying into clouds, the vestibular information is not adequate for maintaining spatial orientation, resulting in a two-dimensional experience.

Saccadian eye movements are jerky movements from one visual fixation point to another, lasting 10 to 100 ms. The amplitude of these movements can vary from a few angular minutes (microsaccadian movements) to many degrees. Angular speed can attain 200–600 degrees per second. This movement has no perception associated with it, contrary to the case when the eyeball is moved by being pressed with one's finger. The new fixation point is held for 0.2 to 2 s. If longer fixation is required, it is perceived as an exertion. During this fixation, the eye is not motionless. It exhibits a fine tremor of 70–90 cycles per second, with an amplitude from 10–15 angular seconds. In addition, the eyes drift with a speed of 0.1 degrees per second from the line of fixation. Microsaccadian movements bring the image back to the point of fixation. These micro movements correct adaptation processes within the retina. With accurate fixation, the perception of the image disappears within fractions of seconds (Troxler phenomenon).

With these pursuit movements, the image of the object is projected onto the fovea centralis, and maximum angular speeds of 80 degrees per second can be achieved. If the object moves faster, corrections are made with saccadian movements. Because of suppression of perception, dynamic visual acuity is diminished. Optical nystagmus is the situation where an evenly paced pattern moves in front of the eye and pursuant movements alternate with retrograde saccadian movements. The effect of moving alternating stripes in front of the eye can be measured, and used for the examination of visual acuity.

Vestibular nystagmus occurs when the semicircular canal system stimulates eye movement. Its task is to maintain the position of visual fixation during movement of the head in order to retain spatial orientation. Larger angles of rotation require corrective action by saccadian movements with appropriate suppression of perception. For this reason, visual acuity decreases with head movements. This is very prominent during vibrations and turbulence in an airplane.

Due to their limited near vision, presbyopics will compensate with increased head movements, thereby further decreasing their visual acuity.

Vision of movement

Closely related to eye movement is the perception associated with visualization of moving objects in space. In both circumstances, pixels change positions on the retina. Nevertheless, the brain knows whether it is the eye or the object that has moved. In order to interpret the retinal image, the brain always consults with the motor centers, the pons and the cerebellum. Lack of such additional information can create miscalculations.

Location change of an object is perceived as movement if the angular speed is at least 1–2°/s. A higher threshold exists if a light spot moves in a dark room. For the perception of movement to occur, the change in position of objects relative to each other is continuously appraised.

Recognition of direction of movement is possible only up to angular speeds of 600°/s. The threshold of movement perception is appropriately higher in the peripheral visual field, but even so it reacts more sensitively.

Head and eye movements are initiated here: for slow movements — the eyes lead, for fast movements — the head precedes the eyes.

This process exhibits adaptation. After sustained visualization of a moving object, a stationary object will seem to move in the opposite direction (successive movement contrast).

Vision performance of the pilot

Daytime vision (scanning technique)

— Characteristics

In order for maximal visual acuity to be achieved, the object is fixated for at least one second by aligning the optical axis of the eye to the object. Outside the range of 5° beyond the line of sight, primary visual acuity is diminished, and only movements further away are noticed.

— Physiological basis

The clearest projection of an object occurs in the central retinal pit, where the highest cone density exists (triangularic mosaic with a minimum dual cone spacing of 2.8–3.0 μm and a cone row spacing of 2.4–2.6 μm). The resolution power of the eye amounts to 1/60°, whereby the minimum distance between two excited cones amounts to 5 μm, and a non-stimulated cone must lie between them.

Nonius visual acuity is decidedly better than point visual acuity, which takes place by way of subsequent complex processing in downstream neural networks.

With diminishing light intensity, a functional enlargement of the receptive field center (for effective excitation summation) takes place in the entire retina.

Negative impacts on daytime vision include: changing visual distances (looking alternatingly at the cockpit instruments and at airplanes in the sky), "stress" due to high performance requirements in the cockpit (mental work), fatigue, poor cockpit layout, performance limitations from external flight-specific causes (oxygen deficiency, acceleration), limited aeronautical training and experience. (The eye unconsciously scans a boundless area outside the cockpit scarcely further than the distance from the instrument panel; therefore a student pilot will see fewer airplanes outside the cockpit than a flight instructor.)

Night vision

— Characteristics

Eccentric fixation: Weakly illuminated objects do not fixate centrally, i.e. the line of sight must be consciously held 10–15° beyond the object. There is no rigid line of sight in such a situation: the image must rove around in various areas of the peripheral retina in order for the object to be depicted.

— Factors influencing night vision and light-dark adaptation

Dark adaptation is complete after approximately 25 minutes, but visual acuity is, nevertheless, substantially reduced. (The light sensitivity of rods is about a thousand times greater than that of cones.)

Local light adaptation takes place via differential illumination of retinal regions.

Hypoxia reduces night vision of the rods above an altitude of 5000 ft; hypoxia also infringes upon daylight vision and restricts the visual field.

Nicotine reduces night vision.

Spatial Orientation and Perception of Motion, Position and Attitude

Physiological basis

Spatial awareness and sense of movement derives informational input from several receptor systems, particularly from the organ of equilibrium (vestibular organ), and from the visual and the proprioceptive systems.

The labyrinthine system consists bilaterally of two macular organs and three semi-circular canals organs. The macular organs translate linear accelerations, primarily gravitational accelerations (gravitational force) and, additionally, the centrifugal accelerations arising during flight. The three semicircular canal organs, which are arranged in three levels perpendicular to each other, translate rotational accelerations. Information derived from these 10 acceleration-sensitive structures creates an image of three-dimensional spatial orientation and movements of the body. Apart from these specific impulses arriving from the vestibular core, motion information from the visual, proprioceptive and other sensory systems also participate. This is why loss of a reciprocal labyrinthine system does not lead to a complete loss of the sense of motion. Additional information concerning head movement arrives particularly from the visual system, and also from the receptors in neck muscles and joint receptors in the cervical spinal column. This convergence enables the nuclei vestibulares to code a wide range of head movement velocities into three dimensions. Furthermore, the vestibular centers have monosynaptic connections to the cerebellum and polysynaptic connections through the thalamus to the cortex. The nuclei of the eye muscles and the spinal cord have rapid connections to these monosynaptic motor projections, which are important for the reflexes involved in standing and locomotion.

These multiple receptor systems and structures involved in spatial awareness and the sense of movement exhibit substantial adaptability, thus limiting the likelihood of misinformation.

Spatial disorientation and illusions of vestibular origin

Illusions caused by stimulation of the semicircular canals (angular stimulation)

— The leans

This is the most well-known form of spatial disorientation. It is the consequences of stimulation above and below sensory thresholds and consists of a false sensation of bank when the aircraft is in level flight. The pilot believes he is flying level when in reality he is in an extended, coordinated turn, and after recovering (usually quite quickly) from this turn, i.e. flying level, again the pilot leans towards the direction of the turn, now erroneously perceiving the bank as the vertical axis. An equally incorrect sensation develops if a roll attitude is undertaken below threshold (usually unintentionally and with less than $2°/s^2$) and then abruptly terminated.

— Illusion of turning

Upon terminating a constant "stabilized" rotation, the sensation of turning in the opposite direction occurs (Somatogyric illusion).

— "Graveyard Spin"

After approximately 30 seconds in a uniform spin, termination of the spin will result in a sensation of spinning in the opposite direction. If the pilot disregards the indications on the flight instruments, (artificial horizon, altimeter, heading indicator, turn and slip indicator, rate of climb indicator), this illusion often leads to a ground impact.

— "Graveyard Spiral"

Flying downward in a coordinated curve is after some time perceived as level flight. When the pilot wants to adjust the low altitude, applying backward pressure on the control stick (pulling up) tightens the turn, but does not result in an altitude gain.

— Coriolis illusion

False information from the semicircular canal receptors on moving the head during rotation may cause cross-coupled or Coriolis illusion. This is the most dangerous of the vestibular illusions, causing an overwhelming feeling of disorientation. It may develop during a sustained turn when the pilot moves his head in an upward or downward direction against the direction of the turning airplane, such as can happen when switches are changed on the side of the pilot seat. Similar effects can be created during a turn when the pilot rotates his head in order to look outside the cockpit. In either case, all semicircular canals are stimulated simultaneously and a feeling of a rolling motion develops, associated with a strong sensation of "rise" or "fall" (tumbling).

Illusions created by the macular organs (linear accelerations)

— Illusion of climbing or descending (somatogravic illusion)

Due to stimulation of the otoliths during inertial changes, an illusion of climbing develops during take-off or when accelerating in straight and level flight. The illusion of descending correlates with negative accelerations, e.g. with landing. Occurring predominantly during instrument or night flight, it can be rapidly corrected by obtaining an outside visual point of orientation.

— The elevator effect (elevator illusion)

During a linear vertical acceleration, there is a corresponding downward movement of the eyes. Updrafts can create this illusion, causing the pilot to move the stick forward to compensate.

Combined visual-vestibular illusions

— The inverted jet phenomenon

This is the illusion of climbing, or even of inverted flight, in passenger or cargo aircraft furnished with locked automatic flight controls (autopilot). Initiating conditions are: instrument flight weather or night flight (horizon not visible), flight into heavy turbulence, poor legibility of the instruments, and technical problems with the autopilot.

— Break-off phenomenon

"Feeling of detachment" or "separation from the reality" appears predominantly in pilots of single-seat aircraft at altitudes over

30 000 ft, but may occur in helicopter pilots at flight altitudes below 1000 ft. Contributing factors are monotony, which can be substantial, and lack of optical stimulation, in addition to the characteristics of high-altitude flight. Consequentially, excitement rises, perception becomes impaired, and fear conditions (phobia) can appear.

— "Flicker Vertigo"

The light of the sun or from an artificial source can be interrupted by the rotation of the rotor or propeller of single-engine aircraft. Crew members have been known to have developed nervousness, nausea, headache, light-headedness, dizziness, spatial disorientation, epileptic convulsions and unconsciousness from such flicker. Recommended counter measures are: changing the direction of flight, changing the rotor or engine speed, wearing non-polarizing sun glasses, switching the position lights to continuous operation, and turning the windshield wipers off.

Vegetative reactions and motion sickness

In principle, humans are not oriented toward dealing with slow and long lasting passive movements. On the other hand, humans have a large repertoire of head and body movements, which correlate with optical, proprioceptive and vestibular afferent activity for proper spatial orientation. Specific interconnecting neurons exist, ranging from the three-neuron reflex (n. vestibularis — connecting from the vestibular nuclei to the alpha-motor neurons of the extra ocular muscle), for the release of rotatory nystagmus. If these afferent activities do not reconcile with each other, such as is the case in moving airplanes (vestibular afferent impulses are excited, optically nothing changes inside the airplane, also proprioception is unchanged), then increased further inquiries between the individual centers create rising neuron activity. Such activities frequently break out over excitatory synapses of brain areas that participate in this coordination. If these unusual excitatory patterns reach the hypothalamus or the central areas of the n. vagus, vegetative reactions, such as nausea, vomiting, drop in blood pressure, and rise of the heart rate, can be induced. This does not relate to protective reflexes of the organism.

This over-stimulation is caused primarily by excitation of the semicircular canals. Purely linear accelerations do not cause motion sickness, as this does not occur in humans with absent bilateral labyrinthine systems. Additionally, infants do not have motion sickness, as the afferent systems necessary for spatial orientation are not yet developed.

Factors that Promote or Prevent Illusions During Flight

Factors that promote illusions during the flight

Objective flight conditions

— Night flight: VFR flight into clouds and fog banks or confusion of natural sources of light (stars, moon) with artificial sources of light, or reflective effects from highly glassed airplane panels (e.g. F-16).
— Alternating flight into and out of clouds: changing the optical perception from flight instruments to surrounding field can lead to conflict situations, which can be worsened by constant light or dark effects.
— Restriction of visibility: rain, snow, sunshine, vapor and fog can further reduce visual capacity to the level of tunnel vision.
— Transition from visual flight to instrument flight (VFR-IFR Transition): during visual adaptation, illusions and spatial disorientation are possible.

Psychological factors

— performance load from other tasks or concerns
— emotional demands, particularly in complicated flight situations
— lack of information
— conflicts within the crew and in relation to employer
— very high motivation and a corresponding need to succeed

— excessive concern with each movement of the airplane, usually due to lack of flight experience and fear of illusions
— diversion of attention from the instruments
— lack of confidence in own capability
— disturbance of mental balance and emotional well-being.

Condition-reducing factors

Sedentary lifestyle, excessive smoking, high consumption of alcohol, acute and chronic lack of sleep, onset of an illness, in particular upper respiratory infections, which can result in Eustachian tube malfunction and cause unilateral vestibular disturbance, as well as recovery from an illness. It should be emphasized that every day fatigue is a very substantial illusion-promoting factor, one that can easily lead to incorrect perceptions of orientation and movement.

Training-related factors

Insufficient experience with instrument flying, lack of knowledge of flight illusions, poor division of attention, intervals between flights greater than two weeks, inadequate proficiency in instrument reading, insufficient training in rapid transition from visual to instrument flight.

Prevention of negative effects of a Coriolis acceleration

— Direct prevention during flight

Confidence in the flight instruments is essential. The unreliability of vestibular and pressure-mechanical information must be consciously considered. Head movements are to be avoided during the execution of rotating motion of the airplane.

Spins must be limited (with beginners never over 5 s, with experienced pilots not over 30 s), a second spin may only be undertaken after the first one has faded away, i.e. after 5–11 seconds.

The execution of anti-g-maneuvers supports the avoidance of illusions by Coriolis acceleration.

— Long-term preventive measures

Physical and mental health as well as concrete knowledge of the physiological effects of flight are critical to avoid illusions. Activities that normally do not involve much in the way of subjective performance limitations can still have negative consequences. In the pre-flight period, exposure to strong sun, sweating, prolonged sitting, oxygen deficiency, alcohol, and fatigue should be avoided, as they can reduce acceleration tolerances. Ingestion of high fat meals and gaseous drinks, such as carbonated beverages, should be avoided before and during flight.

PERFORMANCE AND STRESS LOAD CHARACTERISTICS IN AERONAUTICAL PRACTICE

Temperature Extremes

Hypothermia and functional effects

The primary effects on vital functions are: respiration becomes flatter at body core temperature below 34°C and cease at a core temperature between 16–20°C. Initially the heart rate and blood pressure rise until a core temperature below 34°C is reached, after which the heart rate and blood pressure decrease. Atrial fibrillation develops below a core temperature of 25°C.

Unconsciousness occurs at a body core temperature below 30°C. Even though the metabolic rate decreases with falling body temperature, a relative oxygen deficiency exists due to the increased oxygen consumption in the countermeasure phase at the beginning of hypothermia.

Hyperthermia and heat injury

Heatstroke is a dramatic consequence of the thermal effect and usually occurs due to high ambient temperature in combination with high humidity. Perspiration is suspended when the body core temperature reaches approximately 39°C, and at 41°C loss of consciousness develops.

Stages of the development of a heat stroke:

a) "red stage" — compensatory strong blood circulation in the periphery of the body
b) "grey stage" — cardiovascular collapse
c) death — at a body core temperature of approx. 43.5°C.

Hyperthermia can result in substantial losses of water and electrolytes, indispensable for the smooth operation of biological processes. Average total water absorption amounts to approximately 2.5 L per day, of which 1.3 L comes from ingested fluids, 0.9 L from the water content in the food, and 0.3 L from the water produced in oxidative metabolism. The evaporation from the skin (0.5 L) and the lungs (0.4 L), as well as the water required for the elimination of urine-producing substances (0.5 L), makes it necessary for an adult to drink at least 1.5 L water a day. A negative water balance, caused by decreased water absorption or increased loss of water, creates hypertonic dehydration, resulting in a rise in the osmotic concentration in the extracellular space. This leads to the extraction of liquid from the intracellular space. A loss of more than 20% of body water is related to a rise in body core temperature, anxiety, delirium, coma, and shock.

Heat exhaustion develops at body core temperatures of approximately 39°C, and in severe cases, symptoms of shock will ensue. Furthermore, heat cramps (muscle cramps) can occur due to saline deficiency (esp. in previously strained muscles).

Hyperthermia of the organism and the impairment of psychological functions

There is a certain hierarchy of impairment of psychological performance:

a) decreased ability to perform complex tasks with high cognitive data processing requirements

b) sensory-motor performance decrements of complex activity in the areas of pursuit and compensatory tracking
c) diminished performance in decision-making, and reduced vigilance in visual and auditory discrimination
d) reduced coordination performance which rapidly results in automatic actions
e) diminished simple cognitive performance with minor demands on memory.

Keeping heat level and exposure times equal, the following individual variability can modify the effects of heat load:

a) individual conditions for performance (gender, age, degree of acclimatization, clothing);
b) conditional factors (such as air humidity, motivation and psychophysiological status).

The reduction in performance is dependent on the WBGT (Wet Bulb Globe Temperature), which is derived from weighting environmental dry bulb, wet bulb and globe temperatures, as well as the effects of the air humidity and the exposure time. The tipping point for decompensation is at a WBGT of approximately 36°C and 40 minutes exposure.

Circadian Periodic Functions and Psycho-Physiologic Performance

Physiological fundamentals

There are more than 200 documented physiological, biochemical and psychological functions that follow an approximate 24-hour-rhythm.

As timekeepers for these rhythms, both internal and external factors come into consideration:

1. the pacemaker neuron complex in the hypothalamus, which has developed in the course of evolution, generates a spontaneous

rhythm for the neurophysiological basis of reciprocating membrane conductivity;
2. a neural copy of the external time program, which is acquired by individual experience; and
3. current external interval timers, such as the conscious knowledge of time, perception of well-ingrained daily routines, social contacts, and the rhythm of habit.

The external physical factors primarily originate from bright light (7000–12 000 lux) and/or by the light and dark periodicity of day and night. Light through the eye stimulates the hypothalamus (through nucleus suprachiasmaticus) and has a feedback loop via the sympathetic cervical spinal cord system to the pineal gland, producing more or less melatonin. A reduction of this hormone output indicates an "activity phase" for the body, while an increase in production indicates a resting phase.

Functions with a proven circadian periodicity include: metabolism, heart rate and respiratory rate, arterial blood pressure, body core temperature, electrical skin resistance, blood sugar levels, eyelid blinking rates, and concentrations of various hormones in the blood. Examples of documented performance deficiencies are: variation in reaction times, computational speeds, frequency of error-making, falling asleep at the wheel, and the frequency of reaching the "dead point" during night shift work.

Time intervals associated with high physical and psychological readiness to perform are generally between 6–14 and 16–22. Reduced performance occurs in, with a particularly poor performance period at night 2 and 3. Absolute temporal spacing of the maxima and minima varies for different functions and performances. Performance-critical times also occur when biorhythms are switching between rising and lowering phases. This can cause a temporary instability of timing between systems and lead to an uncoupling of control systems during a time of high energy expenditure.

The circadian periodicity is not held to a strict 24 hour cycle, but rather can be altered into shorter or (usually) longer intervals by the elimination of external time indicators. This can be shown by exposing subjects to isolation tests with interruption of their social contacts, lack of information about local time, and with freely selectable light and dark settings, meal times and rest periods. In most cases, subjects choose a periodicity of around 25 hours. Under the conditions of continuous daylight above the Arctic Circle, certain socially isolated groups have utilized systematically adjustable clocks, where the day is divided into two "halfs" of 10.5 to 13.5 hours. The adjustment of physiological functions within the durations of these 21–27 hour artificial days usually occurs within 2–8 days. This change in duration of the biphasic periodicity is called "free running" or the "unsolicited periodic."

The circadian rhythm can exhibit substantial inter-individual differences in respect to both the intensity and the temporal spacing of the minima and maxima. Thus it gives people options. There are those whose preferred work time is in the morning hours (so called A or morning types), and others whose preferred work time is in the evening hours (so called B or evening types). Further inter-individual differences exist regarding the adaptability to change of temporal regimes.

Shift work

Shift work brings alternating demands into the work environment. The time displacement caused by circadian disturbances has substantial effects on physiological functioning (e.g. energy metabolism) and psycho-physiological fitness. This incongruence between the fitness to perform and the work requirements can cause performance errors and industrial safety problems.

Also affected is the extent of additional demands placed by a number of so-called intervening variables, those which will become effective individually or in combination. These factors cover individual characteristics of the employee such as age, personality structure, "type of rhythm" and the physiological adaptability. Also activity-conditioned factors, such as the amount of the physical or mental load, length of the work time, shift schedules, climatic conditions, noise, and special work materials are to be considered. Also social and domestic issues play important roles, such as the family situation, the number of children, living conditions, and the family's acceptance of the shift work.

Due to the efficiency of external time givers, the shift worker cannot disengage from the time structure of his environment. The conflict between work schedules and daily life rhythms makes the shift worker unable to completely adapt his circadian rhythm. Experiments involving 21 consecutive night shifts have demonstrated that partial adjustments of the biological rhythm affects sleep time, but not work time.

The following recommendations apply to organizations that utilize shift work.

1. Choice of personnel: older workers (over 50 years) should not be given shift work. Those who are "night types" should be preferred.
2. Shift scheduling: very early shifts (beginning before 6:00 a.m.) should be avoided. Night work should generally be kept to a minimum. Long nightshifts of 9–12 hours are only acceptable if no environmental exposure exists.
3. Shift succession: forward rotation of shifts is to be preferred, i.e. the sequence of early shift, late shift and nightshift. Quickly changing shifts, i.e. in groups of 2–3 days, are recommended. One night-free shift should follow nightshifts as often as possible.
4. Participation of the employee: shift workers should be offered as much work time flexibility as is possible, and should participate when work schedules are being planned.
5. Behavior modification: special health education should be given, especially to prevent accidents. Shift workers should engage in moderate physical exercise a few hours before going to sleep.

Jet lag

Jet lag is characterized most commonly by day-time fatigue, insomnia, lengthening of reaction time, and degradation of memory and concentration. Further symptoms may occur, such as increased irritability, listlessness, nausea, headache, inordinate hunger or complete loss of appetite, gastrointestinal and urinary functions at mismatched times, degradation of physical and mental functions, and a generalized feeling of exhaustion. Synonyms for jet lag include "time shift," flight syndrome, and circadian desynchronization. The symptom complex is generated by transmeridian flight over several time zones (>3 time zones), providing a swift relocation from one geographical place to another. This causes a temporary discrepancy between the accustomed individual circadian cycle, which has been shaped by long-term living at the same geographical place, and that which is required at the new place. Temporary health effects and performance limitations are not linked to disease; all symptoms disappear after a few days.

Re-establishment of the normal function and efficiency of the traveler requires about 24 hours for every two hours of time shift. Individual hormonal parameters normalize themselves much more slowly. Eastward flights are more performance-reducing than westward flights, as the internal tendency of humans is to lengthen rather than shorten the circadian period. A flight toward the west requires approximately 20% less recovery time than a flight to the east. Eastward flights over more than two time zones are less problematic for the so-called "evening types" than for the "morning types." The temporary desynchronization of the bodily functions (CNS, hormonal and vegetative) occurs as a physiological reaction in 15–20% of all passengers crossing more than two time zones.

The most important countermeasure for overcoming jet lag is the immediate adjustment to the temporal conditions at the destination. Alcohol and sleeping medications should be avoided. Relaxation techniques, like autogenous training and breathing techniques are preferable. Protein-rich foods for sleep delay and carbohydrates for the promotion of sleep are recommended. Conversion of sleep-wake cycle prior to travel has had only marginal success.

To mitigate the effect of jet-lag, the following are recommended:

— Activity before westward flights: go to sleep at increasingly later times a few days prior to travel

— Activity at departure: change the clock to destination time and adapt to mealtime and sleep cycles of the destination.
— Arrange a one-day layover at half the travel distance during flights to the east (e.g. intermediate stop in Dubai during flight from London to Bangkok)
— After the flight: fight off sleeplessness (take melatonin (5–300 mg/day); use relaxation techniques such as autogenous training
— Remain awake after morning arrivals, soon after landing take a long walk in the open so that melatonin production is inhibited.
— Countermeasures during flight:

1. eat only light food with little salt, fat and sugar;
2. during flights to the west, eat particularly protein-rich food in order to extend wakefulness;
3. drink a lot of fluids, above all mineral waters and fruit juices, but no alcohol
4. do not smoke;
5. take several 20-minute naps, but do not take sleeping pills;
6. walk around in the cabin when possible and compensate for lack of movement by performing in-seat exercises (flex and extend the ankles in particular);
7. after a long transmeridian flight, try not to fall asleep before local bedtime.

Performance Degradation by Alcohol and Drug Abuse

— Frequency of abuse

It is estimated that 2.5–3 million people in Germany (~3.5% of the population) are alcohol dependent; of these approximately 800 000 are admitted to mental hospitals. It is further estimated that 14% of men and 5% of women are in a danger zone, close to becoming dependent on alcohol, approximately 800 000 are dependent on prescription drugs, and approximately 100 000 are dependent on illicit drugs. Within the professional pilot populations, 5–7% alcohol dependence is suspected, and in the USA

7–10% of pilots are assumed to have problems with alcohol, corresponding to a total number of 75 000 pilots (1991). Accident statistics in Germany indicate that 6.5% of aviation accidents have alcohol as a possible cause (1973–1983); in airline aviation, however, so far not one accident has been so caused. In approximately 2% of all fatal aviation accidents, drug use and illness (e.g. cardiac infarct) in the pilot play a role. The United States Air Force determined that alcohol was involved in 15% of fatal accidents, and other drugs were involved in 7% of cases (1973–1984).

The drinking behavior of pilots indicates that 15% use alcohol regularly for "stress management", i.e. to dismantle tensions.

— Effects of alcohol

Because of the impairment of human performance, alcohol should be avoided 24 hours before flight. Simulator studies with experienced pilots have demonstrated a decrease in concentration, vigilance, decision-making abilities, fine-motor coordination, depth perception and coordinated stereoptic activities, beginning at a blood alcohol concentration of 0.25 parts per thousand, and becoming manifest around 0.4 parts per thousand. Furthermore, an increased willingness to take risks and to make unsafe decisions occurs. In routine flying operation, an upper limit of 0.4 parts per thousand is necessary; this corresponds to the blood alcohol limit prescribed in the USA. Nevertheless, the so-called hangover effect is important to keep in mind. Performance degradations can occur with a blood alcohol level of 0.0 parts per thousand, if earlier alcohol ingestion yielded a blood alcohol level of 1.0 part per million. Preventive measures are: 24 hours of sobriety, alcohol breath analysis before each flight, and testing of visual-motoric concentration ability in the cockpit.

REFERENCES

1. Schmidtke H. (1993) Der Leistungsbegriff in der Ergonomie. In H. Schmidtke (eds) Ergonomie, pp. 110–174. Carl Hanser, München Wien.

2. Amendt R. (Hrsg.). (1993) Kompendium der Flugphysiologie, 254 pp. Flugmedizinisches Institut der Luftwaffe, Fürstenfeldbruck.
3. Schmitz I. (1997) Personal information.
4. Wirth D, Volke H-J, Schmitz I, Welsch H, Rudolf M, Buhss U, Meise R. (1999) Untersuchungen zur Minderung mentaler Leistungsvoraussetzungen unter dem Einfluss geringer bis mäßiger Grade atmosphärischer Hypoxie auf der Basis tonischer und evozierter Kohärenzen des EEG. Abschlußbericht an die Deutsche Akademie für Flugmedizin g.GmbH, Lufthansa Basis FRA/PM Frankfurt, 28 pp., 11 Fig., 9 Tab., enclosure. Technische Universität Dresden.
5. Reinhart RO. (1992) Basic flight Physiology, 235 pp. TAB Books, New York *et al.*
6. De Hart RL. (1985) Fundamentals of Aerospace Medicine. Lee & Febinger, Philadelphia.
7. Ruff S, Strughold H. (1957) Grundriß der Luftfahrtmedizin, 263 pp. Barth, München.
8 Papenfuß W. (Hrsg.). (1990) Luftfahrtmedizin, 400 pp. Brandenburgisches Verlagshaus, Berlin.
9 Schulze E, Schröder HJ, Lehweß-Litzmann J, Kressin J. (1990) Flugmedizin, 196 pp. transpress, Berlin.
10. Moser M, Frank P. (1988) Flugmedizin für Piloten, 136 pp. Thieme, Stuttgart.
11. Forth W, Henschler D, Rummel W. (1987) Allgemeine und spezielle Pharmakologie und Toxikologie. BI-Wissenschaftsverlag Mannheim.
12. Bachmann P. (1999) Flugmedizin für Piloten und Passagiere, 222 pp. Pietsch, Stuttgart.
13. Ernsting J, Nicholson AN, Rainford DJ. (Edited by) (2000) Aviation Medicine. Third Edition, 703 pp. Butterworth-Heinemann, Linacre House, Jordan Hill, Oxford OX2 8DP.
14. Grossmann K. (1985) Flugmedizin, 123 pp. Deutscher Ärzte-Verlag, Köln.
15. Jacobson E. (1938) Progressive relaxation. Univ. of Chicago Press.
16. Klinke R, Silbernagel St. (Hrsg.). (2001) Lehrbuch der Physiologie, 842 pp. Thieme, Stuttgart, New York.
17. Landgraf H, Rose D-M, Aust PE. (Hrsg.). (1996) Flugreisemedizin, pp. 351. Blackwell Wissenschaftsverlag, Berlin Wien.

18. Schmidt RF, Thews G. (Hrsg.). (1995) Physiologie des Menschen, 888 pp. Springer, Berlin *et al.*
19. Silbernagel S, Despopoulus A. (1988) Taschenatlas der Physiologie, 371 pp. Thieme, Stuttgart, New York.
20. Wetzig J. (1995) Physiologie, 31 pp. Deutsche Akademie Flugmedizin, Kurs 5 A, Frankfurt.
21. Wirth D, Volke H-J, Rudolf M, Welsch H, Schmitz I. (1998) Kohärenzen des EEG bei Hypoxie in 4000m Höhe. Flug- und Reisemedizin **5**: 35–37
22. Kasprzak B, Wirth D. (1975) Zum Verhalten physiologischer Parameter bei akuter Höhenbelastung mit zusätzlicher Stehprobe in 5000 m NN. Ztschr. f. Militärmedizin **16**: 19–24.

Chapter 6

Cosmic Radiation Exposure of Flight Crews

Lutz Bergau, Rainer Facius and Matthias M. Meier*

INTRODUCTION

With the introduction of jet aircraft in the late 1950's, altitudes were being reached that required a fundamental understanding of the kind and degree of cosmic radiation to which flight crews and frequently flying passengers were now exposed.

While the older piston-driven aircraft could reach maximum altitudes of less than 30000 feet, jet aircraft such as the Boeing 707 regularly achieved altitudes above 40000 feet, and modern business jets such as the Learjet 45 have a maximum operating altitude of 51 000 feet.

Although no conclusive data to date quantify any measurable effect on biological systems of radiation due to flight activities, the aeromedical practitioner needs a good knowledge base in order to deal effectively with the questions their flight crews will confront them with. Fortunately, there is now a considerable database from the findings of dosimetry, as well from the results of epidemiological studies. Already in 1990, the ICRP (International Commission on Radiological Protection) recommended maximum allowable radiation exposures up to 20 mSv (millisievert), annually averaged over five years with a maximum of 50 mSv within one calendar year. The European Basic Safety Standards Directive 29/96 EURATOM

* Corresponding author.
German Aerospace Center (DLR), Cologne, Germany.

has been based on these recommendations and converted into the German Radiation Protection Ordinance concerning flight crews explicitly.

The discussion concerning the potential risks of radiation exposures has, among others, led to demands from interest groups to reduce flight time and maximum flight altitude, as well as much stricter medical surveillance of flight crews.

The following remarks should serve to increase the knowledge and understanding of the topical problems associated with radiation exposures, which is increasingly being expected of aeromedical practitioners.

Natural Radiation

Every human being, as well as the entire biosphere, is constantly exposed to ionizing radiation. This flow of energy has its origin in a variety of sources. The component derived from the atomic cores of the minerals forming rocks is summed up as terrestrial radiation. Ionizing radiation is produced through the decay of long-lived radioactive nuclides, such as uranium-238, thorium-232, and their derivatives in the Earth's crust. The intensity of terrestrial radiation is quite variable, depending on the content of the radionuclides within the Earth's crust. Therefore, some heavily populated regions of Earth, such as Kerala in India, Guarapari in Brazil, Yangjiang in China, and Ramsar in Iran, have radiation levels more than tenfold higher than those measured in most other parts of the world. There are regional variations even within Germany (in northern regions there is only one-third of the terrestrial radiation found in southern Germany). Additional large fluctuations can result from geological formations (granite, gneiss, sandstone) as well as from various building materials.

The radionuclides tritium, carbon-14, and especially the noble gases radon-220 and radon-222 from decay of thorium-232 and uranium-238, are found in the atmosphere, together with their long-lived decay products adsorbed to aerosols. Indoors, in closed rooms, the concentration of radon is 10–30 times greater than outdoors.

Particularly high levels can be measured in the radon-tunnels of Bad Gastein in Austria and Bad Kreuznach in Germany.

This natural radiation exerts its effects via radionuclides, externally onto the biological structures of the human body, and internally via inhaled radioactive dust and gases. Furthermore, drinking water and ingested foodstuffs can contribute to internal radiation exposure from isotopes such as potassium-40 and the previously mentioned tritium and carbon-14.

Civilizational Radiation

The Earth has been exposed to natural radiation since the dawn of time. Not until the last century was this natural radiation augmented by man-made radiation, primarily owing to medical applications, such as X-rays, nuclear medical diagnostic and therapy, and by nuclear energy installations (i.e. nuclear power plants). This additional radiation can be summarized as man-made or civilizational radiation. Added to the sources mentioned are the remainders of the fallout from above-ground nuclear tests in the USA and USSR between 1945 and 1962, in China between 1964 and 1980, and the consequences of the Chernobyl catastrophe in April 1986. Civilizational radiation is responsible for a considerable proportion of today's total human radiation exposure. More than 80% of civilizational radiation originates from medical applications, by far dominated by X-ray diagnostic modalities. The proportion from fallout, the nuclear industry, and even Chernobyl are negligible in comparison. In Germany, medical sources contribute approximately 2 mSv/a in comparison to 2.4 mSv/a from natural sources, thus representing 45% of the total exposure.

Cosmic Radiation

On the surface of the Earth, another contribution to the total amount of radiation is cosmic radiation. This radiation consists of high-energy particles that continually impinge on the Earth from outside the magnetosphere. The origin of this so-called primary radiation is the sun, solar radiation, and supernova explosions in star systems throughout the universe — a main source of galactic radiation.

The composition of the high energetic galactic radiation is as follows: 85% protons, 13.5% alpha particles, and 1.5% heavy atomic nuclei such as C, O, Mg, and Fe, which carry energies from several MeV to 10^{13} MeV.

The radiation originating from the sun is of a similar composition, but these particle energies — in occasional outbreaks — only reach energies of up to 10^4 MeV. The permanent solar wind, which comprises the majority of the total solar radiation, only carries energies of a few keV. The intensity of solar radiation fluctuates widely over time, and is dependent on the sun's activity (see solar flares). Because of its low energy, the permanent solar wind is deflected by the Earth's magnetosphere so that penetration of the atmosphere is prevented.

In contrast, the high-energy particles of primary radiation collide with the atomic nuclei of oxygen and nitrogen and additional components when they penetrate the atmosphere, activating interactions leading to a secondary radiation cascade. During this collision with the atomic nuclei, charged particles are formed, such as alpha particles, protons, and muons, as well as uncharged electric particles, such as photons, and most of all, neutrons. Many of these have enough energy to activate further nuclear reactions. It is estimated that each high-energy proton from the primary radiation can create a million or more secondary particles. Additionally, the interaction of the primary radiation with the aircraft itself can locally create an increase in radiation dosage of 5–10%, the fuel being the main contributor. In practice, this localized effect can be disregarded and the radiation exposure considered equal for all persons on board independent of their position inside the aircraft.

The cascade system in the atmosphere, described above, attenuates the primary cosmic radiation to a considerable degree so that only a minute fraction reaches the Earth itself.

An additional characteristic of galactic cosmic radiation is its isotropy, i.e. that particles strike the Earth equally from all directions of space. The resulting radiation fields are not subject to daily variations.

Altitude dependence

Already at an altitude of 20 km (65 600 ft), corresponding to an air density of 0.088 kg/m^3, proton flux is reduced to nearly half, alpha particles nearly to a quarter, and heavy atomic nuclei to about 3% of the original magnitude.[3] However, at an altitude of 12 km (39 400 ft, air density 0.310 kg/m^3), radiation is still about 100 to 200 times greater than at the surface of the Earth (air density 1.225 kg/m^3).[a]

Due to its extraordinary high biological effectiveness (more details later on), neutron radiation deserves special attention. Its biologically weighted contribution as part of the effective dose of the cosmic radiation on the Earth's surface is only about 3%. At an altitude of 12 km, varying with latitude, one must reckon with a neutron contribution of 50%, reaching a maximum of about 80% at 15–18 km, and declining thereafter.[4]

The data outlined above make it obvious that flight level is the dominant variable determining the degree of radiation exposure. After departure, due to decreasing terrestrial radiation, the overall radiation level is declining up to an altitude of 1000 m (3050 ft). Above this level, radiation intensity increases continuously with altitude, due to the increasing effect of cosmic radiation.

Height Maxima

The nearly linear rise in altitude-related radiation intensity reaches its maximum at approximately 65 000 feet (proton maximum). At this altitude, there is a balance between the build-up of the secondary radiation cascade and its weakening by further penetration down through the atmosphere.[5] During the 27 years the Concorde was flying, cruising at an altitude around 63 000 feet, continual measurements were made by an on-board detection system, demonstrating

[a] Air density according to ICAO Standard Atmosphere, geopotential height.

a doubling of ionizing radiation compared to an altitude of 40 000 feet, which is the usual maximum flight level of subsonic aircraft.[6] Above 140 000 feet (~45 km), the intensity of radiation falls to about 50% of the maximum found at 65 000 feet.

Geographic Latitude

In addition to altitude, the intensity of radiation is to a large extent dependent on latitude. The magnetic field of the Earth has a shielding effect, causing particles of cosmic radiation to be partially deflected. This effect is strongest in the regions of the geomagnetic equator; it diminishes considerably over the poles where the radiation dose at aviation altitudes is about 2–4 times greater than at the equator. At constant altitude, the intensity of radiation begins to rise at a latitude of about 30°N, reaching a maximum plateau at 60°N. The same applies to the southern hemisphere.[7]

SOLAR CYCLES

The surface of the sun continuously ejects low energy subatomic particles, the so-called solar wind. These emissions do not take place at a constant rate, but rather in a cycle, showing a maximum (solar max), respectively a minimum (solar min) every 11 years.

The stronger the particle stream of the sun, the more the interplanetary magnetic field of the heliosphere surrounding the Earth comes to effect, and the greater is the deflection of cosmic radiation from the Earth, thereby varying the intensity of the cosmic radiation reaching the Earth.

At maximal solar activity, we receive a minimum dose rate from galactic radiation, and vice versa, a maximum galactic radiation can be measured at minimal solar activity. At the altitudes where most civil aviation takes place, i.e. between 27 000 and 40 000 feet (~9 and 13 km), the variations between these two extremes can be as much as 60%, and even more at higher altitudes. As stated before, the particles of the solar wind have such a low energy that they are captured by the Earth's magnetic field and have little direct influence on the level of ionizing radiation to which aircraft at typical flight levels are exposed. In 1991, within the 11-year cycle, a solar burst maximum could be determined. The following minimum of solar activity occurred in 1997, and the last (very wide) maximum was observed in 2001/2002. The following minimum occurred in 2008/2009. When considering measurements of radiation intensity, the solar cycle has to be taken into account.[8]

SOLAR FLARES

Huge protuberances occur on the sun at irregular, widely spaced time intervals. These are related to magnetic disturbances, and lead to explosive emissions of optical and particle radiation. These solar streams of particle emissions (solar particle events, or SPE) can in particular cases increase ionizing radiation even at normal flight levels. Latitudes above 60°, i.e. close to the poles, are particularly affected. Between 1956 and 2006, a total of about seven such extreme events were noted, causing the dose rate maximum in some areas to increase by up to 100 times.[9] These fluctuations in solar activity can last from several hours to a day. The likelihood of an aircraft incidentally flying through an area with such elevated radiation is relatively small. The routine measurements, taken by Concorde during 80 000 flights over 20 years, did at no time indicate any excessive elevation of radiation, requiring an emergency descent to lower altitudes.[6]

However, the theoretical possibility of flying into such a region of massively elevated radiation does exist. Consequently, it seems necessary to develop an early warning system for civil aviation. The Space Environment Center of the National Oceanic and Atmospheric Administration (NOAA, USA) can, via satellites, solar telescopes, magnometers, and direct radiation measurements, obtain data, which are forwarded to the FAA in order to generate warnings concerning solar flares.

TISSUE STARS

Research has not been able to clarify the distribution and the biological effectiveness of the so-called tissue disintegration stars. The name of these stars originates from the characteristic star figures that are formed by primary radiation when penetrating a radiation sensitive emulsion. These stars are images of the disintegration reactions forming the radiation cascade mentioned above. This represents, so to speak, the continuation within the human body of the reaction cascade, released by cosmic primary radiation. These stars lead to a relatively high local energy deposition in just a few cells, but do not expose the whole body. The energy distribution of the stars within the tissue is characterized by an extreme non-uniformity. It seems likely that the radiation dose from tissue stars is of little significance.

HEAVY NUCLEI

Heavy nuclei, as part of the cosmic radiation, have a similar minimal effect on the total radiation exposure. Penetration depth by these particles, e.g. those from the iron group of the heavy spectrum, is very limited. The majority of the heavy nuclei is captured within the upper levels of the atmosphere and disintegrated.

Particularly interesting are those heavy ions that are stopped within the tissue, creating regions of very high ionization density around their path. In contrast, fully penetrating particles have less biological effect.

MEASUREMENT OF FLIGHT CREWS' RADIATION EXPOSURE

To date, many measurements and evaluations have been performed in order to quantify the actual amount of radiation to which flight crews are exposed. This research was initiated by the introduction of the passenger jet aircraft, which regularly reached altitudes above 40 000 feet, where radiation levels are several times higher than at the altitudes normally reached in the era of propeller-driven aircraft.

One of the special aspects of the originally planned SST (Supersonic Transport Aircraft) in the USA, followed by the actual flights of the Concorde (manufactured in France and Britain and flown commercially from 1976 to 2003), was the problem of ionizing radiation. This aspect of high altitude flying has given rise to intense investigation activity over the last three decades. Mandated by the Bundesverkehrministerium in Germany (Department of Transportation), Lufthansa German Airlines made measurements on its B-707 flights with the assistance of the Institute of Experimental and Applied Physics at the University of Kiel, Germany.[10]

Accuracy of Measurement

Without going into details about these and other data collected over the past 35 years, it can be ascertained that these data have contributed significantly to the knowledge of radiation exposure of flying personnel. Then, as now, the precise analysis of radiation fields at various flight levels was not an easy task. The "difficulties of applying terrestrially designed and calibrated devices to the measurement of nearly unknown radiation fields at altitude" (Dieter F. Regulla, GSF — Forschungszentrum für Umwelt und Gesundheit — the National Research Center for Radiation, Environment and Health in Germany) still exist.

Despite these uncertainties, there is growing consensus about the average amount of radiation to which flight crews are exposed under normal operational conditions. More difficult to assess are the special conditions, such as solar flares, tissue stars, and heavy nuclei. Transport of insufficiently shielded radioactive cargo is against international rules and is not taken into account here. Between 1991–1992, extensive measurements were undertaken by the GSF (see above) in association with the Workers' Compensation Board and Lufthansa German Airlines.[11] The average annual radiation exposure of flight crews was established to be 3–5 mSv.

Other studies, more recently undertaken, have found similar levels of exposure as those determined by the GSF. A summary of radiation exposure of flying personnel entitled "Determination of flight crews' exposure to cosmic radiation" was published in 1997 by Strahlenschutzkommission, the German Radiation Protection Commission.[12]

Among numerous other studies, further two can be mentioned: "Canadian Aircrew Radiation Environment Study" (THUM *et al.*)[13] and "ACREM — Air Crew Radiation Exposure Monitoring" (Laborbericht der Physikalisch — Technischen Bundesanstalt, August 1999).[14] In the latter study, the extensive measurements undertaken during flights between 1997–1999 were evaluated. A detailed summary of measured and calculated data is given in the report of a working group of the European Dosimetry Group (EURADOS).[15]

Chromosomal Aberrations

Another interesting method of acquiring total body exposure data is the so-called biological dosimetry. On the basis of observed chromosomal structural changes associated with the actual absorbed radiation dose within an organism, the numbers of chromosomal aberrations in human lymphocytes can be determined. Primarily, such biological dosimetry techniques can be successfully applied retrospectively to investigate radiation exposures in cases of radiation accidents when there is limited or non-existent dose information. Indeed, chromosomal aberrations have been investigated in groups exposed to chronic low-level radiation, such as comparing flight crews to ground-based workers. Initial investigations by the Institute of Radiation Biology of the Munster University in Germany have described an elevation in numbers of the so-called dicentric rings, although the number of investigated chromosomes is too small to be of any statistical significance. A further investigation by Romano *et al.* likewise demonstrated an increase in chromosomal aberrations.[16] However, these results could not be confirmed by the Robert Koch Institute in Berlin, which has conducted the largest lymphocyte research to date.[17] In principle, such biologic dosimetry pertaining to chronic radiation exposure can only be utilized if the limited time period of detection of the chromosomal aberrations is taken into account and time-dependent exposure profiles of the subjects are realistically represented.

Summation of Radiation Exposure

The studies undertaken so far provide a clear understanding of the radiation exposure of flight crews. By consensus, total annual radiation exposure of crews on international flights has been estimated to vary between 3 and 6 mSv. In Europe, any radiation exposure in excess of the threshold of 6 mSv per calendar year initiates a legally stipulated examination by a specially qualified and accredited physician in order to monitor the individuals exposed to this level. In flight crews, this is to be expected only in very few and exceptional cases.

BIOLOGICAL EFFECTS

Ionizing radiation produces its biological effects by changing or destroying the integrity of essential molecular structures within living cells. This occurs through direct excitation of atoms or molecules or via ionization, by which electrons are dislodged from their atomic orbits. Additionally, through direct effects on non-essential molecules, such as H_2O, chemically highly reactive radicals are formed, which can cause similar damage to biologically essential molecules by "radiochemical" secondary reactions.

Particularly important are changes to the structures in DNA (deoxyribonucleic acid) as carrier of genetic information. Depending on the amount of absorbed radiation energy, affected cells can either die or exhibit genetic changes if the repair mechanisms fail to provide error-free and complete repairs. Effects of "higher" and "lower" radiation exposures must therefore be differentiated. At low doses, the primary molecular effects are dependent on accidental, isolated radiation encounters within the cell. Regarding the ensuing biological consequences of these so-called stochastic radiation effects, it has been nearly unanimously postulated since the 1950's that there is no threshold for radiation to generate health damage. In other words, the stochastic effect can only be zero for a dose of zero. However, the validity of this postulate has come into question by the results of the radiobiological research in the last two decades. Induction of cancer and genetic damage in subsequent generations is regarded as the most important late consequences of the stochastic radiation effects.

As a rule, the effect of doses of up to one Gy of low-energy ionizing radiation is the breakage of a single strand of DNA's double helix, which can be repaired effectively. With high-energy neutron radiation, even single encounters can produce more severe damage, such as double strand breaks that cannot be fully and correctly repaired. The radiation weighting factor, given in the ICRP-60 recommendations of 1991, is based upon this highly significant radiobiological effectiveness of neutron radiation.

Due to changes of genetic substance, stochastic effects of ionizing radiation may come into effect in the following generation or even in later generations. In complete contrast are the non-stochastic effects, also called deterministic effects. These are the effects from high dose radiation exposure, which via increasing impairment of cellular structure can lead to organ failure and eventually death.

By its nature, the radiation exposure of flying personnel is within the low dose range, so deterministic effects can be excluded, even during exposure to particle storms of solar flares.

RELEVANT ASSESSMENT FACTORS

The following are the most important variables to consider when assessing potential damage due to ionizing radiation:

I. Annual flight hours

Per regulation of the Federal Office of Civil Aviation in Germany, the maximum flight time is 900 hours per year. Surveys by the European Community indicate that for airline pilots, their actual annual flight hours are between 500 and 700 hours. The time spent in ascent to and descent from cruising altitude (approximately 5–20%) must be subtracted from these numbers.

II. Total years of flight

As most pilots end their professional career at age 60, their profession could theoretically result in 40 years of flying. In most cases, the actual number of career years is lower. Since both the International Standards of ICAO (SARPs) and the European regulations (JAR FCL) now allow an age limit up to 65 years, it is possible that average total career flight times will be higher in the future.

III. The preponderance of high altitude flight

A differentiation between short and long haul flights must be made.

IV. Routes predominantly at latitudes above 50 degrees (includes both hemispheres)

RISK ASSESSMENT

The fundamental question is how much being exposed to ionizing radiation in flight increases the risk of cancer in flying personnel above that of the background population. Already in 1992, criteria for scoring this risk were developed by the Department of Transportation and the Federal Aviation Administration (FAA) and published.[18] This work is based on the BEIR-V Report[19] and estimates an additional death rate from radiation-induced malignant tumors of 13–20 per 100 000 after ten years of flying.

More important than these theoretical numbers based on projections, i.e. based on the previously mentioned questionable postulate for stochastic radiation effects, are epidemiological investigations.

EPIDEMIOLOGY

A number of epidemiological studies have been published, which attempt to assess the increased risk of cancer in flight crews. Most older works lack a statistically relevant cohort and a relevant control population. Among these are investigations of a Canadian study group,[20] studies of pilots in British Airways,[21] and unpublished reports of Swissair. The survey of Canadian airline pilots found an elevated incidence of cancer (non-melanoma skin cancer and Hodgkins disease) as well as elevated death rates from brain and rectal tumors. However, the authors recommended a larger cohort study in order to be more confident about these results. Particularly in the case of CNS tumors, the British study concluded that further investigation was required, taking the lifestyles of the pilots into account. Further investigations by Japan Airlines (KAJI *et al.*)[22] encompassed a larger number of subjects; nonetheless, data were too few to allow statistically convincing estimates of mortality rates and cancer incidence. Notable are two other older works: a study published in 1995 by Pukkala *et al.*[23] concerning breast cancer incidence in flight attendants of Finnish airline companies; and the investigation by Gundestrup *et al.*,[24] suggesting that acute myeloid leukemia and other cancers might be caused by in-flight ionizing radiation.

Ballard *et al.*[25] summarized the results of these earlier epidemiological studies in a meta-analysis. For pilots, overall mortality rates were lower for all causes, including lung cancer and leukemia. After correcting for socio-economic variables, pilots were found to have increased rates of two types of cancers. Mortality rates were elevated for malignant melanoma to 1.97 (95% confidence interval 1.02–3.82) and for prostate cancer to 1.45 (95% confidence interval 1.19–2.29). In previous studies, melanoma had not been observed as a potential late consequence of ionizing radiation. Prostate cancer is commonly observed in sedentary occupations, the so-called bus-driver syndrome.

These results, based on findings in single organs, suffer from lack of statistical power. None of the results related to any individual organ system are significant on the 95% confidence level. The likelihood that these cases are the results of chance is further supported by the fact that not a single organ was seen to have an elevated cancer rate in all of the studies. Alone, the combined study of morbidity and mortality of all different kinds of cancer is free of this limitation.

The epidemiological studies by Tveten *et al.*,[26] investigating cancer incidence in Norwegian pilots, and by Zeeb, Blettner *et al.*,[27,28] released in early 2002 (University of Bielefeld, Germany), include cohorts of flying personnel large enough to provide statistically relevant evidence. The study by Blettner *et al.* included a total of 6061 pilots, 16 014 female and 4536 male flight attendants. Both investigations were part of a study sponsored by the European Commission. Noteworthy in these combined European studies[29,30] is that the bias produced by the "healthy worker effect" in both of its main appearances (the healthy worker hire effect and the healthy worker survivor effect) has been reduced or avoided by the study protocol. The results show standard mortality rate (SMR) of the pilots and the female flight attendants to be below the norm for the general population. Overall, the cancer rate for pilots is lower than for the general population. Nonetheless, a few cancers showed a slightly elevated mortality rate; validation of these results requires consideration of the "multiple testing" problem and cannot be finally concluded until after further investigations have been made. In male flight attendants, the SMR is elevated above that of the general population due to specific diseases of the immune system.

In addition to the remarks above, it is important to note that these epidemiological studies do not establish a direct correlation between the results of the mortality studies and the radiation exposure. A number of additional factors could potentially influence the morbidity and mortality rate of flight crews. These include mild hypoxia during flight, circadian rhythm disturbances and their potential effects on the immune competence of the organism, and additional factors found in the specific environment of flying such as low cabin humidity, elevated CO_2 and O_3 levels, and so on. With regard to the frequency of breast cancer in flight attendants, the proven higher incidence of breast cancer in pauci- and nulliparous women must be taken into account, as nulliparity counts to the unique factors that differentiate flight crews from the general population.

LEGAL MEASURES

On the basis of the recommendations of the ICRP (International Commission on Radiological Protection) from 1991[31] the European Union, guided by EU-Regulation 96/29/EURATOM, has determined that all flight crews shall be considered as "occupationally exposed to radiation." Article 42 stipulates special measures to be undertaken if a flight crew member's radiation exposure exceeds the annual threshold value of 1 mSv.[32]

Included are:

- Determination of the amount of radiation exposure of the crew member
- Formulation of duty rosters in order to minimize the total exposure for highly exposed personnel
- Information to employees about potential health hazards
- Special protection of pregnant flight attendants, as determined in Article 10 of the EU regulation

The directive of the European Union, transferred to an amendment of the Radiation Protection Ordinance (Strahlenschutzverordnung, StrlSchV) in Germany, took effect in August 2001 as part of the national legislation. Differing from the ICRP recommendations, a maximum annual limit of 20 mSv was stipulated. When a dose of 6 mSv per calendar year is exceeded, an additional medical examination is required. As mentioned before, in airline operations this is only necessary in rare and exceptional cases.

Upon declaration of pregnancy to the employer, flight attendants are allowed to accumulate 1 mSv until the end of pregnancy. At Lufthansa, however, pregnant crew members have always been exempted from flight duties immediately after declaration of pregnancy. Based on the maternity protection act, pregnant flight attendants are given ground assignments. Other European airlines follow this example.

SUMMARY

Considering the known magnitude of exposure of flight crews and the quality of radiation at relevant altitudes, immediate "deterministic" somatic damages can be excluded. Furthermore, it can be stated with great confidence that direct effects on embryonic development are similarly improbable.

The previously discussed scientific studies, estimating the risk of malignant diseases due to the effect of radiation, are not consistent in their results. The more recent epidemiological publications with large cohort sizes show, nonetheless, that the overall risk of cancer due to cosmic radiation among flight crews is very low. Even with correction for the "healthy worker" effect and other confounders, the cancer rate in flight crews is not higher than in the general population.

REFERENCES

1. Bailey PE. (1982) Neutron radiation dosimetry in high altitude flight personal. *Aviat Space Env Med* **53**(8).
2. Schäfer HJ. (1968) Public health aspects of galactic radiation exposure at supersonic air transport altitudes. *Aerospace Med.*
3. Wallace RW, Sondhaus CA. (1978) Cosmic radiation exposure in subsonic air transport. *Aviat Space Env Med* **49**(4).
4. Schäfer HJ. (1971) Radiation exposure in air travel. *Science* **173**.
5. Upton AC. (1966) *Radiobiological Aspects of the Supersonic Transport.* Health Physics Pergamon Press.
6. Davies DM. (1993) Cosmic radiation in Concorde operations and the impact of new ICRP recommendations on commercial aviation. *Radiation Protection Dosimetry* **48**(1): 121–124.
7. Friedberg W *et al.* (1988) Galactic cosmic radiation exposure and associated health risk for air. *Aviat Space Env Med.*
8. Rossi HH. (1975) Cosmic radiation exposure in supersonic and subsonic flight. *Aviat Space Env Med.*
9. Buley LE. (1969) Provision of solar flare radiation information in support of supersonic transport operations: A review of developments. *Aerospace Med* **40**.
10. Allkofer OC, *et al.* (1962) Untersuchungen über die Strahlen-Gefährdung der Flugbesatzung und des Bodenpersonals von Düsen-Flugzeugen(I). *Atomenergie* **7**(5): 173–178.
11. Regulla D, *et al.* (1991) Equipment, Calibration and Selected Results as used for "Measurements of Cosmic Radiation on Board of German Airlines

on the Major Intercontinental Flight Routes." Bericht des BfS "Stellungnahme zu Berichten über Messungen zur Bestimmung der Strahlenexposition."

12. Kuni H. *Strahlenbelastung in Düsenverkehrsflugzeugen — zur Bewertung aus Medizinischer Sicht.*
13. Schenepel GH. (1996) Die Ermittlung der durch kosmische Strahlung verursachten Strahlenexposition des fliegenden Personals. Berichte der Strahlenschutzkommision des Bundesministeriums für Umwelt, Naturschutz und Reaktorsicherheit, Heft 1.
14. Tome P, *et al.* (1998) Canadian aircrew radiation environmental study. *International Workshop on Cosmic Radiation,* 5–7 February 1998, Charleston, South Carolina.
15. Schrewe UJ. (1999) Air Crew Radiation Exposure Monitoring. PTB-6.31-99-1.
16. Romano E, *et al.* (1997) Increase of chromosomal aberrations induced by ionising radiation in peripheral blond lymphocytes of civil aviation pilots and crew members. *Murar Res* **377**: 89–93.
17. Wolf G, *et al.* (1999) Cytogenetic investigations in flight personnel. *Radiation Protection Dosimetry* **86**(4): 275–278.
18. Friedberg W, *et al.* (1992) Radiation Exposure of Air Carrier Crewmembers (II). DOT/FAA Publication.
19. Beir V. (1990) Committee on the Biological Effects of Ionizing Radiations. Health Effects of Exposure to Low Levels of Ionizing Radiation. National Academy Washington.
20. Band PR, *et al.* Mortality and cancer incidence in a cohort of commercial airline pilots. *Aviat Space Env Med.*
21. Irvine D, Davie SDM. (1999) British Airways flightdeck mortality Study, 1950–1992. *Aviat Space Env Med* **70**: 548–555.
22. Kaji M, *et al.* (1993) Mortality experience of cockpit crewmembers from Japan Airlines. *Aviat Space Env Med* **64**: 748–750.
23. Pukkala E, *et al.* (1995) Incidence of cancer among Finnish airline attendants 1967–1992. *BMJ* **311**: 649–652.
24. Gundestrup M, Storm H. (1999) Radiation-induced acute myeloid leukaemia and other cancers in commercial jet cockpit crew. A populations-based cohort study. *Lancet* **354**: 2029–2031.
25. Tveten U. (1999) Cosmic radiation and airline pilots — Exposure patterns of Norwegian SAS-pilots 1960–1994. IFE/E-99/002.

26. Blettner M, *et al.* Cohort study of German cockpit crew, 1960–1997.
27. Blettner M, *et al.* Mortality from cancer and other causes among airline cabin attendants in Germany, 1960–1997.
28. CRP. (1990) Empfehlungen der Internationalen Strahlenschutzkommission (ICRP 60). Fischer-Verlag.
29. Euratom. (1996) Richtlinie 96/29/Euratom des Rates zur Festlegung der grundlegenden Sicherheitsnormen für den Schutz der Gesundheit der Arbeitskräfte und der Bevölkerung gegen die Gefahren durch ionisierende Strahlung.
30. European Commission. (2004) Radiation Protection 140, Cosmic Radiation Exposure of Aircraft Crew.
31. Ballard T, Lagorio S, deAngelis G, Verdecchia A. (2000) Cancer incidence and mortality among flight personnel: A meta-analysis. *Aviat Space Env Med* **7**(2): 216–224.
32. Blettner M, Zeeb H, Auvinen A, *et al.* (2003) Other causes among male airline cockpit crew in Europe. *Int J Cancer* **106**(6): 946–952.
33. Zeeb H, Blettner M, Langner I, *et al.* (2003) Mortality from cancer and other causes among airline cabin attendants in Europe. A collaborative cohort study in eight countries. *Am J Epidemiol* **158**(1): 35–46.

27. Blettner M [illegible]

[illegible]
29. [illegible]
[illegible]
30. [illegible] der [illegible] der
[illegible]
[illegible]
31. [illegible]
[illegible]
32. [illegible]

Part 4

PREVENTION

Chapter 7

Physiology and Pathophysiology of Nutrition

Herwig H. Ditschuneit*

INTRODUCTION

In western industrialized countries, the leading cause of morbidity and mortality is cardiovascular diseases, statistically at a rate of over 50%. These diseases are overwhelmingly caused by the consequences of atherosclerotic processes of the arterial walls. These processes are not due to arterial wall diseases *per se*, but are caused by reversible reactions to chronic injuries caused by certain risk factors. These are essentially: obesity, metabolic syndrome with hypertension, hyperlipoproteinemia, disorders of glucose metabolism (Type 2 diabetes mellitus), hyperinsulinemia, hyperlipacidemia, and hyperuricemia. A reduction of the growth of these cardiovascular diseases is only possible when treatment is focused on the elimination of the risk factors. Since the occurrence of the risk factors is strongly correlated with changes in nutrition and lifestyle, an effective therapy must be directed at making changes in unhealthy nutrition and lifestyle practices.

The situation among flight crews regarding morbidity is not significantly different from that of the general population. The problem cases in aeromedical practice, just as in general medical practice, are treated principally by addressing the risk factors. Upon presentation

* Albert-Schweitzer-Str. 13, 89134, Blaustein, Germany. E-mail: ditschuneit@medizin.uni-ulm.de; hans-ditschuneit@t-online.de.

of risk factors, the aeromedical examiner (AME) must be particularly diligent in excluding atherosclerotic processes. He must clarify the hazards of the pilot's risk factors in detail, and provide awareness concerning effective preventive and therapeutic measures. Generally, this concerns nutritional changes in order to reduce body weight.

Regarding an individual with an obvious arterial lesion, such as a myocardial infarction, stent or bypass operation, recurrence of symptoms after a subsequent operative intervention must necessarily entail unfitness to fly. Already after the cardinal event, intensive management of risk factors should be initiated. A pilot who clinically manifests circulatory compromise should always be disqualified, because every operative measure is merely rectifying a local disorder without influencing the general underlying pathological process. Nutritional influences upon health should have a high priority in every AME's practice.

THE OPTIMAL DIET

Our diets consist of a variety of chemically defined nutrients. Counted among these are vitamins, minerals, amino acids, and fatty acids, as well as some carbohydrates as fuel supplies. These are absorbed in the diet and ensure well-being and health. Some nutrients are essential; in other words, they must be brought in from outside the body, as the body is not able to manufacture them. Non-essential nutrients can be synthesized from other nutritional components, but can also be ingested and channeled into the metabolic pathways. The metabolic processes are exceedingly complex and have not yet been satisfactorily explained. We still know very little about how nutrients are broken down, transported and utilized, and how they regenerate innumerable specialized tissues so that health can be maintained.

The goal of an optimal diet is to sustain optimal physical and mental fitness. The daily requirements for essential nutrients and energy are dependent upon age, gender, size, weight, metabolism, and physical activity. The recommendations cannot be exactly calculated for each individual; they depend on epidemiological evidence, and a large margin of error must be accepted. Many recommendations rely on broad estimations.

The prerequisite for optimal physical and mental fitness, for health and well-being, and for the preservation of a healthy constitution, is a balanced relationship between energy intake and inergy expenditure; this is of paramount importance. With an increase in calorie ingestion or a reduction in calorie expenditure, weight gain is unavoidable. In contrast, if calorie ingestion lags behind calorie expenditure, then weight loss will supervene. If significant weight gain or weight loss occurs, then the goal of the optimal diet has not been met. In such cases, the only successful procedure to follow in order to rectify the situation is control of food intake with simultaneous monitoring of body weight. In today's society of overabundance, this usually demands strict self-discipline and pronounced willpower. Our genetically determined control system of hunger and satiety has developed over hundreds of thousands of years in such a way that we always want to take in food and always are able to do so, whenever the opportunity presents itself rather than being limited to situations when it is necessary to do so. In times of need, we can also survive without nutrition for extended periods without any significant harm. We have survived for millions of years on scarce food supplies and frequent periods of famine. With the invention of the steam engine 230 years ago, the situation changed dramatically in many parts of the world. Our human productivity has increased manyfold; we have transformed the environment, and exponentially increased the production of foodstuffs while simultaneously reducing the cost. Consequently, many people today ingest far more food than they need, causing a frightening increase in diseases associated with obesity. The genetically determined regulation of hunger and satiety is counterproductive in today's restructured world. We must not follow our inner desires and believe that we are doing right. We must control desires and rationally determine our individual metabolic demands — and live accordingly. This, as it turns out, is extremely difficult, and our attempts to do so are often unsuccessful. For most people, this is a lifelong and difficult battle against the inner self.

NUTRITIONAL DISORDER

Obesity and the Metabolic Syndrome

The greatest nutritional problem stems from the overwhelming supply of delectable foodstuff daily offered to us and the resulting imbalance between energy ingestion and expenditure. A positive energy balance is continuously deposited into fat stores. The results are an increase in adipose tissue via hypertrophic processes and a corresponding weight gain. If the weight gain remains positive over a long period of time and the net weight gain exceeds 60% of the normal weight, an additional hyperplastic process begins, which results in an increase in the quantity of adipose cells.[1]

Most adipose tissue is subcutaneous, while a small portion, about 5–25%, is abdominal. This intraabdominal fat tissue is not uniform; it is distributed in the retroperitoneal and the portal compartment; the latter includes the omentum and the mesenteric tissue and is 70–80% larger than the former. These compartments are substantially different, primarily in that drainage of the portal compartment to the liver via the portal vein gives it metabolic significance which the retroperitoneum does not have.[2–4]

The distribution of subcutaneous adipose tissue is individually variable, but also gender specific. In females, the accumulation of fat is generally greater on the upper thighs, hips, and buttocks. Consequently, females maintain their typical gynoid form with wide hips, in contrast to the males' android form with narrow hips. In the case of a chronically positive energy gain and a large increase of total adipose tissues, the distribution among the various compartments remains fairly uniform in the male. Even the abdominal visceral compartment increases linearly with an increase in total weight. In contrast, an increase in intraabdominal adipose tissue in females occurs only when a total weight gain of approximately 25 kg or menopause is reached.[5,6] In addition to the total adipose mass, also age influences the distribution of fat. In obese men after the second decade of life, a continuous increase of visceral fat in relation to total body fat can be observed, while in women this relative increase occurs generally between the forth and fifth decade of life, after the onset of menopause. In females, the body habitus changes significantly. The typical gynoid shape becomes weaker and takes on android traits. From this point onward, obese women, especially those with visceral adiposity, increasingly develop metabolic disorders. The most significant absolute and relative differences in the amount of visceral adipose tissue are primarily dependent on the degree of obesity and endogenous, genetic factors. However, exogenous factors such as smoking and alcohol abuse also play an important role.

The definition of "android obesity" comprises a degree of visceral adiposity. The diagnosis is not difficult to make when a patient displays obvious abdominal enlargement and a typical habitus. However, since visceral obesity is correlated with metabolic disorders and may develop without an obvious change in habitus, early diagnosis is of great significance.

Obesity and Health

The history of medicine has taught us that there is a close relationship between obesity and certain life-endangering disorders, which have been known to physicians for centuries. In modern times, many prospective studies involving hundreds of thousands of individuals over periods of ten or more years have unequivocally shown that obesity is a risk factor for cardiovascular disease and premature death.

As a parameter for obesity, the body mass index (BMI) or Quetelet index is widely utilized. It compares a person's weight and height and is defined as body weight (in kg) divided by the square of the height (in m): BMI = kg/m^2. It is a relatively good measure of combined adipose mass. From the "American Cancer Society Study," comprising more than 750000 subjects during a period of more than 14 years, the lowest mortality rate was found among individuals with an optimal BMI for males of 19.9–22.9, and for females of 18.6–23.0. A BMI of 30 increases the mortality approximately 150%, and for a BMI of 32 it climbs to 200%.[7–9] In the "The Norwegian Experience," 816000 males and 902000 females were studied over a period of 10 years. The mortality rate of 40–50 year old men with a BMI of 34 and females of 38 was double that of subjects with a BMI of 22–25.[10]

DISTRIBUTION OF ADIPOSE TISSUE IS A GREATER RISK FACTOR THAN THE DEGREE OF OBESITY

The origin of the heightened mortality rate is ultimately reducible to an accelerated atherosclerosis process, which rapidly evolves under the influence of the following risk factors: hypertension, hyper- and dyslipoproteinemia, and diabetes mellitus with hyperinsulinemia, among others. The frequency of these disorders is positively correlated with the degree of obesity (BMI). The prevalence of obesity makes this relationship obvious to every general medical practitioner today. It has also been recognized and described by physicians for many hundreds of years. Early on, it was suggested that a syndrome of obesity, hypertension, diabetes mellitus, and virilization appeared in women in the second half of their lives. Morgagni referred to the "virili aspectu" of these women in his famous book "De sedibus et causis morborum" (1761). This syndrome, combined with an android habitus, was also described by von Achard and Thiers (1921) as *diabètes des femmes à barbe*. In 1947, Vague[11] attempted to objectify these characteristic clinical phenotypes by measuring skin fold and circumferences in upper and lower body areas. With that, he composed his division of "upper-body-obesity" and "lower-body-obesity." Ashwell *et al.*[12] utilized circumferential measurements of the waist and hips, once it became obvious that it was not the degree of obesity, but the distribution of fat in the abdominal area that seemed clinically significant. The index, waist-to-hip ratio (WHR), is a very practical, safe, and inexpensive measurement. Even today, it remains the most commonly utilized parameter for the classification of obesity for clinical and epidemiological evaluations.

A variety of terms are utilized today to describe adipose distribution, but in concept they are all the same: "android obesity or gynoid obesity," "central obesity or peripheral obesity," "upper-body obesity or lower-body obesity"; their different clinical forms are also compared as "apples" and "pears."

The WHR as a measure of intraabdominal fat is not precise enough for many investigations, as the measurement of the circumference does not take into consideration the thickness of subcutaneous fat, nor that of the pelvis and the musculature of the thigh. The size of these parameters can be highly variable in relation to the amount of visceral adipose. An exact determination of intraabdominal fat in relation to the total body mass is only possible with technically difficult and expensive procedures with inherent health hazards. Available today are: CT, MRI, dual photo absorptiometry, or dual energy X-ray absorptiometry.[13] For many investigations, an indirect method of calculating the visceral portion has been by determining the sagittal diameter (D) at a specified height. On the basis of numerous CT examinations, this value was substituted by Sjöström who determined the visceral adipose tissue (VAT) in liters:

$$\text{VAT (L)} = 0.731 \times D - 11.5 \text{ (males)},$$
$$\text{VAT} = 0.37 \times D - 4.85 \text{ (females)}.$$

The aeromedical examiner (AME) can recognize android obesity with relative accuracy without the use of expensive examination instruments. According to J. Vague, a French diabetologist who in 1956 described this risk constellation in detail, android obesity can be recognized by a simple "clinical glance." An objective measure can be accomplished with a tape measure. A waist measurement of less than 94 cm in men and 80 cm in women to a large extent rules out android obesity.

These figures were defined in 2005 by the consensus group of IDF (International Diabetes Federation) for Europids, indicating that in future epidemiological studies of populations of Europid origin, precedence should be given to using both European and North American cut-off points to allow better comparison. For other ethnic groups (not country of residence), other figures are valid, e.g., 90 cm for men and 80 cm for women of South Asian, Chinese and Japanese ethnicity.

Hormonal and Exogenous Factors that Control Visceral Adipose Acquisition

The prerequisite for the development of android obesity is a net energy gain, for which a heightened energy intake is responsible in the first place. The distribution of adipose tissue underlies genetic and neurohormonal control mechanisms. Sex hormones and androgynous steroids play an important role. This is why women have less visceral fat than men. This difference disappears after menopause due to the increased secretion of androgynous steroids. With particularly exaggerated shifts in the spectrum of android and gynoid active hormones toward the android side, the clinical picture of "virili aspectu" (Morgagni) is easily recognizable. Android obesity is not a particular disease, but an expression of the normal aging process, occurring mostly in highly developed countries due to prevailing lifestyles. The formation of android obesity appears to be accentuated by hypogonadism with reduced testosterone secretion in men, and in women by an android hormone constellation. Seidella and others reported in 1990[14] a negative correlation between visceral adipose and testosterone levels in men; Marin and others[15] later (1992) showed that therapeutic testosterone can positively influence visceral adiposity. These earlier observations are gaining renewed interest as prospective longitudinal studies in Finland[16] of 702 men over a period of 11 years showed that the majority of men with initially low levels of testosterone and SHBG (sex hormone-binding globulin) developed metabolic syndrome and Type 2 diabetes mellitus. These observations indicate that hypogonadism may be significant for visceral fat growth, and that hormonal therapy might be indicated in the treatment of metabolic syndrome. However, corresponding prospective studies that would explain such a process have not been carried out yet. Considering the rapid increase in this metabolic disorder, further research into this problem is desirable.

The endpoint of the scale of the hormonal adjustment in the female is embodied in the syndrome of polycystic ovary degeneration. There are no known significant clinical markers of reduced testosterone secretion in the male.

Conspicuous are the results of epidemiological studies, which not only statistically connect WHR, hypertension, stroke, hyperlipidemia, and diabetes mellitus, but also BMI, smoking, and alcohol use.[17–19] From this follows that a reduction of abdominal adipose along with control of exogenous factors such as smoking and alcohol use, can have a positive influence. Corresponding examination results in a large collective of factory workers by Kornhuber *et al.* support these assumptions.[20] The authors reported a significant correlation between gamma-GT, BMI, hypertension, hyperinsulinemia, and glucose intolerance, whereby it was suggested that the variability of gamma-GT within the defined normal range of 6–28 U/L was caused by what is considered in today's terms a "normal" amount of daily alcohol ingestion (< 60 g ~ five units). In the Bavarian idiom, a large stomach is a *Bierbauch*. In France, in prior days, the term *en bon point* was used about the visible sign of prosperity, a nicely rounded abdomen achieved by daily access to a cultivated cuisine complemented with good wine.

Lipolysis in Visceral Adipose Tissue as the Etiology of Associated Diseases

Android obesity is not an illness *per se*, but it leads to illnesses which have been termed "the metabolic syndrome." Pathophysiologically, the enhanced lipolysis of visceral fat with direct drainage into the liver is of central importance. This process leads to hyperlipidemia, which can be verified peripherally.[21] In the case of balanced carbohydrate metabolism with normal glycogen stores in the muscles and liver, a high supply of free fatty acids (FFA) leads to a reduction in glucose utilization with a rise in glucose blood levels and a resultant rise in insulin secretion with concomitant hyperinsulinemia. The experimental proof of this corresponding reduction in insulin sensitivity has been documented in many occupational groups.[22] This insulin resistance is not at the beginning of the chain of events, but rather the consequence of hyperlipacidemia resulting from fat deposition in the portal region. This metabolic situation of elevated fatty acids in the blood in the presence of normal glycogen stores, particularly in an equalized carbohydrate balance, is unique and only appears in android obesity.

Hyperlipacidemia not only increases the oxidation of fatty acids but also the synthesis of triglycerides in the liver and therefore the formation and secretion of VLDL. The consequence is an elevation of triglyceride levels in the blood. The elevated VLDL concentration and its lengthened half-life in the blood disrupt the metabolism of chylomicrons, thereby additionally challenging the exchange process of cholesterol and triglycerides with HDL and VLDL. A decline in HDL-cholesterol and a shift in the spectrum of HDL to triglyceride-rich particles therefore results. A similar shift in the spectrum of LDL-lipoproteins to small particles is likewise related to these processes. The synthesis of apoprotein-B is increased, and the concentration and thereby the amount of LDL particles in the blood is raised.[23] A greater influx of FFA in the liver has further consequences for total metabolism. The clearance of insulin decreases, so that hyperinsulinemia is amplified. Even gluconeogenesis is heightened, which favors a rise in blood sugar following fatty acid dependent reduction in glucose utilization. This hormonal constellation favors the changed metabolic equilibrium always found in visceral obesity. Diseases, such as diabetes mellitus, appear many years later when the participating systems decompensate and the elevated insulin secretion cannot be upheld any longer. Cardiovascular diseases become manifest when the atherosclerotic processes in the arteries have reached a certain degree.

All other associated diseases of the metabolic syndrome can be understood as decompensations of metabolic cycles. The severity of clinical signs and the appearance of obesity manifestations vary significantly and are dependent, not only on the degree of obesity and the length of time it has been present, but also probably on individual different genetic markers. For example, in one case, hypertension might be the primary feature, while in others, it may be diabetic glucose intolerance, hyperlipoproteinemia, or hyperuricemia. In some individuals, the existence of these diseases is only evident after several years of obesity, in others much sooner while some never experience them. A completely healthy obese person is certainly extremely rare. Centenarians are never overweight.

The definition of the diseases mentioned above depends on the proof of specific parameters, which exceed statistically defined normal ranges; however, each abnormal parameter (blood pressure, blood glucose, serum lipid, insulin, uric acid, and others) can exist in healthy persons as well. There are no coexisting subjective complaints or reduction in performance levels associated with them. These parameters are only evident when the consequences of the metabolic syndrome have reached a stage where the accelerated atherosclerosis process interferes with organ perfusion. They then determine the course and clinical markers of the disease, and the fate of the stricken individual.

With the increasing prevalence of obesity, the AME is also more frequently confronted with the problems caused by the metabolic syndrome. With increasing frequency, blood pressures are registered that exceed statistical norms, resulting in a diagnosis of hypertension. Additionally, diabetes mellitus, hyperlipoproteinemia or hyperuricemia are more commonly diagnosed by laboratory testing, although those conditions do not cause any symptoms or reduction in fitness. These findings must not necessarily give rise to the disqualification of a pilot. The AME should take this into consideration and intensively search for signs of atherosclerosis as well as counsel the patient regarding individual risk factors and possible intervention. Obesity and metabolic syndrome are not inescapable fates; they are eminently treatable with the appropriate dietary and physical measures as are their accompanying risk factors. Many captains have been diagnosed with diabetes mellitus on the basis of pathological glucose tolerance tests. The threat of loss of the medical certificate can often be averted with a weight loss of as little as 5 kg. The reduction in body weight leads to a normalized glucose tolerance, the diabetes mellitus is cured and the pilot can keep his medical certificate.

Even younger obese persons, (still) without definitive proof of a metabolic deviation from normal, should have the necessity of weight loss explained to them, especially if the family history gives clues to pertinent diseases. The AME's duty is not limited to provide expert opinion about diseases of regulatory importance; the examination situation should always be used to also give individualized preventative medical advice.

PROBLEMS OF OBESITY THERAPY

Indications

Indication for obesity therapy is not only determined by the degree of obesity, but more often by the associated manifestations of, or anticipation of, metabolic disorders. Whether or not any of these disorders (as understood under the concept of metabolic syndrome — *vide supra*) are to be expected, may be determined with a great degree of certainty from the family history and the type of obesity. The android form of obesity is much more predictive than the gynoid form. Despite a negative family history and regardless of type of obesity, morbid obesity is an indication for therapy due to mechanical overload of the joints, reduction in physical capacity, disturbances of ventilation and/or the Pickwickian syndrome. These patients are rarely approachable.

When indication for treatment is determined to be primarily for the prevention and treatment of a metabolic disturbance and the obesity is mild, all that is needed is diet and exercise, not medications. In rare cases, a reduction in weight may be indicated for someone with a normal body mass.

Influence of Diet on Body Composition

Energy is required by the body primarily for sustaining the basal metabolic rate, thermogenesis, and physical activity. This is provided by direct oxidation of substrates, which are taken up primarily from fat stores. An increase in food intake beyond what is required will lead to an enlargement of fat stores, while a decrease below the required amount will lead to a reduction. A large daily increase in food intake is followed by a rapid raise in body weight, while a small constant increase will result in a slow weight gain. The same dynamics apply when the reduction in food intake falls below requirements; a rapid weight loss can be achieved alone through a severe restriction of energy intake.

The increase in body weight from a positive energy balance consists of 75% fat and 25% fat-free body mass, primarily water. A negative energy balance, however, does not lead to a qualitatively similar loss. Weight loss is qualitatively very variable; it depends on the composition of the body and of the restricted diet.

The principle of dietary therapy can only consist of a reduction of daily energy intake below that which is required. This requirement can vary greatly among individuals, not only through individually variable physical activity, but also by way of metabolic processes, thermogensis, and basal metabolic rate.[24] When energy intake falls below minimum requirements, the organism is forced to digest its fat stores. Together with fat, carbohydrates and proteins are also enlisted for energy acquisition. The stores of carbohydrates, in the form of glycogen and glucose, are relatively small, corresponding to 1000 to 2000 kcal. Protein in the form of muscle mass and other cellular structures are available in much larger amounts. Amino acids can be restructured to glucose via gluconeogenesis, and in this manner oxidative intermediaries can be utilized for energy extraction.

It is difficult, if not impossible, to increase carbohydrate and protein stores by ingesting the corresponding nutrients. When the weight and energy balance is constant, the energy content of a meal, primarily of carbohydrates and proteins, is oxidized and any surplus transformed into fat. The enrichment of a meal with fat, therefore, does not lead to reduced oxidation of carbohydrates and decreased metabolism of protein, because the entire amount of ingested fat will be stored in the fat depots.[25] This process of fat storage costs only about 3% of the calories thus stored. Ingestion of carbohydrates and protein above the immediate requirements will increase the synthesis of triglycerides which will be deposited as fat. However, about

23% of the calories will be transformed to heat.[26] Due to this alimentally induced thermogenesis, energy consumption after a meal rich in carbohydrates and protein is significantly greater than after a fatty meal. This metabolic process is very important for long term dietary therapy.

Requirements for Weight Loss Diets

The composition of weight loss diets has been contemplated by many for a long time and countless diet plans have been pulished during the last 100 years or more. The total cessation of food intake, which has been researched in detail and was recommended by Benedict in 1915, is certainly the fastest, but not the best method.[27,28]

75% of a weight gain consists of fat, while a weight loss through fasting consists primarily of protein while only a small amount of fat is additionally lost. After an initial phase of nutritional deprivation, lasting only a few days and characterized by a rapid decline in protein metabolism,[29,30] a second phase of protein degradation occurs, at a daily rate of about 100 kcal, or 3–5% of the total energy requirement. These two phases of reduced protein metabolism is not only proven to occur in humans, but also in other animals, such as geese,[31] emperor penguins,[32] seals,[33] and rats.[34] The only known exception to this rule is the hibernating bear.[35] A protein loss of 30–50% is life-threatening, and since fasting diets often reach this level prior to the achievement of the desired fat loss, modified diets as alternatives to total fasting have been suggested. All advocate a small amount of protein to counteract protein catabolism occurring from a negative energy balance. Ingestion of protein during a period of negative energy balance does not lead to an increase in the energy budget from increased protein catabolism, but through enhancement of the protein balance by way of anabolic metabolism. After total fasting for several weeks the infusion of a mixture of L-amino acids of high biological grade will only minimally increase the excretion of nitrogen, and with an influx of 30–35 g, a balanced equilibration can be achieved. Orally ingested amino acids or protein have the same effect. With a small amount of biologically high-grade protein, an optimal weight loss diet can be composed, thus preventing protein loss. The protein balance, with respect to high-grade protein, can furthermore be significantly improved by the addition of carbohydrates. Our own studies of protein balance, using egg white protein, has shown that a loss of 1145 g protein, due to total fasting for four weeks, can be entirely compensated by a daily ingestion of 50 g protein together with 25 g carbohydrates. The component of fat in the combined weight loss thereby rises from 43% to 79%, while the loss of protein decreases to 3% (Wechsler *et al.*[26]). A daily ingestion of 50 g protein and 25 g carbohydrates constitutes a maximal value, which will ensure the protein balance even for therapeutic periods of six months and longer. This concept has been confirmed by treatment of hundreds of patients, both ambulatory and hospitalized, and in one extreme case, over a period of 13 months. In most cases *Modifast — Ulmer Trunk7* (three bottles per day) or a conventionally constituted diet restricted to 450 kcal was utilized.

The highest biological grade of water-soluble protein is whey protein[36] which has long been recommended as beneficial during fasting. Already in the *Promptuarium medicinae* (1483), such treatments were recommended, which later developed into the "Schweizereien" in many spa resorts, such as Bad Boll in Württemberg. These modified fasting therapies, with calorie restrictions below 500 calories, offer a further advantage in that after about three days, feelings of hunger disappear whereby compliance is improved.

Daily weight loss is individually variable. While thermogenesis rises during an increase in food ingestion, energy consumption declines when food intake is restricted. This teleological, ingenious and healthy regulatory mechanism is individually variable but is more pronounced in obese than in thin people.[37] Correspondingly, the amount of attainable weight loss differs greatly among individuals. It lies between 200 and 400 g body weight per day. Among those with android obesity, the resulting weight loss occurs more rapidly.

Success from weight loss diets is dependent on many factors. In addition to a diet of protein and carbohydrates, it is important to pay attention to vitamins, minerals, and trace elements when dealing with long term treatment. Vitamin requirements are related to the amount of calories ingested and are of great concern to health-conscious individuals. This also applies to trace elements and minerals, but it should be kept in mind that elimination of these is restricted with decreased food intake, and *vice versa*. Recommendations that have been articulated by a variety of institutions, among others the German Society for Nutrition, should be taken into consideration.

The numerous globally advertised "wonder diets" should be required to prove whether they contain the required amount of proteins, vitamins, minerals, and trace elements. The diet that guarantees this while delivering the minimum amount of calories will result in the fastest weight loss. These treatment modalities, which have been described in the literature as modified fasts, require medical oversight. Additionally, they should document achievement and prevent relapses by incorporating intensive education of the patient about the health hazards of obesity, health improvement through weight loss, nutritional value and energy content of foods, practical instruction regarding food preparation, and the energy budget of the human organism.

Of greater importance than the adjustment of protein balance is an adequate daily fluid intake of at least three liters. Too small a fluid intake leads to an elevated aldosterone secretion and carries a risk of hypokalemia and acidosis due to oliguria. Renal disorders may increase the danger of hyperuricemia. Reduced physical capacity, headache, malaise, and hypotension are evident only when fluid intake falls below three liters and urine production falls below two liters daily.

Nutritional Requirements in Primary Prevention

Everywhere in the animal kingdom where non-natural energy sources abound, particularly fat *ad libitum*, the rate of obesity rises.[38] The same is true for humans. This teleologically healthy reaction to increased food intake was a survival mechanism for hunters and gatherers for thousands of years when access to food was scarce, but is deadly in times where food is available in overabundance. So today the questions arise: What are the dietary possibilities to restrict superfluous energy intake? How can obesity be sucessfully treated? And what recommendations can be made for general prevention of obesity?

Many epidemiological examinations verify that a high fat intake is tightly correlated to obesity. In the USA, for example, calorie expenditure has fallen by 3% over the past 70 years, while fat ingestion has increased by 31% with a corresponding increase in obesity. In the former Eastern Germany, 46% of calories come from ingestion of fat compared with 42% in the old federation. The rates of obesity between the two Germanys vary correspondingly. Experimentally, it has also been verified that over-ingestion of foods rich in fat results in a more rapid weight gain than over-ingestion of foods rich in carbohydrates.[39]

Based on experimental findings about the constancy of glycogen and protein stores, it can be calculated that a daily excess intake of only 100 kcal in the form of fat will increase a person's body weight by 9.3 kg in one year. An excess daily intake of 100 kcal in carbohydrates will also lead to weight gain, but at a slower rate. This is due to the fact that carbohydrates lose 23% and fat only 3% of their energy during the process of fat storage. This process is of great importance in understanding the effect of fat ingestion on body weight. Clinical experiments as well as clinical experience additionally demonstrate that many small meals per day are better than a few larger meals of equal energy content. When dietary fat is replaced with carbohydrates, an automatic increase in meals made from plant fibers will occur. In addition to the favorable effects of these fibers for the treatment of obesity[40] and the prevention of relapse after weight loss, the indigestible soluble fibers of oat bran and fruits with skins are also effective against metabolic disorders related to obesity.[41] They should therefore be eaten daily in the amounts of 40–50 g. For primary prevention, the following formulas are recommended:

1) Reduction of fat ingestion to 20–25% of total caloric intake
2) Distribution of food intake on at least five meals daily

3) Increase in indigestible fibers to 50 g per day, the majority of which should be insoluble
4) Reduction of the amount of animal-derived saturated fat to one third of total fat intake

NUTRITIONAL THERAPY FOR CARDIOVASCULAR DISEASES

The most common cause of death in all industrialized countries is cardiovascular diseases, claiming almost half of all fatalities. These illnesses are based on atherosclerotic changes in the arteries and manifest themselves clinically as coronary heart disease (CHD), myocardial infarction (MI), cerebrovascular accidents, and peripheral and cerebral circulatory deficiencies. The *sclerotic* alteration of the arterial wall, which produces a widening of the lumen and a reduction of elasticity, is a physiological condition of the normal aging process. It leads to a continual further reduction of the elastic function of the aorta and, according to the calculations of Bader, is compatible with a lifespan of 120 years. In contrast, *atherosclerosis* is unrelated to the physiological aging process; it is a reaction of the arterial wall to damage from a variety of stresses, usually referred to as risk factors. The risk factors determine the extent of the atherosclerotic changes and the time at which clinical manifestations appear. Morphologically, it has to do with degenerative changes that initially result in alterations of the intima. The atherosclerotic process is triggered and sustained by these risk factors. Without risk factors, there would be no atherosclerosis. Retrospectively, in terms of cardiovascular diseases, atherosclerosis does not represent an inescapable destiny. In order to successfully tackle the avalanche of cardiovascular diseases, prevention by elimination of risk factors must be pursued.

These risk factors are highly correlated to diet and lifestyle, so the choice of therapy is easy. The practical application, however, is difficult because a successful outcome requires the patient to change diet and lifestyle. This requires self-discipline; the physician can only give advice and make recommendations. No medications exist that can prevent the damage inflicted by an unhealthy diet and lifestyle; whether such medicines can be developed is very questionable.

Clinically, the most important risk factor for vascular diseases is android obesity with the associated metabolic disorders of hyperlipoproteinemia, hypertension, Type 2 diabetes mellitus, hyperinsulinemia, and hyperuricemia. Patients with this metabolic syndrome make up the largest and most important group. In daily clinical practice, we have to treat those with android obesity by eliminating the causal factors and thus prevent the process of atherosclerosis. Only in this manner can we achieve unambiguous success in the fight against cardiovascular disease. Today, we can very effectively treat the symptoms of hypertension, hyperlipidemia, and hyperglycemia with medications, but they must be administered lifelong. Even lengthy treatment does not normalize the underlying pathophysiological disorders. Therefore, for example, medical treatment of Type 2 diabetes mellitus alone will not stop the dangerous progression of atherosclerosis, and the patient's lifespan will not be improved. Likewise, lifelong treatment with anti-hypertensive or antihyperlipidemic medications will not eliminate the dreaded athero-sclerosis and the intrinsic hazards of this metabolic ailment.

The various risk factors should not be evaluated and treated as individual diseases. The diagnosis is based on the aberration of specific metabolic parameters into statistically proven pathological ranges. One should view these as a decompensation of normal metabolic regulation resulting from long-standing overload and not as an independent illness. Therapeutically, one must only eliminate the overload in order to overcome the decompensation and the metabolic derailment.

Those with risk factors related to android obesity exhibit one other anomaly that supports the concept of a generalized metabolic overload: the individual symptoms appear in various strengths, but always together. In patients with hypertension, one finds individually different expressions of hyperlipidemia, glucose intolerance with elevated insulin, fatty acid and uric acid levels. A similar constellation can be observed in patients with Type 2 diabetes mellitus or hyperlipoproteinemia.

All these symptoms can be successfully treated only by elimination of the android obesity.

Nutritional therapy in people with cardiovascular diseases is therefore, first and foremost, dietary restrictions oriented toward the elimination of android obesity (see Section 3.3).

Hyperlipoproteinemia as a risk factor

Disturbances in plasma lipid metabolism are a significant risk factor for rapid and premature development of atherosclerosis. Hyperlipoproteinemia is generally categorized into a primary form, which is genetically determined, and a secondary form, which is the result of a variety of illnesses or of certain medications. The primary form is traceable to a variety of defects that alter the structure, the function, and the concentration of apolipoproteins, as well as to the mobilization of lipid enzymes and receptors. The result is usually an increase, seldom a decrease, in individual lipid fractions. The extent of the lipoprotein increase in the blood is not exclusively genetically determined but is also strongly influenced by exogenous, especially nutritional factors. An important factor is a hypercaloric diet resulting in overweight. The amount and the composition of dietary fat is of great significance, as are dietary cholesterol, carbohydrates, and fibers.

Excess food intake leads to an increase in triglyceride synthesis in the liver and to an elevated delivery of VLDL particles into the bloodstream. When this augmented VLDL production is no longer compensated by a rise in lipolytic activity, the result is an elevated triglyceride level in the blood. Hyperlipacidemia (elevated free fatty acids in the blood), which always accompanies android obesity, is of great significance. During the course of the day, these fatty acids are resynthesized in the liver, leading to a significant rise in the total VLDL production of more than 100 g of triglycerides per day. This endogenous source of driven triglyceride synthesis often considerably exceeds the exogenous intake. The result is that the lipolytic capacity of the blood is exceeded, resulting in an elevated triglyceride level.

Following an increased production of VLDL, and thereby an increased degradation of VLDL into cholesterol-rich LDL, a rise in total cholesterol levels occurs. The less developed the LDL receptor activity, the greater this rise. The LDL receptor activity, by which the elimination of the LDL particle takes place, is inhibited by the continuously elevated supply of saturated fatty acids found in overweight individuals. Often a reduced level of HDL-cholesterol is also found in these individuals. This occurs because the exchange of cholesterol and triglycerides between HDL and VLDL is accelerated, and the larger VLDL-rich triglyceride portion consequently circulates longer in the bloodstream. A direct absorption of HDL into adipose tissue also appears to contribute.

The changes in metabolic regulation found in obese individuals therefore leads to an elevation of triglycerides and LDL-cholesterol in the bloodstream, and a decrease of HDL-cholesterol. On one hand, the extent and relative shift is dependent on the degree of obesity and the amount of ingested animal fat with a high percentage of saturated fats, and on the other hand, it is dependent on genetically determined and individually developed regulatory mechanisms of lipid metabolism.

The Significance of the Type of Dietary Fat

Both quantity and quality of dietary fat are important for the development of hyperlipoproteinemia. In Germany, which in this regard is similar to other highly developed industrial countries, dietary fat comprises 40–45% of total dietary energy ingestion. The majority is of animal origin and has a high concentration of saturated fats. Of all dietary components, these saturated fats exert the greatest effect on the pronounced rise in cholesterol. They especially elevate the LDL particles, of which 50% are composed of cholesterol. Saturated fats reduce the receptor activity of the LDL particles, thereby reducing the catabolism of LDL. Lauric acid (dodecanoic acid – $C_{12}H_{24}O_2$), myristic acid (tetradecanoic acid – $C_{14}H_{28}O_2$), and palmitic acid (hexadecanoic acid – $C_{16}H_{32}O_2$) have the greatest effect. These fatty acids are generally eaten in amounts of 30–60 g daily. Stearic acid (octadecanoic acid – $C_{18}H_{36}O_2$) behaves neutrally as it quickly desaturates to oleic acid (monounsaturated T-9 fatty acid – $C_{18}H_{34}O_2$) which leads to a distinct reduction in total and LDL-cholesterol. It is assumed that oleic acid inhibits the suppression of the LDL receptor by displacing saturated fats. Even triglycerides associated with hypertriglyceridemia are reduced by oleic acid.

Polyunsaturated fats are differentiated between ω-3 and ω-6 fatty acids. The ω-6 FA (with the first double bond in the carbohydrate chain at the sixth C atom from the methylated end) are found primarily in plant oils (linolic, linolenic, and arachidonic acid). In the exchange with saturated fats, these ω-6 acids reduce both total and LDL-cholesterol levels. In addition to the passive dissolution of the receptor suppression, a direct elevation of receptor-dependent absorption of LDL-cholesterol is presumed to be the cause. At high intakes of 12–15%, even the HDL-cholesterol is reduced. This is primarily due to eicosapentaenoic acid (20:5 (n-3)) and docosahexaenic acid (DHA – 22:6(T-3)). These acids inhibit the hepatic synthesis of triglycerides, and thereby diminish VLDL-triglyceride concentration. With a daily ingestion of 1.5–3 g, the triglyceride concentration is reduced by about 25%. This amount can be reached by eating about 150 g of mackerel, herring, tuna, or salmon.

The ω-3 fatty acids are also thought to favorably influence the atherosclerotic process in the arterial wall. ∀-Linolenic acid (ALA – 18:3 (n-3)) is effective only in very large doses, which is not achieved in treatment. Eicosapentaenoic acid is effective in much lower amounts, which is attainable in a normal diet. The ω-3 fatty acids inhibit inflammatory processes and influence the blood clotting through inhibition of platelet adhesion and aggregation. This effect is based upon: 1) the transformation of linolenic acid to arachidonic acid in that the product-inhibition is decreased, and 2) that eicosapentaenoic acid competes with arachidonic acid for the synthesis of eicosanoid, which is dependent on necessary enzymes. In this manner, the formation of the strongly aggregating and vasoconstrictive thromboxane A2 (TXA2 – $C_{20}H_{32}O_5$) is restricted in favor of TXA, which has only a weak effect on aggregation and vasoconstriction. Simultaneously, more PG-I^3 is formed instead of prostacycline-I^2, both of which have anti-aggregating and vasodilating activities. The result is a reduction in the tendency toward thrombosis, an increase in bleeding time, and a fall in blood pressure. Beyond metabolism, eicosapentaenoic acid influences leukotrienes, which are important mediators of inflammation and allergic reaction. Leukotriene B4 (LTB4), which is formed from arachidonic acid, has strong chemotactic and aggregation effects. Because inflammation and thrombogenic processes have great significance in the development of atherosclerosis, it is certain that eicosapentaenoic acid also has an anti-atherogenic effect.

Dietary Cholesterol

The importance of cholesterol in our diet is a favorite topic in lay literature.

Unfortunately, the information given is usually inaccurate. In humans, dietary cholesterol has only a small effect on blood levels. An elevation of 100 mg/day in the diet will only result in an elevation of 2 mg/dL in the blood. This effect is probably caused by a reduction in the catabolism of LDL particles. There is great individual variability.

While most people react only marginally or not at all to an increase in cholesterol ingestion, in some individuals it causes a pronounced increase in the blood level. This variability is related in part to the variability in resorption, which ranges from 20 to 80%. The hypo-responder effectively restricts endogenous cholesterol synthesis during increased ingestion, while the receptor activity is largely unaffected and maintained. The hyper-responder apparently has a genetically underdeveloped regulatory mechanism, or none at all.

The Influence of Carbohydrates

Similar to cholesterol, a high intake of carbohydrates has a variable effect on blood lipids. A caloric exchange of fat for carbohydrates always leads to a rise in triglycerides. Many people have a negligible elevation, while in others, especially in those with a prior elevated triglyceride level, the rise in triglyceride blood levels after an increase in carbohydrate ingestion can be multiples of the base value. This elevation can be particularly pronounced with ingestion of a large amount of mono-and disaccharides. The effect of polysaccharides is less. A diet rich in carbohydrates can initiate a decrease in cholesterol. This effect is dependent on a simultaneous restriction in fat ingestion.

The Influence of Fibers

Fibers have a favorable effect on the serum lipids in that they reduce the level of total cholesterol and LDL. In part, this effect can be attributed to the fact that a high dietary fiber content forces a reduction in the fat and sugar content while increasing the content of starch. Moreover, soluble fibers such as guar, pectin, and the soluble fibers in oats and beans directly reduce cholesterol concentration, as they bind to bile salts and therefore are ot accessible to the enterohepatic circulation. The result is an increase in bile salts, which strengthens the metabolism of the building blocks of cholesterol and thereby reduces the cholesterol pool. In order for this effect to occur, a large amount of fibers is needed, about 120 g oat bran or 100–130 g of beans per day, which may not be a practical diet to follow.

The Significance of the Metabolic Syndrome

The relationship between obesity and the risk factors for atherosclerosis, and therefore cardiovascular disease, has been pointed out in countless publications and many clinical experimental investigations have been based on that relationship. This always involves cross-sections of groups of patients. These kinds of investigations have the disadvantage that groups of patients with a variety of disease processes are summarized, and therefore the progression of metabolic disturbances is not completely discernable. The first results from longitudinal studies in monkeys verified the results from cross-sectional investigations in humans.

Monkeys that had received a diet based on their actual requirements and therefore remained thin, demonstrated a minor rise in blood sugar, a slight decrease in glucose tolerance, and a minor increase in insulin levels with aging. A group of monkeys that received unlimited food during the same study period became obese and developed continuous hyperinsulinemia with a corresponding decrease in glucose tolerance. They eventually developed diabetes mellitus, as the elevated insulin levels could no longer be sustained. The insulin sensitivity continually declined in the setting of augmented food intake, while the condition of obesity continued. The increased insulin production could only be continued for a limited period of time, individually variable. Eventually the production became insufficient, which resulted in manifest diabetes mellitus. Disorders in lipid metabolism developed correspondingly.

The results of the longitudinal animal studies strongly support the general clinical experiences of the last five decades, that cardiovascular disease is caused by excessive fat ingestion. Our endeavors must therefore focus on adjustment of diet and regulation of body weight and not on pharmaceutical regulation of blood sugar, cholesterol, triglycerides, uremic acid, insulin, blood pressure, etc. Body weight is the deciding factor for long term success. Prescribing medications without regard to dietary obesity and the metabolic syndrome is akin to malpractice.

The Principles of Nutritional Therapy of Cardiovascular Diseases

1) The ingestion of energy must be decreased in order to reduce body weight. The ratio of waist-to-hip circumference must be reduced below 1.0 for men and 0.8 for women. In order to achieve this goal within a reasonable period of time, nutrition must be significantly restricted over a period of several weeks or months. The fewer calories ingested, the faster the weight reduction and the sooner the goal will be reached. In order to lose 1 kg fat, about 7500 calories must be eliminated from the diet.

2) The content of fat, especially animal fat, must be reduced to less than 30% of the total intake of calories. Primarily, plant fats and oils should be utilized. Fish with a high content of ω-3 fatty acids (herring, mackerel, tuna, salmon) should be incorporated frequently into the dietary plan (two to three times 100–150 g per week).
3) Nutrients with a high fiber content should be given preference. Mono- and disaccharides are to be avoided. Sweetened drinks must be replaced with water or other calorie-free drinks.
4) The lifestyle should be oriented toward adequate physical activity. Physical exertion should be such that the heart rate attains a rate of at least 170 minus the age (in years) at least twice daily for 10 minutes at a time.
5) As risk factor number one, smoking must be discontinued entirely.
6) The quality of treatment is determined by the resulting body weight, not by the changes in the metabolic parameters in the blood nor in the type and amounts of prescription medications needed.

REFERENCES

1. Faulhaber JD, Petruzzi EN, Eble H, *et al.* (1969) *In vitro* Untersuchungen über den Fettstoffwechsel isolierter menschlicher Fettzellen in Abhängigkeit von Zellgröße: Die durch Adrenalin induzierte Lipolyse. *Horm Metab Res* **1**: 80.
2. Kvist H, Chodhury B, Grangard U *et al.* (1988) Total and visceral adipose tissue volumes derived from measurements with computer tomography in adult men and women: Predictive equations. *Amm J Clin Nutr* **48**: 1351–1361.
3. Sjöström L, Larsson B, Backnan L, *et al.* (1992) Swedish obese subjects, SOS-recruitment to an intervention study and a selected description of the obese state. *Int J Obes* **16**: 465–479.
4. Marin P, Anderson B, Ottosom M *et al.* (1992) The morphology and metabolism of intra-abdominal adipose tissue in men. *Metabolism* **41**: 1242–1248.

5. Sjöström L. (1963) Impacts of body weight, body composition and adipose tissue distribution on morbidity and mortality. In: Stunkard AJ, Waaen TA (eds), *Obesity, Theory and Therapy*, pp. 13–44. Raven Press, New York.
6. Söström L. (1990) Methods for measurement of the total and visceral adipose tissue volume and relationships between visceral fat and disease in 1006 severely obese subjects. In: Oomura Y, Tarui S, Inoue S, Shimazu T (eds), *Progress in Obesity Research*, pp. 323–334. John Libby LTD, London.
7. Lew EA, Garfinkel L. (1979) Variations in mortality by weight among 750 000 men and women. *J Chron Dis* **32**: 563–576.
8. Lew EA. (1985) Mortality and weight: Insured lives and the American Cancer Society studies. *Ann Int Med* **103**: 1024–1029.
9. Van Itallie TB, Lew EA. (1993) Estimation of the effect of obesity on health and longevity. A Perspective for the physician. In: Stunkard AJ, Wadden TA (eds), *Obesity, Theory and Therapy*, pp. 219–229. Raven Press, New York.
10. Waaler HT. (1984) Height, weight and mortality: The Norwegian experience. *Acta Med Scand Suppl* **679**: 1–56.
11. Vague J. (1947): La différenciation sexuelle, facteur déterminant des formes de l'obésité. *Press Med* **55**: 339–340.
12. Ashwell M. (1985) Methodological approaches to the study of the adipose tissues: Their impact on research into the aetiology of obesity. In: Cryer A, Van RIR (eds), *New Perspectives in Adipose Tissue: Structure, Function and Development*, pp. 271–302. Butterworth, London.
13. Van der Kooy K, Seidell JC. (1993) Techniques for the measurement of visceral fat: A practical guide. *Int J Obes* **17**: 187–196.
14. Seidell J, Björntorp P, Kvist H, *et al.* (1990) Visceral fat accumulation is positively associated with insulin, glucose and C-peptide levels but negatively with testosterone levels. *Metabolism* **39**: 897–901.
15. Marin P, Holmäng S, Jönsson L, *et al.* (1992) The effects of testosterone treatment on body composition and metabolism in middle-aged obese men. *Int J Obes* **16**: 991–997.
16. Laaksonen D E, Niskanen L, Punnonen K *et al.* (2004) Testosterone and sex hormone-binding globulin predict the metabolic syndrome and diabetes in middle-aged men. *Diabetes Care* **27**: 1036–1041.

17. Den Tonkelaar J, Seidell JC, van Noord PAH, *et al.* (1990) Fat distribution in relation to age, degree of obesity, smoking habits, parity and oestrogen use — a cross sectional study in 11 853 Dutch women. *Int J Obes* **14**: 753–761.
18. Seidell JC, Cigolini CM, Deslypere J-P, *et al.* (1991) Body fat distribution in relation to physical activity and smoking habits of 38-year-old European men — the European Fat Distribution Study. *Am J Epidemiol* **133**: 257–265.
19. Barneveld T, Seidell JC, Traag N, *et al.* (1989) Fat distribution and gamma glutamyl transferase in relation to serum lipids and blood pressure in 38-year-old Dutch males. *Eur J Clin Nutr* **43**: 809–818.
20. Kornhuber HH, Backhaus B, Kornhuber AW, *et al.* (1989) Risk factors and the prevention of stroke. In: Amery W, Bousser MG, Rose FC (eds), *Clinical Trial Methodology in Stroke*, pp. 191–212. Bailière Trudall, London.
21. Arner P. (1995) Differences in lipolysis between human subcutaneous and omental adipose tissue. *Ann Med* **27**: 335–338.
22. Cary DJ, Jenkins AB, Canpbell LV, *et al.* (1996) Abdominal fat and insulin resistance in normal and overweight women. *Diabetes* **45**: 633–638.
23. Ditschuneit H. (1991) Obesity and related disorders. In: Ailhaud *et al. Obesity in Europe*, pp. 191–2001. John Libbey LTD, London.
24. Danforth E Jr. (1992) Regulation of energy expenditure. In: Belfiore F, Jeanrenaud B, Papalia D (eds), *Obesity: Basic Concepts and Clinical Aspects*, pp. 61–77. Front Diabetes, Karger 11.
25. Flatt JP, Ravussin E, Kevin J, Jequier E. (1985) Effects of dietary fat on postprandial substrate oxidation and on carbohydrate and fat balances. *J Clin Invest* **76**: 1019–1024.
26. Flatt JP. (1988) Energetics of intermediary metabolism. In: Garrow JS, Halliday D (eds), *Substrate and Energy Metabolism in Man*, pp. 8–69. John Libbey & Co Ltd London.
27. Ditschuneit H, Ditschuneit HH, Wechsler JG. (1979) Adipositasbehandlung — Nulldiät oder kalorienreduzierte Diät? *Internist* **20**: 151–153.
28. Ditschuneit H. (1976) Was ist gesichert in der Therapie der Fettsucht? *Internist* **17**: 622.

29. Wechsler JG, Wenzel H, Swobodnik W, Ditschuneit H. (1984) Proteinverlust bei Adipositas während Gewichtsreduktion. In: Ditschuneit H, Wechsler JG (eds), *Ergebnisse der Adipositasforschung.* Perimed Verlagsges Erlangen.
30. Wechsler JG, Ditschuneit HH, Malfertheiner P, Ditschuneit H. (1980) Stickstoffbilanzen während modifiziertem Fasten. *Dtsch med Wochenschr* **105**: 58–60.
31. Le Maho Y, Van Kha HV, Koubi H, Dewasmes G, Girard J, Perre P, Cagnard M. (1981) Body composition, energy expenditure, and plasma metabolites in long term fasting geese. *Am J Physiol* **241**: 342–354.
32. Le Maho, Y, Delclitte P, Chatonett J. (1976) Thermoregulation in fasting emperor pinguins under natural conditions. *Am J Physiol* **231**: 913–922.
33. Nordey ES, Blix AS. (1985) Energy sources in fasting grey seal pups evaluated with computed tomography. *Am J Physiol* **249**: R471–R476.
34. Cherel Y, Bumol AF, Leturque A, Le Maho Y. (1988) *In vivo* glucose utilization in rat tissue during the three phases of starvation. *Metabolism* **37**: 1033–1039.
35. Nelson RA. (1980) Protein and fat metabolism in hibernating bears. *Federatio Proc* **39**: 395–2958.
36. Kofranyi E, Jekat F. (1973) Die Wertigkeit gemischter Proteine. *Hoppe-Seyler's Z Physiol Chem* **354**: 527.
37. Ravassin E, Bumand B, Schutz Y, Jequier E. (1982) 24-hour energy expenditure and resting metabolic rate in obese, moderately obese, and control subjects. *Am J Clin Nutr* **35**: 566–573.
38. Rothwell NJ, Stock MJ. (1981) Regulation of energy balance. *Ann Rev Nutr* **I**: 235–256.
39. Sims EAH, Danforth E. (1987) Expenditure and storage of energy in man. *J Clin Invest* **79**: 1019–1025.
40. Van Itallie TB. (1978) Dietary fiber and obesity. *Am J Clin* Nutr **31**: 543–552.
41. Davidson MH, Dugan LD, Bums HJ, Bova J, Story K, Drennan KB. (1991) The hypocholesterolemic effects of beta-glucan in oat-meal and oat-bran. *JAMA* **265**: 833–839.

Part 5

CLINICAL AVIATION MEDICINE

Chapter 8

Introduction: The Role of Medical Factors in Accident Investigation

Ilse Janicke, Norbert Schauer, Marcus Wieczorek and Reinhard Höltgen*,†

In general aviation, acute illness leading to sudden incapacitation and thereby to fatal accidents is estimated to cause 1.5% of fatal accidents.[1] On the basis of autopsy results from 1000 consecutive fatal accidents in the UK between 1956 and 1995, medical and toxicological factors were found to be causative or contributory in 4.7% of fatal cases, most often in the categories of glider flying and private aviation.[2] From an operational point of view, this is not surprising, as approximately 90% of all pilots engaged in single crew operations belong to these two groups.

The most common medical factor is cardiovascular diseases, causing almost half of all sudden incapacitation accidents. Consequently, the prevention of sudden cardiac events in pilots and the correct risk assessment in those with cardiac conditions are important tasks for the aeromedical consultant. In commercial pilots, cardiovascular events occur less commonly than in the general population, due to stringent selection criteria and regular medical screening of pilots. Fatal accidents with a medical cause rarely occur

* Corresponding author.
† Herzzentrum, Kaiser-Wilhelm-Krankenhaus, Gerrickstraße 21, D-47137 Duisburg, Germany.

Table 1. Medical Factors as Cause of Fatal Aviation Accidents

Category Accidents	Total Number of Causes	Cardiovascular Causes	Other Medical Causes	Total Medical Causes (%)
Glider	67	6	2	8(12)
Private	375	9	17	26(7)
Commercial	114	4	1	5(4)
Military	407	3	5	8(2)
Paraglider/ Hang glider	37	0	0	0
Total	1000	22	25	47(4.7)

in multi-crew operations. The situation is entirely different in general aviation where the pilot pool is very heterogeneous and includes pilots of all ages and socio-economic backgrounds, and where cardiovascular diseases are as common as in the general population.

The current medical requirements (the International Standards and Recommended Practices of ICAO and, in Europe, JAR Class I and II) are based on the so-called 1% rule. After multiple attempts at risk quantification by various aeromedical authorities, this rule became generally accepted in 1984 following the first UK CAA Conference on Cardiovascular Risk and Flying. The rule stipulates that, for Class I certification, the risk of an incapacitating medical event in a pilot engaged in multi-crew operations should not exceed 1% per year (i.e., one event in about 10^6 hours or 100 years). This corresponds to the cardiovascular mortality rate of a 60–65 year old man in northern Europe. The rule is based on the assumption that only one tenth of the flying time (departure, climb, descent and landing) is critical and that the other pilot will be able to sucessfully take over the control of the aircraft in at least 99 of 100 cases. This means that the risk of a medically caused accident in a multi-crew operation is in the order of $1{:}10^9$ flight hours, a very remote risk indeed. This is the justification for the limitation of "valid only as or with qualified co-pilot," used in many countries.

For commercial flights with a single pilot, the 1% rule is not applicable.

In general aviation, the fatal accident rate is in the order of 1:40 000 flight hours,[3] mostly due to human error, a rate that is 20–25 times higher than that of commercial aviation. If one assumes that not more than 1:25–50 of the fatal cases are caused by medical events (for Class I 1:100), then the limits for Class II can also be determined, so that the acceptable event rate of 1% per year or $1:10^6$ flight hours (1 to $25 \times 4 \times 10\,000$) is not exceeded. Unlimited Class II requirements are therefore more or less identical with the requirements for limited Class I medical certification "valid only as or with qualified co-pilot = OML (Operational Multi-crew Limitation)."

In selected cases, medical certification of pilots with a greater than 1% risk may be possible for Class II with limitations, such as "valid only with safety pilot = OSL (Operational Safety Pilot Limitation)" or "valid only without passengers." Certification is individually assessed in such cases.

Since 1976, the number of aeromedical review cases has risen sharply in Germany, reaching an average of 150/year (range: 130–250/year) between 1991 and 2000. Eye diseases and cardiovascular conditions (ischemic heart disease, approximately 40%; arrhythmia and conduction defects, about 30%) are the foremost causes. Cases involving CPL and PPL applicants are about 45% each, and those involving glider pilots are about 10%. In the last 20 years, the upper age of pilots who have applied for special consideration because of cardiovascular diseases has been between 50 and 70 years. Approximately 60% of these applicants have been successful in obtaining a special issuance through the review process. Of these, approximately one third are allowed to fly only with OML/OSL limitations.

Age is the greatest risk factor for cardiovascular diseases.[4] On the basis of autopsy results, 18% of the age group between 30 and 50, and 43% of those over 50 years of age have aeromedically relevant coronary artery disease. For this reason, pilots over the age of 60 are not allowed to fly as pilot-in-command of aircraft engaged in international air transport operations with the exception of multi-crew operations where the other pilot is younger than 60. Although this is an international rule, its application differs somewhat from one country to another.

After the age of 65, pilots may no longer fly as ATP. The older the pilot, the more frequent and extensive the cardiovascular evaluation should be, especially if other risk factors are present.

The aeromedical examiner's principal responsibility is to perform the required examinations and evaluations to the best of his ability, but not so far as to go beyond the 1% marker, thereby subjecting the pilot to overly rigorous diagnostic screening. The second most important duty of all aviation medicine practitioners is prevention. Additionally, the medical examiner should be in a position to advise a pilot with a disqualifying medical condition, especially with regard to the circumstances under which a special issuance can be obtained. This handbook describes all the aeromedically relevant cardiovascular diseases and outlines situations where medical certification is possible despite disqualifying conditions or disorders. In this respect, the medical examiner is in partnership with the pilot.

REFERENCES

1. Booze CF. (1989) Sudden in-flight incapacitation in general aviation. *Aviat Space Env Med* **60**: 332–335.
2. Cullen SA, *et al.* (1997) Role of medical factors in 1000 fatal aviation accidents: Case note study. *Br Med J* **314**: 592.
3. General aviation accident review. (1987) CAP542. Cheltenham, Civil Aviation Authority.
4. Cooke JNC. (1999) The ageing pilot: Is increased scrutiny justified? *Eur Heart J* **1**(Suppl. D): D48–D52.

Chapter 9

Cardiovascular Risk Factors

Norbert Schauer*

HYPERLIPIDEMIA

With the pharmaceutical intervention in lipid metabolism possible today, hyperlipidemia is presumably the most controllable risk factor after smoking. The prevalence of hyperlipidemia in the United States and Europe is an important risk factor for the development of atherosclerotic vascular disease, whether in the heart, the brain, or in the peripheral vasculature of the human body.

It is important to understand that not only is cholesterol brought into the body through diet, but that all body cells can synthesize it. High density lipoprotein (HDL) carries cholesterol to the liver, where it is metabolized into bile salts.

Hyperlipidemia is defined as

Total cholesterol over 200 mg/dL.

Hypertriglyceridemia is defined as

Triglyceride over 200 mg/dL.

Although not all processes of lipid metabolism are fully understood, it is known that low density lipoprotein (LDL) cholesterol is responsible for the development and progression of atherosclerotic vascular disease. HDL cholesterol (otherwise known as "good

* Maria Theresiastraße 22/1, A-6020 Innsbruck, Austria.

cholesterol") is a protective element of cholesterol, and as an antagonist of LDL, it reduces the risk of development of CAD.

It is noteworthy that an exaggerated response of the angiotensin II-ATI receptors occurs under the effects of hypercholesterolemia. This leads to a further increase in vasoconstriction, renewed cellular growth, and the release of free radicals.[1]

HYPERTRIGLYCERIDEMIA

The predictive value of hypertriglyceridemia is not as clear as that of hypercholesterolemia. The literature is full of controversial viewpoints regarding possible cellular damage caused by triglycerides. Fortunately, measures to lower hypercholesterolemia, such as nutritional adjustments, increased physical activity, and cholesterol-lowering agents, also improve triglyceride levels, presumably further reducing the risk.[2,3]

From a preventative perspective, it is very important that every applicant for pilot certification has his or her total cholesterol, HDL cholesterol, and triglycerides measured. These tests are inexpensive and require minimal effort. Elevated cholesterol is not a disqualifying feature *per se*, but it does require attention because of its significant therapeutic and prognostic implications.

Therapy

There are two important treatment options available. First and most importantly lifestyle modification, and secondly medical therapeutics.

Lifestyle modification includes weight loss, increased physical activity, a low fat diet, and adequate control of other cardiovascular risk factors (see below).

Weight loss

Overweight is defined as weighing more than the so-called normal weight or being over the normal body mass index. The reference is: normal weight in kg (according to Broca): body height in cm minus 100; or the Body Mass Index (BMI) or Quetelet index: body weight (kg) divided by height in m^2.

A woman of normal weight will have a BMI of 23, a man 24. A BMI of 27.3 and 27.8 respectively, should be categorized as serious. Weight loss will reduce the cholesterol level and blood pressure, and will reduce the risk of coronary artery disease.

Physical activity

The AHA (American Heart Association) recommends three to four exercise periods per week, at a minimum of 30 minutes of intensive activities such as cycling, running, or cross country skiing.

Morris *et al.* reported in the 1950's that coronary artery disease is less common among conductors and mail carriers than in inactive bus drivers[4] (so flight attendants should have less heart disease than pilots). Many studies have supported these findings. In a meta-analysis of 27 observational studies, it was shown that physical inactivity doubled the risk of heart attack.[5] Prospective long duration studies have also unequivocally shown that women as much as men can protect themselves from the risk of coronary artery disease by increasing their physical activity.[6–8] Additionally, physical activity is linked to a reduction in the risk of stroke, naturally derived from the positive effects from weight loss, reduced blood pressure, lowered cholesterol, and improvements in glucose tolerance.[9,10]

Diet

Dietary measures encompass a reduction in the total number of calories ingested in order to attain normal weight. Additionally, the percentage of fat should not exceed 30% of the total caloric intake, and primarily polyunsaturated fatty acids should be used. Daily ingestion of cholesterol must remain below 300 mg (for comparison, an egg contains 280 mg). 60% of calories should come from complex carbohydrates. A moderate amount of alcohol is beneficial.

Practically speaking, this means that protein in the form of ocean fish is desirable over meat. Animal fat, especially butter, should be replaced by alternative plant oils, especially olive oil. Fruit, salads, vegetables, and whole wheat products should be the basis of a healthy diet. Noteworthy are the so-called "new age" foods with phytosterine additives. Phytosterines are similar to cholesterol, are in an esterified form, and inhibit cholesterol absorption in the gut by a competitive mechanism. Indeed it was possible to demonstrate that phytosterine additives led to a 10% reduction of LDL cholesterol. This is an effective non-pharmaceutical and inexpensive tool, although there are no data demonstrating long-term benefits based on hard data points.[11]

Medical therapeutics

The greatest therapeutic breakthrough in cardiology in the last 15 years has been the introduction of statins.

The effectiveness of statins was demonstrated in large randomized studies, finished in 1998. In the 4S Study (Scandinavian Simvastatin Survival Study), it was shown that a 34% reduction of risk in coronary artery patients could be achieved by reducing total cholesterol from 188 to 121 mg/dL.

The West of Scotland Coronary Prevention Study (WOSCOPS) demonstrated similar results with regard to primary prevention. Pravastatin was shown to reduce average LDL cholesterol levels from 197 mg/dL to 142 mg/dL, which reduced serious coronary artery events by 31%.

With this in mind, the classic lipid-lowering agents such as colestyramine, niacin, and probucol as well as bezafibrate and beta-sitosterol have lost dominance in clinical practice.

What lipid values should be targeted?

We recommend that high-risk patients requiring primary prophylaxis maintain their LDL below 130 mg/dL, and for secondary prophylaxis, a level below 70 mg/dL is preferred. The literature provides enough examples to show that the benefit of lowering cholesterol is not a linear effect. In WOSCOPS, a reduction in LDL of 24% was optimal, i.e., maximum effect with minimum side effects, so "the lower the better" is not always true.

SMOKING

Smoking is the only absolutely modifiable risk factor for coronary artery disease. In the United States smoking is the primary cause of over 400 000 preventable deaths each year. It is unfortunate that even non-smokers who inhale smoke produced by others (passive smoking) similarly carry an elevated coronary risk. Long-term studies since 1950 have shown that smoking 20 cigarettes per day increases the risk of coronary artery disease two to three times.

The thrombotic potential of oral contraceptives is synergistic with smoking. Additionally, this does not only increase the risk of myocardial infarction but also the rate of sudden cardiac death, the development of aortic aneurysms and peripheral vascular disease, as well as the risk of cerebral vascular events. Etiologic causes include an increased oxidation of LDL-cholesterol and a decline in HDL-cholesterol. Smoking also suppresses endothelial vasodilatation, enhances detrimental hemostatic effects, raises CRP and fibrinogen, and induces spontaneous platelet aggregation along with adhesion of monocytes to endothelial cells.

Chronically, but also acutely, smoking facilitates coronary vasospasm as well as reduces the threshold for ventricular arrhythmias.

Smoking cessation reduces the risk of the first heart attack by nearly 65%.[66]

While it is important to note that the cardiovascular risk declines distinctly after smoking cessation, the risk of lung, pancreas and stomach cancer continues for another 10 years; so does the risk of developing chronic obstructive pulmonary disease. The use of nicotine patches or gum may facilitate abstinence.

HYPERTENSION (SEE ALSO SECTION 3)

In contrast to smoking, hypertension is not a visible risk factor, and it is often not recognized and therefore not treated. Pilots are particularly reticent to accept blood pressure medications, as they have a general attitude against medical therapeutics (perceived as incompatible with their careers).

High blood pressure correlates strongly to an elevated risk of stroke and heart infarction. A 7 mmHg elevation in blood pressure correlates to a 27% increased risk of heart attack and a 22% increased risk of a cerebral vascular event. As stated in the section on hypertension, any reduction of hypertension has a significant risk-lowering effect on coronary events.

INSULIN RESISTANCE IN DIABETES MELLITUS

Patients with diabetes have a three-to-five-fold increased risk of future cardiovascular events, women more so than men.[12,13]

Insulin resistance alone without manifestations of diabetes is strongly associated with the development of microvasculature disease. This can occur well before diabetic manifestations appear.[14]

It is known that diabetics develop substantial changes in their endothelium and in the function of smooth muscle.[18,19] Additionally, there is an increased leukocyte response to the vascular endothelium, which has huge implications in the development of atherosclerotic vascular disease. Along these lines, diabetic nephropathy develops (microalbuminuria), which the aforementioned process facilitates, and microalbuminuria in Type II diabetes is apparently a predictor of elevated mortality caused by cardiovascular events.[20,21]

At this point in time we understand the correlations, but it is not yet known whether reducing blood glucose levels alone is adequate to reduce cardiovascular risk. Until now, most studies have demonstrated improved microvascular circulation, but there has not yet been any evidence of a significantly reduced cardiac risk.[22]

Therefore, physical activity, diet, weight loss, and the control of all other possible risk factors are still important, even prior to manifestations of Type II diabetes.

PHYSICAL ACTIVITY AND OVERWEIGHT

Numerous studies have shown a relationship between physical activity and reduced vascular events and mortality.[23–30]

In terms of overall mortality, it can be shown that it is not only lifelong physical activity that reduces cardiovascular risk but also sport activities begun in the middle and later years. It is important to note that parallel to this there is a concomitant reduction of risk of cerebral vascular events, and this is independent of arterial hypertension.[31,32]

Commercial pilots, who have demanding occupational duties, often combined with considerable mental stress, but who nonetheless could serve as poster children for physical inactivity, would be well advised to comply with the American Heart Association recommendations: a balanced diet of 2000 calories per day and physical activity three and a half to four hours per week, preferably as a daily exercise period of 30 minutes.

The correlation between physical activity and reduction in cardiovascular risk is not entirely understood. It is assumed that the causes are multifactorial, as there is a reduced risk associated with hypertension management, weight control, and normalization of lipid profile and glucose levels.[33–36] Furthermore, physical activity improves the function of the endothelium, increases fibrinolysis and reduces platelet aggregation, leading to a reduction of in-situ thrombi.[37–39]

Dietetic measures should always be undertaken along with physical activity, and vice versa, as the benefits of each potentiates the other. In the Nurses' Health Study, a direct linear relationship existed between Body Mass Index and the risk of coronary artery disease (upper end of normal being 25).[40]

Noteworthy is also the fact that the adipose distribution is a separate risk factor, and short-term studies have found that the waist-to-hip ratio is an independent marker for vascular risk for both elderly men and women.[41,42]

Whether being overweight is an independent risk factor for cardiovascular disease or is a mediator of the development of glucose intolerance, insulin resistance, hypertension, impediment to physical activity, or the development of hyperlipidemia, continues to be controversial.

STRESS AS A CARDIOVASCULAR RISK FACTOR

It is easy to imagine that emotional stress can elevate myocardial demand (rise in blood pressure and heart rate) and precipitate local myocardial ischemia. It is also well known that patients with a predilection for coronary vasospasms can initiate this in stressful situations, and more easily so with atherosclerotic disease. Additionally, the catecholamine response can lead to a hyper-coagulable state.

The consequences of these mechanisms (sudden cardiac death in the setting of assault with a weapon or natural disasters) are currently being epidemiologically evaluated.[43] It is not yet known whether mental stress leads to atherosclerosis, but it seems possible.[44]

Enough evidence exists to support the inclusion of emotional stress to the list of coronary risk factors. Stress management counseling should be a cornerstone in the treatment of flight crew members.

FIBRINOGEN

Plasma fibrinogen influences platelet aggregation as well as blood viscosity. In combination with thrombin, it facilitates the last step toward thrombus formation. A direct correlation exists between elevated fibrinogen and overweight, age, smoking, diabetes, and high LDL cholesterol. An inverse correlation exists between high HDL cholesterol, ingestion of alcohol, and physical activity.[45,46]

Not surprisingly, the Framingham Study showed a positive correlation between elevated fibrinogen and the risk of future infarction. Because of individual differences in plasma fibrinogen levels, interpretation difficulties, and problems with measurement techniques, fibrinogen levels are not routinely utilized as an estimation of risk.

LIPOPROTEIN (a)

Lp(a) possibly inhibits endogenous fibrinolysis. It is found together with fibrin in atherosclerotic lesions.[47,48] Apo(a), a component of Lp(a), has chemotactic activity toward monocytes in the endothelium.[49]

Multiple retrospective studies have provided evidence for an association between Lp(a) and elevated cardiovascular risk. Newer prospective studies concerning this controversial result have not yet shown whether the determination of Lp(a), which is attached to an LDL particle, is generally of predictive value.

In all at-risk patients with an elevated Lp(a), the LDL cholesterol value should be added to that of Lp(a), and through dietary measures or medication (statins), this combined value should be reduced. To date it has not been determined whether niacin (vitamin B_3), which reduces Lp(a), has any clinical benefit.

HOMOCYSTINE

Homocystine levels above15 mmol/L are considered mild to moderate elevations. In population and retrospective studies, correlations between mild to moderate elevations of homocystine levels and atherosclerosis have been found.

It would be reasonable to obtain homocystine levels among certain groups of patients with marked premature atherosclerosis who do not have any other risk factor. Ingestion of 400 μg of folic acid reduces the level of homocystine by about 25% (the concurrent ingestion of vitamin B leads to a further 7% reduction). Distribution of vitamin B is much more economical than screening the entire population. Currently there is no randomized prospective study underway to determine whether a decrease in homocystine levels is correlated with a reduction in coronary artery disease risk. General screening of the population is not recommended, nor should screening be part of the routine medical evaluation of pilots.

FIBRINOLYTIC ACTIVITY

Disturbance of fibrinolysis can result from the imbalance of thrombolytic enzymes: tissue activated plasminogen (tPA), plasminogen activators of the urokinase type (u-PA), and the endogenous inhibition principally of plasminogen activator Inhibitor-1 (PAI-1). Numerous studies have also shown a relationship between this imbalance and an elevated coronary artery risk. Despite relatively good analysis, the clinical relevance of this risk marker is questionable, especially since both the collection, handling, and measurement are extremely difficult, if not impossible, because of very large variations with circadian rhythm, platelet degranulations after the blood draw, etc.)

INFLAMMATION AS A PREDICTOR OF VASCULAR EVENTS

It is known that inflammation, as indicated by high sensitivity C-reactive protein (hs-CRP), intercellular adhesion molecule (ICAM-1) or interleucine 1 (IL-1), accompanies all aspects of atherosclerosis.[50,51] It can also be demonstrated that numerous markers serve as minor systemic indicators of cardiovascular risk.[52] Included are the aforementioned hs-CRP and ICAM-1 together with IL-6 and Tumor Necrosis Factor, which may reflect possible inflammation processes within the region of the arterial wall.

Despite numerous studies, the exact pathophysiological mechanisms have not been elucidated and the question of the chicken and the egg (atherosclerosis due to inflammation or inflammation due to atherosclerosis) has not been resolved.

Regarding markers of inflammation, hs-CRP is the most clinically relevant, as it is easily and inexpensively measured in the serum. Many studies have shown that hs-CRP is a predictor of coronary artery disease among healthy men and women, as well as in older patients, in smokers, and in patients with stable or unstable angina pectoris.[52–60] Interestingly, hs-CRP represents a moderately elevated cardiovascular risk. It has also been shown that the administration of low dose ASA will lower an increased risk in those with a low grade inflammation level.[61] It is also possible that a reduction in lipids by use of statins helps reduce inflammation.

It is evident that lipid levels should be reduced and tissue inflammation suppressed as this may stabilize plaques and thus entail a reduced risk of coronary events. Above all, it is interesting that weight loss and physical activity both can reduce coronary artery risk and CRP levels.[62–65]

As mentioned before, it is not yet clear whether infections *per se* play an etiological role in atherosclerotic development. Studies regarding use of antibiotics and anti-inflammatory agents are currently underway.

DIRECT PLAQUE DEVELOPMENT

In addition to the coronary risk factors discussed above are certain parameters related to inflammation. Direct plaque formation and calcification can be measured with CT angiography, which allows a coronary artery calcium score (CACS) to be obtained. Currently, there are a series of studies evaluating the relationship between high-risk patients and high CACS.[67,68] The discussion concerning predictive value in the clinical setting continues to be controversial. It is not yet known whether those soft plaques, which are not calcified and therefore unstable and highly rupture-prone, might be missed on coronary artery CT evaluations.

New studies show that hs-CRP elevations double the risk of plaque rupture at all levels of CACS.[69] A further prospective study of asymptomatic individuals with at least one coronary risk factor has shown that a high CACS is predictive of myocardial infarction and death from coronary heart disease. A high CACS can modify predicted risk obtained from usual risk factors alone, especially among patients in the intermediate-risk category in whom clinical decision making is most uncertain.

It is possible that the best approach to stratification of coronary risk may be obtained by the often used and readily available method of measuring the thickness of the intima media of the carotid arteries by use of ultrasound.

REFERENCES

1. Nickenig G, Sachinidis A, Michaelsen F, *et al.* (1997) Up-regulation of vascular angiotensin II receptor gene expression by low densitiy lipoprotein in vascular smooth muscle cells. *Circulation* **95**: 473–478.
2. Hodis HN, Mack WJ. (1995) Triglyceride rich lipoproteins and the progression of coronary artery disease. *Curr Opin Lipidol* **6**: 209–214.
3. Hokanson JE, Austin MA. (1996) Plasma triglyceride level is a risk factor for cardiovascular disease independent of high-density lipoprotein cholesterol level: A meta-analysis of population-based prospective studies. *J Cardiovasc Risk* **3**: 213–219.
4. Morris JN, Heady JA, Raffle PAB, *et al.* (1953) Coronary heart disease and physical activity of work. *Lancet* **2**: 1035–1057, 1111–1120.
5. Berlin JA, Colditz GA. (1990) A meta-analysis of physical activity in the prevention of coronary heart disease. *Am J Epidemiol* **132**: 612–628.
6. Folsom AR, Arnett DK, Hutchinson RG, *et al.* (2007) Physical activity and incidence of coronary heart disease in middle-aged women and men. *Med Sci Sports Exerc* **29**: 901–909.
7. Leon AS, Myers MJ, Connett J. (1997) Leisure time physical activity and the 16-year risks of mortality from coronary heart disease and all-causes in the Multiple Risk Factor Intervention Trial (MRFIT). *Int J Sports Med* **18**(Suppl 3): 208–215.
8. Rosengren A, Wilhelmsen L. (1997) Physical activity protects against coronary death and deaths from all causes in middle-aged men. Evidence from a 20-year follow-up of the primary prevention study in Göteborg. *Ann Epidemiol* **7**: 96–75.
9. Lee IM, Hennekens CH, Berger K, *et al.* (1999) Exercise and risk of stroke in male physicians. *Stroke* **30**: 1–6.
10. Lee IM, Paffenbarger RS Jr. (1998) Physical activity and stroke incidence. The Harvard Alumni Health Study. *Stroke* **29**: 2049–2054.
11. Westrate JA, Meijer GW. (1998) Plant sterol-enriched margarines and reduction of plasma total- and LDL-cholesterol concentration in normocholesterolaemic and mildly hypercholesterolaemic subjects. *Eur J Clin Nutr* **52**: 334–343.

12. Kannel W, McGee D. (1979) Diabetes and glucose tolerance as risk factors for cardiovascular disease: The Framingham Study. *Diabetes Care* **2**: 120–126.
13. Manon JE, Colditz GA, Stampfer MJ, *et al.* (1991) A prospective study of maturity-onset diabetes mellitus and risk of coronary heart disease and stroke in women. *Arch Intern Med* **151**: 1141–1147.
14. Nathan DM. (1993) Long-term complications of diabetes mellitus. *N Engl J Med* **328**: 1676–1685.
15. Reaven GM. (1997) Banting Lecture 1988. Role of insulin resistance in human disease. *Nutrition* **13**: 65; discussion 64, 66.
16. Panahloo A, Yudkin JS. (1997) Diminished fibrinolysis in diabetes mellitus and its implication for diabetic vascular disease. *J Cardiovasc Risk* **4**: 91–99.
17. Kannel WB, D'Agostino RB, Wildson PW, *et al.* (1990) Diabetes, fibrinogen and risk of cardiovascular disease: The Framingham experience. *Am Heart J* **120**: 672–676.
18. Stehouwer CD, Nauta JJ, Zeldenrust GC *et al.* (1992) Urinary albumin excretion, cardiovascular disease, and endothelial dysfunction in non-insulin-dependent diabetes mellitus. *Lancet* **340**: 319–323.
19. Johnstone MT, Creager SJ, Scales KM, *et al.* (1993) Impaired endothelium-dependent vasodilation in patients with insulin-dependent diabetes mellitus. *Circulation* **88**: 2510–2516.
20. Neil A, Hawkins M, Potok M, *et al.* (1993) A prospective population-based study of microalbuminuria as a predictor of mortality in NIDDM. *Diabetes Care* **16**: 996–1003.
21. Valmadrid CT, Klein R, Moss SE, Klein BEK. (2000) The risk of cardiovasular disease mortality associated with microalbuminuria and gross proteinuria in persons with older onset diabetes mellitus. *Arch Intern Med* 160, 1093–1100.
22. Sandvic L, Erikssen J.Thaulow E, *et al.* (1993) Physical fitness as a predictor of mortality among healthy, middle-aged Norwegian men. *N Engl J Med* **328**: 533–537.
23. Paffenbarger RS Jr, Hyde RT, Wing AL, *et al.* (1993) The association of changes in physical-activity level and other lifestyle characteristics with mortality among men. *N Engl J Med* **328**: 538–545.

24. Paffenbarger RS Jr, Hyde RT, Wing AL, *et al.* (1986) Physical activity, all-cause mortality, and longevity of college alumni. *N Engl J Med* **314**: 605–613.
25. Sandvic L, Erikssen J, Thaulow E, *et al.* (1993) Physical fitness as a predictor of mortality among healthy, middle-aged Norwegian men. *N Engl J Med* **328**: 533–537.
26. Rosengren A, Wilhelmsen L. (1997) Physical activity protects against coronary death and deaths from all causes in middle-aged men: Evidence from a 20-year follow-up of the primary prevention study in Goteborg. *Ann Epidemiol* **7**: 69–75.
27. Morris JM, Calyton DG, Everitt MG, *et al.* (1990) Exercise in leisure time: Coronary attack and death rates. *Br Heart J* **63**: 325–334.
28. Blair SN, Goodyear NN, Gibbons LW, Cooper KH. (1984) Physical fitness and incidence of hypertension in healthy normotensive men and women. *JAMA* **252**: 487–490.
29. Leon AS, Connett J. Jacobs DR Jr, Rauramaa R. (1987) Leisure-time physical activity levels and risk of coronary heart disease and death: The Multiple Risk Factor Intervention Trial. *JAMA* **258**: 2388–2395.
30. Ekelund LG, Haskell WL, Johnson JL, *et al.* (1988) Physical fitness as a prevention of cardiovascular mortality in asymptomatic North American men. *N Engl J Med* **319**: 1379–1384.
31. Lee IM, Paffenbarger RS Jr. (1998) Physical activity and stroke incidence: The Harvard Alumni Health Study. *Stroke* **29**: 2049–2054.
32. Lee IM, Hennekens CH, Berger K, *et al.* (1999) Exercise and risk of stroke in male phyisicans. *Stroke* **30**: 1–6.
33. Kokkinos PF, Narayan P, Colleran JA, *et al.* (1995) Effects of regular exercise on blood preasure and left ventricular hypertrophy in African-American men with severe hypertension. *N Engl J Med* **333**: 1462–1467.
34. King AC, Haskell WL, Young DR, *et al.* (1995) Long-term effects of varying intensities and formats of physical activity on participation rates, fit intensities and formats of physical activity on participation rates, fitness, and lipoproteins in men and women aged 50 to 65 years. *Circulation* **91**: 2596–2604.
35. Helmrich SP, Ragland DR, Leung RW, *et al.* (1991) Physical activity and reduced occurrence of non-insulin-dependent diabetes mellitus. *N Engl J Med* **325**: 147–152.

36. Lynch J, Helmrich SP, Lakka TA, *et al.* (1996) Moderately intense physical activities and high levels of cardiorespiratory fitness reduce the risk of non-insulin-dependent diabetes mellitus in middle-aged men. *Arch Intern Med* **156**: 1307–1314.
37. Clarkson P, Montgomery HE, Mullen MJ, *et al.* (1999) Exercise training enhances endothelial function in young men. *J Am Coll Cardiol* **33**: 1379–1385.
38. Stratton JR, Chandler WL, Schwartz RS, *et al.* (1991) Effects of physical conditioning on fibrinolytic variables and fibrinogen in young and old healthy adults. *Circulation* **83**: 1692–1697.
39. Kestin AS, Ellis PA, Barnard MR, *et al.* (1993) Effect of strenuous exercise on platelet activation state and reactivity. *Circulation* **88**: 1502–1511.
40. Manson JE, Colditz GA, Stampfer MJ, *et al.* (1990) A prospective study of obesity and risk of coronary heart disease in women. *N Engl J Med* **322**: 882–889.
41. Rexrode KM, Carey VJ, Hennekens CH, *et al.* (1998) Abdominal adiposity and coronary heart disease in women. *JAMA* **280**: 1843–1848.
42. Rimm EB, Stampfer MJ, Giovannucci E, *et al.* (1995) Body size and fat distribution as predictors of coronary heart disease among middle-aged and older US men. *Am J Epidemiol* **141**: 1117–1127.
43. Leor J, Poole WK, Kloner RA. (1996) Sudden cardiac death triggered by an earthquake. *N Engl J Med* **334**: 413–419.
44. Krantz DS, Sheps DS, Carney RM, *et al.* (2000) Effects of mental stress in patients with coronary artery disease. *JAMA* **283**: 1800–1802.
45. Scarabin PY, Aillaud MF, Amouyel P, *et al.* (1998) Associations of fibrinogen, factor VII and PAI-1 with baseline findings among 10 500 male participants in a prospective study of myocardial infarction — the PRIME Study. Prospective Epidemiological Study of Myocardial Infarction. *Thromb Haemost* **80**: 749–756.
46. Margaglione M, Capucci G, Colaizzo D, *et al.* (1998) Fibrinogen plasma levels in an apparently healthy general population — relation to environmental and genetic determinants. *Thromb Haemost* **80**: 805–810.
47. Loscalzo J, Weinfeld M, Fless GM, *et al.* (1990) Lipoprotein(a), fibrin binding, and plasminogen activation. *Arteriosclerosis* **10**: 240–245.
48. Dangas G. Mehran R, Harpel PC, *et al.* (1998) Lipoprotein(a) and inflammation in human coronary atheroma: Association with the severity of clinical presentation. *J Am Coll Cardiol* **32**: 2035–2042.

49. Poon M, Zhang X, Dunsky KG, *et al.* (1997) Apolipoprotein(a) induces monocyte chemotactic activity in human vascular endothelial cells. *Circulation* **96**: 2514–2519.
50. Ross R. (1999) Atherosclerosis — An inflammatory disease. *N Engl J Med* **340**: 115–126.
51. Libby P. (1995) The molecular bases of the acute coronary syndroms. *Circulation* **91**: 2844–2850.
52. Ridker PM, Hennekens CH, Burning JE, *et al.* (2000) C-reactive protein and other markers of inflammation in the prediction of cardiovascular disease in women. *N Engl J Med* **342**: 836–843.
53. Koenig W, Sund M, Froelich M, *et al.* (1999) C-reactive protein, a sensitive marker of inflammation, predicts future risk of coronary heart disease in initially healthy middle-aged men: Results from the MONICA (Monitoring Trends and Determinants in Cardiovascular Disease) Augsberg Cohort Study, 1984 to 1992. *Circulation* **99**: 237–242.
54. Roivainen M, Viik-Kajander M, Palosuo T, *et al.* (2000) Infections, inflammation, and the risk of coronary disease. *Circulation* **101**: 252–257.
55. Ridker PM, Burning JE, Shih J, *et al.* (1998) Prospective study of C-reactive protein and the risk of future cardiovascular events among apparently healthy women. *Circulation* **98**: 731–733.
56. Tracy RP, Lemaitre RN, Psaty BM, *et al.* (1997) Relationship of C-reactive protein to risk of cardiovascular disease in the elderly: Results from the Cardiovascular Health Study and the Rural Health Promotion Project. *Asterioscler Thromb Vasc Biol* **17**: 1121–1127.
57. Kuller LH, Tracy RP, Shaten J, *et al.* (1996) Relation of C-reactive protein and coronary heart disease in the MRFIT nested case-control study, Multiple Risk Factor Intervention Trial. *Am J Epidemiol* **144**: 537–547.
58. Haverkate F, Thompson SG, Pyke SD, *et al.* (1997) Production of C-reactive protein and risk of coronary events in stable and unstable angina European Concerted Action on Thrombosis and Disabilities Angina Pectoris Study Group. *Lancet* **349**: 462–466.
59. Liuzzo G, Biasucci LM, Gallimore JR, *et al.* (1994) The prognostic value of C-reactive protein serum amyloid A protein in severe unstable angina. *N Engl J Med* **331**: 417–424.

60. Morrow DA, Rifai N, Antman EM, *et al.* (1998) C-reactive protein is a potent predictor of mortality independently of and in combination with troponin T in acute coronary syndromes: A TIMI 11Asubstudy. Thrombolysis in Myocardial Infarction. *I AM Coll Cardiol* **31**: 1460–1465.
61. Ridker PM, Cushman M, Stampfer MJ, *et al.* (1997) Inflammation, aspirin, and the risk of cardiovascular disease in apparently healthy man. *N Engl J Med* **336**: 973–979.
62. Smith JK, Dykes R, Douglas JE, *et al.* (1999) Long-term exercise and atherogenic activity of blood mononuclear cells in persons at risk of developing ischemic heart disese. *JAMA* **281**: 1722–1727.
63. Visser M, Bouter LM, McQuillan GM, *et al.* (1999) Elevated C-reaction protein levels in overweight and obese. *JAMA* **282**: 2131–2135.
64. Cushman M, Meilahn EN, Psaty BM, *et al.* (1999) Hormone replacement therapy, inflammation and hemostasis in elderly women. *Arterioscler Thromb Vasc Biol* **19**: 893–899.
65. Ridker PM, Hennekens CH, Rifai N, *et al.* (1999) Hormone replacement therapy and increased plasma concentration of C-reactive protein. *Circulation* **100**: 713–716.
66. Manson JE, Tosteson H, Ridker PM, *et al.* (1992) The primary prevention of myocardial infarction. *N Engl J Med* **326**: 1046–1416.
67. Kelan PC, Bielak LF, Ashai K, *et al.* (2001) Long-term prognostic value of coronary calcification dedected by electrom-beam CT in patients undergoing coronary angiographie. *Circulation* **104**: 412.
68. Achenbach S, Ropers D, Phole K, *et al.* (2002) Influence of lipid lowering therapy on the progression of coronary artery calcification: A prospective evaluation. *Circulation* **106**: 1077.
69. Park R, Detrano R, Xiang M, *et al.* (2004) Combined use of computed tomography with Framingham score for risk prediction in asymptomatic individuals. *JAMA* **291**: 210.
70. Greenland P, LaBree L, Azen SP, *et al.* Coronary artery calcium score combined with Framingham score for risk prediction in asymptomatic individuals.

71. Hodis HN, Mack WJ, LaBree L, *et al.* (1998) The role of carotide arterial intima-media thickness in predicting clinical coronary events. *Ann Intern Med* **128**: 262.
72. O'Leary DH, Polak JF, Kronmal RA, *et al.* (1999) Carotid artery intima and media thickness as a risk factor for myocardial infarction and stroke in older adults. Cardiovascular Health Study Collabotrative Research Group. *N Engl J Med* **340**: 14.

Chapter 10

Arterial Hypertension

Norbert Schauer*

ESSENTIAL ARTERIAL HYPERTENSION

Twenty-five percent of the adult population have arterial hypertension, which is defined as a blood pressure measuring > 140 mmHg systolic and > 90 mmHg diastolic. Hypertension leads to an elevated incidence of non-fatal and fatal coronary events, stroke, renal parenchymal diseases, and elevated mortality from other causes.

Pilots and flight crews are not exempt from this. In more than 90% of cases, the hypertension is essential, only 2–5% have an identifiable cause. Professional flight crews are generally quite young at their first physical examination, allowing identifiable causes to be found and treated (see below).

What is elevated blood pressure?

Table 1. Definition of Blood Pressure Stages in Applicants not Taking Antihypertensive Medication[1,2]

Stage	Systolic (mmHg)	Diastolic (mmHg)
Normal	< 120	< 80
Prehypertension	120–139	80–89
Hypertension		
– Stage 1 Hypertension	140–159	90–99
– Stage 2 Hypertension	≥ 160	≥ 100

* Maria Theresiastraße 22/1, A-6020 Innsbruck, Austria.

"White Coat Syndrome"

This is a situationally induced elevation of blood pressure to 20% above normal — which should result in a series of self measurements and, if necessary, should initiate Life Style Modification.

Pseudo-Hypertension

This is a mis-measurement due to an extremely rigid brachial artery (in the event that the blood pressure cuff cannot compress the artery). Suspect Pseudo-hypertension if the cuff is inflated well above the arterial pressure, yet the radial pulse is palpable (Osler's sign). Objective measurements can only be obtained by invasive techniques.

Clinical Evaluation of Blood Pressure

History: age, family history; duration of high blood pressure condition, weight, and other cardiovascular risk factors (such as diabetes, nicotine, hyperlipidemia, sedentary lifestyle) should be elicited.

SECONDARY HYPERTENSION

This is hypertension secondary to renal artery stenosis, renal parenchymal disease, primary hyperaldosteronism, pheochromocytosis, aortic isthmus stenosis, hyperthyroidism, alcohol abuse, or of pharmacologic origin.

THE EVALUATION OF SUSPECTED ARTERIAL HYPERTENSION

Clinical examination with blood pressure measurements of the upper and lower extremities. Fundoscopy, examination of peripheral vessels, neurological and thyroid examination.

Laboratory examination: red and white blood cell count, electrolytes, particularly potassium if there has been no prior diuretic therapy,

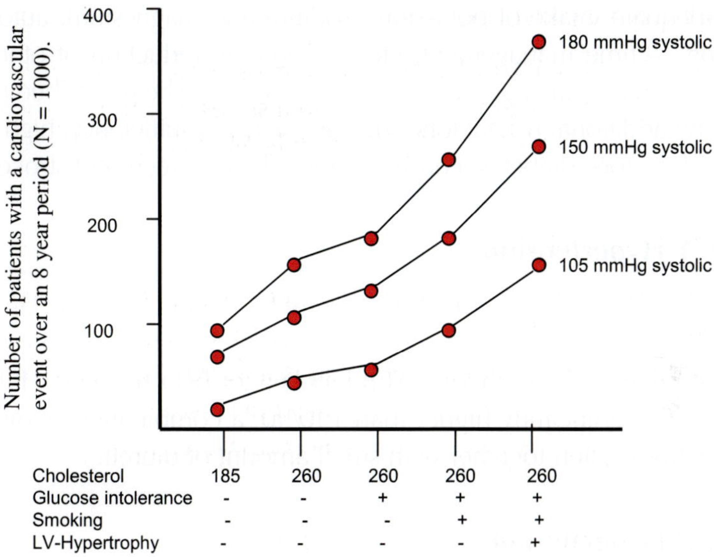

Figure 1. Importance of arterial hypertension in the evaluation of cardiovascular risks: For a given blood pressure level (*right*), the risk of a cardiovascular event increases with the other factors mentioned — observation of cardiovascular events in 1000 patients over 8 years (after Ref. 22).

fasting blood glucose and lipid panel. Possibly homocystine and Lp(a). Calcium as a marker of hyperparathyroidism. Uric acid before diuretic therapy, urinalysis including microlbuminuria. ECG and echocardiogram to identify target organ damage.

The most important target organs are the cerebral vascular system (carotid duplex sonography), the cardiovascular system (echocardiography), the retina (fundoscopy), the kidneys, and the peripheral vascular system.

TREATMENT OF HYPERTENSION

Prehypertension

"Life Style Modification": Weight loss if overweight, reduction or cessation of alcohol use, regular aerobic exercise, reduction of table salt, adequate intake of potassium, sodium and magnesium, autogenic training — time management, etc. In addition, reduction of other risk factors (smoking, fat ingestion). Medications should be prescribed if indicated by additional risk factors, such as cardiac insufficiency, high coronary risk factors, diabetes, chronic kidney disease, recurrent stroke.

Stage 1 Hypertension

When blood pressure is over 140/90 mmHg: Continuation of "Life Style Modification". Initiation of adequate monotherapy medication (particularly in pilots, ACE inhibitors, AT-II blockers or beta blockers). If blood pressure is significantly higher than 140/90, a combination of different preparations, often together with small amount of diuretic.

Stage 2 Hypertension

When blood pressure is equal to or above 160/100 mmHg: 2–3 medications in combination. Trials of BID-TID therapeutic dosing. If pseudo-hypertension or situational hypertension can be ruled out, increase dosage, excluding the use of similar class medications. Intensive evaluation in the direction of secondary hypertension (exogenous pro-hormone (Superdrol®-methasteron), volume overload, NSAIDs, cortisone therapy, mineralocorticoid use, contraception, caffeine, nicotine).

TAB 1 HYPERTENSION

Myocardium as Target Organ

Left ventricular hypertrophy (LVH) is an independent, strong predictor of morbidity and mortality (sudden cardiac death, heart attack, stroke). Much of this knowledge comes from the Framingham Heart Study. Numerous antihypertensive pharmaceuticals (but not vasodilators)[3,4] have been demonstrated to bring about a regression of LVH.

In aviation medicine, antihypertensive therapy relies in particular on several studies that recommend ACE inhibitors (initially, and if necessary, with addition of a low dose diuretic) because of their excellent regressive effect on the left chamber. Clonidin, ditiazem or prazocin are less effective and therefore less used. These central acting antihypertensives are not compatible with aeromedical certification.

One should not forget that there are studies which show that life style modification, such as weight loss, limitation of table salt and aerobic exercise can also lead to a reduction in LVH.

When pronounced LVH is diagnosed in a pilot, efficacy of treatment by documenting LVH regression is necessary. This requires time, both for the therapy to be effective and for repeated sonographic examinations to be conducted over a length of time.

Additional comments regarding antihypertensive therapy

In principle, it is generally a good idea to use diuretics and beta blockers as first line therapy. According to Table 1, one must consider potential or actual accompanying diseases when making a choice of therapeutic modalities. Because of the particularities of aviation duties, the aviation medicine practitioner is best advised to choose ACE inhibitors as first line therapy in pilots, while reserving mild diuretics and beta blockade as second choice, due to polyuria and dehydration.

Situational hypertension (White Coat Hypertension)

In order to determine whether a situational arterial hypertension needs to be treated or not, echocardiogram (LVH) and duplex sonography of the extracranial circulation (intima media thickness) can be utilized. If the target organs are pathologically changed, then there is indication for treatment.

Life style modification (when blood pressure is between 140–158 systolic and 90–99 diastolic) should be undertaken for six months; thereafter medication should be initiated if necessary.

Target blood pressure for pilots

On the basis of graphs, many observations and epidemiologic studies, "the lower the better" could be the focus of blood pressure optimization. However, studies have shown that for blood pressure values >139 / 79 and <119 / 64, the risk of cardiovascular and non-cardiovascular mortality rises, not linearly, but the risk of cardiovascular events rises as a J-curve.[5,6] In the large Hypertension Optimal Treatment (HOT) study[7] with over 18000 patients in three groups (goal BP < 90, < 85, < 80), it was shown that the lowest risk of cardiovascular events occurred at a diastolic pressure of 82.6 mmHg and the lowest risk of cardiovascular mortality was at 86.5 mmHg. From this can be deduced that a blood pressure goal of 139/85 mmHg (which in our situation has the advantage of having few side effects on the basis of lower dosage of antihypertensive medication) is entirely adequate.

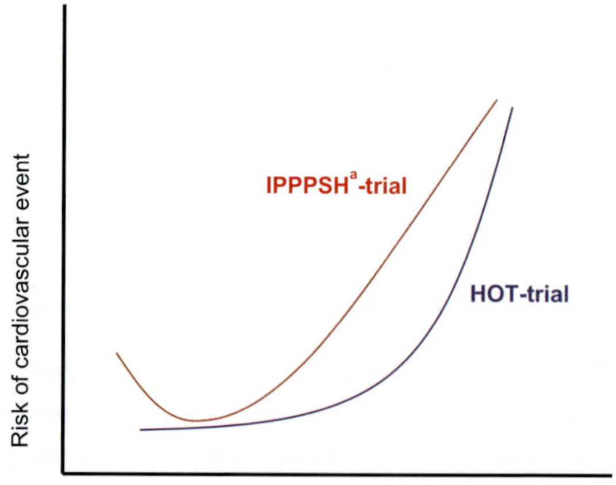

Figure 2. The relationship between risk of cardiovascular event and degree of hypertension according to two large studies.

[a] International Progressive Primary Prevention Study in Hypertension.

MEDICAL THERAPY OF ARTERIAL HYPERTENSION

ACE Inhibitors

The ACE inhibitors block the angiotensin converting enzyme (ACE) and thereby the transformation of angiotensin I to angiotensin II, resulting in blood pressure reduction. We recommend them on the basis of good tolerance in flight crews. Endless studies have shown the effectiveness in flight crews with minimal psychiatric, neurological, ophthalmological and vestibular side effects.[8,9] ACE inhibitors induce a cough in about 2–4% of cases. As indicated in Table 1, ACE inhibitors can reduce the progression of renal insufficiency, particularly in patients with diabetic tendencies.

Angiotensin II Receptor Antagonists

The angiotensin II receptor antagonists are the successors to the ACE inhibitors. The blood pressure reducing effect of this substance is due to the blockage of the AT-I receptors.[10] Angiotensin II leads to vasoconstriction, to an increase in sodium resorption in the kidneys, as well as secretion of aldosterone.

Theoretically, the angiotensin receptor blockers are superior to the ACE inhibitors,[11] as they block the vasoconstrictive AT-I receptors, and simultaneously stimulate the vasodilatation effects of AT-II receptors. Altogether, the ACE inhibitors and the AT-II blockers are presumably equally effective[12]; the main advantage lies with the lack of cough as a side effect, which occurs relatively frequently with the ACE inhibitors.

Beta Blockers

Like ACE inhibitors, beta blockers can also be used as first choice medications. They are particularly suitable for patients with a hyperdynamic circulatory profile, which is occasionally observed in flight crews. Sometimes prescribing very low doses will adequately lower blood pressure, while avoiding side effects.[13] Beta blockers are contraindicated in sinus bradycardia, high grade AV blockade, as well as in chronic obstructive pulmonary disease, bronchial asthma, and severe arterial occlusive disease. Beta blockers can have an additional advantage in individuals with migraine.

Calcium Channel Blockers

There are three therapeutic groups:

1. Dihydropyridine: such as amblodipin, nimodipin
2. Benzothiazepine: diltiazem
3. Phenylalkylamine: verapamil

The blood pressure lowering effect of calcium channel blockers occurs through the inhibition of calcium influx into the smooth muscle cell with consequential vasodilatation. In recent years, calcium channel blockers have been used particularly in heart insufficiency and CAD.[14] It has been found that low doses of the long acting dihydropyridine in hypertension is particularly effective in older patients[15–17] and have reduced the number of coronary events.

Diuretics

Diuretics inhibit the NaCl resorption in the renal tubules, with the further effect of reduced plasma volume, cardiac output and renal blood flow. This alone is not responsible for the blood pressure lowering effect. Within 6–8 weeks, the extracellular fluid volume and cardiac output normalizes.[18,19] Nonetheless, peripheral vascular resistance remains lower. It is possible that this lowered peripheral vascular resistance is due to an effect on the potassium channel activity.[20]

Diuretics are divided into four large groups: first are those that have an effect on the proximal tubule — carbonic anhydrase inhibitors; second are the loop diuretics; third the thiazide diuretics; and fourth are the potassium sparing diuretics. Usually the thiazide diuretics are the first choice, occasionally in combination with a potassium sparing diuretic. Diuretics should be administered in the

Table 2. Indications and Effects of Oral Antihypertensive Pharmacotherapy Metabolic and Physiological Effects

Class	Indication	Chol.	Trigl.	HDL	K	Mg	UA*	Insulin Resistance	Regression of LVH**	Secondary Cardio-Protection
ACE inhibitors	Diabetes mellitus with nephropathy, post infarction, CHF***									
Angiotensin II antagonists	Same as above									
β-blockers without ISA¶	Post infarction, migraine, tachycardia									
β-blockers with ISA	Same as above									
Calcium channel blockers	Older patients, CAD¶¶, renal insufficiency									Possible with diltiazam and verapamil
Diuretics	Same as above									

(*Continued*)

Table 3. (*Continued*)

Class	Indication	Chol.	Trigl.	HDL	K	Mg	UA*	Insulin Resistance	Regression of LVH**	Secondary Cardio-Protection
Centrally acting α-blockers	Sedative effect, if desired									
Peripherally acting α-blockers	Diabetes mellitus, hyperlipidemia, benign prostatic hypertrophy									
Vasodilators	Peripheral arterial disease, vasculitis									

*: UA = uric acid
**: LVH = left ventricular hypertrophy
***: CHF = congestive heart failure
¶: ISA = intrinsic sympathomimetic activity
¶¶: CAD = coronary artery disease

smallest possible dose, especially in flight crews. Patients with glucose intolerance, diabetes mellitus or a history of gout should not receive diuretics. Lipid profiles and glucose tolerance can be unfavorably influenced.

Alpha Blockers

The centrally acting alpha blockers (e.g. doxazosin) have a strong sedating side effect and should therefore be avoided in pilots. Peripherally acting alpha blockers block the effects of peripheral post-synaptic alpha adrenergic receptors, and are less likely to lead to a reflex tachycardia than the direct vasodilators. Cardiac volume and plasma volume are not changed, so that they can be used in combination with other medications. They are particularly recommended with coexisting metabolic disorders as they have a tendency to improve insulin sensitivity.[21] Should the alpha blockers be used in flight crews, dosage should be increased slowly to avoid syncope.

Direct Vasodilators

Direct vasodilators (such as minoxidil) should not be used due to their side effects (reflex tachycardia, induction of autoimmune disorders). Additionally, they lead to direct vasodilatation and do not reduce LV hypertrophy.

REFERENCES

1. The Seventh Report of the Joint National Committee on Prevention, Detection, Evaluation and Treatment of High Blood Preasure. NIH Publication No. 03 52 33, 2003.
2. Guidelines Subcommittee: 1999 World Health Organization International Society of Hypertension guidelines for the management of hypertension. (1999) *J Hypertens* **17**: 151.
3. Schmiederer RE. (1996) A meta-analysis of randomized double-blind studies. *JAMA* **275**(19): 1507–1513.

4. Schmiederer RE, Schlaich MP, Klingbeil AU, Martus P. (1998) Update on reversal of left ventricular hypertrophy in essential hypertension (a meta-analysis of all randomized double-blind studies until December 1996). *Nephrol Dial Transplant* **13**(3): 564–569.
5. IPPSH Collaborative Groups (1985): Cardiovascular risk and risk factors in a randomized trial of treatment based on a beta-blocker oxprenolol: The International Prospective Primary Prevention Study in Hypertension (IPPSH). *J Hypertens* **3**: 379.
6. Cruickshank IM. (1988) Coronary flow reserve and the J curve relation between diastolic blood pressure and myocardial infarction. *BMJ* **297**: 1227.
7. Hansson L, Zanchetti A, Carruthers SG, *et al.* (1998) Effects of intensive blood pressure lowering and low-dose aspirin in patients with hypertension: Principal results of the Hypertension Optimal Treatment (HOT) randomised trial. *Lancet* **351**: 1755.
8. Amroliwalla FK. (1994) Angiotensin converting enzyme (ACE) inhibitors in hypertensive aircrew. *Aviat Space Environ Med* **65**(11): 1054–1057.
9. Rhodes DB, Howe B. (1997) Lisinopril for the treatment of hypertension in USAF aircrew (abstract). *Aviat Space Environ Med* **68**(7): 628.
10. Burnier M, Brunner HR. (1998) Angiotensin II receptor antagonists in hypertension. *Kidney Int* **54**: S107.
11. Bell TP, DeQuattroV, Lasseter KC, *et al.* (1999) Effective dose range of candesartan cilexetil for systemic hypertension. *Am J Cardiol* **83**: 272.
12. Hansson L, Lindholm LH, Niskanen L, *et al.* (1999) Effect of angiotension-converting-enzyme inhibition compared with conventional therapy on cardiovascular morbidity and mortality in hypertension: The Captopril Prevention Project (CAPPP) randomised trial. *Lancet* **353**: 611.
13. Serlin MM, Orme MLE, Baber N, *et al.* (1980) Propranolol in the control of blood pressure: A dose-response study. *Clin Pharmacol Ther* **27**: 588.
14. Psaty BM, Heckbert SR, Koepsell TD, *et al.* (1995) The risk of myocardial infarction associated with antihypertensive drug therapies. *JAMA* **274**: 620.
15. Staessen JA, Ragard R, Thijs L, *et al.* (1997) Randomised double-blind comparison of placebo and active treatment for older patients with isolated systolic hypertension. *Lancet* **350**: 757.

16. Liu L. Wang JG, Gong L, *et al.* (1998) Comparison of active treatment and placebo in older Chinese patients with isolated systolic hypertension. *J Hypertens* **16**: 1823.
17. Hansson L, Zanchetti A, Carruthers SG, *et al.* (1998) Effects of intensive blood-pressure lowering and low-dose aspirin in patients with hypertension: Principal results of the Hypertension Optimal Treatment (HOT) randomised trial. *Lancet* **351**: 1755.
18. Brater DC. (2000) Pharmacology of diuretics. *Am J Med Sci* **319**(1): 1–9.
19. Puschett JB (2000) Diuretics and the therapy of hypertension. *Am J Med Sci* **319(**1): 1–9.
20. Pickkers P, Huges AD, Frans G, *et al.* (1998) Thiazide-induced vasodilation in humans is mediated by potassium channel activation. *Hypertension* **32**: 1071.
21. Lehy D, Walmsley P, Levenstein M. (1996) Principal results of the hypertension and lipid trial (HALT): A multicenter study of doxazosin in patients with hypertension. *Am Heart J* **131**: 966.

Chapter 11

Heart Diseases and Disorders

Norbert Schauer*

MYOCARDITIS (INFLAMMATORY CARDIOMYOPATHY)

One of the most difficult diagnoses to make in the living person is myocarditis. Often it remains clinically silent, is self-limiting within the circulatory system, or is diagnosed very late following a long progression. Myocarditis has no characteristic pathognomonic laboratory findings. Myocardial biopsy can be very helpful in establishing the diagnosis.

We know that cardiotropic viruses exist; the most common one affecting the heart is Coxsackie B virus. It is not necessarily the virus itself, but rather the immune response to the virus within the heart muscle that causes the typical myocarditis disorders.[1–5]

- Invasion of the pathogen
- Production of heart muscle damaging agent
- Immune-mediated myocardial damage

Histologically, florid myocarditis is demonstrated by infiltration of the myocardium by T-lymphocytes and macrophages. The extent of myocarditis is directly dependent on the intensity of immunologic response of the organism. Biopsy monitoring of myocarditis has shown that myocardial function almost always improves after the immunological processes abates.

* Maria Theresiastraße 22/1, A-6020 Innsbruck, Austria.

Because the therapeutical possibilities are almost non-existent, many centers forgo performing myocardial biopsies.

Myocarditis has a variety of clinical presentations: one of the main symptoms is tachycardia associated with performance limitations, often following a flu-like illness. Subsequently conduction defects may develop, sometimes all the way to third degree AV block. Even atrial fibrillation may occur.

Chest pain with or without dyspnea is not uncommon, ranging from organ sensation to angina pectoris suspicious of infarction, depending on the degree of impairment of left ventricular function.

Arrhythmia caused by AV conduction disturbances may lead to pronounced palpitations or syncope. Sudden cardiac death can be the first symptom.

The clinical examination may demonstrate tachycardia, arrhythmia, fever and changes in cardiac heart sounds. Corresponding to a reduction in LV function, typical signs of left heart insufficiency may appear.

In addition to sinus tachycardia, the ECG shows a negative deflection in the T waves in multiple leads. Also the development of Q waves is possible, which can simulate infarction when corresponding symptoms are present. "Long QT syndrome" and low voltage can likewise be an expression of myocarditis.

Laboratory results show an elevated sedimentation rate 60% of the time. There is leucocytosis in only 25% of cases. An elevation in CK-MB and CK is evident in only 12% of patients. Viral IgG titers can be elevated to four times normal. Chest X-ray can demonstrate an enlarged cardiac silhouette, corresponding to the above mentioned symptoms as an indication of left heart insufficiency. In early florid myocarditis, the left ventricle is normal or only minimally enlarged, but nonetheless abnormal wall motion and mural thrombosis may occur (even with still relatively good LV function). Hypertrophy of the heart muscle may develop from inflammatory edema in the acute stage.

Heart catheterization, while not a standard procedure for the evaluation of myocarditis, can measure elevated end-diastolic pressure.

If biopsied, which by some cardiologists is considered without therapeutic benefit, at least six specimens must be taken from the right ventricle.

According to the **Dallas criteria**, active myocarditis exists if inflammatory infiltrates with necrosis or degenerative changes of the affected myocytes are visualized, as they are not typical of ischemic changes from coronary artery disease. A "borderline myocarditis" exists when only minimal inflammatory infiltration without myocardial damage is evident. In the future, gallium scans or MRI will be able to support the diagnosis of myocarditis.

If myocarditis is diagnosed based on the above mentioned indicators, therapy is directed toward treatment of heart insufficiency (sodium restriction, diuretics, digitalis, ACE inhibitors and angiotensin II inhibitors), balanced with limitation of physical activity. If the disease progresses, aggressive treatment with catecholamines and mechanical assistance, such as the intra-aortic balloon pump and assistive devices, as a "bridge to transplant" are indicated. This is only when there is no other alternative, as the heightened immune response of myocarditis patients increases the risk of transplant rejection. Not to be forgotten is anticoagulation, as even with minimally reduced LV function, there is a risk of mural thrombosis with consequential arterial embolism.

Rhythm disturbances are treated in the usual fashion, and if necessary, with the assistance of a pacemaker. The benefit of immune suppressive therapy is still unclear and remains generally within the realm of specialty centers performing controlled studies. If hospitalization if necessary, symptomatic treatment (β-blockers, ACE inhibitor, diuretics, antiarrhythmics, etc.), and complete bed rest with oxygen supplementation are indicated.

In severe refractory cases, heart transplantation should be considered. Non-steroidal anti-inflammatory medications (NSAIDs) are contraindicated in the acute phase.[6–8] Immune suppressive drugs are not recommended.

Naturally there are also other causes besides viral. Worth mentioning are the connective tissue diseases, vasculitis, radiation myocarditis, chemical and toxic myocarditis, and post streptococcal myocarditis caused by release of endotoxins.

The pericardium commonly participates in myocarditis with the corresponding symptoms of pericarditis (see above).

Prognostically significant is that the myocarditis usually resolves and heals. In a small portion of cases, reduced ventricular function, progression to dilated cardiomyopathy, arrhythmia or sudden cardiac death results.[9,10]

The diagnosis of myocarditis leads to disqualification for all classes of medical certification for at least six months. For recertification, a complete recovery must be demonstrated. This involves stress testing with normal cardiopulmonary performance, an echocardiogram in which the EF must be at least 50%, no significant regional wall motion disturbances, a 24 hour ECG with no significant arrhythmias, and semi-annual cardiology evaluations.

Certification for Class I should be limited to one year and multi-crew operations only. Also for Class II restrictions should be applied.

Heart transplant is permanently disqualifying for all classes of medical certification.

PERICARDIAL DISEASES

The pericardium surrounds and stabilizes the heart and the great vessels. The visceral and parietal pericardium limits the sudden dilatation of the heart and thus assists in atrial filling.

Acute Pericarditis

Acute pericarditis is characterized by chest pain, pericardial friction rubbing, characteristic ECG changes (ST elevation, low voltage, atrial extrasystole, and atrial fibrillation), pericardial effusion, tamponade, and pulsus paradoxus. An elevated creatine kinase muscle and brain isoenzyme (CK-MB) indicates an associated epimyocarditis.

Echocardiography most often shows a pericardial effusion. During inspiration, a tamponade produces an increase in the right ventricular diameter and a decrease in the left ventricular diameter.[10]

The right ventricular wall collapses. The effusion consists primarily of an exudate, which is hemorrhagic if from tuberculosis or from a tumor (rarely so with rheumatic fever). Depending on the severity, the volume of the effusion may be between 200 and 2000 mL.

Bed rest and continuous observation for indications of pericardiocentesis is necessary.[11,12] Care must be taken with anticoagulation, as the danger of a hemorrhagic pericardial effusion exists.

Viral or Idiopathic Acute Pericarditis

If no evidence of viral illness can be identified, such as viral antibodies, which can certainly be difficult to determine, one speaks of an acute cryptogenetic or idiopathic pericarditis. Hospitalization is generally for one to four weeks. A quarter of the patients can experience up to four recurrences. Granulocytosis followed by lymphocytosis is common.

Viral or idiopathic pericarditis usually disappears within one month. Rare causes for pericarditis are syphilis, fungal infections, and parasites (amebiasis, toxoplasmosis, echinococcus, trichinosis), as well as a malignancy.[13]

Chronic Pericarditis

All examinations that could identify tuberculosis must be undertaken, as tuberculosis is treatable and serious consequences can be expected. Chest X-ray, examination of all organ systems, TB skin test, cultures and smears of gastric secretions, pleural and pericardial fluids, eventually even thoracotomy for pericardial effusion analysis, and in the case of caseous necrosis, anti-tuberculosis treatment are indicated.

Further etiologies for chronic pericardial effusion include myxedema, lupus erythematosus, rheumatoid arthritis, neoplasm, mycosis, radiation therapy, pyogenic infections, severe chronic anemia, and rarely chylopericarditis. Hemorrhagic effusions are usually caused by neoplasm, tuberculosis, uremia, or a rupture of an aortic aneurysm into the pericardium.

Treatment

Prior to the initiation of treatment, one should always determine whether procainamide, hydralazine, isoniazid, and minoxidil is being taken, as these can be causes of pericarditis.

There is no specific treatment for pericarditis. Bed rest is recommended, and ASA 500 mg every three to four hours or indomethacin 50–100 mg every six hours should be administered. In the event of severe pain or pain lasting more than 72 hours, steroids can be added (80 mg/day), which should also suppress the clinical manifestations. Prior to the administration of steroids, tuberculosis or purulent pericarditis must be ruled out. Tuberculosis skin testing should not be neglected.

Post-traumatic heart syndrome occurs after trauma, surgery (post-cardiotomy syndrome), and following infarct (Dressler syndrome), and is characterized by leukocytosis, an elevated sedimentation rate, and pericarditis-associated ECG changes. Therapy consists of NSAIDs, and possibly glucocorticoids in tapering dosages.

Chronic constrictive pericarditis

Following inflammation, the pericardial space can be obliterated by granulomatous tissue. This hinders ventricular filling when the elasticity of the pericardium is reached (during active effusion, ventricular filling is hindered during the entire diastole). Clinical presentation is dependent on the consequences of right heart insufficiency caused by the massive congestive influx from exudative enteropathy due to the impaired lymph drainage of the small bowel — pulmonary edema rarely occurs. Note: there is a danger of confusion with cirrhosis of the liver — look for jugular venous distention! Tricuspid stenosis can also simulate chronic constrictive pericarditis.

Therapy

Sodium restriction and administration of diuretics are required, but in the end, pericardial resection is the only definitive therapy, as long as the pericardial changes have not affected the myocardium.

Pericardial cysts are harmless and usually occur in the right cardiophrenic angle.

Pilots with acute aseptic pericarditis should be temporarily disqualified. After three months and full recovery, limited recertification is acceptable for Class I with multi-crew limitation, and for Class II with a safety pilot or "no passenger" restriction, as long as stress testing and normal cardiopulmonary function can be documented. An echocardiogram with an EF of at least 50% and with no significant regional wall motion disturbances is necessary, as well as a 24-hour ECG without significant rhythm disturbances. Semi-annual evaluations by a cardiologist with the previously mentioned tests should probably be continued for at least two years. An angiogram should only be performed if there is question regarding the results of the non-invasive tests.

CARDIOMYOPATHY

The cardiomyopathies are diseases of the heart muscle itself. In order to arrive at this diagnosis, other primary causes of heart muscle diseases must be ruled out. The term cardiomyopathy is best avoided when referring to ventricle dilatation due to coronary artery disease.

For aeromedical purposes, division into the functional classes (dilated, restrictive, hypertrophic) is helpful. Two uncommon forms are worthy of mention: arrythmogenic right ventricular dysplasia and the non-classifiable forms. (International Society and Federation of Cardiology (ISFC).)

The specific cardiomyopathies are: ischemic, valvular, hypertensive, and the inflammatory cardiomyopathies (see below).

Myocardial biopsy is reasonable in the context of evaluation for heart transplantation and in the event of anthracycline toxicity, but is not of any value regarding aeromedical certification.

Dilatative Cardiomyopathy

Idiopathic dilatative cardiomyopathy

Dilatative cardiomyopathy is defined as an enlargement of the left ventricle or both ventricles, combined with a decreased LV pump function.[14] In 20–30% of cases, a familial cluster of cardiomyopathy is evident.[15,16] The rest consists of sporadic idiopathic or secondary dilatative cardiomyopathy. Macroscopic evidence, as suggested by the definition, consists of enlarged cardiac cavities and frequent mural thrombi, whereby the heart valves and coronary arteries remain unchanged. Microscopic findings include perivascular and interstitial fibrosis, cellular infiltrates and necrosis of individual myocardial cells. The symptoms of dilatative cardiomyopathy are the same, whether familial, sporadic, or secondary in origin[17] so that the diagnosis is usually one of exclusion.

The symptoms of dilatative cardiomyopathy range from a limited left heart insufficiency to pronounced biventricular insufficiency; the latter carries a five year survival rate of only 40%. This is the most common indication for heart transplantation. Non-lethal and lethal rhythm disturbances can complicate the course of dilatative cardiomyopathy and, not infrequently, an automatic internal defibrillator is implanted as a "bridge to transplant."

Alcoholic cardiomyopathy

This is the most common form of secondary dilatative cardiomyopathy in the western world. After alcohol cessation, the disease can stagnate or even improve. Otherwise it carries a poor prognosis — less than one fourth survive three years.

Tachyarrhythmias, particularly atrial fibrillation but also ventricular tachyarrhythmias and the development of LVH in association with arterial hypertension, may be consequences of chronic alcohol abuse. Diastolic compliance disorders progressing to pulmonary edema can occur.

Arrythmogenic right ventricular dysplasia

This condition occurs in familial clusters in genetically predisposed individuals. Triggered by myocarditis, it most commonly affects the right ventricle (fatty and fibrotic degeneration of the myocardium). Occasionally the left ventricle is involved, producing a clinical picture of dilatative cardiomyopathy. Often VES and VT originate from the right ventricle. Sudden cardiac death is not uncommon.

An established dilated cardiomyopathy or arrythmogenic right ventricle dysplasia is disqualifying for all classes of medical certification. In the rare case of recovery from cardiomyopathy, proof of complete recovery from the condition must be made in order for recertification to be considered (the assumption being made that the correct diagnosis was myocarditis).

This involves stress testing showing normal cardiopulmonary performance, an echocardiogram demonstrating an EF of at least 50%, no significant regional wall motion disturbances, a 24-hour ECG without significant arrhythmias, and semi-annual evaluations by a cardiologist. Class I limited to one year and multicrew operations, and restricted Class II may be possible.

Hypertrophic Cardiomyopathy

Hypertrophic cardiomyopathy consists of a concentric hypertrophy of the left ventricle, in one fourth of the cases involving the septum (previously placed in the foreground and therefore carrying its own diagnostic name). The origin of this disease is uncertain.[14] It is associated with an increased incidence of sudden cardiac death, also in the families of effected patients.

A disturbance of calcium transfer is thought to lead to calcium overload in the cells and therefore to diastolic compliance disorders.[18,19] Systolic function is most often not affected, except in the late stages of the disease.

Echocardiographic characteristics are not discernable in childhood but become possible in adolescence at the earliest.

In the event that hypertrophic cardiomyopathy is definitively diagnosed, the applicant is not aeromedically qualified if there are rhythm disturbances, ECG changes, and unambiguous reports of symptomatology typically associated with hypertrophic cardiomyopathy (such as diastolic insufficiency).

If suspicion for this disorder exists, then an applicant may obtain Class I certification limited to one year and multicrew operations and restricted Class II, as long as stress testing indicates normal cardiopulmonary performance, echocardiogram demonstrates an EF of at least 50% without significant wall motion, significant arrhythmias, and semi-annual evaluations are performed by a cardiologist.

In the event that there is any doubt, angiography should be included in the evaluation. Sustained or non-sustained ventricular tachycardia, as well as dizziness of unclear etiology, is not compatible with medical certification.

Obliterative and Restrictive Cardiomyopathy

Obliterative and restrictive cardiomyopathy from any cause carries a decidedly poor prognosis and, once diagnosed, is permanently disqualifying.

Treated hemochromatosis of the heart is compatible with Class I certification, limited to one year and multicrew operations and restricted Class II as long as stress testing indicates normal cardiopulmonary performance, echocardiogram demonstrates an EF of at least 50% without significant wall motion disturbances, the septum is measured at less than 20 mm, a 24-hour ECG is without significant arrhythmias, and semiannual evaluations are performed by a cardiologist. In the event that there is any doubt, angiography should be included in the evaluation.

SARCOIDOSIS

Sarcoidosis is an inflammatory granulomatous disease of unknown etiology. In most cases the lung parenchyma is affected; however, the lymph nodes, joints, musculature, liver, kidneys, skin and, in 27% of affected patients, the heart may also be involved.[20]

Despite cardiac involvement, the cardiac symptoms are often less pronounced than the pulmonary symptoms, so that cardiac sarcoidosis often goes undiagnosed. Affection of the heart by granulomatous infiltrates (particularly the anterior wall, the septum and the apical region of the left ventricle) primarily leads to conduction disturbances, ventricular arrhythmias and finally to a clinical picture of dilatative cardiomyopathy with all the symptoms of heart insufficiency. Pulmonary hypertension can appear due to pulmonary fibrosis. There are reports that sarcoidosis of the heart is sensitive to steroids, but no certain data are available.[21]

In that sarcoidosis can also manifest itself as vasculitis of the large and small vessels (in the region of the aorta, may be confused with Takayasu's arteritis). Suspicion in pilots necessitates coronary angiography.

Sarcoidosis requires a symptom-limited stress test with normal cardiopulmonary performance measurements. There must not be any stress-induced coronary insufficiency; scintigraphy may be helpful for future comparison studies. The resting ECG shall not indicate any conduction abnormalities.

In the event of any doubt of myocardial involvement, MRI is helpful. Echocardiography must demonstrate an EF of at least 50% without any evidence of wall motion abnormalities. Coronary angiography is indicated if vasculitis or ischemia is suspected. A 24 hour ECG may not show any significant rhythm or conduction disturbances. We recommend cardiological follow-up every six months with serial ECG and Doppler echocardiograms as well as Holter monitoring. As long as complete healing is documented, restricted certification may be considered.

REFERENCES

1. Muckelbauer JK, Kremer M, Minor I, *et al.* (1995) The structure of coxsackievirus B[3] at 3.5 Å resolution. *Structure* **3**: 653–667.
2. Rückert RR, Fields BN, Minor I (eds). (1990) Picornaviridae: The viruses and their replication. In: *Virology*. Lippincott-Raven, Phildaelphia, pp. 609–654.
3. Kandolf R, Kirschner P, Ameis D, et al. (eds). (1988) Enteroviral Heart Disease: Diagnosis by *In Situ* Hybridization. New Concepts in Viral Heart Disease. Springer, Berlin, Heidelberg, New York, Tokyo, pp. 337–348.
4. Kandolf R, Kirschner P, Ameis D, *et al.* (1987) Cultured human heart cells: A model system for the study of the antiviral activity of interferons. *Eur Heart J* **8** (Suppl J): 453–456.

5. Kandolf R, Klingel K, Zell R, *et al.* (1993) Molecular pathogenesis of enterovirus-induced myocarditis: Virus persistance and chronic inflammation. *Intervirology* **35**: 140–151.
6. Peters NS, Poole-Wilson PA. (1991) Myocarditis — a controversial disease. *J R Soc Med* **84**: 1 ff.
7. Peters NS, Poole-Wilson PA. (1991) Myocarditis — continuing clinical and pathologic confusion. *Am Heart J* **121**: 942 ff.
8. Olinde KD, O'Connel JB. (1994) Inflammatory heart disease: Pathogenesis, clinical manifestations and treatment of myocarditis. *Annu Rev Med* **45**: 481 ff.
9. Ainger WH, Lorell BH. (1989) Challenge of cardiomyopathie. *J Am Coll Cardiol* **13**: 1219–1239.
10. Horowitz MS, Schultz CS, Stinson EB. (1974) Sensitivity and specificity of echocardiographic diagnosis of pericardial effusion. *Circulation* **50**: 239–247.
11. Eisenberg MJ, Oken K, Guerrero S, Saniei MA, Schiller NB. (1992) Prognostic value of echocardiography in hospitalized patients with pericardial effusion. *Am J Cardiol* **70**: 934–939.
12. Klopfenstein HS, Cogswell TL, Bernath GA, Wann LS, Tipton RK, Hoffmann RG, Brooks HL. (1985) Alterations in intravascular volume affect the relation between right ventricular diastolic collapse and the hemodynamic severity of cardiac tamponade. *J Am Coll Cardiol* **6**: 1057–1063.
13. Permanyer-Miralda G, Sagrista-Sauleda J, Soler-Soler J. (1985) Primary acute pericardial disease: A prospective series of 231 consecutive patients. *Am J Cardiol* **56**: 623–630.
14. WHO/ISFC (1996) Report of the 1995 World Health Organization/International Society and Federation of Cardiology Task Force on the definition and classification of cardiomypathies. *Circulation* **93**: 841–842.
15. Keeling PJ, Gang Y, Smith G, et al. (1995) Familial dilated cardiomyopathy in the United Kingdom. *Br Heart J* **73**: 417–421.
16. Dansky HM, Buttrick PM. (1994) Unravelling the genetic basis of dilated cardiomyopathie, *Heart Failure* **10**: 5–10.
17. Michels VV. (1993) Genetics of idopathic dilated cardiomyopathy. *Heart Failure* **9**: 87–94.

18. Kawai C, Yui Y, Hoshino T. (1983) Myocardial catecholamines in hypertrophic and dilated (congestive) cardiomyopathie: A biopsy study. *J Am Coll Cardiol* **2**: 834–840.
19. Brush JE, Eisenhofer G, Garty M. (1989) Cardiac norepinephrine kinetics in hypertrophic cardiomyopathy. *Circulation* **79**: 836–844.
20. Silverman KJ, Hutchins GM, Bulkley BH. (1978) Cardiac sarcoid: A clinicopathologic study of 84 unselected patients with systemic sarcoidosis. *Circulation* **58**: 1204–1211.
21. Shimad T, Shimada K, Sakane T, *et al.* (2001) Diagnosis of cardiac sarcoidosis and evaluation of the effects of steroid therapie by godolinium — DTPA-enhanced magnetic resonance imaging. *Am J Med* **110**: 520.

Chapter 12

Coronary Artery Disease

Ilse Janicke*

ICAO STANDARDS AND RECOMMENDED PRACTICES

The applicant shall not possess any abnormality of the heart, congenital or acquired, which is likely to interfere with the safe exercise of the applicant's licence and rating privileges. There shall be no significant functional or structural abnormality of the circulatory system.

MEDICAL REQUIREMENTS (JAR-FCL 3)

Applicants with suspected cardiac ischemia shall be investigated. Those with asymptomatic minor coronary artery disease requiring no treatment may be assessed as fit by the Aeromedical Section. A stress ECG shall be performed and, if necessary, supplemented by a radionuclide study or stress echocardiogram and/or coronary angiogram. Symptomatic coronary artery disease is disqualifying.

Class I: *Examination of serum lipids, including cholesterol, is required to facilitate risk assessment at the examination for first issue of a medical certificate, and at the first examination after the 40th birthday.*

Class II: *If two or more major risk factors (smoking, hypertension, diabetes mellitus, obesity, etc.) are present in an applicant, estimation of serum lipids and serum cholesterol is required at the examination for first issue of a medical certificate and at the first examination after the 40th birthday and on clinical indications.*

* Heart-Center Duisburg, Duisburg, Germany. E-mail: ilsejanicke@t-online.de.

Multiple risk factors shall require review, investigation, and supervision by the Aeromedical Center or Aviation Medical Examiner in conjunction with the Aeromedical Section.

DEFINITION, EPIDEMIOLOGY AND PATHOPHYSIOLOGY

Cardiovascular diseases are the most common cause of morbidity and mortality in men over 40 and women over 50 years of age in the western world. The prevalence in middle aged men is close to 2%. Coronary artery disease (CAD) is the leading cause of loss of licence in industrialized nations and is the most common cause of subtle and overt "sudden incapacitation." CAD as a manifestation of systemic atherosclerosis often overlaps with other vascular diseases of aeromedical significance such as cerebrovascular diseases, which carry an increased risk of stroke as high as 30–40% (Doppler screening required); conversely, people with peripheral arterial occlusive disease and claudication symptoms have a 40–50% risk of significant CAD.[1]

A causal relationship with CAD is probable for a number of cardiovascular risk factors. It is possible to differentiate between influenceable and non-influenceable risk factors (see Chapter 9 on Cardiovascular Risk Factors). The complex pathophysiology of CAD rests primarily on the processes of atheroma development and platelet activation with thrombosis, which are responsible for such clinical events as angina, myocardial infarction, and sudden cardiac death. Plaque formation leads either to a limitation of coronary arterial reserve and angina pectoris (large, hard plaques) or to sudden plaque rupture followed by significant cardiac events that are unrelated to the degree of underlying stenosis (soft plaques filled with lipids and with thin caps). Less common causes of non-atherosclerotic coronary artery stenosis include congenital coronary anomalies, coronary artery dissection, vasculitis (collagen-vascular disease), storage diseases, and spontaneous coronary artery thrombosis.

CLINICAL PICTURE, SYMPTOMS, AND DIFFERENTIAL DIAGNOSIS

Initial Manifestation of CAD

In 55% of cases, angina pectoris (AP) is the first symptom of CAD. In 25% myocardial infarction (MI) and in 20% sudden cardiac death is the first manifestation. Silent myocardial ischemia is common (about 30% of cases), particularly in diabetics, the elderly, and smokers. Typical angina pectoris (sudden onset; reproducible with similar intensity; mostly retrosternal, radiating pain; initiated by physical or mental stress, by cold weather or by strong wind; lasting several minutes, relieved with nitroglycerine) is due to incongruity between oxygen delivery and demand. Angina pectoris entails disqualification for all classes of medical certification, regardless of control by medication and underlying etiology such as coronary artery stenosis, aortic valve stenosis, anemia, hyperthyroidism, or fever.

CANADIAN CARDIOVASCULAR SOCIETY ANGINA SCORE (CCS)

CCS I: No angina with normal activity, occurs only with high level of continuous physical exertion.

CCS II: Slight interference with normal activity (cold weather, rapidly climbing stairs, etc.).

CCS III: Significant limitation with normal activities (donning or doffing clothing, light housework, walking 100 meters or one flight of stairs).

CCS IV: Angina with every physical movement or at rest.

Other angina equivalents are dyspnea on exertion; reduction in endurance; nocturnal angina; gastro-cardiac syndrome; walk-through angina (pain only at the start of physical activity, then disappearing); and atypical chest pain.

In typical angina, about 80–95% of men and 45–95% of women are affected by CAD.

Atypical chest pain is related to an increased CAD risk, in men 43–70% and in women 15–45%, depending on other risk factors. Consequently, coronary angiography may be necessary in pilots with a questionable cardiac diagnosis. Commercial pilots and private pilots who are passionate about flying usually present themselves as very fit with regard to their cardiac status, and are generally unwilling to disclose any cardiac symptoms. The clinical skills of the medical examiner are therefore critical.

REQUIRED EVALUATIONS IN CAD

Ischemia Cascade (Fig. 1)

Besides a careful history, the evaluation of the pilot requires a functional evaluation with standardized dynamic or pharmacological stress testing

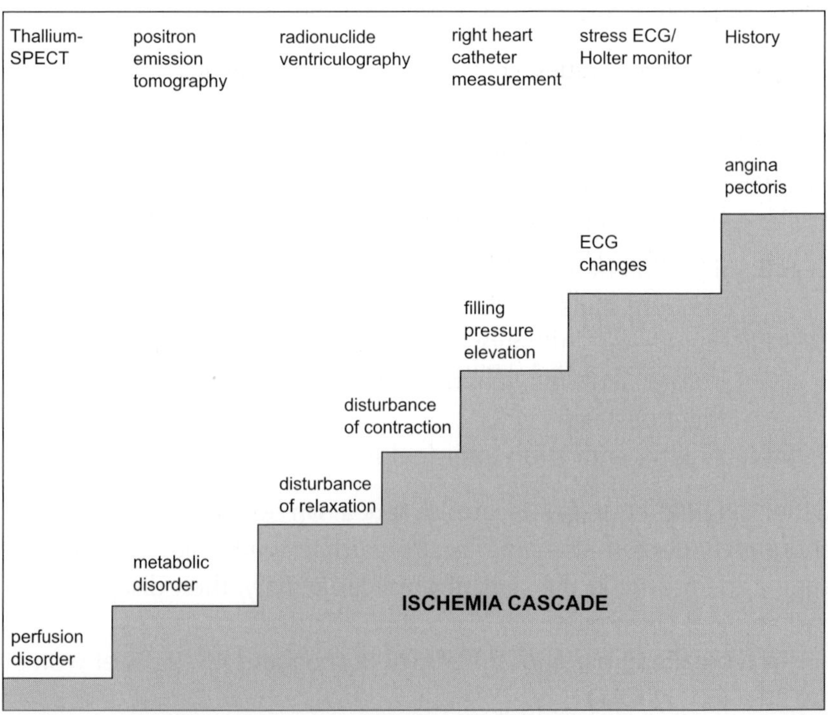

Figure 1. Ischemia cascade and position of the individual examination steps.

in order to assess hypoperfusion and reduced cardiac contractility. A better understanding is offered by the so-called "ischemia cascade": More than 50–60% of coronary artery stenosis results in perfusion homogeneity to the detriment of the post-stenotic supply area. This can be shown by perfusion scintigraphy (such as Thallium-SPECT), which is highly valuable in evaluating the prognosis. Dependence on substrate demand during physical stress leads to an increasing perfusion deficit and metabolic changes in cellular tissues, demonstrable by positron emission tomography (PET). Hemodynamically relevant stenosis (≥70%) can be determined by assessing systolic contraction defects with stress echocardiography or stress MRI. Contractile deficits involving the entire left ventricle will alter the hemodynamic function. Only at the end of the ischemic cascade do ECG changes and eventually angina pectoris symptoms develop.

Clinical Evaluation

A search for indirect clues, i.e. clinical signs that may be relevant to CAD:

- Body Mass Index = weight (kg)/height (m^2). A BMI > 27 defines over-weight, and >30 is obesity.
- Waist-to-hip ratio: abdomen to hip circumference ratio >1 in men and >0.8 in women correlates with an elevated CAD risk.
- Xanthelasmata, arcus lipoides (arcus senilis), even with normal cholesterol and young age.
- Signs of nicotine use (yellow fingertips).
- Increased blood pressure (measure both arms).
- Anemia (conjunctivae, nail beds).
- Peripheral arterial diseases: pedal pulse, vascular auscultation (bruits).
- Cardiac auscultation to determine other causes of chest pain.

Resting ECG

ICAO standards and recommended practices

Class I: *Electrocardiography shall form part of the heart examination for the first issue of a Medical Assessment. Electrocardiography should*

be included in re-examination of applicants between the ages of 30 and 50 no less frequently than every two years and thereafter annually.
Class II: *Electrocardiography should form part of the heart examination for the first issue of a Medical Assessment and at the first examination after the 40th birthday and at each aeromedical examination thereafter.*

JAR-FCL 3 certification requirements

Class I: *A standard 12-lead electrocardiogram and report are required at the examination for first issue of a medical certificate, then every five years until age 30, every two years until age 40, annually until age 50, and at all revalidation or renewal examinations thereafter and on clinical indication.*
Class II: *A standard 12-lead electrocardiogram and report are required at the examination for first issue of a medical certificate, at the first examination after the 40th birthday and at each aeromedical examination thereafter. Exercise electrocardiography is required only when clinically indicated.*

ECG: Interpretation of Normal Variants

Because resting ECG's can produce many variations that can be incorrectly interpreted as indicating organic heart disease, leading to expensive, invasive testing with negative results, the ECG with its normal variations will be described. First of all, extracardiac influences (positional changes, neurovegetative tone) may be identified as variations of normal ECG.

P wave

- In all leads, the P wave should be positive except in avR, III (possibly negative, biphasic in V1).
- Sympathetic tone: peaked P in II, III, and aVF.
- Increased vagal tone: widened P in II, III, and aVF.
- Tall in pectus excavatum.

PQ interval

- Long PQ interval >210 ms is a normal variant in sinus bradycardia and when the vagal tone is increased.
- Shortened PQ interval with sympathetic tone.

QRS complex

- Diagnostically significant deviation I, II, III, V1, V6, normal width 70–110 ms.
- In pectus excavatum QRS splitting (rsr′, rSr′-type in V1) (Fig. 2).

Q wave

- Physiological, if < ¼ of the R amplitude, usually in V4–V6.
- In III, often in left axis deviation, obesity, and diaphragmatic herniation.

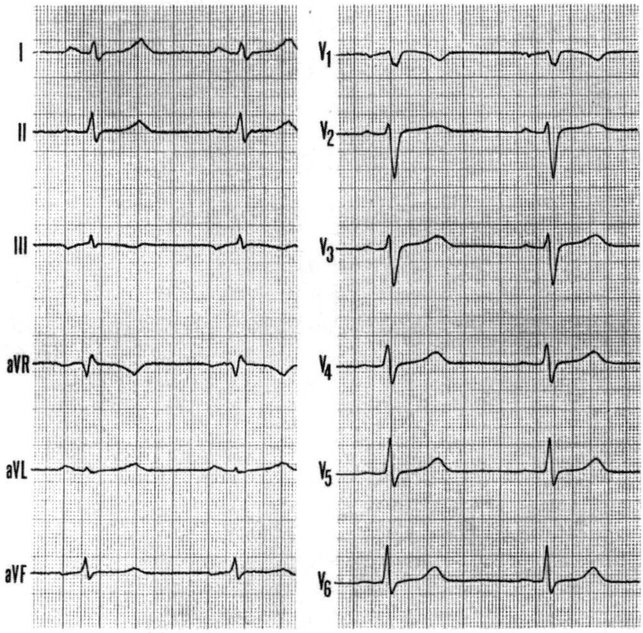

Figure 2. Pectus excavatum: Right axis deviation and indicating right bundle branch block.

- *Note:* After posterior infarction, pathologic Q waves are seen not only in III, but also in II and aVF (> ¼ R wave).
- In left axis deviation, positive deflection at inspiration and negative at expiration and vice versa. This is particularly impressive in III in incomplete left axis deviation.

R wave

- Elevated in V1: *Situs inversus,* reversal of leads (Fig. 3).
- High amplitude in V 5/6: thin person (pseudohypertrophy), athletic heart.
- Low amplitude: obesity, emphysema.

ST segment

- Duration from the end of the S wave to the beginning of the T wave. In the extremities and left precordial leads, the ST segment

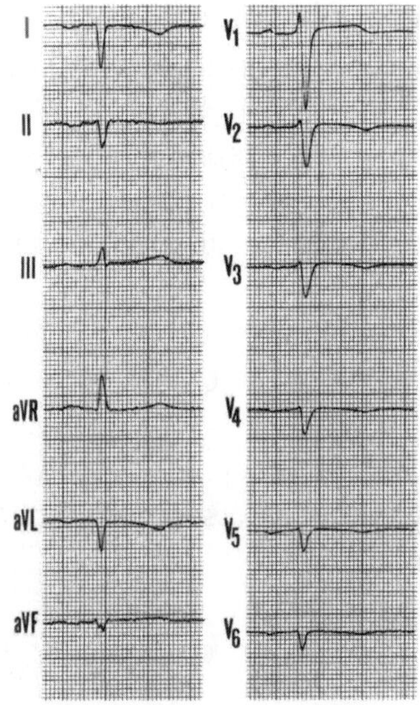

Figure 3. Situs inversus: I and aVL are mirror images, right precordial large positive deflection in contrast to normal ECG.

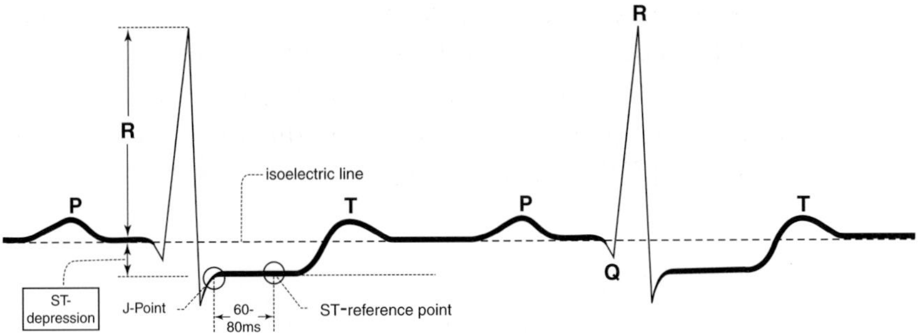

Abb. 10: Messpunkte für R-Zacke, J-Punkt, ST-Strecke. Horizontale ST-Strecken-Senkung.

Figure 4. Horizontal ST segment depression and measuring points for R waves, J point, ST segment.

is isoelectric or maximally displaced 0.1 mV from the null line (in relation to the PR segment).

- Sympathetic tone: slight ST depression, ascending progression (II, III, aVF, V4–6), J point depression (first point of ST interval behind QRS complex, Fig. 4).
- With an absent S, the ST is often elevated and concave from the drop-off from R.
- Increased vagal tone: early repolarization syndrome = ST elevation from a J point elevation in athletically trained young adults, often together with other vagal signs. Disappears with atropine (Fig. 5).
- Orthostatic reaction: ST depression, T wave flattening, or vacillating T wave: negative while standing, normal when supine (delayed counter regulation after change to vertical position).
- Hypokalemia: minimal ST depression, negative/biphasic T wave.
- Tachycardia: Very high T waves with J point elevation or ascending ST depression are possible (Fig. 6).

T wave

- Normally positive, in concordance with QRS deflection except in III, possibly very variable. In V1, the T wave may be negative,

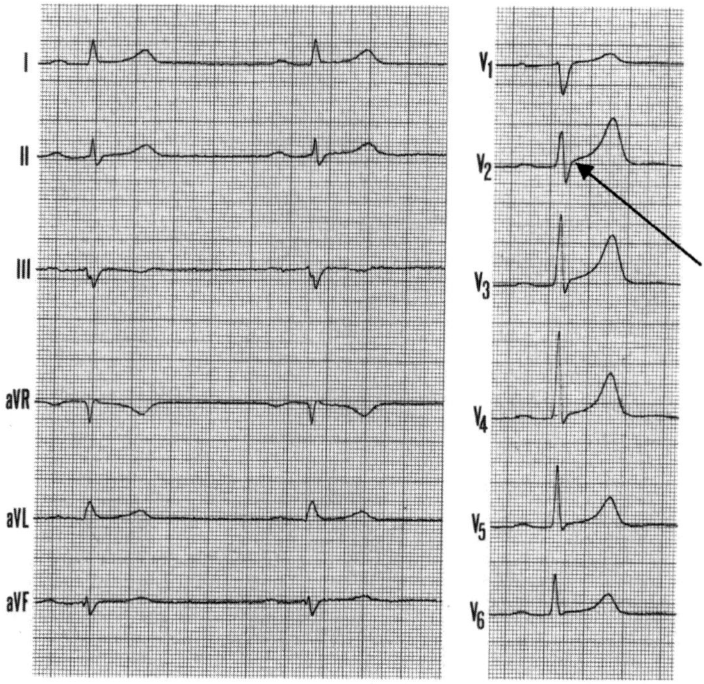

Figure 5. J-point and ST-elevation, bradycardia.

isoelectric, biphasic, or positive; this is also the case in V2 in healthy adults up to age 25. In women, occasionally negative T wave in V1/2 until age 35.

- Increased vagal tone: high broad T wave (in almost all leads), occasionally slight ST elevations.
- Sympathetic tone: T wave flattening, isoelectric or preterminal negative T.
- Immediately after eating: in V2–V5 a flat or flat-negative T wave, normal while fasting and after ingestion of KCl.

U wave

- If present, the U wave is seen after the T wave with same polarity as the T wave; the U wave is positive in II and V3/4.

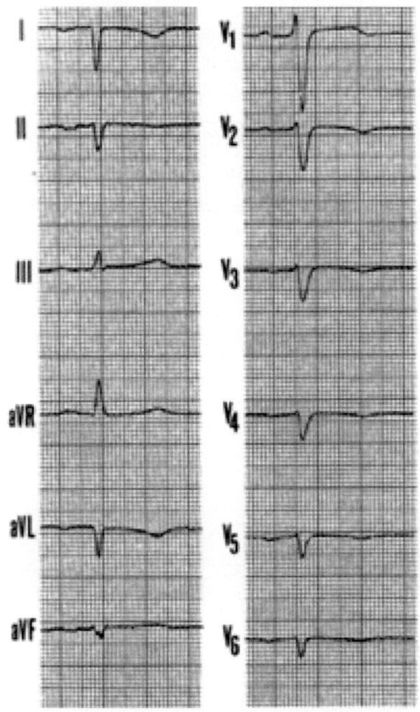

Figure 6. Sinus tachycardia (150/min) in hyperthyroidism.

- U waves occur in hypokalemia and when the vagal tone is increased (Fig. 7).

QT interval

The QT interval is measured from the beginning of the Q wave to the end of the T wave; it is frequency dependent, therefore a QT interval correction is calculated according to the Bazett formula: QTc = uncorrected QT/√RR. Normal: 350–430 ms. It is important to estimate the risk of arrythmogenic events and not to disregard antiarrhythmic therapy.

Except in case of organic heart disease, most sympathetic and parasympathetic effects on the resting ECG disappear at rest, after beta-blockade or on small doses of atropine. Tachycardia may cause even the experienced clinician some difficulty, in that the ST-T segment can demonstrate significant changes based on purely sympathetic tone, from which conclusions about pathological effects

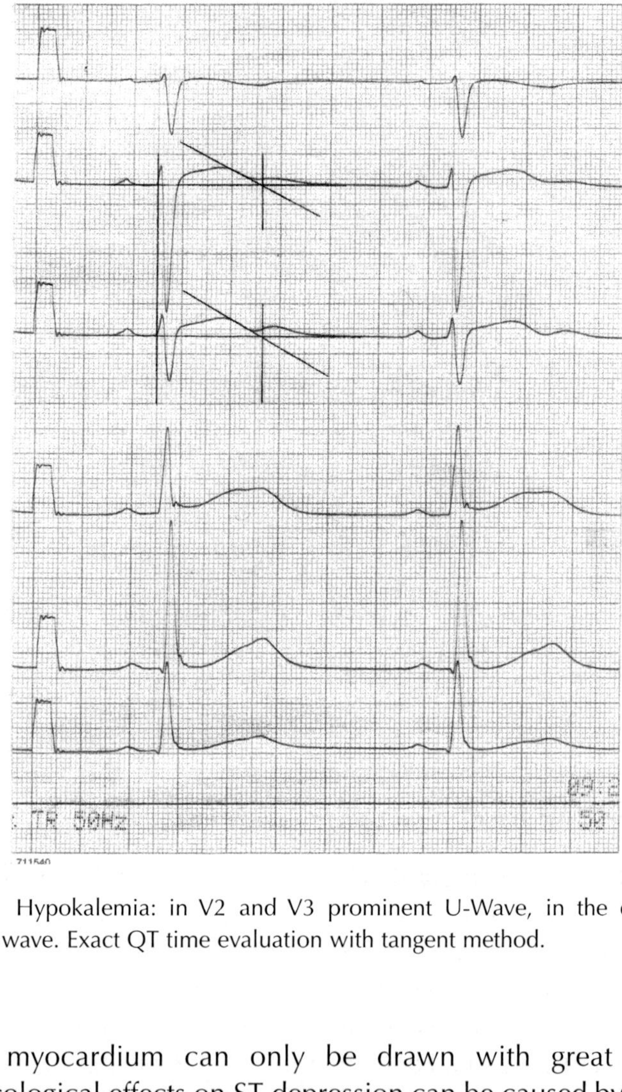

Figure 7. Hypokalemia: in V2 and V3 prominent U-Wave, in the other leads TU fusion wave. Exact QT time evaluation with tangent method.

on the myocardium can only be drawn with great caution. Pharmacological effects on ST depression can be caused by digitalis, antiarrhythmic, antidepressive, and cytostatic agents.

The resting ECG will show changes in 2–3% of asymptomatic male pilots, most commonly affecting the ST segment and the T wave. They have little predictive value with regard to CAD, but nonetheless increase with increasing age and the number of risk factors. In order to clarify such resting ECG changes, or in case of clinical signs of CAD, stress ECG and, if necessary, further cardiological investigation should be undertaken.

STRESS TESTING

Stress ECG

ICAO Standards and Recommended Practices: *For guidance on exercise electrocardiography, see Manual of Civil Aviation Medicine, Part III. Medical Assessment. DOC 8984.*

JAR-FLC 3 Certification Requirements: *Exercise electrocardiography (symptom-limiting, 12-channel ECG to Bruce Stage IV or equivalent loading) shall be required:*

(1) *when indicated by signs or symptoms suggestive of cardiovascular disease;*
(2) *for clarification of a resting electrocardiogram;*
(3) *at the discretion of an aeromedical specialist acceptable to the AMS;*
(4) *at age 65 and then every four years for Class 1 (revalidation or renewal).*

Indication and Predictive Value

Stress testing serves to clarify CAD and the course/therapy of hypertension, coronary insufficiency, valve disease, and pulmonary disease. Because of its low specificity (true negative results over total number without the disease) of only 90%, it is not useful as a general screening tool for asymptomatic individuals under the age of 40 without risk factors. For this group, the stress ECG is false positive in 10% of males and 30% of females. From a cardiological perspective, exceptions include those individuals for whom their occupations in principle present a risk to others, such as airline pilots.

Consideration of the benefit to the pilot and consequential safety issues must be carefully weighed against the risk of an unjustified disqualification resulting in loss of licence and livelihood.

The indication for stress testing should be liberally applied by the medical examiner, especially to those pilots who are over 40 years of age and have atherosclerotic risk profiles. For the majority of asymptomatic older pilots >50 years without risk factors, no further diagnostic evaluation is required if the maximal stress testing is negative. The prognosis in those cases regarding the underlying coronary artery anatomy is good.

The ST segment of the stress ECG is not useful as a solitary discriminating tool for pilot certification, due to its limited specificity. Only with consideration of individual pre-testing probability for CAD (age, gender, symptoms, risk factors, etc.) does the predictive value of stress testing become diagnostically helpful. The predictive value is greatest when pre-test probability lies in the range of 30–70% (Bayes' theorem). The stress ECG provides some diagnostic help in men >40 years with atypical angina and in women with atypical angina >55 years. In higher risk groups (men over 40 with typical angina), stress ECG provides little further diagnostic advantage as 90% have angiographically relevant CAD but does provide information regarding localization and severity.

The sensitivity (true positive results over total number with the disease) of stress ECG depends on the extent of the CAD. Most often stress ECG is positive in three vessel disease or main stem stenosis of 90%, whereas it is negative in 50% of cases with single vessel disease. The greater the ST segment depression, the greater the likelihood of multi-vessel disease.

If an ST segment depression is determined on stress ECG, there are two possibilities:

- It might be a false positive that must be clarified.
- It might be a true positive, and the risk of future cardiac events must be determined through further diagnostic evaluation.

Indications of imminent cardiac events include limited performance (<75 W), angina pectoris during stress testing, ST depression >0.2 mV at low inclines, sustained ST depression in the recovery phase, poor blood pressure response >130 mmHg such as drop in blood pressure, ST elevations with stress load, and complex ventricular arrhythmias.

Technical Application

In the United States, standardized stress testing within aviation medicine is carried out by means of a treadmill and following the Bruce protocol (with stepwise increase in treadmill speed and inclination). In Europe, seated or semi-reclining bicycle ergometry is primarily utilized (Table 1). For comparison of treadmill test with bicycle ergometry, the conversion factor of metabolic equivalent (MET) is used. This comprises a linear relationship between load and O_2-uptake. 1 MET = O_2 uptake of 3.5 mL/min/kg body weight.

Required Precautions

- Contraindications and termination procedures should be well known and emergency equipment must be available.
- Anti-ischemia medication should be discontinued (nitroglycerine 24 h, Ca-antagonists 24 h, beta-blockers three days, and digoxin/digitoxin 10–21 days) prior to testing.

Table 1. Comparison of Treadmill and Bicycle Stress Testing

Treadmill	Bicycle
Shorter protocol duration	Longer protocol duration
Running is a physiologic loading method	Economic, steady
Better cardiovascular load through use of larger muscle mass	
Better detection of ischemia in obesity	Sitting does not stress muscle adequately in obesity
Worse recording of blood pressure and ECG	Better recording of blood pressure and ECG

- Five-minute rest period, at room temperature of 18–22°C, prior to testing.
- Nothing per os two hours prior to testing.

ECG Procedure: 12-lead ECG (according to Mason and Likar) is recommended. Application of the limb leads on the trunk will minimize movement artifacts. Good contact requires removal of hair and application of skin emollient; suction electrodes are best. Continuous recording of six leads with brief switching to the remaining leads. The chest leads are of greatest importance, with lead V5 having the highest accuracy. The sensitivity of stress testing can be increased by use of additional right precordial leads.[2]

Cardiovascular Load

Step-wise increase in workload until symptom-limited maximal peak load is attained with demonstrable exhaustion ($W_{max.}$ = max. O_2-consumption $V_{O_2max.}$), but no more than 15 minutes in order to avoid premature muscle fatigue. Blood pressure, heart rate, and ECG recording during the last 30 seconds of each load increase.

Rule of Thumb for Maximal Performance

Men (20–30 years of age): Maximal performance 3 W/kg, 10% reduction per decade of life.
Women (20–30 years of age): Maximal performance 2.5 W/kg, 8% reduction per decade of life.

With obesity, there is a corresponding reduction in performance. Clinical endpoint of maximal symptomatic performance (heart rate = 220 – age in years) are fatigue, angina pectoris, muscle pain, or objective findings such as ST depression and blood pressure elevation. The higher the work load, the greater the likelihood of discovering discrete circulatory compromise. In pilots, maximal performance should normally be reached. ECG changes are quite common in the recovery phase, which should continue for at least six minutes.

Table 2. Treadmill Test Following the Bruce Protocol

Stage	Speed (km/h)	Incline (%)	Length (min)	Workload (MET)
1	2,75	10	3	5
2	4,0	12	3	7
3	5,5	14	3	10
4	6,75	16	3	13
5	8,0	18	3	16
6	8,85	20	3	
7	9,65	22	3	

Table 3. Standardized Bicycle Stress Test

Prephase	5 min
Initial stage	50–75 W (4, 0–5, 0 MET)
Length of time at each stage	2 min
Increase of load at each stage	50 W, at higher work loads 25 W
Total duration	At least 6 min, 3 stages, maximally 12–15 minutes
Max. symptomatic load	HF_{max} = 220 — Age (years) (8, 5–11 MET)
Recovery phase	6 min

Differentiation Criteria

What changes are normally seen during stress testing?

P wave	Becomes wider and amplitude increases, but vector remains the same
PR interval	Slight delay
R wave	Amplitude advances to left precordial
QRS duration	No change
S wave	Negative amplitude (right precordial) increases, terminal QRS vector rotates to the right and upward
J point	Depression to 0.1 mV
ST segment	Rapidly increasing depression
T wave	Flattening, often to the isoelectric line

Evaluation of the ST Segment

Two points are analyzed: the J point and a second measurement point 60–80 ms later.

The ST segment ascends when the J point is depressed greater than the second measurement point, and descends when the opposite occurs as the J point is only slightly depressed and the second measurement point is strongly depressed (Fig. 4).

Evaluation of ischemia

- Depression of the second measuring point of at least 0.1 mV with horizontal or descending progression: chest leads 0.1–0.2 mV, limb leads 0.05–0.1 mV, at least three complexes in a row (Fig. 8).
- With small R amplitudes, an ST depression of 0.05 mV is pathological. At high R amplitudes, ST depression is pathological only above 0.1 mV.
- Slow ascending ST depression with depression of the second measurement point of at least 0.2 mV indicates in 1/3 of cases that CAD exists. Critical review, in ischemia mostly are found in adjacent leads horizontal/descending ST depression (Fig. 9).
- J point depression of more than 0.2 mV is probably pathological.
- In women, pathological findings are often false positive, and the limit for ischemia can be 0.2 mV.
- ST elevation >0.1 mV is certainly pathological. If there is no prior infarct, an ST elevation is due to proximal stenosis or coronary artery spasm. After myocardial infarct, an ST elevation indicates segmental wall motion disorder such as an aneurysm.
- In 20% of cases, CAD exists with increase of ST-T changes from rest (toward positive and negative) and non-specific T-wave changes.[3]
- In young asymptomatic individuals, a positive change of a negative T wave can be interpreted as sympathetic tone.
- Previous ST-T wave changes, for example in hypertrophy, bundle branch block or pre-excitation syndrome, are not predictive of CAD.

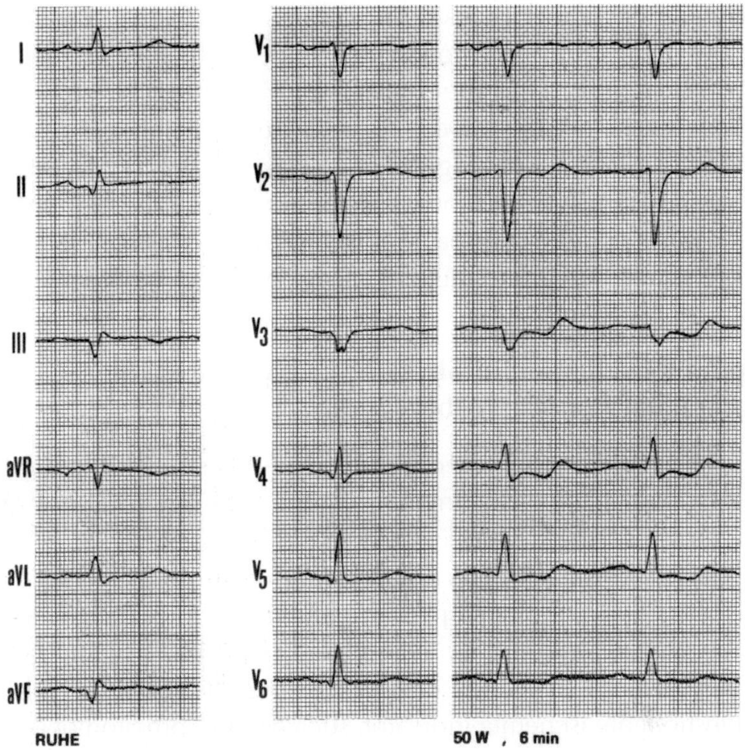

Figure 8. Inferior wall scar and ischemic ST depression of V3–V6 of 0.2m at 50 Watt.

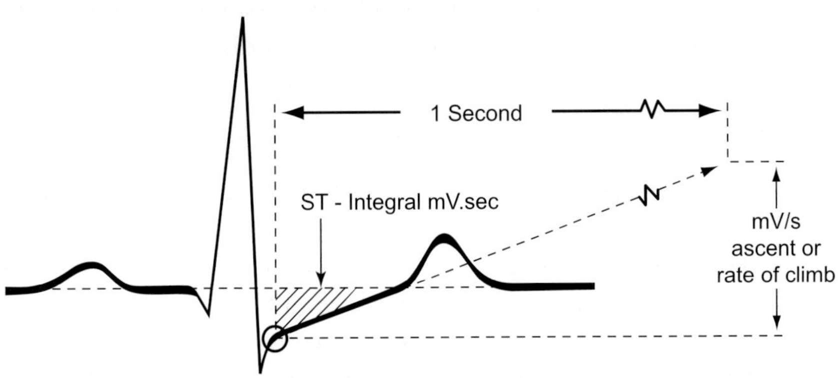

Figure 9. Slow ascension of ST depression.

- Left bundle branch block (LBBB) under stress testing is prognostically unfavorable. Although not necessarily typical for CAD, LBBB can indicate a rate-induced bundle branch block.
- Appearance of a negative U wave or negative changes of a positive U wave are pathological.
- Typical ST depression four to six minutes after the beginning of stress testing, as a late reaction, is often an expression of a severe three-vessel CAD and must be taken seriously.

Simplified Evaluation of Stress Testing with Regard to Individual Pre-test Probabilities

1. Confirmed coronary artery insufficiency on stress testing if there is typical or atypical angina pectoris and development of ST depression >0.1 mV.
2. Probable coronary artery insufficiency on stress testing if there is ST depression or angina pectoris; angina pectoris and ST depression with hypertrophy or left bundle branch block.
3. Possible coronary artery disease on stress testing if there is one questionable ischemia indicator, such as ST depression of 0.3 mV on digitalis.
4. Unlikely coronary artery insufficiency on stress testing if there is ST depression of 0.1 mV on digitalis without symptoms. Questionable symptoms of angina pectoris.
5. No coronary artery insufficiency on stress testing if there is no ST depression and no angina pectoris with exertion.

Misinterpretation of Stress ECG (False Positive)

ST depression without CAD may be seen as a consequence of

— Hyperventilation, resting tachycardia.
— Effect of medication: digitalis, diuretics, antiarrhythmics, α-methyldopa, tricyclic antidepressants.
— Myxedema, hypoxia, hyperglycemia, hypokalemia, anemia.

— Hypertension-induced LVH, pre-excitation syndromes, syndrome X.
— Mitral valve prolapse, high-grade mitral valve insufficiency.
— Hemodynamically significant organic heart defect.

In order to differentiate false positive from true positive results, a repeat evaluation should be undertaken after sublingual nitroglycerine; if the changes disappear, the pilot must undergo further cardiological evaluation before medical certifcation can be considered.

Computerized Analysis of Stress ECG

Those who do not regularly read stress ECG tracings may be well advised to rely on computer analysis. The ECG recording is converted by a particular algorithm into numerical values. The measurement point (J point and a point 60–80 ms afterwards) must be correctly pre-assessed and marked.

Advantage: Certain artifacts (such as baseline shift, and 50/60 Hz cycle interference) are corrected electronically. Disadvantage: In case of signal perturbations, inaccurate analysis can occur.

Stress Testing After Myocardial Infarct

After six months, with the assistance of the cardiologist, the AME should arrange a stress testing in order to advise the pilot whether it is reasonable to initiate the strenuous and expensive certification process regarding special issuance ("waiver"). In order not to overlook potential problems, stress testing should be performed without anti-arrhythmic or anti-anginal medications.

Goals

(1) identification of ischemia, exercise-induced coronary insufficiency, and load performances.

(2) identification of patients with unfavorable prognosis, risk evaluation.
(3) identification of arrhythmia tendency (particularly polymorphic ventricular extrasystoles, couplets, salvos), repeat stress testing without beta blockade.

Assessment

- Inadequate/absent blood pressure response (<50 mmHg), inadequate heart rate increase, dyspnea, sweating, and pallor correlate with a poor prognosis (warning signs!).
- Ischemic reaction should be assessed only in leads without infarct-related QRS, ST and T wave changes.
- Following posterior wall infarct, stress testing has a high predictive value for ischemia in the anterior wall; the reverse case of ischemia detection on stress testing following anterior infarct is less predictive.
- ST elevations or T wave inversions in the area of prior infarct are not a sign of coronary insufficiency, but rather a consequence of wall motion disturbance (such as dyskinesis indicating a large infarct area).
- When still evident two months post infarction, stress-induced ST elevations are prognostically unfavorable signs carrying an annual mortality rate of about 8%.[4]
- ST depression on stress testing after infarction carries an even worse prognosis.

In questionable cases, myocardial scintigraphy or stress echocardiography is indicated.

Stress Testing after Myocardial Infarct

Symptom-limited stress testing without medications should take place six months after coronary by-pass surgery; prior to that, ECG changes due to surgery could still be present, and exercise performance may not yet be maximal. Subsequently, annual stress testing should be performed as well.

Goals

Evaluation of functional results and exercise performance after surgery. Evaluation of risk of cardinal events ("sudden incapacitation").

Assessment

- Stress testing should be normal.
- Pathological results signify incomplete or unsuccessful revascularization (sensitivity 90%).
- Isolated ST depression of 0.1–0.2 mV without symptoms and arrhythmia at maximal load should be followed up with coronary arteriography (by-pass restenosis usually occurs within the first three months) but may be compatible with restricted certification.
- If there are no symptoms, mildly positive postoperative stress testing results (in contrast to strongly positive preoperative results), associated with inconspicuous findings on further non-invasive tests may not require a second coronary arteriogram.

Stress Testing after Coronary Angioplasty (PCI/Stent)

Stress testing should be performed six months after intervention as most re-stenosis occurs within the first six months; stress testing in the first few weeks following angioplasty is often false positive.

Goals

Evaluation of therapeutic intervention.

Assessment

- Detection of restenosis should normally be determined by maximal symptom-limited stress testing.

- Positive predictive values of restenosis are relatively rare (33%), sensitivity and specificity are only about 60% (better with scintigraphy or stress echocardiography).
- Comparison of pre- and post angioplasty stress testing results.
- A slight ST depression of 0.1–0.2 mV does not necessarily mean restenosis; pilots should, however, undergo a secondary coronary arteriography in order to assess fitness for flight.

Prognostic Evaluation

The value of stress testing in predicting sudden incapacitation is not high. Nonetheless, stress testing allows determination of subgroups with less than 1% risk of cardiac events. If there are no risk factors and age-appropriate maximal stress testing provides negative results, the coronary event rate is 0.2 to 0.4% per year. Repeated positive stress testing results together with cardiovascular risk factors carry a coronary event rate of >5% per year[9] (based on examination of 4015 asymptomatic healthy males at age 45). If an additional negative chronotropic reaction occurs, the prognosis is less favorable. A good understanding of stress ECG testing analysis and ability to distinguish between normal and abnormal is a prerequisite for the medical examiner and a sine qua non for a high quality evaluation, the aim of which is to protect the health of the pilot, to determine the risk of future cardiac events as well as to limit unnecessary testing.

Stress Echocardiography

Predictive value

In case of ambiguous medical history, inconclusive stress testing, or suspected CAD, and especially if the pre-test probability is intermediate (e.g. males with atypical angina pectoris and normal stress testing; men without angina pectoris with pathological stress testing; and women with typical angina pectoris and normal stress testing), the non-invasive, non-radionuclide stress echocardiography has a significantly greater sensitivity and specificity (each about 85%) in diagnosing CAD than stress ECG testing. The value of stress echocardiography in precise risk stratification and prognostication has been proven[6–8] and has particular importance within the field of aviation medicine.

In case of stress-induced ischemia (at least 70% stenosis), where new regional wall motion disturbances (hypokinesis, akinesis, dyskinesis) are evident, the target coronary vessel is likely to be the site of the culprit lesion. The absence of stress-induced wall motion disturbances largely rules out myocardial ischemia but not necessarily an underlying coronary artery disease.

In occupational groups with particularly high safety requirements such as airline pilots, the entire coronary morphology must be understood. When referring a pilot for stress echocardiography, the medical examiner should be aware that the predictive value of the method used is dependent to no small degree on the particular skill and experience of the evaluator.

Indications

- **CAD primary diagnosis:** Ischemia screening with known CAD (degree of stenosis? localization?)
- **Ambiguous stress ECG results:** Positive, without symptoms; with hypertension; digitalis; after PCI/CABG. Negative with symptoms; with bundle branch block, WPW, pacemaker.
- **Risk factor stratification after myocardial infarction:** Exercise-induced wall motion disorders represent an appreciable risk of cardiac event and may entail permanent disqualification if revascularization is not possible.

  Evaluation of ejection fraction (<50% is disqualifying) and an ischemia-induced valvular dysfunction (e.g. mitral valve insufficiency).
- **Functional results after intervention, CABG surgery:** Examination after six months provides information regarding medium-term success of revascularization, best compared with pre-operative stress echocardiography. Functional coronary diagnosis has

a higher prognostic value, so that medical certification can be based on an optimal examination without need of post-operative angiography.

- **Tissue viability** before surgery or intervention (no benefit of revascularising a scar).
- **Prognostication:** It is possible to differentiate between patients with low and high risk by stress echocardiography. Patients with typical or atypical angina pectoris symptoms and pathological treadmill have a good prognosis if the stress echocardiography is unremarkable.

Technical Procedure

Emergency equipment, termination procedures, and contraindications are similar to stress testing; method-specific termination includes new wall-motion disturbances in a minimum of two adjacent segments.

During stress testing, a continuing left-sided transthoracic echocardiography (video documentation) is performed, along with continual ECG and blood pressure monitoring.

By way of computer assisted synchronized imaging and by comparing images at rest with images during exercise (special computer program with a multi-screen monitor "quad screen" format), a direct comparison of segmental contraction of the left ventricle can be accomplished during and after stress testing. The entire time required for preparation, examination, and post-testing observation is in the order of one hour.

Proper examination can proceed if (a) patient information is available 24 hours prior to the test, (b) no anti-anginal medications are used, and (c) beta-blockers are withheld for 48 hrs. Any use of stress medications should be noted.

Whether a patient should be physically or pharmacologically stress tested is determined by the clinical symptoms and the problems to be addressed. Dynamic stress testing is accomplished on a bicycle ergometer with left lateral application of the echo transducer. There are disadvantages of monitoring during physiological stress testing: motion artifact diminishes the quality of the echo signal so that images of very short lived ischemia may be lost. Consequently, pharmacological stress testing has been standardized for pilots, preferably with use of dobutamine, dipyridamol, or adenosine. While dipyridamol and adenosine produce ischemia via the "steal effect," dobutamine is used in low doses to increase heart rate via the cardiac beta-1 receptors. It can be titrated up to 40 μg/kg/min or to the onset of elevated heart rate, blood pressure and myocardial O_2 demand so that schemia, if present, will be visible. The effect of dobutamine is quickly blocked by i.v. beta-blockade, and that of dipyridamol/adenosine by theophylline.

Side Effects

The bicycle stress echocardiogram is favored in cardiology practice as a rapid, low risk procedure. The limitations of these examinations should not be underestimated. Pharmacological stress testing

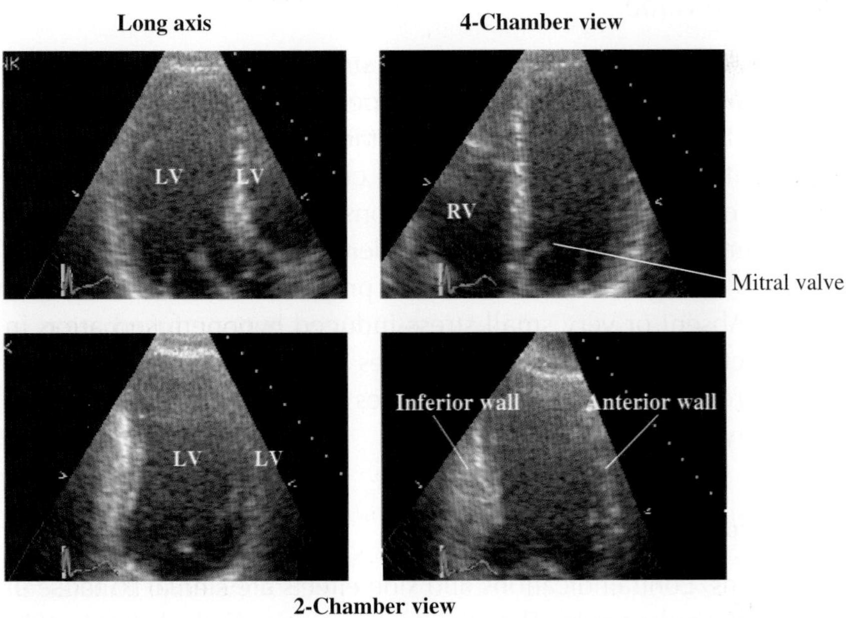

Figure 10. Stress echo-four view format.

with dipyridamol/adenosine often has slight side effects such as thoracic complaints, headache, dizziness, etc., frequently necessitating termination of the examination before the target heart rate has been attained, while with dobutamine, the target heart rate and loading is usually achieved. Serious side effects (couplets, non-sustained VT, atrial fibrillation) are rare and usually only appear in high dosage protocols. They disappear within minutes after beta-blocker infusion.

Even though these pharmacological stress echocardiography techniques are relatively safe methods of examination with a satisfactory side effect profile, they should be used exclusively by experienced cardiology clinics/practices, where resuscitation is possible and serious cardiac complications can be well managed.

NUCLEAR MEDICINE PROCEDURES

Myocardial Scintigraphy

Predictive value

Another objective and non-invasive stress test, myocardial perfusion scintigraphy, utilizes radioisotopes and has been used since the 1970's. After i.v. injection of a radioactive material that distributes itself through the myocardial circulation, coronary arterial stenosis of 50% or more can be demonstrated even before it results in ischemia and contractile disorders (see ischemia cascade). The test is highly valuable in the prediction of future cardiac events. Absent or very small stress-induced hypoperfused areas in good picture quality carry event rates under 1%, whereas pathological results leading to event rates up to 7.4% annually are disqualifying.[9,10]

Indications

Indications, contraindications and side effects are similar to those of stress echocardiography. The rate of false positive findings (up to 30%

in women) should be taken into consideration. Scintigraphy is not of predictive value with:

1. Left bundle branch block
2. Pacemaker
3. Pre-excitation syndrome (WPW)
4. Dilated/hypertrophic cardiomyopathy
5. Coronary microangiopathy from diabetes
6. Morbid obesity/large breasts (inferior ischemia artifact).

Technical procedure

Maximal dynamic or pharmacological stress testing (with dobutamine, dipyridamol or adenosine) is carried out after at least four hours of fasting and after discontinuation of all anti-anginal medications. Shortly before stress testing, a radioisotope (thallium-201chloride, Tc-99m-MIBI or tetrofosmine) is injected. It is rapidly absorbed into the myocardium, reaching saturation within minutes and allowing for imaging of the hypoperfused areas for the next 15–30 minutes. The myocardial distribution of the radioisotope is recorded by single photon emission tomography (SPECT) or, less commonly, with the much more expensive positron emission tomography (PET). It is triggered by ECG recordings, and tracer distribution is shown in cross sections according to the standard heart axes.

The stress recordings are compared with the resting images over similar timeframes and in comparable cross sections. The images can be produced in black and white or in color. Color looks very nice but perfusion homogeneity can be over-interpreted by excessive contrast.

Critical interpretation

- No evidence for fixed or reversible ischemia = normal finding.
- Fixed perfusion defect under stress and at rest = myocardial scar, may be compatible with medical certification in certain circumstances.

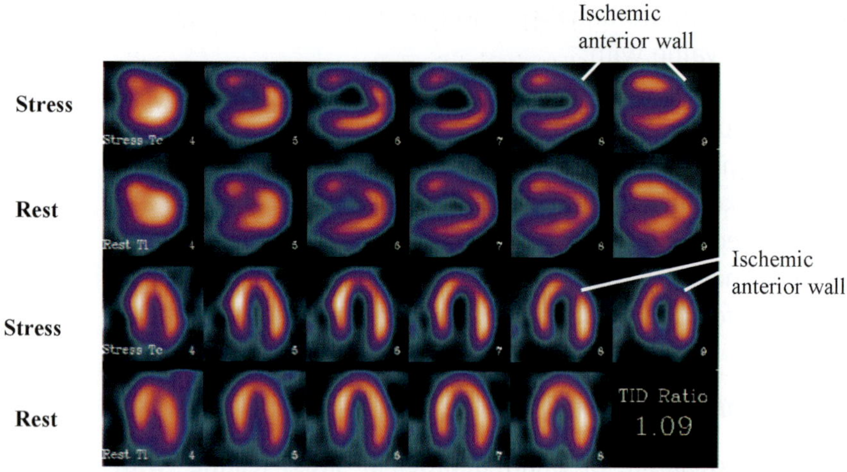

Figure 11. Technetium SPECT myocardial scintigraphy: Reversible perfusion defect in anterior wall and apex.

- Reversible perfusion defect = adequate perfusion at rest, inadequate under load. Not compatible with medical certification as the myocardium is at risk and electrical instability may develop (Fig. 11).
- Ambiguous results are often due to a diaphragmatic artifact, which appears as non-homogenous perfusion, and require further evaluation.

Prognostication

On the basis of numerous and in some cases very large studies, myocardial scintigraphy plays an important prognostic role in many cases of CAD. The number and expansion of reversible perfusion defects, transient left ventricular dilatation, and left ventricular ejection fraction influence future cardiac events. The diagnostic predictive value follows Bayes' theorem.

- *Asymptomatic individuals*

If stress testing and nuclear studies are negative, the annual incidence of angina, infarction, and death are less than 1%. If stress testing is positive and the nuclear study is negative, the annual incidence of angina rises to 1.8%, while significant cardiac events remain at less than 1%. If both studies are abnormal, the annual incidence of coronary events is between 2 and 6%. Pilots whose profile indicates a substantial risk of CAD should undergo coronary angiography.

- *Assumed or known CAD*

If stress testing and scintigraphy are normal, the annual incidence of infarction and death is 0.8%; if both tests are abnormal, it increases to well over 1%. On the basis of a meta-analysis of six studies between 1989 and 1994, an annual event rate of only 0.9% was found with known mild CAD disease, provided maximal stress scintigraphy was normal. This correlates with the general population.

- *Scintigraphy after infarction*

With perfusion scintigraphy it is possible to differentiate persons with high risk of cardiac events from those with low risk. The mortality rate is 0% in one year and 1% in two years in cases with small completed infarction, fixed perfusion defect, and with an ejection fraction >50%. This is compatible with the 1% rule. The mortality rate is 2% in case of reversible perfusion defect which thus is not compatible with the 1% rule.

- *Scintigraphy after myocardial revascularization (PCI/CABG)*

Scintigraphy in this situation can be ambiguous. In general, it is valid: in the case of no reversible perfusion defects, the rate of relevant cardiac events is less than 1% per year. There are studies, however, that show the annual rate of infarct or death to be about 1.5% despite normal scintigraphy after infarct.[8] This method should not solely be used to estimate prognosis.

- *Prognostic value of different tests in combination*

Scintigraphy and stress echocardiography provide complementary information for prognostication that is vital in the context of aviation. The combination of clinical parameters, stress testing, scintigraphy, and coronary angiography unambiguously increases the prognostic predictive value in a stepwise fashion. The value of myocardial scintigraphy additional to gender and stress testing is actually higher than that of coronary angiography.[11] After a myocardial infarct, however, other evaluations are required to estimate the prognosis.

- *How often shall pilots undergo scintigraphy?*

Coronary atheromas can develop differently over time. The recommendation for pilots is as described in (Ref. 9): persons without risk factors for CAD and without a history of revascularization should undergo scintigraphy every two years. In the case of cardiovascular risk factors or a history of revascularization, annual scintigraphy is recommended. If the findings change, coronary angiography is indicated.

Positron Emission Tomography (PET)

Positron emission tomography is the best nuclear medical procedure for imaging the function and pathophysiology/pathobiochemistry on a molecular basis. With the assistance of specific perfusion markers (positron emission), the diagnosis of ischemia by means of pharmacological stress testing is of higher accuracy than that provided by stress echocardiogram or SPECT scintigraphy. The metabolism marker of F-18 FDG-glucose can differentiate between the metabolic activity of the heart muscle and scarred yocardium (in the past, the gold standard in the evaluation of vital tissue). An elective revascularization only results in an improvement of cardiac function if performed on vital myocardial tissues. Due to high costs, logistical problems and limited availability (of the positron emission device), and the increased establishment of cardiac MRI centers, PET is not routinely used for diagnosis of cardiac ischemia.

Magnetic Resonance Imaging (MRI) with Stress

In the1970's, the first magnetic resonance images of the human anatomy were made, utilizing the special nuclear characteristics of the electron spin of hydrogen following radiofrequency irradiation. In recent years, cardiac MRI has become a complimentary procedure to echocardiography in the assessment of the morphological and functional characteristics necessary to diagnose illnesses of the heart and the great vessels.

On the basis of rapid image sequencing, brief measurement intervals and rapid resolution, moving organs such as the heart can be pictorially represented. Advantages over echocardiography are better picture quality, reproducibility, and the capability to measure wall thickness changes.

Indications

Assessment of the essential global functional parameters and calculations of right and left ventricular volume parameters as well as cardiac output. Cardiac MRI (CMRI) has become the gold standard for the evaluation of left ventricular function in CAD and the cardiomyopathies. For pilots, this is of particular importance, as they need a minimum of 50% ejection fraction for certification.

For the prediction of flow-limiting coronary artery stenosis, there are two CMRI possibilities: 1) Dobutamine or adenosine-stress MRI with analysis of any new appearances of regional contractile disturbances. This is a technique that can also be used in those who are difficult to evaluate by echocardiography (sensitivity and specificity 85–90%).[12] 2) The second non-invasive method is MR first-pass-perfusion imaging, with sequence at rest and during infusion of adenosine. An i.v. bolus of an MR-contrast medium (gadolinium-DTPA) is given at rest followed by pharmacological stress testing over 60–80 cardiac cycles (sensitivity 87–90% and specificity about 85%).

MR first-pass-perfusion imaging can be considered a clinical standard for non-invasive evaluation of coronary artery stenosis.

Cardiac MRI has replaced PET as the gold standard for viability testing due to the "late enhancement effect," where extracellular MR medium concentrates in the enlarged interstitial areas in necrotic myocardial tissue.

Technical requirements

A magnetic strength of 1.5 tesla (3.0 tesla in clinical trials), a special gradient system, and special software are required for cardiac assessment. Indispensable prerequisites for cardiac MRI is the triggering ECG. Adequate evaluation and, in particular, the implementation of the stress test are only possible when radiologists and cardiologists work together. During stress testing, the necessary emergency equipment must be MR compatible and immediately available.

Current disadvantages and pitfalls of CMRI

All CMRI examinations must be accomplished during breath holding. Problems include artifacts from breathing, the need of an ECG trigger, and patient movements. The handling of possible complications, occurring while the patient is in the MRI "tube," can give rise to problems. Comparison of a particular plane at rest and under stress can result in an erroneous accordance of the planar position, as when the heart shortens under stress loading. A significant disadvantage is that CMRI is not yet performed in real time. Contraindications include pacemakers and defibrillators, ferromagnetic metallic implants, and some heart valve prostheses.

With regard to cardiac evaluation, rapid MRI has been developed with the goal of becoming a "one-stop-shop," in that the morphology (coronary or by-pass stenosis, plaque morphology) as well as the main functional aspects (segmental wall thickness, wall thickness changes during stress loading, evaluation of perfusion, and metabolism of the myocardium) can be depicted with a single MRI examination. This will be meaningful to pilots, because early diagnosis of CAD and evaluation of therapeutic modalities can be accomplished without need of further invasive or non-invasive diagnostic endeavors.

Diagnostic Coronary Imaging

Great strides have been made during the last decades in the field of non-invasive coronary diagnostics. Despite statements to the contrary, frequently encountered in the lay press, no method can currently replace coronary arteriography as the gold standard for CAD diagnosis. For pilots with risk factors, the non-invasive screening methods still represent the future.

Electron Beam Computed Tomography (EBCT)

Developed in the 1970's, EBCT found its way into clinical cardiology in 1983. EBCT is synonymous with Ultra-fast CT and Cine-CT.

Technical principles

EBCT utilizes a linear accelerator to create an electron beam which is focused on a semi-circular wolfram target around the patient. The X-rays created penetrate the patient, and their intensity is measured by detectors. A significant advantage is the minimal time (<100 ms) required to acquire a cross-section, and a spatial resolution of <0.5 mm^2. The fast production of images (17 images/s) allows the heart to be imaged in a series of planes and triggered to specific phases in the cardiac cycle. The radiation exposure is comparatively modest, corresponding to ten chest X-rays.

Indications

1. Quantitative assessment of coronary calcification.
2. Immediate visualization of coronary artery lumen by contrast enhanced 3D surface reconstruction.

Predictive value

1. EBCT is a validated quantitative method to assess accumulation of coronary calcium. Calcification is a specific expression of coronary atherosclerosis and can be found in early stages of CAD. Soft non-calcified plaques cannot be identified. A positive result does not indicate coronary stenosis (low specificity), but does indicate the presence of CAD. From the individual calcium plaques, a total score is determined (Agatston),[13] the value of which is a measure of cardiovascular risk over the next two to five years.[14] The calcium index score rises with the number of traditional risk factors.

   The independent prognostic potential of calcium load is still unclear. The following recommendations are based on current knowledge: The calcium index score should be considered together with age and gender. If the calcium index score is higher than the cohort's average, then an elevated coronary risk should be assumed.[15,16] For example, an Agatston score above the 75th percentile is associated with a 12-fold increased mortality risk. A pilot should not be disqualified on the basis of this result, but it should lead to further evaluation. With proof of coronary calcification, secondary prevention is recommended.

The American Heart Association has developed the following guidelines for EBCT:

- EBCT is not a substitute for stress testing in patients with angina pectoris.
- EBCT as a screening tool for patients with risk factors is not yet well defined.
- EBCT is not indicated in asymptomatic patients without risk factors.
- A negative finding does not entirely exclude atherosclerotic plaques, but the likelihood of relevant stenosis is quite low.
- A positive finding indicates a medium-elevated risk of cardiovascular disease in the next two to five years.

2. By means of the technically intensive, time-consuming, and expensive 3D surface reconstruction, a direct, contrast strengthened, non-invasive representation of the coronary arteries is possible.

   Sufficiently good image quality in the proximal and middle sections of coronary arteries and by-pass grafts is only possible in 75% of cases. The clinical application of this method is limited after stent insertion/revascularization.

Disadvantages:

- 20% of images are not valid, particularly in the elderly and those with severe calcification. Respirations and motion artifacts can interfere in right coronary artery evaluation.
- Examination is possible only in stable sinus bradycardia.
- Amount of contrast medium is greater than in coronary angiography.
- Very high initial equipment costs.
- Very high examination costs that are often not covered by insurance.
- The level of predictive value of coronary angiography is not achieved.

Multi-Slice CT (MSCT)

The multi-slice CT is a further development of spiral CT. A detector circles around the patient, who is slowly transported through the scanner while measurements are taken. Numerous ECG-triggered levels can be simultaneously scanned, out of which all possible images can be reconstructed without significant motion artifact. Currently (2008), MSCT with 64 lines (time resolution of 165 ms, and a maximal image resolution of 0.42 mm) is considered the standard. The dual source technology is the newest generation.

The above-mentioned Agatston score and modified volume scores for evaluating coronary calcium is utilized with MSCT, although the

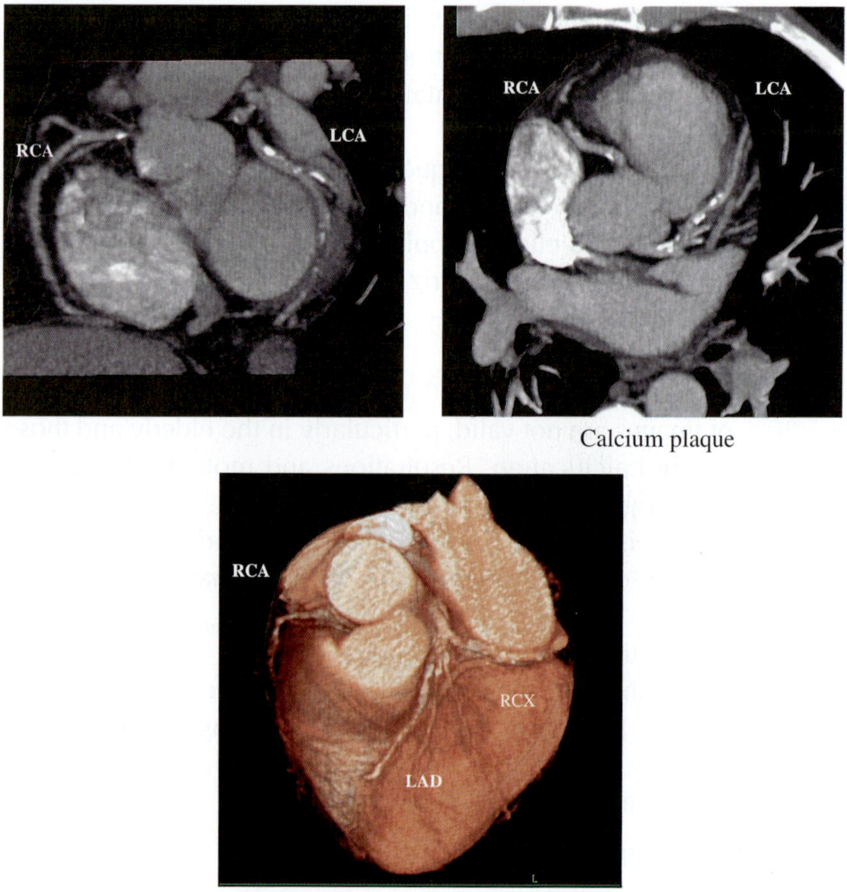

Figure 12. Multidetector CT angiography with 3D-reconstruction.

determination of calcium index scores as a screening method should not be employed, not even in pilots, due to uncertainty in interpretation, the radiation exposure, and contrast medium burden. CT angiography is also unable to detect non-calcified coronary artery plaques. There is a good correlation with invasive coronary angiography regarding the evaluation of proximal and mid-coronary sections, the patency of by-pass vessels, and the detection of coronary artery anomalies.

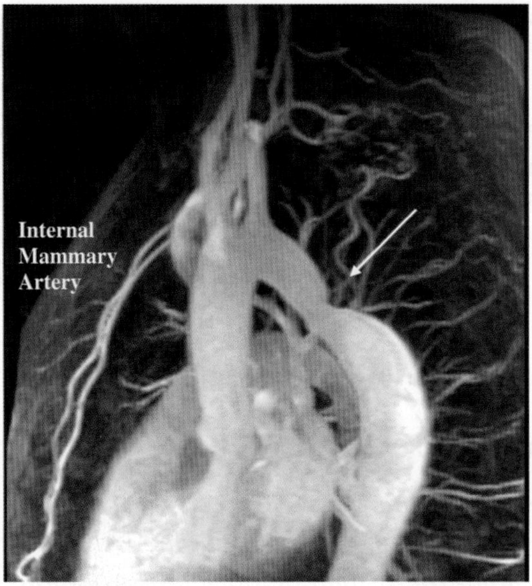

Figure 13. MR-angiography: Aortic isthmus stenosis.

Evaluation after stent implantation does not appear to be entirely reliable. Similarly, there is no reliable evaluation method for severe coronary artery calcification.

Relative disadvantages include a significant radiation exposure and contrast medium load (100 mL). The requirement of a heart rate below 70/min often necessitates the use of beta-blockers to reduce the heart rate in order to optimize the examination.

Magnetic Resonance (MRCA)

The established indications for cardio-MRI are diseases of the great vessels, inherited cardiac anomalies, tumors, and peri-myocarditis.

MR coronary angiography (examination time 20 minutes) is afflicted with significant uncertainties. With the different techniques (T2-weighted frequency at breath holding, contrast enhanced 3D-MRCA at breath holding), hemodynamically significant coronary artery stenosis can only be detected in the proximal sections with a sensitivity of 80%. This is inadequate for coronary artery diagnosis. Problematic are the limitations of resolution in the small caliber tortuous coronary arteries, the contrast between the coronary arteries from their surrounding tissue, and the compensation of movement of the heart and respiration.

MR coronary angiography does not currently hold a place in routine cardiac diagnostics. Exceptions are coronary anomalies and by-pass imaging. CT angiography of the coronary vessels is therefore superior.

Coronary Angiography

Medical Requirements (JAR-FCL 3): *A coronary angiogram obtained around the time of, or during, the ischemic cardiac event shall be available. There shall be no stenosis of more than 50% in any major untreated vessel, in any vein or artery graft, or at the site of an angioplasty/stent, except in a vessel leading to an infarct. More than two stenosis between 30% and 50% within the vascular tree should not be accepted. An untreated stenosis greater than 30% in the left main or proximal left anterior descending coronary artery should not be acceptable. The angiogram must be made available to the AMS.*

Diagnostic coronary angiography, with a resolution of 0.3 mm, was accidentally discovered by Sones in 1959, and is the gold standard for evaluating anatomy and morphology of the cardiac vessels. Together with ventriculography for determining left ventricular function, it represents one of the most important independent prognostic parameters. Selective coronary angiography in experienced hands today carries a minimal risk of less than 0.1%, and it can be performed on an out- or in-patient basis. By optimizing the instrumentation and imaging techniques, which is best accomplished digitally, the radiation exposure has become relatively small (corresponding to about 100 chest X-rays). After local anesthesia, the femoral artery (Judkins technique) or cubital artery in the arm (modified Sones technique) is punctured, and a preformed diagnostic catheter is inserted over a sheath. Together with ventriculography, the entire amount of contrast volume used is usually less than 100 mL. If the arterial access site is percutaneously closed or a small diameter sheath (4 F) is utilized, the patient can stand up after four hours.

Indications for coronary angiography (Guidelines according to ACC/AHA Commission[17] customized for evaluation of pilot fitness):

Asymptomatic individuals

— Suspicion of CAD on the basis of non-invasive tests (such as evidence of ischemia).
— Condition after myocardial infarction (at least six to nine months after the event).
— Condition after by-pass operation or angioplasty/stent six to nine months after intervention.
— Condition after by-pass operation or angioplasty/stent after five years for evaluation of ischemia.
— Males >35 years or females >40 years prior to heart valve surgery.
— Condition after thoracic trauma.
— Heart rhythm and conduction disorder suspicious of CAD in non-invasive tests.
— Complete left bundle branch block in individuals >40 years.
— Clarification of cardiomyopathy.
— Clarification of congenital heart disease prior to surgery.

Symptomatic individuals

— Clarification of atypical chest pain with ambiguous non-invasive tests.
— Stable/unstable angina.
— Clarification of left ventricular function disorders.
— Acute coronary syndrome, acute myocardial infarction (transmural/non-transmural).
— Condition after cardiac resuscitation.

Predictive value

The large epicardiac coronary arteries are the left main (LM), the circumflex (LCX), left anterior descending (LAD), and the right coronary artery (RCA) (see Fig. 14). Most often, co-dominant blood supply types are differentiated from the left dominant or right dominant blood supply types. The severity of the CAD, and therefore the prognosis, depends, among other things, on whether one, two or three vessels are involved, and whether there is relevant stenosis of the left main stem vessel.

The sensitivity and specificity of coronary arteriography for coronary artery stenosis is exceedingly high, and the gradation of the stenosis vacillates between examiners by c.20%. Because the images are captured briefly, the prognosis regarding future infarct is not reliable,

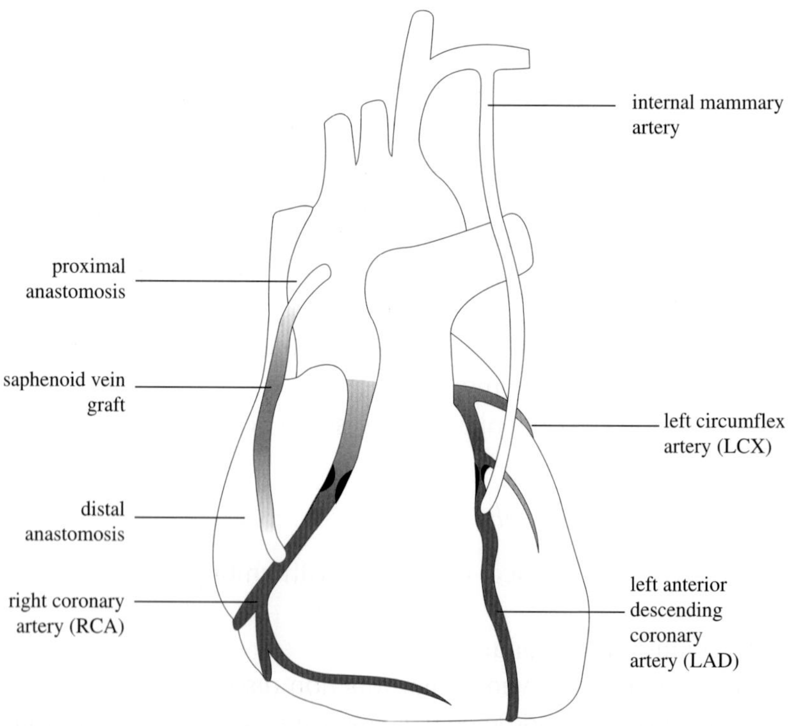

Figure 14. The large epicardiac coronary arteries, saphenous vein graft to RCA and IMA graft to LAD.

although large studies in the 1970's delivered good correlations between angiography and clinical course data.[18] Minimal stenosis during rapid plaque growth or more commonly a rupture of a soft plaque in situations with middle grade stenosis may result in an infarct.

Zero vessel CAD

Some of those pilots who, because of typical or atypical angina pectoris, undergo coronary angiography, do not have any stenosis in the large epicardial vessels but are found to have "small vessel disease." The prognosis is excellent, independent of the clinical picture. Even with coronary artery spasm, the prognosis is excellent.

Coronary artery sclerosis

Mild coronary lesions <30% indicate the onset of coronary atherosclerosis along with the corresponding prognostic consequences for pilots. Changes in the lumen <30% carry a 10-year cardiac event rate (including cardiac death, infarct, progression) of 13.8%; if the senotic changes are between 30 and 50% of the lumen, an event rate of 30% over ten years can be expected. Therefore, JAR-FCL-3 limits prognostically important main stem and proximal LAD stenosis to <30%.

Coronary artery disease

Coronary artery disease is defined as a stenosis greater than 50%. Depending on the morphology of the stenosis, this grade can be hemodynamically relevant.

Single vessel CAD

Single vessel CAD has a relatively good prognosis dependent on the location of the stenosis. The five-year survival rate varies between 92 and 100%.[18] Lesions of the proximal LAD have the highest mortality, similar to two-vessel CAD; isolated RCA lesions have the best prognosis. With good collateralization, complete obstruction may be asymptomatic and may not diminish left ventricular function. If there is no evidence of ischemia by scintigraphy/stress echocardiography, restricted medical certification may be possible.

Two vessel CAD

The survival rate over five years varies between and 87 and 100%, slightly worse than with single vessel disease. The average rate of infarct or death over five years is 4.3%. The prognosis is worse with main stem stenosis (eight years survival rate of 43%); consequently, main stem stenosis of 50% or more should be corrected surgically.

Three vessel CAD

Three vessel CAD, especially with proximal lesions, entails permanent disqualification as long as there is no revascularization. The five-year rate of infarct/death is at least 5.5%.

Left ventricular angiography

Left ventricular function is a very important independent prognostic parameter. The more severe the CAD, the more likely there is a decrease in LV function. Single vessel CAD with normal LV function carries a five-year survival rate of 89%, in contrast to 77% with reduced LV function. Medical certification (special issuance) can only be awarded if the ejection fraction of the left ventricle is shown to be ≥50% by echocardiography, left ventriculography, etc. (normal >60%), without significant wall motion disturbances and normal right ventricular function.

Aeromedical disposition

A small portion of pilots with significant CAD have a low risk of future cardiac events. Optimal risk stratification requires that non-invasive and invasive examinations are evaluated in the light of all clinical data and risk factors. Because even mild CAD can rapidly progress, annual evaluation by a cardiologist, including stress testing and possibly another coronary arteriogram, may be necessary. Pilots should be disqualified if symptoms or non-invasive test results indicating CAD develop.

Therapies Regarding Flight Fitness and Prognosis

ICAO standards and recommended practices

An applicant who has undergone coronary bypass grafting or angioplasty (with or without stenting), or other cardiac intervention, or who has a history of myocardial infarction, or who suffers from any other potentially incapacitating cardiac condition shall be assessed as unfit unless the applicant's cardiac condition has been investigated and evaluated in accordance with best medical practice and is assessed to not likely interfere with the safe exercise of the applicant's licence or rating privileges.

JAR-FCL 3 certification requirements

Applicants with symptomatic coronary artery disease, or with cardiac symptoms controlled by medications, shall be assessed as unfit. After an ischemic event (defined as a myocardial infarction, angina, significant arrhythmia or heart failure due to ischemia, or any type of cardiac revascularization), initial Class I certification is not possible. At revalidation or renewal, a fit assessment may be considered by the AMS if the investigations in paragraph 6 Appendix 1 to Subpart B are completed satisfactorily. Class 2 certification may be considered by the AMS if the investigations in paragraph 6 Appendix 1 to Subpart B are completed satisfactorily.

After an ischemic cardiac event, including revascularization, applicants without symptoms shall have reduced any vascular risk factors to an appropriate level. Medication, when used only to control cardiac symptoms, are not acceptable. All applicants should be on acceptable secondary prevention treatment. At least six months from the ischemic event, the following investigations shall be completed:

a) *an exercise ECG (symptom limited) to Bruce Stage IV, or equivalent, showing no evidence of myocardial ischemia nor rhythm disturbance;*
b) *an echocardiogram (or equivalent) showing satisfactory left ventricular function with no important abnormality of wall motion (such as dyskinesia or akinesia) and a left ventricular ejection fraction of 50% or more);*
c) *in cases of angioplasty/stenting, a myocardial perfusion scan or stress echocardiography (or equivalent test), which shall show no evidence of reversible myocardial ischemia;*
d) *further investigations, such as a 24-hour ECG, may be necessary to assess the risk of any significant rhythm disturbance.*

Follow-up shall be yearly (or more frequently if necessary) to ensure there is no deterioration of cardiovascular status. It shall include exercise ECG and cardiovascular risk assessment.

After coronary artery vein by-pass grafting, a myocardial perfusion scan (or equivalent) shall be performed if there is any indication, and in all cases, within five years from the procedure.

In all cases, coronary angiography, or an equivalent test, shall be considered at any time if symptoms, signs, or non-invasive tests indicate cardiac ischemia.

Successful completion of the six-month review will allow Class I applicants to fly multi-pilot (OML). Class II applicants, having fulfilled the above criteria, may fly unrestricted at the discretion of the AMS.

MYOCARDIAL INFARCTION[19]

The high incidence of cardiovascular disease in the western world (77/100 000 inhabitants/year) and the significant improvement in acute heart attack treatment with acute percutaneous coronary intervention (PCI) with 90% opening of the affected vessel within 90 minutes, along with significant reduction in mortality, has led to an increased interest in risk factor stratification.

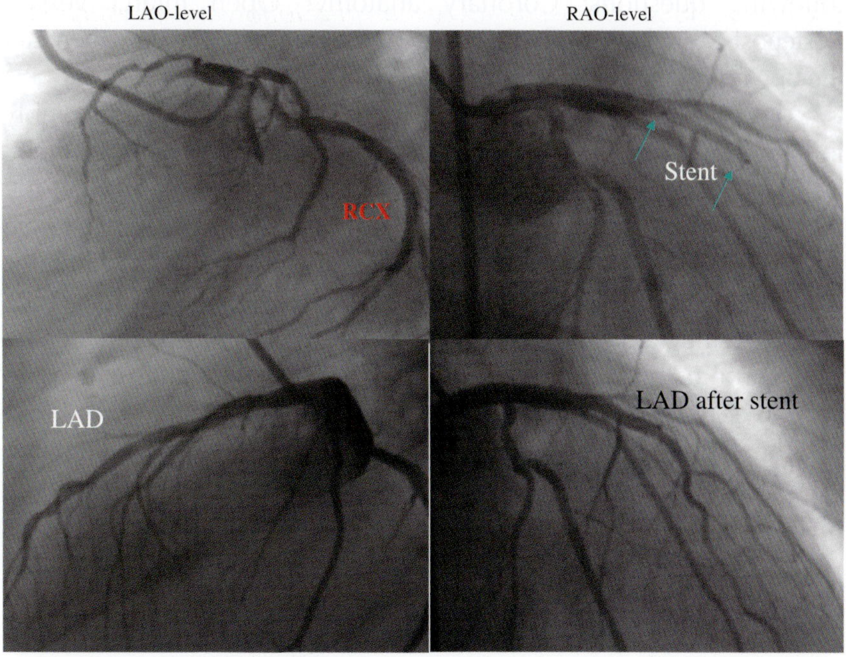

Figure 15. LAD-occlusion with acute recanalization and stent insertion.

A prognostic determinant is the time between the onset of pain and the opening of the affected vessel, which should be as short as possible, thereby minimizing the myocardial scar and the subsequent reduction in LV function.

The AME should provide preventive education to pilots with risk factors.

The long-term prognosis after infarct is determined by such events as re-infarction, recurrent ischemia, significant arrhythmias, and cardiac insufficiency. These risks must be assessed individually, utilizing all available parameters. After myocardial infarction, the medical examiner, in collaboration with the cardiologist, should accurately counsel the pilot with regard to prognosis and outlook for certification, and inform about anticipated examinations. After myocardial infarction in asymptomatic young people and pilots, the prognostic indication for coronary angiography should be based on answers to the following questions: Coronary anatomy? Open infarct vessel? Restenosis? Single or multiple vessel CAD? LV-function? Only then can therapy and prognosis be determined.

The elevated mortality risk after infarct appears to be favorably influenced by opening the diseased vessel (reduction in peripheral ischemia, post-infarct LV dilatation, and electrical instability at the edge of the infarct region). Regarding pilots, the decision to open vessels in an infarcted area should be made individually and liberally. By utilizing prior functional examinations of prognostic relevance (such as scintigraphy, stress echocardiography, etc.), which can identify vital chronically ischemic myocardium, those areas that can profit from later revascularization can be identified.

The ejection fraction (EF) is an important prognostic parameter, on which the prognosis of the underlying cause is dependent. An EF of about 50% in the setting of CAD and limited infarct carries a 10-year survival rate of about 91%, which clearly declines with reduced heart function. Through the combination of a number of non-invasive stress tests, the "prognostic power" can be raised, so that six months after infarct/PCI/revascularization, routine coronary arteriography is no longer necessary. Through the rapid development of non-invasive coronary arteriography (MSCT, MR-coronary arteriography), invasive tests can be substituted on an individual basis in the future. Regarding the question of rhythm stability, especially in the edge area of myocardial scar, Holter monitoring, which should be reviewed in its entirety by the physician (no computer interpretation), and the use of signal averaging ECG are helpful.

Interventional Therapy

Balloon angioplasty (PTCA = percutaneous transluminal coronary angioplasty, PCI = percutaneous coronary intervention), first used in the heart in 1977 by Grüntzig, eliminates stenosis through compression of the atherosclerotic plaque, rupture of the plaque and vessel intima along with local stretching of the vessel wall. The primary success rate, dependent upon the morphology of the stenosis, is above 95% and results in reduction of the stenosis to less than 50% of the reference diameter. The rate of fatal complications is 0.5–1%, depending on the patient's stability. After interventional coronary artery treatment (angioplasty, stent) a pilot is deemed disqualified and may be assessed as fit after investigation.

The main problems of interventional coronary artery treatment is acute coronary artery obstruction, which can lead to an emergency by-pass operation and entails a restenosis rate of up to 30% in the first six months. An increased utilization of intracoronary stents (stainless steel, tantalum, platinum, nitinol) could reduce the number of emergency by-pass operations, decrease infarct and fatal complications to 0.3–1.0%, and restenosis to 16–20%. Early stent thrombosis can be reduced to 0.5–1% by optimal utilization of anti-thrombotic strategies (ASA, clopidogrel, etc.) Utilization of the newer stents, which release proliferation inhibitors and/or immune suppressive drugs from a polymer coating, could achieve a highly significant reduction in the incidence of restenosis[20] (<10%) (such as Cypher™-Stent with Sirolimus or Taxus™-Stent with Paclitaxel) and are indicated for particularly small coronary arteries and long lesions. The rate of renewed catheterization can be reduced through the implantation of DES (drug eluting stents). In countries where these cost-intensive stents are covered by health insurance, the DES are implanted in a majority of cases (60% of cases in Switzerland, and 80% in the USA). Long-term results are still awaited, as the routine use of DES in pilots as well as the duration of the two anti-thrombotic regimens (ASA and Clopidogrel) are currently being assessed. It is to be noticed that a meta-analysis (ESC 2006) described a higher rate of late stent thrombosis after completion of dual anti-thrombotic regimens. Other interventional methods, such as atherectomies (Simpson), rotablation, and laser treatments have fallen to the background.

Indication for coronary dilatation

Domains include single and double vessel disease with:

1) Angina pectoris and/or evidence of ischemia and relevant stenosis.
2) Marginal stenosis with pronounced ischemia.

3) Relevant stenosis in larger coronary arteries even without obvious angina pectoris/ischemia (prognostic indication):

— prior to non-cardiac operations
— in risk-related occupations (pilots/bus drivers)
— when collateral perfusion is threatened
— in case of stenosis/closure after infarct ("open artery" hypothesis).

With three-vessel CAD, PCI is indicated when stenosis morphology is favorable for PCI, LV function is normal, and the patient is non-diabetic. In individuals with multiple vessel CAD, the cardiac risk and particularly the rate of restenosis in relationship to the number of treated lesions is higher after six months.

On the basis of multi-variant analysis, the risk of significant cardiac events after angioplasty lies below 1.0 % per year, provided: single vessel CAD, age <60, no heart insufficiency, EF >50%, no diabetes or hypertension, and angina pectoris CCS Class 0-II.

Course after stent implantation/restenosis detection

A planned stent implantation in a single native coronary artery can be expected to reduce the annual mortality rate to under 1%; the risk of restenosis, however, is about 16–20%. In contrast, stent implantations in vein grafts provide only short-term favorable results.[21] Higher rates of in-stent restenosis can be expected in primary unstable angina pectoris, restenosis after PCI, diabetes mellitus, recanalization of chronic occluded vessels, LAD stenosis, as well as implantation of multiple stents in one or more vessels. This elevated restenosis rate can, as clearly indicated by previous studies, be reduced by utilization of drug eluting stents. After multiple interventions, recertification should be considered with caution and must be individually assessed. In the case of a special issuance, complete revascularization must be proven and restenosis must be verified.

Success following intervention can be defined by symptomatic criteria (angina pectoris) and by a variety of functional tests with variable predictive capabilities.

- Recurrence of angina pectoris within the first month after angioplasty suggests insufficient dilatation of the vessel or angina from another affected vessel.
- Angina between one and six months after angioplasty usually indicates restenosis.
- Angina six months after intervention suggests a significant stenosis at another site. Indeed, silent restenosis, which affects prognosis, occurs in up to 33% of cases.

Consequently, functional tests to detect restenosis are a requirement for recertification. Stress ECG carries approximately a 45% positive predictive value for restenosis detection, and is higher if the stress testing is not performed immediately after PCI. Myocardial scintigraphy has a significantly higher predictive value for restenosis detection.

In our own study of 150 individuals undergoing restenosis detection after six months following intervention, the history had a positive predictive value (precision rate) of 77%, and stress ECG one of 84%, with a marginal sensitivity of 50% but with acceptable specificity. The dobutamine stress echocardiography had a positive predictive value of 87% with significant better sensitivity and specificity. This was the case for atypical angina pectoris and/or non-diagnostic or pathological stress ECG. Similar data are valid also for stress MRI, which is much less subjective. Through a combination of a variety of tests, one can sufficiently accurately estimate the prognosis of cardiac events.

Coronary angiography is the most reliable method of proving/disproving a restenosis after coronary artery intervention. Pilots with single vessel CAD following PCI/stent and proven absence of restenosis have a cardiac event risk under 1% per year and therefore the best prospect for recertification.

SURGICAL THERAPY

Coronary artery by-pass operation using venous grafting was introduced in 1968 by Favorolo.[22] Due to improvements in the technique, anesthesia, and especially through the utilization of mammary arteries, the prognosis and rate of successful revascularization (despite longer operating time) has been significantly improved. By-pass operation is conducted under hypothermia and under cardioplegia. Venous by-pass grafts, most often the great saphenous vein, are implanted between the aorta and a coronary artery segment distal to the stenosis. The currently routinely used left internal mammary artery (IMA) is mobilized out of its tissue bed, the side branches ligated, and the distal end joined with the LAD. Complete arterial revascularization is the goal.

Indications for CABG Operation:

1) Significant (>50%) left main stem stenosis or left main equivalent (>70% proximal LAD and proximal circumflex).
2) Three vessel CAD, particularly in patients with reduced systolic LV function (<50%).
3) Two vessel CAD with proximal LAD stenosis and EF <50%, or by evidence of ischemia.

Venous grafting is followed by early thrombotic closure at a rate of 10% in the first year, so the outcome must be verified prior to recertification. In the following years, the annual closure rate is 1–3%. After five years, 80% of venous grafts are still open, and after 10 years, 60% remain open. These data are pooled from studies that include patients with reduced LV function. Mammary arteries remained open 95% of the time after 10 years. The survival rate of three vessel CAD was 89% if the LAD was supplied by IMA grafting, in comparison to 71% when venous by-pass was used alone.[23] The surgical mortality rate of patients with bilateral IMA-grafting is somewhat higher than with unilateral application.

Minimally invasive by-pass operations of single vessel CAD, joining the left internal mammary artery and the LAD through a left thoracic intercostal incision can be accomplished on a beating heart without the use of a heart-lung by-pass machine. Because of distal anastomosis stenosis, surgical success should be verified by coronary angiography prior to recertification.

Today, by-pass operations requiring sternotomy are performed even on the beating heart without heart-lung by-pass machines; the heart is stabilized with a holding device so that the by-pass can be sutured. This MIDCAB (Minimally Invasive Direct Coronary Artery By-pass) technique is particularly advantageous for high-risk patients.

ANGIOPLASTY/PCI VERSUS CORONARY ARTERY BY-PASS GRAFT SURGERY (CABG)[24]

Numerous randomized studies of multiple vessel CAD have compared the by-pass operation with PCI (BARI, CABRI, RITA, GABI, EAST, and ERACI).

Regarding infarct and mortality, these therapeutic strategies are equivalent, except for diabetics, where by-pass is better. The relative effect of PCI over CABG on the five-year mortality rate in patients with a range of severity of CAD was evaluated in the Duke study[25] (Cox model hazard rations). In severe single vessel CAD, including proximal LAD stenosis and moderate two-vessel CAD, PCI and CABG were equal in retrospective analysis over five years. In contrast, in severe two-vessel CAD, including left main stem and in all three-vessel CAD, particularly with restricted LV function (<50%), by-pass should be considered for the long term. After surgery,

Table 4. Comparison of Annual Cardiovascular Mortality over Five Years (Duke Study)

	PCI	CABG	Medications
1-CAD	0.55 %	1.0%	0.67%
2-CAD	1.12%	0.7%	1.57%
3-CAD	2.87%	1.02%	3.45%

an improvement in LV function can occur, so that the ejection fraction of >50%, which is indicated for recertification, can be achieved.

Coronary artery intervention, directed toward symptomatic treatment, can result in more frequent re-interventions (since the introduction of DES this has been reduced), resulting in repeated disqualification. In certain situations, the riskier by-pass operation may result in an improved long-term prognosis and more often in complete revascularization (88% versus 51% with PCI). Regarding pilots, the performance of the revascularization procedure (intervention or surgery, eventually DES) should influence the decision.

Prognosis

The long-term course following CABG depends on clinical variables and the treatment of risk factors. Predictors of perioperative mortality are emergency surgery, repeated surgery, age, female gender, diabetes, renal sufficiency, peripheral atherosclerotic vascular disease, COPD, limited LV function, hypertension, advanced CAD, and other co-existing cardiovascular diseases (Coronary Artery Surgery Study).[26] Because of the initial selection, the professional pilot differs from the general population in two ways: co-existing diseases are rare and hypertension, if present, is well controlled. From a medical perspective, the heterogeneous group of private pilots is closer to the general population.

The control of risk factors strongly influences the long-term course after every revascularization procedure. The risk of cardiac event for a normal man aged 30–59 is 0.3–1.0% per year. The risk of sudden incapacitation in patients with the clinical characteristics of a pilot after by-pass operation (without myocardial infarction) is about 1.6% per year. If the pilot does not smoke and is not hypertensive, the annual risk falls to 0.4%.

After by-pass surgery with an IMA graft, a pilot with normal LV function and optimal cholesterol values, who does not smoke and has a healthy lifestyle with physical activity, can expect a five-year course that is comparable to an asymptomatic individual of similar age and gender.

Recommendations/Requirements

The choice of revascularization procedure for pilots with coronary artery disease, particularly with regard to prognosis, should be executed as discussed above. Complete revascularization is necessary for recertification. Because by-pass surgery with heart-lung machines can lead to neurological complications ranging from subtle intellectual and functional changes to significant stroke, neurological and psychological rehabilitation must be demonstrated to be entirely complete. Through a combination of clinical examinations and a variety of non-invasive tests, such as stress ECG, scintigraphy, stress echocardiography etc., it is possible to estimate the degree of functional revascularization, the prognosis, and the risk of cardiac events following by-pass surgery. Prior to recertification, perfusion scintigraphy or an equivalent test should be performed, and in any case a perfusion scintigraphy should take place after five years. In case of symptoms or a pathological non-invasive test, a coronary angiogram must be performed. The question of post-CABG early occlusion can, in the future, be determined by Multi-Slice CT examination (MSCT) of the newest generation as a non-invasive alternative to coronary angiography. In the context of complete revascularization, a repeat coronary angiogram in five years is not entirely necessary.

MEDICAL THERAPY

ICAO Standards and Recommended Practices: *An applicant for any class of Medical Assessment shall be required to be free from any effect or side-effect of any prescribed or non-prescribed therapeutic, diagnostic, or preventive medication taken, such as would entail a degree of functional incapacity that is likely to interfere with the safe operation of an aircraft or with the safe performance of duties. Use of herbal medication and alternative treatment modalities requires particular attention to possible side effects.*

JAR-FLC 3 Certification Requirements: *Holders of medical certificates shall not take any prescription or non-prescription medication* *or drug, or undergo any other treatment, unless they are completely sure that the medication, drug, or treatment will not have any adverse effect on their ability to safely perform their duties. If there is any doubt, advice shall be sought from the AMS or an AMC or an AME.*

Many medications available without prescription are pain killers such as Aspirin® and ibuprofen, anti-allergic medicines such as antihistamines, and stimulants. Those that contain ingredients that end with *-ine*, such as chlorpheniramine, phenylpropanolamine, ephedrine, or phenylephrine can potentially influence pilot performance. A general rule: if a pilot suffers from an illness or condition that requires treatment, this is cause enough to consider the condition incompatible with safe flying.

Acetylsalicylic Acid (ASA) and Clopidogrel

In all patients with stable or unstable angina pectoris, post myocardial infarction, angioplasty/stent, and by-pass surgery, the prognosis is significantly improved by daily intake of 75 to 325 mg ASA, which causes a reduction in incidence of infarct, restenosis, graft occlusion, etc. This is also the case for mild coronary wall changes <30% and for myocardial bridges. Generally 100 mg/day is administered. In the case of intolerance, there are entero-soluble formulations in capsules, which are dissolved in the small intestine. The bleeding time, over the long term, is not significantly elevated. Newer thrombocyte inhibitors using other mechanisms, such as clopidogrel or ticlopidin, are similarly suitable for prognosis improvement after infarct. Due to increased side effects and hematopoietic changes, clopidogrel is preferred to ticlopidin. Fitness to fly is not affected.

β-BLOCKERS

Propranolol was the first approved β-blocker for pilots, but should be avoided today as it has greater side effects than other β-blockers. Numerous large studies have shown a reduced reinfarction and mortality rate with the use of β-blockers after myocardial infarct. The ISIS-I study of atenalol use in about 16 000 patients *(Lancet 1986/88)* was the most extensive. Metoprolol and bisoprolol (50 mg daily) are preferred in pilots due to the hydrophilic characteristics and minimal CNS side effects. This recommendation is based on evaluations by the Flugmedizinisches Institut der Luftwaffe in Fürstenfeldbruck (Aviation Medicine Institute of the Air Force in Fürstenfeldbruck) and other military medical facilities.

ACE Inhibitors and AT_1- Receptor Antagonists

Both ACE inhibitors and AT_1 blockers lead to vasodilatation through angiotensin II inhibition, and thereby a to reduction in left ventricular after-load and blood pressure. AT_1 blockers, in contrast to ACE inhibitors, do not have a bradykinin effect (cough reflex). The ACE inhibitors are also preferred in heart insufficiency and post infarct.

In all studies, ACE inhibitor therapy following infarct leads to a decrease in the progression of heart insufficiency, and to reduced hospitalization, cardiovascular mortality, and total mortality (AIRE, TRACE, Consensus II, ISIS-4, GISSI-3). In the SAVE study, captopril reduced the mortality rate by 20% and the re-infarct rate by 25%. When administered within the first 48 hours after infarct, this effect could be demonstrated even with long-acting ACE inhibitors. This substance group appears to have no significant CNS effects and is therefore compatible with medical certification. Therapeutic monitoring, especially initially, is obligatory. The dose should be reduced in the case of sodium and volume depletion, such as with dehydration, diarrhea, etc.

Diuretics

Potassium sparing diuretics are well tolerated and compatible with safe flying. The metabolic side effects, such as increase in lipids, uric acid, and worsening of glucose metabolism should not be overlooked. Loop diuretics are not compatible with medical certification, due to their side effects, such as electrolyte disturbance and their relative consequences and short therapeutic effects.

Angiotensin Receptor Antagonists and Calcium Channel Blockers

See Section 3, Arterial Hypertension.

Lipid Lowering Agents

The treatment of hypercholesterolemia with statin lowering agents (HMG-CoA-reductase inhibitors) is a major development in recent years. This treatment leads to a significant improvement in the prognosis of CAD with a significant reduction in mortality, in particular from less risk of myocardial infarction and less need of emergency by-pass operation. This is also the case for patients with normal LDL cholesterol, the target being 100 mg/dL. Please also see Chapter 9: Cardiovascular Risk Factors.

Anti-Anginals

Medications such as nitrates and molsidomin for the treatment of symptomatic angina pectoris are disqualifying. The medications required after by-pass surgery can usually be discontinued prior to recertification.

Recommendations regarding secondary prevention for patients with CAD and other atherosclerotic vascular disease

Following the AHA/ACC Guidelines for Secondary Prevention for Patients with Coronary and Other Atherosclerotic Vascular Disease: 2006 Update (Smith SC (2006) J Am Coll Cardiol **47:** 2130–39) and the recommendations of the Deutsche Gesellschaft für Kardiologie — Herz- und Kreislaufforschung (German Society of Cardiology — Heart and Circulation Research).

Table 5. Recommendations

Goal of Risk Intervention	Recommendations
Smoking: Complete cessation of smoking, avoidance of smoking environments	Ask questions regarding smoking at every visit. Include partner or family; make agreement regarding smoking cessation. Referral for further consultation, reference material (patient literature), nicotine substitutes and smoking cessation programs. Quitting smoking is the single most important measure for patients with vascular disease.
Nutrition: Low fat anti-atherogenic food	Calorie balanced, high fiber (>20 g/day, low fat diet (<30% of total energy consumption), with only a small portion of saturated fats (<10% calories) and cholesterol (<300 mg/day). The consumption of meat and animal fat should be reduced; ocean fish meals are desirable. The diet should be rich in whole wheat products, fresh fruits, and vegetables. Moderate alcohol consumption (about 15 g/day) has no deleterious effects on the cardiovascular and total risk. At >30 g/day, risk increases. In women, lower thresholds apply.
Overweight: Attaining a normal body weight (BMI <25) and elimination of abdominal adipose	Calorie restricted diet. Identification of the causes of being overweight: alcohol, hidden fats in sausages, cheese and prepared foods, chocolate, cakes, over indulgence in fruit (calories!). Appropriate physical activity (see below) is particularly important in patients with elevated blood pressure, elevated triglyceride, and diabetes mellitus. Initial goal of weight reduction should be 10% of the initial weight. Further intervention follows success.
Hyperlipidemia: Ideal-goal: LDL-Chol <100 mg/dl (2.5 mmol/l)	Achieving normal weight is desirable, and also regular physical activity, particularly when HDL <40 mg/dl (1.0 mmol/L). Reduction of unsaturated fatty acids <7% of total calories, and cholesterol <200 mg/d, elevation of omega-3 fatty acids in the form of fish or capsules (1 g/d).

(Continued)

Table 5. (*Continued*)

Goal of Risk Intervention	**Recommendations**		
Secondary goal: HDL-Chol >40 mg/dl (1 mmol/l) Triglyceride <190 mg/dl (<5 mmol/l) In case of Triglyceride >200 mg/dl, non-HDL-C should be <130 mg/dl	LDL <100 mg/dl: No therapy With ACS LDL <70 mg/dl is reasonable	LDL >100 mg/dl: Additional to strict diet, statins should be considered, especially if HDL <40 mg/dl.	LDL >100 despite drugs: Increase LDL-lowering drug therapy. For triglyceride >500 mg/dl eventually fibrate or niacin.
Sedentary lifestyle: Goal: Minimally 30 Min. activity at least 5 times weekly, better 7 days/week	30–60 min moderately intensive activity five times weekly (walking, jogging, bicycling, or other arduous activity) supports an active lifestyle; going for a walk during work breaks, climbing stairs rather than taking elevators, gardening. Medically supervised program for mid to high-risk patients (coronary exercise groups). The heart rate during physical activity should always be kept in predetermined non-ischemic and asymptomatic ranges. Every physical activity beyond normal daily activity carries a beneficial effect.		
Elevated blood pressure: Goal of <140/90 mm Hg, in diabetes II <130/80 mmHg	Lifestyle modification: Weight control (1 kg weight reduction leads to 2 mmHg blood pressure decrease), regular aerobic activity, permanent limitation of alcohol consumption to <30 g alcohol/day (women <20 g/day), salt restriction. Supplementation with blood pressure medication, individualized by age and other conditions (β-blockade, ACE inhibitors), when blood pressure >140 systolic or >90 diastolic.		
Aggregation inhibitors	ASA 75–162 mg/day. Post CABG, ASA 100–325 mg/d within 48 h post-op. Additional Clopidogrel 75 mg/d with ACS and after PCI for 12 months in combination (>1 month for bare metal stent, >3 months for		

(*Continued*)

Table 5. *(Continued)*

Goal of Risk Intervention	Recommendations
	Sirolimus-eluting stent and >6 months for paclitaxel-eluting stent. Eventually higher ASA dose to 325 mg/d. Anticoagulation with INR goal 2–3 after infarct, when indicated (atrial fibrillation, thrombus).
ACE-Inhibitors after infarct	For prevention and treatment of heart insufficiency with limited ventricle function (EF <40%). For prevention of coronary events in diabetics and patients with elevated risk.
β-blocker	In all patients after myocardial infarct, ACS or left ventricular dysfunction, exertional ischemia — with regard to the usual contraindications. Or when ACE inhibitors are contraindicated.
Estrogen	While the introduction of hormone replacement therapy cannot be recommended during secondary prevention, prior hormone replacement therapy under gynecological supervision for at least two years can be continued.
Other measures	No secondary effect is proven for measures not pointed out in these recommendations, such as vitamins and antioxidants.

General

Through the implementation of secondary preventive measures, an improvement in prognosis and flight performance of patients with coronary artery disease can be demonstrated. This is where the patients have the possibility to actively influence their disease.

REFERENCES

1. Aronow WS, *et al.* (1994) Prevalence of coexistence of coronary artery disease, peripheral arterial disease, and atherothrombotic brain infarction in men and women <62 years of age. *Am J Cardiol* **74**: 64–65.

2. Michaelides AP, *et al.* (1999) Improved detection of coronary artery disease by exercise electrocardiography with the use of right precordial leads. *N Engl J Med* **340**: 340–345.
3. Robb G, *et al.* (1975) Appraisal of the double two test. A long-term follow-up study of 3325 men. *JAMA* **234**: 722–727.
4. Bruce RA, *et al.* (1987) Unusual prognostic significance of exercise induced ST elevation in coronary patients. *J Elektrocardiol* **20** (Suppl 1): 84–88.
5. Bruce RA, *et al.* (1987) Exercise enhanced assessment of risk factors for coronary heart disease in healthy men. *J Electrocardiology* **20** (Suppl.1): 162–166.
6. Nescovic AN, *et al.* (1995) Positive high-dose dipyridamole echocardiography test after acute myocardial infarction is an excellent predictor of cardiac events. *Am Heart J* **129**: 31–39.
7. Crouse L, *et al.* (1991) Exercise echocardiography as a screening test for coronary artery disease and correlation with coronary arteriography. *Am J Cardiol* **67**: 1213–1218.
8. Severi S, *et al.* (1994) Diagnostic and prognostic value of dipyridamole echocardiography in patients with suspected coronary artery disease. *Circulation* **89**: 1160–1173.
9. Underwood SR. (1999) Myokardial perfusion imaging and pilot certification. *Eur Heart J* **1** (Suppl. D): D84–D93.
10. Iskander S, *et al.* (1998) Risk assessment using single-photon emission computed tomographic technetium-99m sestamibi aging. *J Am Coll Cardiol* **32**(1): 57–62. Review.
11. Hachamovitsch R, *et al.* (1998) Incremental prognostic value of myocardial perfusion single photon emission computed tomography for the prediction of cardiac death: Differential stratification for risk of cardiac death and myocardial infarction. *Circulation* **1797**(6): 535–543.
12. Nagel E, *et al.* (1999) Noninvasive diagnosis of ischemia induced wall motion abnormalities with the use of high-dose dobutamine stress MRI: Comparison with dobutamine stress echocardiography. *Circulation* **99**: 763–770.
13. Agatston AS, *et al.* (1990) Quantification of coronary artery calcium using ultrafast computed tomography. *J Am Coll Cardiol* **15**: 827–832.

14. Detrano R, *et al.* (1996) Prognostic value of coronary calcification and angiographic stenoses in patients undergoing coronary angiography. *J Am Coll Cardiol* **27**(2): 285–290.
15. Raggi *et al.* (2000) Identification of patients at increased risk of first unheralded acute myocardial infarction by electron-beam computed tomography. *Circulation* **101**(8): 850–855.
16. Wayhs R, *et al.* (2002) High coronary artery calcium scores pose an extremely elevated risk for hard events. *J Am Coll Cardiol* **39**(2): 225–230.
17. Scanlon PJ. (1999) ACC/AHA Guidelines for coronary angiography: Executive summary and recommendations. *Circulation* **4**; **99**(17): 2345–2357.
18. Bruschke AVG, *et al.* (1992) The natural history of angiographically demonstrated coronary artery disease. *Eur Heart J* **13** (Suppl. H): 70–75.
19. Baldus S, *et al.* (1999) Patency of the infarct-related artery: Prognostic considerations. *Eur Heart J* **1** (Suppl D): D63–D66.
20. Sousa JE, *et al.* (2001) Sustained suppression of neointimal proliferation by sirolimus-eluting stents: One-year angiographic and intravascular ultrasound follow-up. *Circulation* **104**: 2007–2011.
21. deFeyter PJ, *et al.* (1993) Balloon angioplasty for treatment of lesions in saphenous vein grafts. *J Am Coll Cardiol* **21**: 1539–1549.
22. Favorolo RG. (1968) Saphenous vein autograft replacement of severe coronary artery occlusion. *Ann Thorac Surg* **5**: 334–339.
23. Kirklin JW, *et al.* (1989) Summary of a consensus concerning death and ischemic events after coronary artery by-pass grafting. *Circulation* **79** (Suppl 1): 81.
24. Chua TP, *et al.* (1999) What is acceptable revascularization of the myocardium in the context of certification to fly? *Eur Heart J* **1** (Suppl. D): D78–D83.
25. Mark DB, *et al.* (1994) Continuing evolution of therapy for coronary artery disease: Initial results from the era of coronary angioplasty. *Circulation* **89**: 2015–2025.
26. Coronary Artery Surgery Study (CASS) Principal investigators and associates (1984): Myocardial infarction and mortality in the Coronary Artery Surgery Study (CASS) randomized trial. *N Engl J Med* **310**: 750–758.

Chapter 13

Cardiac Valve Disease/Valve Replacement

Isle Janicke*

ICAO Standards and Recommended Practices: *The applicant shall not possess any abnormality of the heart, congenital or acquired, which is likely to interfere with the safe exercise of the applicant's license and rating privileges. There shall be no significant functional nor structural abnormality of the circulatory system.*

Medical Requirements (JAR-FCL 3): *Applicants with significant abnormality of any of the heart valves shall be assessed as unfit. Applicants with minor cardiac valvular abnormalities may be assessed as fit by the AMS. Unidentified cardiac murmurs shall require evaluation by a cardiologist acceptable to the AMS and assessment by the AMS. If considered significant, further investigation shall include at least 2D Doppler echocardiography. Applicants with implanted mechanical valves shall be assessed as unfit. Asymptomatic applicants with a tissue valve who at least 6 months following surgery shall have satisfactorily completed investigations which demonstrate normal valvular and ventricular configuration and function may be considered for a fit assessment by the AMS.*

HEART MURMURS]

50% of all healthy hearts have heart murmurs, most easily heard in young, thin individuals. One must differentiate between functional

* Herzzentrum, Kaiser-Wilhelm-Krankenhaus, Gerrickstraße 21, D-47137 Duisburg, Germany.

heart murmurs in hyperdynamic conditions (pregnancy, tachycardia, anemia), which are accidentally discovered but prognostically favorable, and pathological heart murmurs caused by disease. Murmurs without organic origin are typically heard in early-midsystole and found at the left parasternal border, ending before the second heart sound, low in frequency, short and soft (1/6 to 2/6 = soft, but immediately audible), do not radiate and vary with position and activity. They usually arise from the aortic or pulmonic outflow tracts. Pansystolic, late systolic, diasystolic, and continuous murmurs almost always have organic origins and must be further evaluated by a cardiologist.

In a first-time applicant, it is wise to have a heart murmur evaluated by a cardiologist with a very sensitive 2D-Doppler echocardiogram before the applicant embarks on expensive training. This is imperative in 3/6 systolic ejection murmurs and even more so when associated with ECG changes.

AORTIC VALVE

Bicuspid Valve

Medical Requirements (JAR-FCL 3): *Bicuspid aortic valve is acceptable without restriction if no other cardiac or aortic abnormality is demonstrated, but requires biannual review with echocardiography.*

The bicuspid aortic valve is the most common congenital heart valve abnormality, found in 1–2%, following mitral valve prolapse. It occurs more commonly in men than in women and is more susceptible to endocarditis. Frequently accompanying congenital abnormalities are the patent ductus arteriosus (Botalli) and aortic coarctation, which can easily be determined by bilateral Doppler pressure measurements of the arms and legs at rest and after exertion. The risk of an aortic dissection appears to be elevated, particularly with coexisting aortic dilatation (>4.0 cm). A lesser grade of aortic root dilatation can be compatible with medical certification. In this congenital fusion of two commissures with turbulent flow, 30% develop secondary calcified aortic stenosis, 30% develop aortic insufficiency,whereas the rest develops no changes.

Significant stenosis or insufficiency usually develops in the fifth decade of life and can be identified in time with annual echocardiography.

Aortic Stenosis (AS)

Medical Requirements (JAR-FCL 3): *Aortic stenosis (left ventricular function must be intact) with a mean pressure gradient of up to 20 mmHg may be assessed as fit. Those with a mean pressure gradient above 20 mmHg but no greater than 40 mmHg may be assessed as fit for Class 2 or Class 1 OML limitation. A mean pressure gradient up to 50 mmHg may be acceptable, at the discretion of the AMS. Follow-up with 2D Doppler echocardiography will be determined by the AMS.*

Aortic stenosis is the most common primary organic heart defect in adults in central Europe; it is more common in men than in women. Secondary calcified bicuspid aortic stenosis occurs most often and manifests itself in the fourth to fifth decade of life. In individuals over the age of 70, senile degenerative calcified aortic stenosis predominates, predisposed by diabetes mellitus, hypertension, and hyperlipidemia. Rheumatic aortic stenosis rarely appears isolated and is decreasing in frequency. The normal aortic valve opening area is between 2.6–3.5 cm^2, corresponding to a flow velocity of 0.9–1.8 m/s (assuming a normal cardiac output) according to the guidelines of AHA-Task Force Report 2006.[1]

AS	Surface Area	Velocity	Mean Pressure
Mild	> 1.5 cm^2	< 3 m/s	< 25 mmHg
Moderate	1–1.5 cm^2	3–4 m/s	25–40 mmHg
Severe	< 1.0 cm^2	> 4 m/s	> 40 mmHg

Individuals with mild and moderate aortic stenosis are usually asymptomatic for a long time; if so, the prognosis is very good and the rate of sudden cardiac death is <1%.

The typical symptoms of angina pectoris, left heart insufficiency, and syncope, appear more often when valve surface areas are less than 1.0 cm^2, and without surgical correction are associated with a worse prognosis (sudden cardiac death 15–20%). Severe aortic stenosis is associated with microemboli causing cerebral vascular accidents.

Examination

Pilots will not necessarily admit to typical symptoms. Auscultation: at least medium strength, rough, low frequency 3/6 systolic ejection murmur (can even be sensed by a hand on the chestwall) with a crescendo-decrescendo characteristic, best heard at the right second intercostal space in sitting position and during exhalation, radiating into the carotids. The louder the systolic murmur and the later the maximum intensity, the worse the aortic stenosis. Volume can decrease with critical aortic stenosis or worsening heart function.

ECG: ST-T changes can develop prior to signs of left ventricular hypertrophy (LVH). Signs of LVH (left axis deviation, positive Sokolow-Lyon-index) are present in 85% of severe AS. T wave inversions appear in moderate to severe stenosis (Fig. 1). It should be noted that ECG progression over time to LVH and ST-T wave changes are a sign of increasing stenosis.

Stress ECG testing is not contraindicated in asymptomatic individuals. It requires evaluation of exercise capacity, blood pressure response (decreasing), and stress induced symptoms.

2-D Doppler echocardiography has a key function in the diagnosis of aortic stenosis. It provides: morphological assessment of valve, LV-hypertrophy (>11 mm), LV function, reliable determination of pressure gradients and valve opening area and, if necessary, planimetry of the valve opening area and the transvalvular flow velocity. An erroneous high gradient can be measured in situations with a high cardiac output. Severe aortic stenosis exists with a P mean > 40 mmHg (P max. > 80 mmHg). This correlates well with invasively measured values.

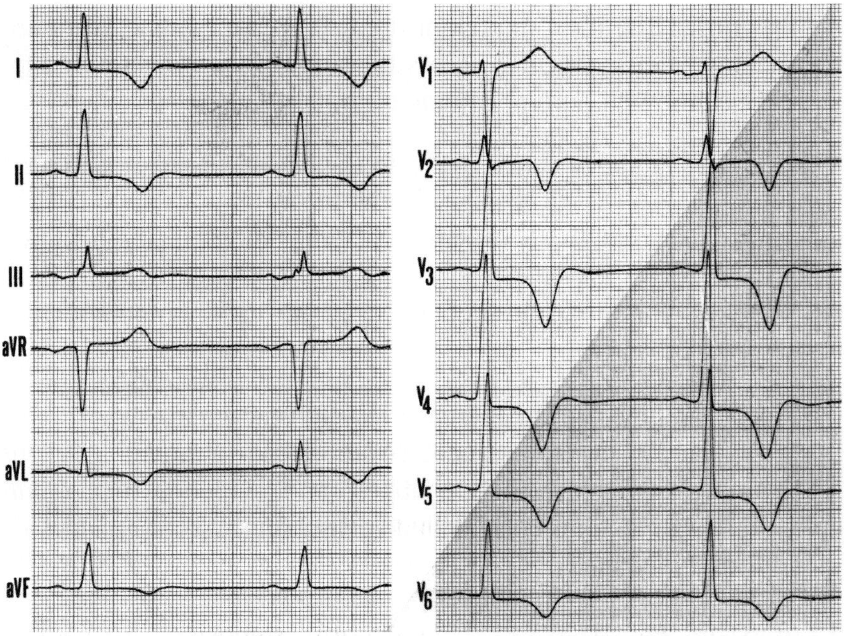

Figure 1. ECG in severe aortic stenosis.

Cardiac MRI: If the echocardiogram is ambiguous due to poor acoustic quality, an MRI should be undertaken.

Cardiac catheterization is indicated in case of significant aortic stenosis or symptoms not yet associated with significant aortic stenosis for further therapeutic determination (associated with CAD?).

Therapy: If the AS is asymptomatic in spite of being hemodynamically significant and the LV function is good, surgery is not absolutely indicated as the natural risk is lower than the peri-/postoperative risk. Nonetheless, there are disqualifications that can be lifted following appropriate surgery (see below), allowing restricted certification. Indications for surgery in the asymptomatic state include but are not limited to: reduced LV function, accompanying CAD, ventricular tachycardia, and excessive LV hypertrophy >15 mm. In single valve replacement, the in-hospital mortality rate is 1.5–5.6%. Aortic valvuloplasty is associated with a high restenosis rate, a severe complication that may lead to disqualification in the long run.

Prognosis: The most important predictors of a cardiac event are the maximal flow velocities across the aortic valve, determined by Doppler echo, with normal cardiac output:

- < 3.0 m/s: in the next five years, no cardiac events are anticipated (<1%).
- 4 m/s: 50% probability of symptoms or death within the next two years.
- 3–4 m/s: intermediate probability of the development of the symptoms.

The symptoms are an increase in left ventricular hypertrophy, decrease in LV function, increase in mean pressure gradient >50 mmHg, significant ECG changes, and evidence of cerebral emboli. These symptoms entail definitive disqualification for all classes of medical certification.

Aortic Valve Insufficiency

Medical Requirements (JAR-FCL 3): *Aortic regurgitation may be acceptable for unrestricted certification only if trivial. There shall be no demonstrable abnormality of the ascending aorta on 2D Doppler echocardiography. Annual review shall be carried out by a cardiologist acceptable to the AMS.*

In 70% of the cases, chronic aortic insufficiency (AI) is due to disease of the aortic valve (bicuspid aortic valve, endocarditis and other inflammatory diseases, post-rheumatic fever, etc.); the remaining 30% are due to diseases of the aortic root (aneurysm, dissection, connective tissue disorder such as Marfan's syndrome, arthritis disorders like Reiter's disease, Bechterew's disease, lupus, rheumatoid arthritis, etc.).

The increased stroke volume, caused by regurgitation, leads to left ventricular overload, later to exertional hypertrophy and dilatation with reduction in LV function, initially during exertion, later also at rest.

Individuals with chronic AI are often asymptomatic for many years, until exertional dyspnea is reached. A high blood pressure amplitude (cannonball pulse) is typical in moderate to severe AI. If the diastolic blood pressure is reduced (softening of the Korotkoff sounds) and/or pulsatile phenomena exist (such as visible capillary pulse following fingernail pressure), then significant AI and, consequently, a disqualifying condition exists.

Auscultation: During the diastole, a high frequency "blowing" decrescendo murmur is best heard at the left third intercostal space in patients leaning forward. Every murmur in a pilot must be evaluated with echocardiography.

ECG is not a good predictor for significant organic heart defect or LV hypertrophy. Findings may include left to extreme left axis deviation, accentuated Q-waves as expression of volume hypertrophy, evidence of left ventricular hypertrophy, inverted T-waves (developing late), and non-specific intraventricular conduction delay.

2D-Doppler echocardiography may provide proof of AI and indication of severity with high sensitivity and specificity, if interpreted by experienced cardiologists. Determination of the etiology of AI is usually possible with trans-esophageal echocardiography. Dilatation of the ascending aorta >40 mm is incompatible with medical certification. In the event of poor echo windows or discrepancy between clinical signs and echocardiography, a radionuclide ventriculography or cardiac MRI examination must be added.

The systolic LV size and function, which is determined by serial echocardiographic examinations, is decisive for the prognosis in the asymptomatic stage. An ejection fraction <50% and an end-systolic left ventricular diameter > 55 mm (parasternal) indicates an unfavorable prognosis. In the presence of LV dysfunction, 25% of cases develop symptoms each year, and valve replacement is usually necessary two to three years later. The time for invasive diagnostics and surgery has arrived. A slight enlargement of the end-diastolic LV diameter in the setting of normal end-systolic diameter is compatible with certification, limited to OML Class I (JAR-FCL3). A parasternal end-diastolic LV dilatation > 60 mm leads to disqualification.

The prognosis is very good for asymptomatic individuals with chronic AI and a normal LV function, as mortality is only 0.2% per year. If there is evidence of LV functional disorders, the mortality is

1.3% per year. In case of an EF <50% and heart insufficiency, disqualification should stand and further diagnostics be undertaken, due to the significantly elevated mortality.

Medical therapy: In the case of mild AI without LV dilatation other than from endocarditis, no specific therapy is indicated. Definitive recommendations for vasodilatation in mild to moderate asymptomatic aortic insufficiency and normal LV function cannot be determined on the basis of available data. Because of the increase of regurgitation in the setting of increased diastole, ß-blockers are not helpful.

MITRAL VALVE

Mitral Stenosis (MS)

Medical Requirements (JAR-FCL 3): *Rheumatic mitral valve disease shall normally be assessed as unfit.*

The normal mitral valve area is in the range of 4–5 cm^2. An area between 2.5 cm^2 and 1.5 cm^2 indicates mild mitral valve stenosis. Symptoms (dyspnea) can appear during stress or physiological load. The most common cause of acquired mitral stenosis is rheumatic fever 10–30 years earlier and frequently not remembered, affecting females in two-thirds of the cases. In asymptomatic or minimally symptomatic individuals, the survival rate is >80% in 10 years.

Significant flight safety problems include systemic emboli (endocarditis or intermittent atrial fibrillation), which develops in 20% of cases and is lethal in 10–15% (high relapse rate), and atrial fibrillation (up to 50%). The latter can be the initial symptom of mitral stenosis and is a result of the elevated left atrial pressure. This abruptly leads to a decrease in cardiac output of 20%, to pulmonary edema, and often causes emboli, which, among other things, can cause syncope. Eventually this leads to permanent disqualification. The diagnosis of MS is determined by the history, typical auscultory findings in the left lateral decubitus position (loud first heart sound, mitral opening sound after the second heart sound, followed by a low frequency diastolic murmur, chest X-ray, and ECG (biphasic P-wave in lead II, atrial fibrillation, later right axis deviation). 2D-Doppler echocardiography provides direct evidence of MS with dependable gradation and determination of mitral valve area, on the basis of highly reproducible morphological, functional, and hemodynamic parameters. For hemodynamic evaluation of mild MS, a dynamic stress echocardiography is reasonable, among other studies. Applicants with a mild mitral stenosis (mitral valve area $>2.0\ cm^2$ and continuous sinus rhythm may be assessed as fit at the discretion of the medical assessor. A 72-hour Holter monitor serves to rule in or rule out intermittent atrial fibrillation, which can lead to disqualification.

Therapy: In mild, asymptomatic MS and sinus rhythm, there is no specific therapy. Atrial fibrillation, emboli, and atrial enlargement (>55 mm measured parasternally), are indications for anticoagulation with warfarin or phenprocoumon, which *per se* is disqualifying. For interventional and operative therapies of mitral stenosis from a perspective of flight fitness, please see the section on *Valve Surgery*.

Mitral Valve Prolapse (MVP)[2]

Medical Requirements (JAR-FCL 3): *Asymptomatic applicants with isolated mid-systolic click may need no restriction. Applicants with uncomplicated minor regurgitation may need to be restricted to multi-pilot operations, as determined by the AMS. Applicants with evidence of volume overloading of the left ventricle demonstrated by increased left ventricular end-diastolic diameter shall be assessed as unfit. Periodic review and assessment as determined by the AMS is required.*

Mitral valve prolapse (synonyms: Barlow-syndrome, mid-systolic click/late-systolic murmur syndrome, floppy valve syndrome, etc.) variously prolapses a portion of one or both mitral leaflets during ventricle systole over the mitral valve ring level into the left atrium. MVP syndrome is defined when other symptoms exist simultaneously.

Primary etiology: Along with mucopolysaccharide acid storage disease, the enlarged mitral leaflet leads to a thickening of the leaflets and destruction of the mitral ring = myxomatous valve degeneration. It is often familial (25–50%), with possible associations with Marfan, Ehlers-Danlos syndrome, WPW (pre-excitation), skeletal abnormalities (pectus excavatum, flat chest, ectomorphic habitus, high palate, long arms, hyperflexive joints), hypertrophic cardiomyopathy, migraine, congenital QT syndrome, and other congenital cardiac anomalies.

Secondary etiology: Atrioventricular tissue is pathomorphologically inconspicuous, such as with CAD, ischemia, rheumatic diseases, cardiomyopathy, myocarditis, LV dilatation, etc. With regard to aeromedical relevance, close attention should be paid to primary or idiopathic MVP, as this condition is often not discovered during normal examinations.

Prevalence: Between 20 and 60 years of age, the prevalence is 1–2.5%. Often the diagnosis is made in older patients and may be due to questionable echocardiographic criteria. Individuals with mild to moderate ballooning of one or both thickened mitral leaflets (in four-chamber views) with normal coaptation points and with physiological or absent mitral insufficiency should be considered healthy (Fig. 2).

Symptoms: Most patients with MVP are asymptomatic. Possible symptoms are uncharacteristic non-exertional chest pains, easy fatigability, dyspnea, dizziness, syncope, and unspecified palpitations.

ECG: Nonspecific ST changes and T wave inversions in II, III, aVF, and left lateral leads, PVC's and PAC's, supraventricular tachycardia, associated with QT prolongation, and WPW (Fig. 3).

Mitral valve prolapse usually carries a good prognosis (cardiac events <1%/year). There is a sub-group of individuals that carries a higher risk of cardiac events. From an aeromedical perspective, because of increased complications in the long run, these need to be identified. Echocardiography plays a key role in identifying them.

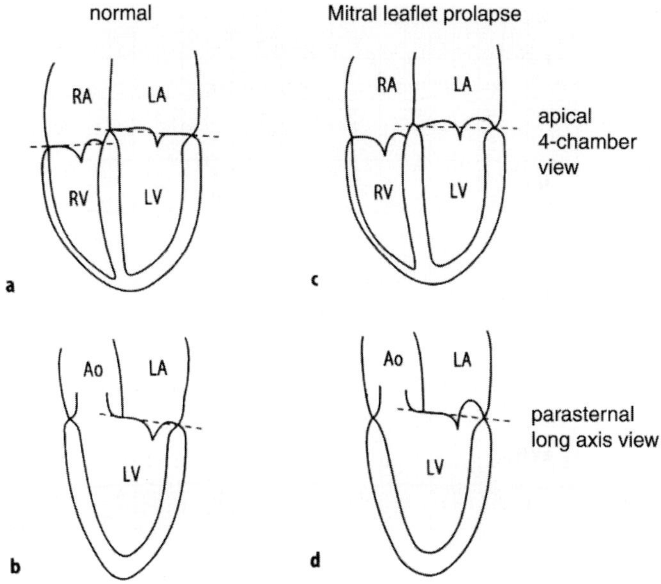

Figure 2. Mitral leaflet position in normal and in mitral leaflet prolapse subjects. The posterior leaflet rises above the level of the valvular ring by over 2 mm.

The following abnormalities necessitate particular observation and evaluation:

1. Auscultatory mid-systolic clicks and late systolic murmurs → inspection: distinctive skeletal features, marfanoid habitus, family history → echocardiography in two Doppler planes: in case of overlapping of leaflets directed to LA of at least 2 mm and leaflet thickening >5 mm, documented mitral insufficiency, lengthened leaflet cords and ring dilatation, aortic valve and tricuspid valve prolapse (25–50%) should be considered. LV diameter measurements should be less than 60 mm at end-diastole.

   Echocardiography should be repeated annually, and the aeromedical disposition should be made in consultation with the medical assessor of the Licensing Authority. Significant enlargement of the left ventricle is disqualifying.

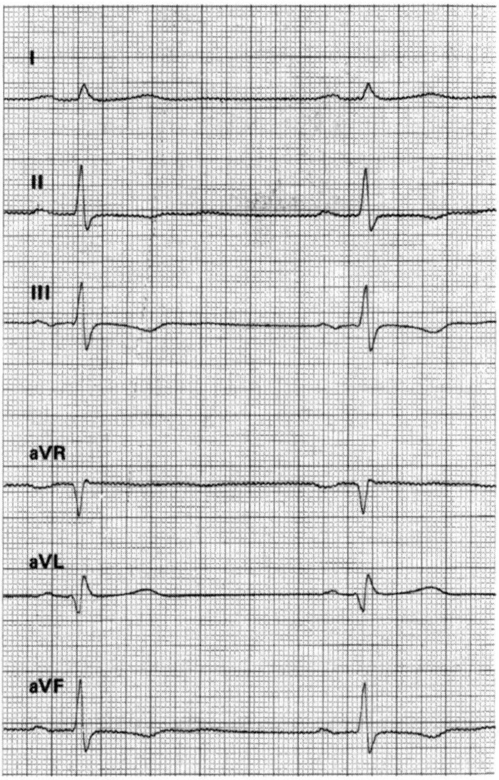

Figure 3. Preterminal negative T in II, III and aVF in Mitral leaflet prolapse.

2. If MVP has been diagnosed and resting ECG shows pathology with prolonged QT interval, T wave inversions or ST segment abnormalities inferiorly and laterally, ventricular arrhythmia and sudden cardiac death are more common (around 1% per year, frequently in the familial form). As simultaneous CAD is possible, pilots should be further evaluated with examination of function and, if necessary, coronary angiography and 72-hour Holter monitoring. ECG changes can often be normalized with ß-blockers.
3. Stress ECG testing is false positive in 50% of cases. Currently even scintigraphy can be false positive. Consequently, liberal use of coronary arteriography is indicated.

4. Symptoms are palpitations, dizziness, syncope, and arrhythmia (atrial and ventricular extrasystoles — accessory pathways are often not recognizable on ECG), and AV nodal reentry tachycardias. VT and VF as etiologies of sudden cardiac death are possible with an estimated frequency of 1.9 per 10 000 patient-years, but the true incidence is unclear.

   72-hour ECG, showing ventricular and supraventricular tachycardia, may possibly necessitate electrophysiological evaluation and ablation, after which recertification is possible. With a normal ECG, the risk of sudden cardiac death is very low. ß-blockers reduce symptoms.
5. Chest pain is often atypical with sub-mammary location, non-exertional, and lasting longer than angina pectoris.

   CAD should be ruled out. ß-blockers reduce symptoms.
6. Embolic events such as TIA, stroke, and amaurosis fugax occur with a rate is 4% in six years. In cases with myxomatous valve changes, fibrin emboli are particularly common. Lesions in cranial CT and larger emboli are permanently disqualifying. Normal CCT with absence of embolus source and thin mitral leaflets in trans-esophageal echo-cardiography may be compatible with restricted certification (OML/OSL), as long as it is related to TIA or amaurosis fugax and the applicant has been treated with thrombocyte inhibitors (ASA or clopidogrel) for six months without any further embolic events.
7. Mitral valve insufficiency: Clinical manifestation of MI (mitral insufficiency) in MVP usually occurs in the third to fourth decade, and a significant MI (≥ Grade III, progression 15% in 15 years), which usually is due to the rupture of the chordae tendineae or the development of atrial fibrillation, is disqualifying. Men >50 years of age and those with marfanoid habitus are particularly affected.

   Annual echocardiography is indicated and should be carried out by an experienced cardiologist. Significant MI entails unfitness for all classes of certification. If valve surgery is considered, mitral valve reconstruction should be preferred, so that future certification may become possible.

Definitive mitral valve prolapse is not compatible with military flying. If the diagnosis is made after military training has begun, full flying status is allowed provided the prolapse is minimal and asymptomatic and ECG is normal. In such cases, full certification is also possible for civilian pilots. Moderate prolapse requires limitation to OML. Acceleration >+2.5 G and Valsalva maneuvers should be avoided.

Mitral Insufficiency (MI)

Medical Requirements (JAR-FCL 3): *see mitral valve prolapse.*

The most common causes of chronic mitral valve insufficiency are mitral valve prolapse and inflammatory valve diseases (i.e. bacterial endocarditis, rheumatic endocarditis, Libman-Sacks endocarditis). Rheumatic MI is disqualifying. Secondary mitral valve insufficiency appears in all dilatative diseases of the left ventricle (CAD, ischemia of the papillary muscles, cardiomyopathy, and congenital aortic diseases, which are disqualifying *per se*).

Diagnosis: Leading symptoms are exertional dyspnea and performance limitations. Rapid atrial fibrillation worsens these symptoms and is disqualifying. Diagnosis is made by auscultation (high frequency, holosystolic ejection murmur immediately following the first heart sound, best heard over the apex, radiating into the axilla), ECG (prolonged P wave, left hypertrophy etc.). Chest X-ray and 2D-Doppler echocardiography allows direct observation of MI and semi-quantifiable evidence of the etiology of the insufficiency (prolapse, vegetations, cardiomyopathy, rupture of chordae tendineae and papillary muscle), determination of LA/LV size and systolic LV function, and estimation of pulmonary artery pressure.

Aeromedical Disposition

1) Asymptomatic individuals who meet the following criteria may be certified:
   a) mild MI, LV not enlarged (end-systolic <45 mm parasternal)
   b) no evidence of LV dysfunction (EF > 60%)
   c) no evidence of pulmonary hypertension

d) sinus rhythm on ECG
e) symptom limitations on graded exercise testing to Bruce Stage IV, and no other health problems exist.

Cardiological evaluations with echocardiography, stress ECG testing and Holter monitoring are required every six to 12 months. Limitation to OML for Class I is necessary.

2) More than minimal grade MI, non-rheumatic in origin, may carry the limitation "only with safety pilot," OSL.
3) Significant (even asymptomatic) MI, equal to or greater than Grade III, with volume overload of the left ventricle, enlarged end-diastolic left ventricular diameter (>60 mm) and/or end-systolic diameter >40 mm and/or post-transient ischemic attack, is disqualifying for all classes of medical certification.
4) The decision when to operate in the asymptomatic state is difficult. In cases where the disease is worsening, surgery to maintain valve function should be made early on to increase the possibility of recertification. Decisive predictors for post-operative prognosis is the pre-operative ejection fraction. With a significant MI, the LV should be hyperkinetic.

   A normal EF with a significant MI indicates LV dysfunction. In the asymptomatic state, surgery is indicated in patients in NYHA[a] classes I and II with significant MI, EF ≤ 60%, and end-systolic diameter of >40 mm.
5) The type of valve surgery that can be recommended and which is compatible with flight certification is discussed in the following section.

VALVE SURGERY

Medical Requirements (JAR-FCL 3): *Applicants with implanted mechanical valves shall be assessed as unfit. Asymptomatic applicants with a tissue valve (or valve reconstruction) who at least six months following surgery shall have satisfactorily completed investigations that*

[a] NYHA: New York Heart Association.

demonstrate normal valvular and ventricular configuration and function may be considered for a fit assessment by the AMS, as judged by:

- *a satisfactory symptom limited exercise ECG to Bruce Stage IV or equivalent, which a cardiologist acceptable to the AMS interprets as showing no significant abnormality. Myocardial scintigraphy/stress echocardiography shall be required if the resting ECG is abnormal and any coronary artery disease has been demonstrated;*
- *a 2D Doppler echocardiogram showing no significant selective chamber enlargement, a tissue valve with minimal structural alterations and normal Doppler blood flow, and no structural nor functional abnormality of the other heart valves. Left ventricular fractional or shortening shall be normal;*
- *the absence of requirement for cardioactive medication; a follow up with annual cardiologic review by a cardiologist acceptable to the AMS with exercise ECG and 2D Doppler echocardiography.*

A Class I fit assessment shall be limited to multi-pilot operation (Class I OML). A fit assessment for Class 2 applicants may be applicable without a safety pilot ("OSL").

Valve Reconstruction

The possibility of reconstructive surgery should not be withheld from the pilot who is considering recertification in cases such as AV valve insufficiency and aortic valve insufficiency. The medical assessor together with an accredited cardiologist should identify a qualified center with significant experience in valve reconstruction. On the basis of the anatomy, restoration of insufficient tricuspid and mitral valve performance is possible. Certain morphological changes are particularly suitable for surgical correction (e.g., MVP, chordae tendineae rupture, perforation of the mitral leaflet, rheumatic MI in children and youths, dilatation of the mitral annulus, etc.). In specialty centers, even aortic valve reconstruction is possible with increasingly good outcomes, especially in case of insufficient bicuspid aortic valves or aortic insufficiency due to aortic root dilatation.

Mitral valve reconstruction with or without suturing an artificial valve ring into place (annuloplasty, valvuloplasty) is surgically sophisticated and only possible if no extensive deformation, calcification, or destruction of the valve apparatus exists. It carries a good long-term outcome and is compatible with medical certification under the proviso that no relevant mitral regurgitation exists, that the left atrial appendage is operatively ligated (source of emboli), the applicant is in sinus rhythm, is six months post-operative, and the valve is demonstrated to be stable by echocardiography.

Young patients with degenerative or rheumatic mitral insufficiency and normal left ventricular ejection fraction without atrial fibrillation profit the most from valve reconstruction, because the surgery is performed before irreversible myocardial damage takes place. Preservation of subvalvular mitral valve apparatus leads to improved post-operative LV function and a more favorable life expectancy. The main advantage, in contrast to valve replacement, is the lower rate of embolism (<0.8% per year) and that anticoagulation is unnecessary in the majority of cases. The rate of infectious endocarditis corresponds to the acquired mitral valve disorder, necessitating corresponding endocarditis prophylaxis for dental, gastrointestinal, and urogenital operations. The incidence of second operations in mitral valve prolapse syndromes approximates 1.6% per year. The 10-year survival rate on average is above 90%.

Percutaneous balloon valvuloplasty for mitral valve stenosis usually comes into question with rheumatic MS only. On the basis of the high rate of abrupt onset of atrial fibrillation and cerebral embolism, this diagnosis *per se* entails permanent disqualification.

Bioprostheses (Fig. 4)

Since 1965, the bioprostheses in use include:

- *Xenografts (= Heterograft):* Prostheses derived from denatured porcine aortic valves, supported by stents (e.g. Hancock,

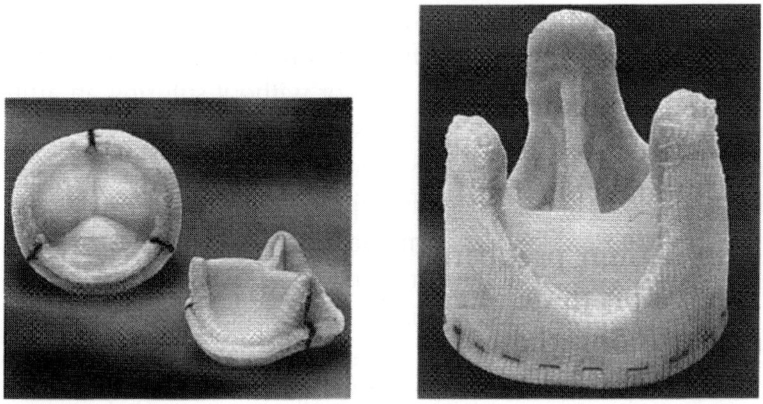

SJM stent mounted bioprosthesis

Porcine stentless tissue valve

Figure 4. Different tissue valves.

Carpentier Edwards Bioprosthesis with suture annulus and metal support).

- *Homografts (= Allograft):* Cryo-conserved aortic valves from human cadavers, without sewing flange and metal support (limited availability, technically difficult surgery).
- *Bovine pericardial bioprosthesis:* (Lonescu-Shiley prosthesis), seldom involves structural valve destruction as with above-mentioned xenografts (after 15 years 77% are functional).
- *Autografts:* Autotransplantation of the patient's own pulmonic valve in aortic position, pulmonic valve replaced by homograft or heterograft (Ross procedure with excellent survival rate and good hemodynamic features).
- *Heterografts (without metal supports):* Stentless with better characteristics, better prognosis, such as (Medtronic®, *SJM*®).

The hemodynamic characteristics and the valve areas of all valve prostheses are, without exception, not as good as those of natural valves, especially with regard to parabolic flow profile. The flow characteristics consist of a more or less significantly pronounced jet flow with turbulent shear forces and dead water zone with problems mentioned below. The shear forces near the walls in bioprostheses are in general lower than in mechanical prostheses, except for the St. Jude Medical bileaflet valve prosthesis.

Aeromedically Relevant Characteristics of Bioprostheses

- Bioprostheses are less thrombogenic than mechanical valves. The incidence of thromboembolic complications per 100 patient years nonetheless amounts to 0.5–4.4, with aortic bioprostheses to only 0.6–1.5 per 100 patient years. Anticoagulation is only required during the first three months post-operatively; thereafter, lifelong treatment with 100 mg ASA daily is required.
- All bioprostheses are prone to more or less rapid degeneration from calcification. Consequences are stenosis and insufficiency, sudden tears of portions of valves, paravalvular leaks, and susceptibility to vegetations. The degree of degeneration correlates to time from implantation, and is worse in the mitral valve with young patients and with increased calcium metabolism. Second surgery after 10 years is needed in 20–30% of cases. Only 15% of aortic homografts will need re-operation after 10 years,[3] so that homografts should be given preference in pilots who are usually under 70 years of age.
- The risk of endocarditis is elevated; the cumulative risk after five years lies between 3 and 6%.

Implications for Pilots

The aortic prosthesis of first choice should be the one with the lowest complication rate. Longest durability has the stentless homograft prosthesis, but its availability is the limiting factor. After implantation of a Carpentier Edwards bioprosthesis, Hancock bioprosthesis or comparable prosthesis, certification may be considered under certain circumstances as described above. After implantation of a mitral bioprosthesis, aeromedical certification must be critically evaluated with focus on durability and embolism rate. Slowly progressive degeneration of the bioprosthesis will have the above-mentioned consequences and echocardiographic evaluations must be conducted, initially annually and after the fifth post-operative year semi-annually, in some cases complemented with trans-esophageal echocardiography. Comparison with earlier post-operative echocardiographies is very helpful, particularly as the course of pressure gradients over time provides information about the function of the prosthesis. An embolic event entails permanent disqualification.

Pilots with organic heart defects necessitating surgery should receive good preoperative advice. From a purely medical perspective, younger and middle-aged patients are less suitable for implantation of a bioprosthesis because of its tendency to degenerate. Usually secondary surgery will later become necessary and it carries a high mortality rate. With mechanical prostheses, on the other hand, permanent disqualification is unavoidable due to the necessary anticoagulation.

MECHANICAL HEART VALVES

Medical Requirements (JAR-FCL 3): *Applicants with implanted mechanical valves shall be assessed as unfit. Systemic anticoagulation therapy is disqualifying.*

The reasons for unfitness are the rate of thrombosis and thromboemboli and a significant risk of bleeding due to anticoagulation treatment with phenprocoumon/warfarin/coumadin, which is permanently necessary and is the cause of 75% of the complications following valve replacement. Mechanical prostheses (metal, carbon, or polyester) vary by the valve mechanism and the hemodynamics. The danger of thrombosis is greatest with tricuspid valves and least with aortic valves.

The oldest mechanical heart valves, the Starr-Edwards ball and cage and the Björk-Shiley tilting-disk, which were introduced in the 1960s, are permanently disqualifying for all valve positions, due to their high thromboembolism rate and unfavorable hemodynamics.

Significant reduction in thrombogenesis was achieved with the introduction of the currently utilized heart valves made from pyrolite. The widely used third type of mechanical prosthesis, the bileaflet valve prosthesis, has a particularly favorable flow profile (somewhat better than bioprostheses) and the lowest gradient. The most reliable and least problematic is the St. Jude-Medical Prosthesis (SJM), which was introduced in 1977 and today (2008) is the most commonly used artificial heart valve with over 800 000 implantations.

In the long run, isolated SJM replacement is in one study[4] stated to have a rate of thrombosis, thromboembolism, and significant bleeding of less than 1%. The incidence of thromboembolism/100 patient-years is 0.6–0.7% for aortic position and 0.9–3.9% for mitral position. The bleeding rate from anticoagulation is additional. The optimal anticoagulation for SJM prosthesis for aortic position lies in the INR (international normalized ratio) range of 2.7–2.8, and for mitral position, 2.9–3.1. The reduction of the level of anticoagulation and the introduction of INR-determinations, (with the advent of comparable, laboratory independent measurements instead of the PT) has reduced the risk of bleeding from anticoagulation. It is now about 1–2% per patient/year, highest in the first months of therapy. The amount of bleeding complications could be further reduced through the introduction of INR self-testing and low dose anticoagulation after mechanical valve replacement (ESCAT Study = early self controlled anticoagulation trial).[5] In this study, the INR goal for aortic prosthesis is in the range of 1.8–2.8, and for mitral prosthesis, 2.5–3.5. 76% of the measurements were in the therapeutic range, and the incidence of significant bleeding was 0.74% versus 1.2% with conventional anticoagulation, while the thromboembolic rate was very low at 0.18%.[6] The international guidance recommends permanent disqualification after mechanical valve replacement. In our opinion, this may not always be necessary; in very special individual cases with INR self-testing, restricted certification (OML or OSL) may be possible, as it is already practiced in the USA.

REFERENCES

1. Bonow RO, *et al.* ACC/AHA 2006 practice guidelines for the management of patients with valvular heart disease: Executive summary *J Am Coll Cardiol* **48**(3): 598–675.
2. Webb-People MM. (1992) Mitral leaflet prolapse: Aspects of fitness to fly. *Eur Heart J* **13**(Suppl. H): 117–129.

3. Doty DB. (1996) Aortic valve replacement with homograft and autograft. *Sem Thor Cardiovas Surg* **8**: 249–258.
4. Remadi JP, *et al.* (1998) Mitral valve replacement with the St. Jude medical prosthesis: A 15-year follow-up. *Ann ThoracicSurg* **66**(3): 762–767.
5. Koertke H, *et al.* (2003) INR self-management permits lower anticoagulation levels after mechanical heart valve replacement. *Circulation* **9**(108 Suppl.1): 1175–1178.
6. Koertke H, *et al.* (2005) Low-dose international normalized ratio self-management: A promising tool to achieve low complication rates after mechanical heart valve replacement. *Ann Thorac Surg* **79**: 1909–1914.

Chapter 14

Cardiac Rhythm and Conduction Disturbances

Reinhard Höltgen*,† and Marcus Wieczorek†

ICAO STANDARDS AND RECOMMENDED PRACTICES (ANNEX 1 — PERSONNEL LICENSING, 10TH EDITION, 2006)

- 6.3.2.5.2 An applicant with an abnormal cardiac rhythm shall be assessed as unfit unless the cardiac arrhythmia has been investigated and evaluated in accordance with best medical practice and is assessed not likely to interfere with the safe exercise of the applicant's licence or rating privileges.
- 6.3.2.6 Electrocardiography shall form part of the heart examination for the first issue of a Medical Assessment.
- 6.3.2.6.1 Electrocardiography shall be included in re-examinations of applicants over the age of 50 no less frequently than annually.
- 6.3.2.6.2 Recommendation — *Electrocardiography should be included in re-examinations of applicants between the ages of 30 and 50 no less frequently than every two years.*
- *Note 1 — The purpose of routine electrocardiography is case finding. It does not provide sufficient evidence to justify disqualification without further thorough cardiovascular investigation.*

* Corresponding author.

† Heart Center Duisburg, Clinic for Cardiology and Angiology, Herzzentrum Duisburg, Gerrickstrasse 21, 47137 Duisburg, Germany.

Atrial Fibrillation

Atrial fibrillation (AF) is a common cardiac arrhythmia caused by disorganized electrical activity in the atria, more often in the left with passive activation of the right atrium. Pathophysiologically, the left atrium is usually the initiator of the paroxysms, but the right atrium plays a role in the disarray.[3]

The majority of paroxysmal atrial fibrillations is initiated through foci in the pulmonary veins. High frequency focal electrical activity in these foci with conduction into the left myocardium along with simultaneous appearance of 4 to 6 micro-reentry cycles in the atria, leads to destabilization. Depending on the so-called atrial substrate (i.e., atrial size, degree of fibrosis, refractory times, etc.), spontaneous cessation of the paroxysms after variable latency periods is common. In case of solitary pulmonary vein foci where the atrial substrate to perpetuate the paroxysms is not available, the paroxysms are typically of shorter duration but have a tendency to recur. If significant atrial dilatation coexists, for example as a consequence of hypertensive heart disease, the paroxysms tend to persist and lead to chronic or persistent atrial fibrillation.[3,18]

Epidemiology

Atrial fibrillation is a rhythm disturbance which increases with age.[21] Men are affected significantly more often than women. The incidence of chronic atrial fibrillation in men younger than 65 is between 1 and 2%.[27]

There are no good data regarding the frequency of paroxysmal atrial fibrillation. Patients with paroxysmal AF are typically younger than patients with chronic AF and are less likely to have a structural cardiac anomaly.

The long time, usually years, between paroxysms is one reason that there are no reliable epidemiological data. The self-limiting nature of rhythm disturbances (within hours) is another.

Definitions

Idiopathic atrial fibrillation: AF without an identifiable cardiac etiology. The cardiological diagnosis is without a pathological cause (ECG, echocardiogram, stress-ECG, if necessary cardiac angiogram). It is essential to exclude hyperthyroidism. Patients with idiopathic AF often have the above-mentioned pulmonary vein foci as documented by electrophysiological testing.

Paroxysmal atrial fibrillation: Sudden onset of episodic AF which usually converts spontaneously after a variable period of time.

Persistent atrial fibrillation: AF without spontaneous termination, although it can be terminated by cardioversion.

Permanent atrial fibrillation: Chronic, continuous AF which can no longer be terminated.

"Lone atrial fibrillation" exists, if no identifiable cause for the AF and also no structural defects can be found.

Mechanisms which can lead to "sudden incapacitation" in atrial fibrillation

Hemodynamic changes

Hemodynamic changes may be less pronounced in the sitting (pilots) than in the standing positions. The sudden shift from a normal sinus rhythm to a rapid and irregular ventricular rhythm without mechanical atrial systole can, in individual cases, lead to significant hemodynamic changes with a sudden drop in systolic blood pressure and a simultaneous rise in the left atrial pulmonary artery pressure. These hemodynamic changes are usually rapidly compensated by the autonomic nervous system through measurable adaptation responses, for example peripheral vasoconstriction. Failure or delay of adaptation responses can, in individual cases, lead to syncope or pre-syncope. In the sitting position (pilots), hemodynamic changes will be less pronounced.

In AF, the acute hemodynamic compromise of a patient's cardiovascular system is not correlated to the degree of cardiac disease. It is often associated with a positive reaction at the tilt table test.[13,20] The abovementioned acute hemodynamic changes are usually observed during paroxysmal AF. These changes are less obvious in patients with chronic AF, though hemodynamic worsening of sinus rhythm can be documented and a decline in stress coping capacity is evident.

Embolic complications

The risk of thromboembolic complications in patients with AF (and atrial flutter) is primarily correlated with the patient's age and the degree of underlying structural cardiac abnormalities. Patients with chronic AF and patients with paroxysmal AF have a comparable risk of emboli as long as age and underlying etiology are identical. The most common clinical manifestation of a thromboembolic event is a cerebral insult with corresponding neurological deficits. Depending on the abovementioned clinical parameters, the risk of a neurological insult can be as high as 5% per year.

In comparison with patients in sinus rhythm, patients with idiopathic AF (paroxysmal or chronic) and younger than 65 do not have an increased risk of thromboembolism. Therefore, they do not require anticoagulation.[2] The risk of thromboembolism in all other patients with AF increases significantly after a period of two days, and is the highest in patients with a prior embolic event.

The level of anticoagulation therapy is determined by the individual risk of embolic events due to AF: High risk groups (prior emboli, mitral stenosis, valve prosthesis) should be effectively anticoagulated with Marcumar (phenprocoumon) or Coumadin (warfarin) to a level of 2.0–3.0 (International Normalized Ratio — INR) in order to minimize the risk of thrombosis while accepting a bleeding risk of 3 to 10% per year.

According to the ACC/AHA/ESC Guidelines 2006 (European Heart Journal 2006: 27, 1979–2030), therapy can consist of either ASA 100 mg or warfarin/phenprocoumon, when the risk factors are moderate (age >75 years, hypertension, heart insufficiency, diabetes).

In both cases the risk of embolism is probably more than 1% per year, and treatment with warfarin or phenprocoumon carries a bleeding risk of 3–10% per year, so aeromedical certification is not possible.

Subjective symptoms

Independent of the acute hemodynamic consequences of AF, the subjective impairment caused by palpitations can be so pronounced as to interfere with concentration. This occurs more often with paroxysmal AF and less so for patients with chronic AF.

Aeromedical Dispositions

The following are recommendations for aeromedical assessment of pilots with atrial fibrillation:

Basically, at first evidence of atrial fibrillation, the pilot must be disqualifed. Further evaluation should be accomplished through targeted diagnostics and individual evaluation to decide if, and under what circumstances, aeromedical certification may again become possible.

Regarding paroxysmal and chronic AF, the following principles apply:

A) Disqualification is mandatory if there is evidence of structural cardiac anomalies; therefore the following disorders must be considered:

- Primary cardiomyopathy (hypertrophic of dilated)
- Arterial hypertension with hypertensive heart disease
- Coronary heart disease with evidence of ischemia
- Valvular disease.

In all of these, the likelihood of an incapacitating cardiovascular event is substantially greater than 1% annually.

B) Pilots with AF (paroxysmal or chronic) without evidence of structural anomalies (the so-called idiopathic AF) should be disqualified if they are older than 65 years of age and not anti-coagulated. In this group, the statistical risk of thromboembolic complication is above 1% per year.

The goal of pharmacotherapy is suppression of paroxysmal episodes and control of heart rate. Because of possible central nervous system and proarrhythmic side effects, certain medicines cannot be utilized in pilots. These are, among others, clonidine, flecanaide, propafenone, amiodarone and disopyramide.

For prevention of AF recurrence and/or control of heart rate in chronic AF, the following medicines are acceptable:

- β-receptor blockers
- sotalol (which is not favorable from an aeromedical perspective)
- verapamil
- digitalis glycoside.

The absence of side effects that could impair flight performance must be confirmed individually (if applicable, in a flight simulator). It must be pointed out that the use of β-blockers and verapamil can increase AV conduction time. The effect of these substances is based on the fact that a reduced heart rate during paroxysmal AF can increase the likelihood of spontaneous conversion. The digitalis preparations are also primarily similar. Nonetheless, their effect under adrenergic influence can be severely reduced. Sotalol is quite effective but exhibits a potential to increase the repolarization period (QT interval) and, in certain cases, has proarrhythmic effects, ranging from tachycardia to torsade de pointes.

Due to the requirement that there shall be no significant functional nor structural abnormality of the circulatory system, medical certification of applicants with AF can be considered under the following conditions:

- Normal ECG (12 leads): resting heart rate less than 90/min and during stress testing less than 220/min, even under AF.
- Normal stress testing without evidence of ischemia (as much as can be determined under medication).

- Normal findings on myocardial scintigraphy or dobutamine-echocardiography.
- Echocardiography with biventricular ejection fraction over 50%.
- Normal ventricular diameter (2D echocardiography).
- Maximal left atrial diameter of 4.5 cm.
- If applicable, coronary angiography without evidence of significant coronary artery stenosis.
- Holter monitoring: 48 hours continuous ECG monitoring on three different occasions with an interval of four weeks, without evidence of AF in patients who have experienced a singular episode or have a paroxysmal form.
- No pauses longer than 2.5 seconds during the day, not even after cardioversion to sinus rhythm.
- In patients with chronic AF: documentation of the shortest RR interval over 300 ms, and the longest RR interval under 3.5 seconds.

It is evident that only pilots who are in the low risk group (such as lone atrial fibrillation and age under 65 years with about 0.5% risk of embolism per year) are fit for medical certification.

Medically indicated Marcumar (or Coumadin) therapy in pilots with AF implies an elevated cardiovascular risk and entails a significant risk of bleeding; it is therefore always disqualifying.

Special cases

After a single episode of AF with an identifiable cause (excessive physical activity with electrolyte imbalance, following excessive alcohol consumption, thyreotoxicosis), a first-time applicant can be issued a Class I medical certificate if the likelihood of recurrence is low (JAR-FLC3). This can be difficult to determine in individual cases. With recertification or renewal cases, certification can be determined by the abovementioned criteria. It is necessary to add restrictions to multicrew duties or "without passengers." After two years, restrictions can be lifted as long as no further episodes of symptomatic AF have occurred. Implantable closed-loop recorders have become available in recent years. These can recognize and record arrhythmias and, upon interrogation, provide exact evidence of a patient's individual arrhythmia burden.

Incomplete arrhythmia suppression carries some residual risk for the development of an embolic event, probably less than 1% per year. Three unremarkable 48-hour ECGs do not entirely exclude intermittent paroxysmal AF. This is to be taken into account when certificating pilots and calls the recommendation for Holter monitoring in question.

From this follows that pilots with AF should be limited to multicrew duties. Essentially, the deciding factor is the symptomatology during the paroxysms, because symptoms can be so pronounced that they temporarily impair the pilot's cognitive performance. From the clinical symptomatology experienced with AF during daily activities, it can be difficult to extrapolate to the cockpit situation. Therefore all pilots with paroxysmal AF, despite medication, should be disqualified. Flexibility may be possible if, in individual cases over an appropriate period of time, it is possible to demonstrate that the clinical symptomatology of AF is well tolerated and the paroxysms are rare.

Pilots with chronic AF ("lone AF")

The risk of embolic events is similar to that of paroxysmal AF, under 1% per year. Permanent presence of this rhythm disturbance, in contrast to the paroxysmal form, carries a reliable prognosis as well as a predictable clinical symptomatology, primarily a reduction of the cardiopulmonary function. The clinical impression can be validated any time through flight simulation. Under the specifications of an appropriate examination frequency, limited medical certification (multicrew) is possible. Cardiological evaluations with Holter monitoring and echocardiography are required semi-annually. Commercial single-crew aircraft operation may not be possible.

Invasive electrophysiological diagnostics and therapy

In the event that antiarrhythmic therapy does not entirely suppress the arrhythmia, and/or the symptomatology of episodes is distressing, curative therapy should be considered. Invasive surgical and electrophysiological therapeutic options are currently in the midst of rapid development.

In order to inhibit perpetuation of macro and micro reentry cycles, ablation procedures utilizing radiofrequency or microwave and ultra sound techniques or cryoablation are available. These were initially considered adjuncts to the original operative procedures (Maze I/Maze II). With a variety of techniques, application of these surgical ablation procedures on other indications were soon established as independent methods, primarily in cardiac surgery[11] where the minimally invasive right-sided thoracotomy approach with a heart-lung bypass machine was used.[22] Following that, epicardial ablation emerged as the primary minimally invasive intervention procedure, using a right-sided mini-thoracotomy approach, without the need for a heart-lung bypass machine. The application of electrophysiological catheter procedures has subsequently undergone significant development. Today, a variety of techniques have to be considered for any catheter-interventional procedure.

Following the electrical isolation of the arrythmogenic pulmonary vein focus, radiofrequency or cryoablation is initiated.[17] Observation for possible development of symptomatic scar-induced pulmonary vein stenosis is necessary for a period of time following this procedure.[16] The most likely cause for stenosis is that the initial ablation energy was administered into the pulmonary vein, which is why these techniques have been modified. By isolating the pulmonary vein on the atrial side or by limiting the ablation to the elimination of electrophysiologically identified connections between the pulmonary vein and the atrial myocardium (pulmonary strain), pulmonary vein stenosis can be prevented. Special catheters (such as the "lasso catheter") have been developed, which can determine with precision the topographic position of such connections by means of multiple, precisely spaced electrodes.

The so-called left atrial substrate modification originates from a different philosophy, namely the assumption that the preservation of atrial fibrillation in the region of the pulmonary vein ostia requires localized areas of reentry phenomenon (so-called "rotors") which perpetuate AF.[26] This atrial trans-septal approach results in a compartmentalization of the left atrium through encircling of the pulmonary vein ostia via a line of ablation, through which the serial rows of ablation points are realized. Depending on the operator, additional connection lines (such as a connection between the encircling of the right and left pulmonary vein ostia in the atria or a line from the left encircling to the mitral valve annulus) are applied. Visualization of the individual atrium as well as the introduced ablation line requires an electro-anatomical mapping procedure (NavX or CARTO).

In general, the success and safety of these methods have been shown by retrospective scientific analysis. Currently, there is a 6% "severe complication" rate, including intra- and peri-procedural death. An increasing number of reports indicate that an atrio-esophageal fistula may possibly appear later.

The therapeutic goal of this invasive method is not necessarily the definitive cessation of arrhythmia (achievable in favorable cases), but rather a significant reduction of arrhythmia episodes. While freedom from arrhythmia without arrhythmia therapy can be expected in about 85% of patients, recent reports indicate that in order to achieve no recurrences, more intensive aftercare is needed. The operative procedure can therefore be considered as an alternative, resulting in long-term sinus rhythm for about 90% of patients, without sternotomy or antiarrhythmic medications.

Decision regarding if and under what circumstances aero medical certification is possible can be evaluated six months postoperatively. Certification requires freedom from symptoms and semi-annual cardiological examinations for up to two years after such an intervention.

It is important to note that the catheter ablation procedure for AF is not to be considered as an alternative to warfarin/phenprocoumon treatment. Anticoagulation must be considered independently of a successful ablation and, because of bleeding risk and risk of embolism, will entail unfitness.

Atrial Flutter

Atrial flutter, in contrast to atrial fibrillation, is a rhythm disturbance exclusively of the right atrium,[10] if indeed a typical atrial flutter exists (Fig. 1). Many patients reveal atrial flutter and fibrillation in their medical histories, which are transitions from one rhythm disturbance to another. These are well documented and verify the strong relationship of these arrhythmias to eachother. Only in a few cases does one or the other rhythm disturbance exist exclusively

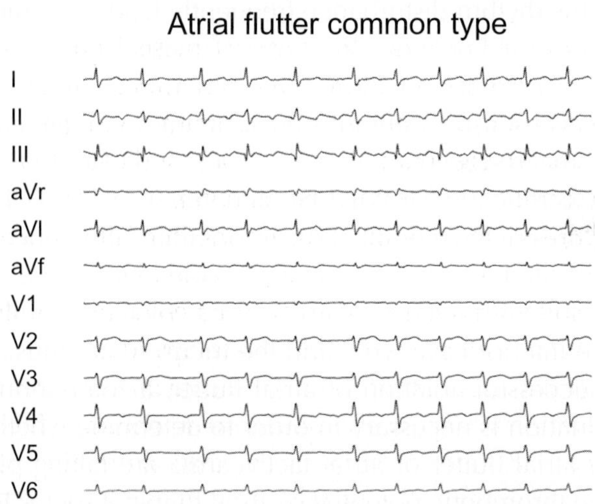

Figure 1. Atrial flutter common type. The figure shows a 12-lead electrocardiogram of typical atrial flutter (counter clockwise: activation of the right atrium) with 2-3:1-conduction ratio to the ventricle. It reveals an undulating baseline with recurring identical flutter waves of characteristical "sawtooth" shape, as an expression of permanent atrial electrical activity. These "F-waves" ("F" for flutter) are negative in II, III and aVF, positive in V1. They can be observed best during the phases of 3 (and more):1-conduction, so that the QRS-complex does not overlap most of the parts of the ECG representing the atrial activation. As an evidence of continuous atrial activation, the lack of an isoelectric interval between the flutter waves can be observed, as long as all the 12 ECG-leads are taken into consideration.

over a long period of time. Considering that the recurrence of atrial flutter can be suppressed by means of catheter ablation, these observations have many significant practical consequences. However, the afflicted patient has a not insignificant risk of experiencing further episodes of atrial fibrillation or atrial tachycardia within a 12-month time frame.

The cascade of these events has been studied[14] and should therefore be considered. Only in a few cases is typical atrial flutter the only, and in the greater context, the sole atrial rhythm disturbance. The appearance of atrial flutter is often observed in patients with structural heart disease, of which hypertensive heart disease is the most common. Atrial flutter is rarely observed in individuals with healthy hearts.

With regard to symptoms and therapy, these patients are treated similarly to patients with atrial fibrillation. On the basis of the high atrial rate, this rhythm disturbance frequently leads to symptoms and therefore to disqualification. In contrast to atrial fibrillation, potentially curative catheter ablation plays a dominant role[6] in that the integrated cavotricuspid isthmus flutter circuit no longer can enter in this form of macro-reentry.

Limited certification (OML/OSL according to JAR.FCL3) is then possible. Unrestricted certification is possible after one year, provided a repeated electrophysiological evaluation demonstrates a favorable result with regard to bidirectional blockade of the isthmus between the inferior caval vein and the tricuspid annulus.

Upon successful ablation of atrial flutter, a semi-annual cardiological evaluation is necessary in order to determine whether further episodes of atrial flutter or atrial tachycardia are taking place. With regard to the thrombotic potential of atrial flutter, it seems to be comparable to that of atrial fibrillation, with only minor differences,[9] for which the reader is referred to the corresponding chapter.

AV Node Reentry Tachycardia (AVNRT)

Pathophysiology

Patients with AVNRT (approximately 60% of those with with paroxysmal supraventricular tachycardia) typically have two functionally different conducting AV node structures: the so-called fast AV node pathway which, by its rapid antegrade conduction velocity, masks the other so-called slow conducting AV node pathways. Whether these pathways are part of an integrated AV node system or should be considered as paranodal atrial myocardial structures is a topic of on-going scientific discussion. On the basis of the differing refractive periods — long effective refractive period (ERP) of the fast pathway, short ERP of the slow pathway — these two conduction connections can be distinguished from each other, for example, through the appearance of extrasystoles. The atrial extrasystole is so premature that it cannot be conducted via the fast tract and therefore is conducted into the chambers via the slow AV node pathway. This is seen in the ECG as a lengthening of the PR interval after atrial extrasystoles. During persistent tachycardia, the P wave is typically no longer recognizable (Fig. 2).

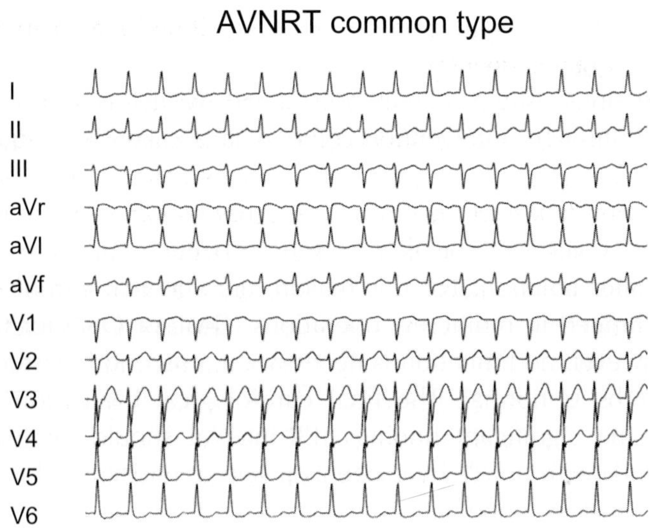

Figure 2. Atrioventricular nodal reentrant tachycardia. The figure shows a 12-lead electrocardiogram of a typical ("slow-fast") atrioventricular nodal reentrant tachycardia (AVNRT). It is the most common regular tachycardia of supraventricular origin, and as such, shows QRS-complexes of normal duration and contour. As atria and ventricles are depolarized nearly simultaneously, the P-wave is buried in the QRS-complex and therefore not recognizable.

The simultaneous activation of atria and ventricles in tachycardia can lead to pronounced cardiovascular effects, including syncope. Until compensatory mechanisms come into play, an AVNRT has been found by way of invasive examination to be between 95 and 260 beats per minute.

An association between AVNRT and cardiovascular disease does not exist. This rhythm disturbance is observed in healthy hearts as well. Women are more often affected than men.

The clinical symptomatology with the appearance of tachycardia in individual cases is difficult to predict (well tolerated until sudden incapacitation occurs) as it is modulated through numerous vegetative influences. Consequently, pilots with untreated AVNRT are unfit for all classes of medical certification.

On the basis of the special therapeutic recommendations by national and international specialty groups, the first line of therapy in patients with symptomatic AVNRT is the execution of a potentially curative catheter ablation of the so-called slow AV node pathway.[1] With the application of radiofrequency energy to the area of the coronary sinus ostium, elimination of the AVNRT is nearly always achieved. In larger intervention centers, pacemakers are required in less than 1% of cases. The recurrence rate is considered to be up to 7%, so that a repeat of the intervention may be necessary in individual cases. Over 95% of all recurrences occur within the first six months after ablation. For this reason, aeromedical certification is initially limited to multicrew operations (OML or OSL) for the first year. However, no limitation is necessary if a second EPS study after two months is normal. The final cardiological evaluation should result in no significant findings (PR-interval should be less than 0.2 seconds with no AV blockage as a sign of undisturbed functioning of the fast AV node pathway).

If there is evidence under isoproterenol that the tachycardia has not been extinguished, a second invasive electrophysiological evaluation is highly recommended, but could be limited in the future to patients who either have significant symptomatic episodes and/or infrequent paroxysms. In the latter case, the usual time frame of follow-up intervals is not adequate to evaluate the success of the ablation.

In the literature, it has been disputed whether or not patients who, at the end of evaluation, do not show evidence of complete elimination of the slow pathway (about 40%), will in general have a higher rate of recurrences.[8,15] With this in mind, recommendations have been made to allow unrestricted certification only when complete elimination of the slow pathway can be demonstrated by electrophysiological testing. Patients who merely demonstrate a modulation of slow pathway and who at final examination demonstrate a singular AV node echo, were recommended to undergo another invasive examination prior to unrestricted certification. Meanwhile, the modulation of the slow pathway of the AV node, so that only one single echo common type is left but the former inducible AVNRT cannot be reinduced, is an accepted endpoint of the ablation procedure and has the same outcome in the long run as a complete elimination of the AVN slow pathway.[25]

Medical prophylaxis of recurrences has been pushed into the background by the success of catheter ablation. The efficacy of medical prophylaxis is not very predictable and the significant recurrence rate and many side effects of medication render such treatment incompatible with safe flying.

WPW Syndrome

All pilots with symptomatic preexcitation syndromes are unfit for medical certification. In terms of accessory conduction tracts, patients with narrow and wide complex QRS tachycardias fall into this category, as well as patients with atrial fibrillation.

Three variations of rhythm disturbance are characteristic of WPW syndrome:

1. The so-called orthodrome circus movement tachycardia, which is impressive in its narrow QRS complex. The re-entry cycle consists of antegrade conduction via the AV node and the retrograde conduction is via the accessory connection back to the atria.
2. The so-called antidrome circus movement tachycardia, with a wide QRS complex as a consequence of antegrade conduction

over the accessory tract and retrograde conduction over the AV node (generally less common).

3. Tachycardia with alternating wide QRS complex as a consequence of atrial fibrillation and simultaneous antegrade conduction over AV node and accessory connection.

Evidence of a delta wave (Fig. 3) in the ECG can be subtle, particularly in "left sided," localized accessory pathways (with the electrical conductibility between left atrium and left ventricle). The left sided localization has the largest topographical distance from the AV conduction system, because the duration of the intra- and inter-atrial impulse propagation has a comparable late atrial arrival via the accessory pathway in comparison with the

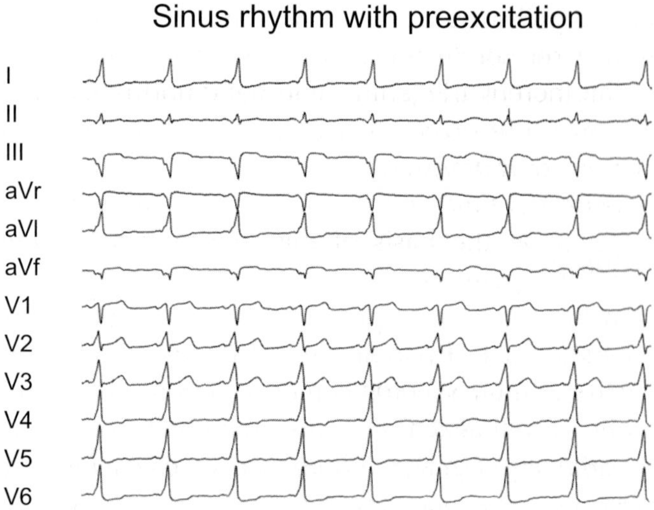

Figure 3. Preexcitation in WPW syndrome. The figure shows a 12-lead electrocardiogram of a patient with an accessory pathway. In this case, it is located in a diverticulum of the proximal coronary sinus. Electrical activity coming from the atrium depolarizes parts or the whole ventricle earlier than would be expected if the impulse traveled along the normal conduction system (AV-node and His-Purkinje-system). This premature ventricular activation causes an alteration in the QRS-complex, an ECG abnormality called "Delta-wave."

arrival of the compact AV node. The delta wave, in any case, is evidence that this accessory connection conducts in an antegrade direction.

A slight conduction capacity of this accessory tract can be assumed to exist when the delta wave is evident only intermittently and/or disappears during stress loading or at higher frequencies. An absent delta wave does not exclude a preexcitation syndrome, in that certain accessory pathways have the capacity to conduct retrograde, i.e. from the ventricle back to the atrium. This phenomenon is not recognizable in a superficial ECG during sinus rhythm (the so-called concealed WPW syndrome).

Antegrade conducted accessory pathways (open WPW syndrome) with high conductivity of the bundle (= short effective refractory period) are particularly dangerous.[29]

The appearance of atrial fibrillation (in 2% of cases with existing accessory pathways) creates the danger that atrial fibrillation impulses will be conducted as a rapid salvo onto the ventricle myocardium, thereby triggering ventricular fibrillation. Ventricular fibrillation therefore does not develop due to the rapid irregular atrial rhythm being transmitted "1:1" into the ventricle or over a lengthy period of time with hemodynamic problems as a consequence. Death on the basis of this mechanism has been well documented in patients with WPW syndrome, but is quite uncommon.[29]

The majority of tachycardic heart rhythm disturbances on the basis of preexcitation syndrome manifest themselves in the third decade of life. The potential for extrasystoles to trigger circus movements increases with age and may eventually lead to clinical appearance of this congenital anomaly.

After successful ablation treatment, medical certification is initially limited to multicrew operations. Unlimited certification is possible after a year, or after two months following a second EPS study. After one year, ongoing cardiological evaluations are no longer necessary.

The asymptomatic patient

A preexcitation pattern, shown by 12-lead ECG (frequency 0.25%) in an asymptomatic pilot, justifies a limitation to multicrew operations. The following are required for assessment:

- Normal stress ECG without evidence of coronary ischemia.
- Normal myocardial scintigraphy or stress echocardiography particularly when a delta wave is evident, and also when repolarization disturbances in the ECG are found regularly.
- Normal echocardiogram with biventricular EF over 50% and normal diameter.
- Invasive electrophysiological studies (EPS) demonstrates an effective refractory period of the accessory tract of over 300 ms and an HV-interval <70 ms, or an intermittent WPW pattern on ECG which disappears with exertion.
- Regular cardiology evaluations including 24-hour Holter must be maintained.

An initial Class I applicant with asymptomatic delta waves is only fit for certification if an electrophysiological examination including adequate medical stimulation of the autonomic nervous system excludes an inducible reentry tachycardia and multiple accessory conduction tracts. A Class II pilot can obtain an unlimited certificate if the required EPS studies are performed.

Although the prognosis in this asymptomatic group is very good,[29] nonetheless there exists a statistically increased risk of supraventricular tachycardia (about 2% per year). This is the rationale for the abovementioned restrictions with regard to medical certification.

It seems reasonable, particularly on the background of the required invasive EPS, to terminate the accessory pathways with a targeted catheter ablation, in order to:

1. Obtain unlimited medical certification (see AVNRT).
2. Deal early on with the risk of symptomatic tachycardia.

3. Avoid permanent disqualification after documentation of a short ERP.

"Prophylactic" catheter ablation in asymptomatic patients should only be undertaken after considering that particular ablation techniques can be associated with significant complications in individual cases:

Risk of AV blockade with ablation of right anteroseptal, midseptal and also posteroseptal accessory bundles.

Aeromedical disposition after successful catheter ablation in preexcitation syndromes is nearly the same as after ablation for AVNRT:

Limited medical certification Class I (OML) for 12 months, unless another EPS after two months demonstrates a favorable result. In the absence of long term favorable results, OML cannot be lifted. This requirement (according to JAR-FLC3) is valid also for Class II; here the limitation OSL or OPL (valid only without passengers) may be necessary.

Medical prophylaxis does not play a relevant role in decisions regarding medical certification.

The appearance of tachycardia in the up to now asymptomatic patient entails disqualification.

Special cases

Patients with only retrograde conducting accessory connections with short refractory periods and/or serious clinical symptomatology during tachycardia: The potential for recurrence cannot be determined by ECG and should therefore be evaluated by electrophysiology in the post ablation period. Initially, only restricted certification is possible.

Symptomatic preexcitation syndrome

As every symptomatic preexcitation syndrome results in disqualification, medical certification can only be reconsidered after successful performance of a curative catheter intervention.

The rate of success of treating preexcitation syndrome is dependent on the localization of the accessory tract and is between 90 and 99%. Right sided conduction tracts show a significantly higher recurrence rate than left sided cases, which can have practical consequences in the follow-up period.

Several special types of the classic preexcitation syndrome exist, whereby the accessory tracts exhibit characteristics that can significantly differ from that of the classic Kent bundle. The particular conduction characteristics of these tracts determine, inter alia, the clinical picture of the patient. On the basis of these variations, patients with corresponding symptomatology should have an EPS in order to determine the patient-specific electrophysiological characteristics of the accessory tracts and, if applicable, undergo an ablation procedure. These types of preexcitation are known as Lown-Ganong-Levine (LGL) or Mahaim syndromes.[4] Mahaim fibers are accessory tracts which are almost exclusively right sided. Their ventricular insertion is not near the tricuspid valve annulus, but rather in the area of the apex of the right ventricular myocardium. They demonstrate only decremental antegrade conduction, so that the conduction behavior is more similar to that of the AV conduction system than that of the Kent bundle. This type of accessory bundle allows only antidrome tachycardia, and the open preexcitation shows a left bundle branch block (LBBB) deformation of the QRS complex on a surface ECG. Therefore it is imperative to define this frequency-dependent LBBB, as this has significant therapeutic consequences. In contrast to the Mahaim fibers, which show an increasingly wide QRS complex, the frequency-dependent LBBB in general suddenly develops blockade at a critical frequency.

Atrial Tachycardia

Atrial tachycardia is usually linked to structural cardiac disease, therefore seldom encountered in the practice of aviation medicine.

Unambiguous evidence of atrial tachycardia entails unfitness. Medical certification requires a search for underlying cardiac disease; if found, permanent disqualification is the rule.

In addition to pharmacotherapy, curative therapy utilizing catheter ablation is a possibility after exclusion of underlying cardiac disease. If successful, certification needs limitation unless a repeat EPS verifies a normal finding. Due to the generally increased risk of recurrence of this type of supraventricular tachycardia, a corresponding invasive EPS should follow. Otherwise, the process is the same as described for successful catheter ablation of other supraventricular rhythm disturbances.

Ventricular Extrasystoles

Ventricular extrasystoles are common; if infrequent and unifocal, they are generally harmless in healthy hearts.

Evidence of frequent (>2% of QRS complexes), repetitive and/or polymorphic ventricular extrasystoles (<5 seconds in duration with a frequency of >120/min) is not a normal finding and requires further cardiological evaluation before medical certification can be considered. The goal is to find evidence of or exclude a structural cardiac disease. In the absence of structural cardiac disease, this distinctive rhythm feature is considered to carry a good prognosis in most cases.

In younger patients, especially those with electrocardiological clues for a right sided source of the extrasystoles, it is necessary to search particularly for signs of arrythmogenic right ventricular disease (in these cases an MRT evaluation of the right ventricle should be performed).

Evidence of a structural disease generally rules out medical certification. If there is uncertainty regarding the prognostic significance of the ventricular extrasystoles, EPS with corresponding stimulation maneuvers at baseline or under isopreterenol can be helpful in certain cases, even when the specificity is diminished in patients with coronary heart disease and completed infarct.

The value of the so-called signal average ECG regarding complex ventricular extrasystoles is controversial. It has its place in the area of non-invasive risk factor stratification, with regard to the appearance of sustained ventricular tachycardia in post infarct patients.[5,19] This is true even more so when a restriction in the left ventricular pump function exists. The evidence of high frequency and low amplitude signals at the end of the signal average QRS complex is associated pathophysiologically with a so-called "arrhythmia substrate." In this substrate, one finds an inhomogenous and generally slowing depolarization, which has a favorable predisposition for the emergence of reentry tachycardia in the ventricles.

BRADYCARDIA AND CONDUCTION DISTURBANCES

Sinus Node Dysfunction and SA Blockade

Differentiation between normal heart frequency modulation and "physiological" arrhythmia from real disorders of the sinus node or manifestation of sinus node disease can be especially difficult in young and otherwise healthy people. In the area of aeromedical certification, this can nonetheless have particular significance as the diagnosis of a pathological sino-atrial function results in disqualification for all classes of medical certification.

Physiological sinus node function and arrhythmia without pathological significance

The definition of normal sinus frequency is not unproblematic and must take into consideration the age as well as the physical condition of the patient. Sinus bradycardia of 40/minute in healthy and physically fit people in a relaxed state is not pathological. Sinus bradycardia under 40/minute in aerobically untrained people during the day may at least be a suspicious finding, particularly when symptoms associated with bradycardia are found in the history.

Pronounced fluctuation in sinus frequency with respiration in young patients is entirely physiological; in some cases it is an expression of high vagus tone.

Sinus pauses up to 2.5 seconds is found in 10% of the healthy population and pauses to two seconds in about 20% of athletes. Pauses greater than 2.5 seconds require further investigation, particularly for evidence of symptoms, whereas pauses over 3.5 seconds are to be considered pathological.

Chronotropic competence

Analysis of the variability of sinus node function as a response to physical loading is a decisive examination tool in the evaluation of sinus node function.

In many cases it is possible by stress testing to differentiate patients with vegetative modulating sinus bradycardia at rest and high normal frequency adaptation from sinus node function disturbances (so-called intrinsic sinus node dysfunction), due to inadequate heart rate.

Chronotropic competence during stress testing not only measures the attained heart rate at a particular stress level, but also the acceleration of the heart rate (i.e., heart rate over time).

Typically the increase in heart rate in some patients with sick sinus syndrome (SSS) is normal; however, the absolute heart rate at each individual stress testing level is reduced in comparison to the norm. Therefore it is important for the diagnosis of this group to determine the maximally achieved heart rate and compare it to the norm (for example 215 minus the age). The reproducibility of chronotropic competence is generally possible, limited by the individual vagal tone.

There is thus a sensible method for the evaluation of chronotropic competence by determining the measured heart rate acceleration and the individual maximally achieved heart rate. Healthy hearts should achieve the maximally achievable heart rate during stress testing in order to classify for medical certification.

P-wave morphology

In sinus rhythm, the P-wave duration is normally up to 100 ms in healthy hearts. As a rule, leads I, II, III and aVF exhibit a positive P-wave with the highest amplitude in II and aVF. The terminal negative vector portion in lead V1 is minimal. Diversions from this in certain circumstances indicate an intra-atrial conduction disturbance and should be classified as pathological.

Abnormal sinus node function

Sinus node dysfunction manifests itself electrocardiographically and/or clinically. It is slowly progressive and evolves benignly over many years. Sinus node syndrome consists of a variety of individual anomalies.

1. Significant, inadequate and persistent sinus bradycardia.
2. Sinus arrest with corresponding pauses and eventual evidence of junctional or atrial ectopy as escape rhythms.
3. Paroxysms or chronic atrial fibrillation as a result of sinus bradycardia or long pauses.
4. A variety of sino-atrial blocks.
5. Chronotropic incompetence.

It is evident that sinus node dysfunction consists of a heterogeneous group of rhythm anomalies that are not exclusively due to disturbed sinus node function, but more often related to a disorder of the sino-atrial transition and intra-atrial conduction.

Consequences for aeromedical certification

Pilots with symptomatic sinus node syndrome are disqualified.[19] For questions regarding aeromedical certification following pacemaker implantation, please see the section on pacemaker therapeutics.

Pilots who are asymptomatic, but have clues regarding sinus node function disorders (such as obvious sinus bradycardia less than 40/minute) should obtain close (semi-annually) cardiological oversight. Limitation of certification should be taken into consideration. All the cardiological evidence pertaining to supraventricular tachycardia can be utilized and should result in normal findings. Pauses over 2.5 seconds should not appear on Holter monitoring.

Diagnostic options

- Holter monitoring (heart rate variability, pauses, etc.), eventually loop recorder as external storage for retrospective analysis and activation by the patient.
- Stress ECG: chronotropic competence, pauses from SA blockade, arrhythmias.
- In individual cases: invasive EPS with determination of sinus node recovery period and the sino-atrial conduction time (this test had moderate sensitivity and high specificity, therefore an inconspicuous EPS does not rule out the existence of a significant sinus function disorder).
- Pharmacological tests such as autonomic blockade with atropine and β-blockade.
- Valsalva maneuver and orthostatic provocation test (evaluate different autonomic reflexes).

AV Blocks

Significant pacemaker disturbances of the heart — and the higher AV blocks are included — are disqualifying. Second (Mobitz type II) and third degree AV blocks are pathological findings and require further examination. They are disqualifying for flight.

A thorough cardiac/internal medicine evaluation is necessary. Only in a few cases will evidence of structural heart disease be compatible with aeromedical certification, even after treatment with a pacemaker implant.

As mentioned above, AV blocks are considered *a priori* to be pathological and are therefore incompatible with aeromedical certification. The aeromedical decision is practically not influenced by the existence or lack of clinical symptoms.

Exceptions

Individual, early subsiding, non-conducting P-waves and/or evidence relating particularly to the appearance of alternating long and short AV intervals during the night.

The appearance of very early single occurrences of supraventricular extrasystoles without conduction (early P-wave without a succeeding QRS complex) can be an expression of suppression of the antegrade conduction capacity of the AV node, or the transfer of conduction through a slow AV node bundle and is not the same as the diagnosis of "intermittent AV block." The differentiation is problematic, and can, in individual cases, be resolved with electrophysiological examination.

Intermittent second degree AV block — Wenckebach's phenomenon (Mobitz I)

This type of blockade during high vagal tone (therefore nocturnal) is often a normal variant in otherwise asymptomatic individuals with healthy hearts. This is particularly the case in very young people. In older people, restricted certification should be considered. Evidence of Wenckebach's block of short duration and with narrow QRS complexes have been shown to lead to a progression of higher grade AV block. In order to issue unlimited certification, pathological changes causing blockade must be excluded by additional cardiological evaluation, preferably including EPS.

First degree AV block

Here, there is actually no block, but rather a delay greater than the norm at the level of the AV node. Simultaneous bundle branch block should be excluded, as this could be an infranodal conduction delay, which carries an unfavorable prognosis. An invasive EPS is therefore recommended from an aeromedical perspective. Evidence of pathological Hissian or infra-Hissian conduction times rule out all classes of medical certification.

If all other cardiological evaluations are normal, unrestricted medical certification is possible.

Especially with regard to stress testing, it should be noted whether an increase in the PR interval occurs under exertion, which can likewise be considered pathological and should entail a limitation in certification.

The shortening, even at rest, of a clearly lengthened (up to 400 ms) PR interval is an expression of the functionality of the dual input to the AV node and should be further evaluated. Shortening to 0.20 s during stress testing or with atropine infusion is required in order to be considered favorable for certification.

In case of doubt, an electrophysiological evaluation should be undertaken. Normal findings are compatible with certification.

AV node duality (existence of two different conducting AV node pathways).

The only conspicuous finding is that, in certain phases of physical exertion, a sudden lengthening of the PR interval appears, because the ERP of the fast AV node pathway has been reached. This could be misinterpreted as a variant of AV block on the ECG. In the case of dual AV input, sudden lengthening of the PR interval is present. In the case of AV conduction block, one finds fluid transition of the PR interval change. AV node duality is found even without evidence of AV node tachycardia in about 6% of the general population. One should inquire about a history of palpitations, with respect to performing an adenosine provocation test.

14.2.3 Pacemaker Therapy and Aeromedical Certification

Pacemaker therapy is a rather rare occurrence in aeromedical evaluations. Pilots who have received a pacemaker can obtain certification (limited: OML Class I) under the following conditions:

- No evidence of cardiac disease, which *a priori* would be disqualifying.[12]
- Implantation of a bipolar pacemaker (minimizing potential influences of external sources on the pacemaker).
- No pacemaker dependency (such as complete AV block with unstable intrinsic rhythm less than 30/minute).
- Pacemaker failure rate is less than 1% per year (manufacturers information in relevant reports, available in international journals such as PACE).

These conditions are based on the assumption that pacemakers are implanted for intermittent AV block.

At the earliest, medical certification can be considered after a post-operative observation period of three months. Regular (six months) pacemaker evaluations are necessary and should be carried out by a physician with special training in pacemakers.

Hemiblock

Left anterior hemiblock (LAH) is found in 1 to 2% of the general population. An LAH that has been in existence for a long time is associated with a good prognosis and is compatible with medical certification, provided this is an isolated finding. A new LAH should prompt an evaluation for myocardial ischemia including a stress test. An already long-time existing incomplete LBBB (QRS to 120 ms) should be assessed as a chronic LAH, as long as a structural underlying heart disease is ruled out. A new appearance of an incomplete LBBB should be evaluated similar to a complete LBBB (see that section).

Left posterior hemiblock (LPH) is diagnosed less commonly. The limited data available suggests that, after excluding structural disease, a good prognosis is to be expected. A newly developed LPH requires an evaluation for myocardial ischemia by stress testing.

REPOLARIZATION ANOMALIES AND HEREDITARY DISEASES

QT Prolongation

QT prolongation is sporadically found among flight crews. On rare occasions this is an expression of a genetic disorder in the form of Jerwell-Lange-Nielsen syndrome in association with deafness, or the Romano-Ward syndrome which is an autosomal dominant genetic disorder.[28]

In many of these cases the QT prolongation is very obvious (>550 ms) and/or associated with morphological changes of the T wave. Because of the high risk for malignant ventricular arrhythmia, this constellation is disqualifying. However, subtle forms do exist.

More commonly, more moderate QT prolongation is encountered (QT over 440 ms), which require further evaluation:

- family history (cases of sudden cardiac death)
- exclusion of structural heart disease
- medication history (even antibiotics)
- if applicable, electrophysiology and genetic evaluation.

Hereditary Diseases

By now, a number of hereditary diseases are known which exhibit a primary electrical or myocardial etiology. These are related to an elevated risk for the development of malignant arrhythmias and are therefore disqualifying for all classes of medical certification. Examples of such hereditary diseases are:

- hypertrophic cardiomyopathy
- arrythmogenic right ventricular cardiomyopathy
- long QT syndrome
- short QT syndrome
- Brugada syndrome
- idiopathic ventricular tachycardia.

As these disorders are uncommon, there are no prospective or randomized studies for this group. In secondary prevention studies (AVID, CIDS, CASH), only a few of these patients could be included. Retrospectively, the consensus of the experts is that in order to survive sudden cardiac death, ICD implantation should be undertaken. The decision for ICD implantation for primary prophylaxis requires follow-up by an electrophysiology center. Defibrillator implantation is incompatible with all classes of medical certification. The individual risk factor stratification is, for the time being, still an object of ongoing research.

With regard to hypertrophic cardiomyopathy, risk factor stratification includes examples of risk factors such as:

- syncope of unknown etiology
- family history of elevated death rate

- abnormal blood pressure response to stress testing (increase <20 mmHg)
- multiple or long non-sustained VT on Holter ECG
- septal thickness ≥ 30 mm (alone a sufficient indication for ICD implantation; over 25 mm septal thickness is disqualifying).

There is no known prospective randomized study regarding arrythmogenic right ventricular cardiomyopathy (ARVC). In these cases, the risk factors exist on the basis of significant right ventricular dysplasia; occasionally, there is left ventricular participation such as is evidenced by a family history of sudden death. Further procedures depend on the individual profile, and a prophylactic ICD implantation is possible. Without the existence of significant RV dysplasia, catheter ablation or medical evaluation of inducibility of ventricular tachycardia should be considered. In the event that a diagnosis is secured (often difficult), disqualification follows.

Idiopathic ventricular tachycardia, also monomophic right or left ventricular tachycardia without any evidence of structural cardiac disease, should primarily initiate catheter ablation which, if successful, can be considered curative. Standard clinical and Holter electrocardiographic follow-up — at least for a period of six months — can help determine whether permanent therapeutic success has been achieved.

Syncope

Syncope is defined as a transitory condition of unconsciousness in association with a generalized loss of muscle tone, followed by spontaneous recovery.

A broad palette of diseases may cause such failure of blood pressure regulation; among these are some cardiac diseases:

- syncope on the basis of brady- and tachycardic disturbances
- syncope due to organic heart disease with extensive congenital heart disease (such as aortic stenosis)

- orthostatic syncope
- neurogenic syncope, among others.

A syncope entails disqualification. Exceptions to this rule may be considered only in certain situations:

Notable situations are corrected bradycardic rhythm disturbances such as with pacemaker therapy (see that section) or curative catheter ablation of tachycardic heart rhythm disturbances (see supraventricular tachycardia). Syncope on the basis of ventricular activity generally leads to disqualification, as in most cases a structural heart disease is responsible and the prognosis unfavorable.

There exists in rare cases an idiopathic ventricular extrasystole or tachycardia (for example with a focus in the right ventricular outflow tract in the area of the left ventricular interventricular apical septum). The life-long prognosis is favorable if structural heart disease cannot be discovered. The elimination of the responsible focus with electrophysiological evaluation followed by catheter ablation can be considered potentially curative. Further syncopal episodes following successful catheter ablation are not to be expected. A tilt test should nonetheless be performed in order to rule out a generalized baroreflex dysfunction.

Evidence of structural heart disease eliminates any basis for medical certification of any type. This is also the case if the etiology of the syncope is not identifiable and syncopal attacks occur without clear prior warning signs.

A limited certification (OML/OSL) can be considered, initially for six months, in individual cases (in accordance with JAR-FCL3) if an extensive cardiological evaluation is conducted (symptom limiting stress testing, such as myocardial scintigraphy or stress echocardiography, 2D echocardiography, 24-hour Holter ECG, tilt testing and neurological evaluation). Unrestricted certification is possible if, after five years, there have been no presyncope or syncope.

Syncope on the basis of a hypersensitive carotid sinus probably occurs very seldom in flight crews. Usually arterial hypertension of long standing is noted.

With targeted pressure on the carotid sinus, the patients develop symptomatic asystole or bradycardia (cardio-inhibitor type) and/or a fall in blood pressure of more than 50 mmHg systolic (vasodepressor type). In most cases, there is a combination of disorders. Pacemaker therapy is particularly effective for the cardio-inhibitor component of this disorder, and is minimally effective in patients with a dominant vasodepressor component. The likelihood of recurrent syncope in this patient group is high; medical certification is in most cases not possible.

Neurocardiogenic syncope[24] in patients without structural heart disease generally carries a good prognosis and can be demonstrated in otherwise healthy people. Recurrence rate over the long term is nonetheless notable, and unfortunately cannot be accurately predicted by any testing (such as a negative tilt test under medication). Neurocardiologenic syncope in pilots is generally disqualifying.

REFERENCES

1. Aguinaga L, Anguera I, Eizmendi I, *et al.* (1998) Long term outcome of radiofrequency catheter ablation in patients with atrioventricular nodal reentrant tachycardia. *Rev Espan Cardiol* **51**: 383–387.
2. Akhtar W, Reeves WC, Movahed A. (1998) Indications for anticoagulation in atrial fibrillation. *Amer Fam Physician* **58**: 130–136.
3. Allessie MA, Konings K, Kirchhof CJHJ, Wijffels M. (1996) Electrophysiologic mechanisms of perpetuation of atrial fibrillation. *Am J Cardiol* **77**: A10–A23.
4. Anderson RH. (1998) Mahaim pathway. *J Cardiovasc Electrophysiol* **9**: 448.
5. Andresen D, Bruggemann T, Behrens S, Ehlers C. (1997) Risk of ventricular arrhythmias in survivors of myocardial infarction. *Pace Pac Clin Electrophys* **20**: 2699–2705.
6. Arribas F, Gil ML, Cosio FG. (1998) Atrial flutter ablation: Role of endocardial mapping. 339–359.
7. Brembilla-Perrot B, Suty-Selton C, Houriez P, *et al.* (2000) Prolongation of the averaged QRS complex: A simple prognostic factor in patients with post-infarction bundle branch block and a history of syncope. *Arch Mal Coeur Vaisseaux* **93**: 1285–1289.

8. Carim Y, Daniels J, Obel IWP. (1998) Radiofrequency ablation of the slow pathway for treatment of atrioventricular nodal re-entrant tachycardia: Experience of the first 93 patients treated at Milpark Hospital. *S Afr Med J* **88**: C214–C219.
9. Corrado G, Sgalambro A, Gentile F, *et al.* (1999) Thromboembolic risk in atrial flutter: Preliminary results of the Italian multicenter FLASIEC study (Vol. 98, p. 3694, 1998). Circulation **99**: 328.
10. Cosio FG, Lopez-Gil M, Goicolea A, Arribas F. (1992) Electrophysiologic studies in atrial flutter. *Clin Cardiol* **15**: 667–673.
11. Cox JL, Sundt TM. (1997) The surgical management of atrial fibrillation. *Annu Rev Med* **48**: 511–523.
12. DeBacquer D, DeBacker G, Kornitzer M. (2000) Prevalences of ECG findings in large population based samples of men and women. *Heart* **84**: 625–633.
13. Doi A, Miyamoto K, Uno K, *et al.* (2000) Studies on hemodynamic instability in paroxysmal supraventricular tachycardia: Noninvasive evaluations by head-up tilt testing and power spectrum analysis on electrocardiographic RR variation. *Pace Pac Clin Electrophys* **23**: 1623–1631.
14. Emori T, Fukushima K, Saito H, *et al.* (1998) Atrial electrograms and activation sequences in the transition between atrial fibrillation and atrial flutter. *J Cardiovasc Electrophysiol* **9**: 1173–1179.
15. Fuji E, Kasai A, Omichi C, *et al.* (2000) Electrophysiological determinants of persistent dual atrioventricular nodal pathway physiology after slow pathway ablation in atrioventricular nodal reentrant tachycardia. *Pace Pac Clin Electrophys* **23**: 1916–1920.
16. Haissaguerre M, Shah DC, Jais P, *et al.* (2000) Mapping-guided ablation of pulmonary veins to cure atrial fibrillation. *Amer J Cardiol* **86**: 9K–19K.
17. Haissaguerre M, Jais P, Shah DC, *et al.* (1998) Spontaneous initiation of atrial fibrillation by ectopic beats originating in the pulmonary veins. *N Engl J Med* **339**: 659–666.
18. Jais P, Shah DC, Haissaguerre M, *et al.* (2000) Atrial fibrillation: Role of arrhythmogenic foci. *J Interv Card Electrophysiol* **4**: 29–37.
19. Kappenberger L, Schlaepfer AJ. (1999) Sino-atrial disease: Prevalence, diagnosis and outcome. *Eur Heart J Suppl* **1**: D105–D108.

20. Kato H, Masutani S, Hoshiyama M, *et al.* (1996) Neurally mediated syncope complicated with paroxysmal atrial fibrillation. *Acta Paediat Jpn* **38**: 695–698.
21. Kottkamp H, Hindricks G, Breithardt G. (1998) Atrial fibrillation: Epidemiology, etiology, and symptoms, 135–151.
22. Kottkamp H, Hindricks G, Hammel D, *et al.* (1999) Intraoperative radiofrequency ablation of chronic atrial fibrillation: A left atrial curative approach by elimination of anatomic "anchor" reentrant circuits. *J Cardiovasc Electrophysiol* **10**: 772–780.
23. Littmann L, Symanski JD. (2000) Hemodynamic implications of left bundle branch block. *J Electrocardiol* **33**: 115–121.
24. Malik P, Koshman ML, Sheldon R. (1997) Timing of first recurrence of syncope predicts syncopal frequency after a positive tilt table test result. *J Am Coll Cardiol* **29**: 1284–1289.
25. McElderry HT, Kay GN. (2006) Ablation of atrioventricular nodal reentry by the anatomic approach. In: Huang SKS, Wood MA (eds.), Catheter Ablation of Cardiac Arrhythmias, Saunders, Philadelphia, pp. 325–346.
26. Pappone C, Rosario S, Oreto G, *et al.* (2000) Circumferential radiofrequency ablation of pulmonary vein ostia: A new anatomic approach for curing atrial fibrillation. *Circulation* **102**: 2619–2628.
27. Singer DE. (1996) Anticoagulation for atrial fibrillation: Epidemiology informing a difficult clinical decision. *Proc Assoc Am Physicians* **108**: 29–36.
28. Vincent GM. (1998) The molecular genetics of the long QT syndrome: Genes causing fainting and sudden death. *Annu Rev Med* **49**: 263–274.
29. Wellens HJ, Rodriguez LM, Timmermans C, Smeets JL. (1997) The asymptomatic patient with the Wolff-Parkinson-White electrocardiogram. *Pace Pac Clin Electrophys* **20**: 2082–2086.

Chapter 15

Congenital Heart Diseases[1]

Ilse Janicke*

ICAO Standards and Recommendations: *The applicant shall not possess any abnormality of the heart, congenital or acquired, which is likely to interfere with the safe exercise of the applicant's license and rating privileges.*

Medical Requirements (JAR-FCL 3): *Applicants with congenital conditions, including those surgically corrected, shall normally be assessed as unfit unless functionally unimportant and no medication is required. Cardiology assessment by the AMS shall be required. Investigations may include 2D Doppler echocardiography, exercise ECG, and 24-hour ambulatory ECG. Regular cardiology review shall be required. Restriction to multi-crew (Class I 'OML') and safety pilot (Class 2 'OSL') operation may be required.*

INTRODUCTION

Congenital heart diseases are found in 1% of all live births and are usually diagnosed early in childhood; in countries with good pediatric care they are surgically corrected. Due to extreme advances in diagnostic techniques, and particularly in the operative and interventional therapies (at an increasingly young age) in the last 40 years, today 80% of these patients achieve adulthood without medical

* Herzzentrum, Kaiser-Wilhelm-Krankenhaus, Gerrickstraße 21, D-47137 Duisburg, Germany.

problems and with a relatively good prognosis. Particularly critical evaluation is indicated here, especially after correction of complex heart defects. Special experience with congenital heart defects in adulthood with corresponding echocardiographic knowledge is necessary. At initial application for a medical certificate and prior to starting a long and expensive training process, the proper authorities should be consulted in all cases of heart operation/intervention in infancy or childhood.

For full unrestricted certification, the risk of sudden incapacitation from a cardiac event during the period of validity of the certificate may not be higher than in individuals of similar age and gender, and chronic impairment should be minimal. For restricted certification, the 1% rule applies. Long-term experience is limited but a full pilot career cannot be expected.

Owing to the following problems, permanent disqualification is the rule after surgical correction of complex heart defects in infancy:

- Disturbances of heart rhythm: potentially dangerous and in the long term increasingly common, such as atrial fibrillation after atrial switch operation in transposition of the great vessels, or ventricular tachycardia after ventriculotomy in the correction of the tetralogy of Fallot.
- Pathological hemodynamic situation including LV dysfunction, pulmonary hypertension, residual shunt, and outflow tract obstruction, even if asymptomatic.
- Necessary specific cardiac medications, in particular anticoagulation therapy.

Currently, only non-corrected or surgically corrected heart anomalies which can be shown, on the basis of current experience, to be nearly free of events, are compatible with certification.

The seven most common heart defects, which comprise 75% of all congenital heart anomalies, are:

1. Ventricular septal defect (30%)
2. Atrial septal defect (10%)

3. Patent ductus arteriosus (Botalli) (10%)
4. Coarctation of the aorta (7%)
5. Pulmonary stenosis (7%)
6. Aortic and subaortic stenosis (6%)
7. Tetralogy of Fallot (6%)

VENTRICULAR SEPTAL DEFECT (VSD)

VSD appears isolated or combined with other congenital anomalies. 75% of all VSD, especially the small ones, spontaneously close before the fifteenth year of life. At the initial aeromedical examination, the pilot should be asked about a childhood heart murmur, and if affirmative, should undergo echocardiography.

Closure is not indicated in small VSD (loud holosystolic murmur on auscultation) with minimal left-to-right shunt <30% (which remains stable), normal heart size on chest X-ray, and no pulmonary hypertension. Endocarditis prophylaxis and periodic echocardiographic examinations are indicated. Special attention should be paid to commercial pilots flying to countries with poor hygiene as they have an increased risk of endocarditis. Surgical intervention should be considered for a left-to-right shunt of 30–50% or muscular VSD.

Following surgical closure of a larger VSD (shunt >50%), recertification is more problematic. The 30-year survival rate is 82%, lower than in age and gender matched individuals, but increases to 88% with early surgical intervention (before the second year of life) and with normal pulmonary vascular resistance.[2] The rate of sudden death (from post-operative conduction disturbance or ventricular rhythm disturbance) is minimal, less than 0.24% per year.[3,4] After successful operative closure, certification (with OML or OSL restriction) can be considered under the following conditions:

- Normal physical examination
- Normal 2D-Doppler echocardiogram
- Normal pulmonary artery pressure/resistance
- No conduction disturbance other than right bundle branch block
- No arrhythmias (especially ventricular) in 24-hour ECG

One year after patch closure, a VSD without a residual shunt no longer requires endocarditis prophylaxis.

ATRIAL SEPTAL DEFECTS

Patent Foramen Ovale (PFO) with or without Atrial Septal Aneurysm (ASA)[5,6]

In 25–30% of humans, the foramen ovale remains open without hemodynamic consequences (as long as no complex congenital heart defects exist), and no primary pathological findings need to be considered. There is an association between cerebral ischemia of "unknown etiology" and the existence of PFO in younger patients under the age of 50–55, although paradoxical embolism or the fulfillment of a variety of diagnostic criteria are rarely evident. Other sources of emboli (arrhythmias, atherosclerosis of the aorta or carotid arteries, left heart disease) are less common in this age group. The current examination method of choice is trans-esophageal echocardiography with contrast for the assessment of right-to-left shunt and the size of the defect during Valsalva or cough. On the basis of the high recurrence rate of emboli (3–4% per year), secondary prevention is necessary. The choice of therapeutic strategies is debatable: medical treatment with ASA or anticoagulation, incurring a risk of bleeding from anticoagulation, results in an annual thromboembolism recurrence rate between 1.9 to 14%, precluding aeromedical certification. Surgical PFO closure is a technically developed and safe intervention, which carries a very low embolism recurrence rate in selected patients. In specialty centers today, catheter procedures to effect PFO closure with a PFO closure device under angiography and echocardiography guidance in the cath lab carries a relatively low risk and has a high success rate (complete closure in 98% of cases after one year), and is preferred over open heart surgery once CAD has been excluded. Prospective controlled studies comparing PFO closure with conservative therapy are underway. Complications (about 1%) are embolism from device fragments, thrombus formation on the closure devices, and more rarely endocarditis. Supraventricular rhythm disturbances or atrial fibrillation appears in up to 10% of cases early after intervention and usually resolve spontaneously. Thereafter, medical treatment consists of ASA and, initially, additional clopidogrel. Recurrent emboli occur at a rate of 0–2% per year, but usually not with complete closure. Restricted certification may be possible, at the earliest six months after cessation of treatment with ASA.

OSTIUM SECUNDUM DEFECT (ATRIAL SEPTAL DEFECT, ASD II)

ASD II, at 70%, is the most common atrial septal defect, and lies in the area of the fossa ovalis in the middle atrial septum. Women are affected three times more often than men.

Echocardiographic examination is required to look for accompanying congenital anomalies such as mitral valve prolapse, pulmonary stenosis, and mitral stenosis (TEE). Initial symptoms (performance limitation, dyspnea on exertion, cough) appear in relationship to the size of the defect and usually occur in late youth or early adulthood. Commonly, there is a systolic (pulmonic) heart murmur with splitting of the second heart sound in childhood, and the ECG shows an incomplete (80%) or rarely a complete RBBB and right axis deviation.

40% of affected individuals develop pulmonary vascular disease before turning 40. Morbidity and mortality clearly rise after age 40, caused by right heart insufficiency and pulmonary hypertension. Diagnosis is made with trans-esophageal echocardiography with contrast. Isolated ASD II carries a very low risk of endocarditis, and prophylaxis is not necessary.

Small ASD II with a left-to-right shunt ≤ 1.5:1 and a normal RV volume carries an excellent prognosis and should not be surgically closed. In as much as there are no accompanying congenital anomalies and absent pulmonary hypertension, unrestricted Class I and II certification is possible. If the possibility of a paradoxical cerebral embolus exists through increased pressure in the right atrium via the right-left shunt (coughing, Valsalva, diving), this singular defect can be closed without cardiac surgery through a heart catheterization procedure. Medical fitness for certification must then be determined on an individual basis in consultation with an experienced cardiologist (see PFO).

A larger ASD II with a shunt >1.5:1 (>10 mm) should be closed as soon as possible (preferably before the fifth to tenth year of life), as long-term results are better. Medical certification is usually possible. If closure occurs prior to the age of 24, life expectancy is not much less than for a comparable normal person. Delayed surgery, which also carries a good long-term prognosis, may give rise to age-related problems such as increasing supraventricular rhythm disturbances and a risk of fatal cerebrovascular events,[7] so that certification may no longer be possible. The risk of late arrhythmias makes regular cardiology examinations necessary whether surgery/intervention has occurred or not.

OSTIUM PRIMUM DEFECT (ASD I)

Ostium primum defect, with a frequency of 15% of all ASD's, lies in the lower portion of the septum at the level of the AV valve. It is frequently associated with split formation of the anterior mitral leaflet, resulting in mitral insufficiency, and is a part of the complex of AV channel defects (as a rule, surgery is carried out in infancy). The ECG typically shows a pathological, extreme left axis deviation.

The risk of sudden cardiac death, even after surgical repair, cannot be clearly defined. With the frequently associated rhythm disturbances, the 10-year survival rate is only about 80%. This is not compatible with medical certification for flying. In individual cases, certification with limitation Class I OML can be considered if, after surgical correction, there has been no significant MI, no conduction disturbance or other heart rhythm disturbance, no residual shunt, and normal pulmonary vascular resistance. 2D echocardiography must be performed at least annually, and supplemented with trans-esophageal echocardiography and 24-hour Holter ECG, if necessary.

SINUS VENOSUS DEFECT

Sinus venosus defect, 15% of all ASD's, lies near the vena cava's superior entry into the right atrium, and is almost always associated with an abnormal location of the entry of the pulmonary vein. The main problem is the high incidence of heart rhythm disturbance, which is not reduced by surgery, but rather increased. With small defects where surgery is not indicated, limited certification for Class I OML can be considered, if no relevant or complex sinus node or conduction defects exist. Surgical correction normally rules out certification, unless multiple 24-hour ECG's do not disclose significant heart rhythm disturbances. At least annually, 2D-Doppler echocardiograms and multiple 24-hour ECG's are necessary.

PATENT DUCTUS ARTERIOSUS (BOTALLI)

The fetal connection between the pulmonic artery and the thoracic descending aorta remains patent in 10% of live births. In 15% of these cases, further congenital anomalies such as ASD, VSD, coarctation of the aorta, aortic/pulmonic stenosis, bicuspid aortic valve and aortic root disorder exist, which can become aeromedical problems.

The diagnosis is usually made in infancy. Girls are two to three times more often affected than boys. Because of the significant risk of endocarditis (10%), nearly all defects, even small ones, are closed (usually with interventional coils/spirals, etc.) One year after complete closure, endocarditis prophylaxis is no longer necessary. A closed defect is compatible with unlimited certification. Small patent defects in adulthood may be compatible with limited certification (OML), provided a cardiovascular evaluation rules out other congenital defects.

COARCTATION OF THE AORTA (AORTIC ISTHMUS STENOSIS (see Figure 13 of Chapter 12)

This narrowing of the aorta lies between the departure of the left subclavian artery and the beginning of the descending thoracic aorta. Depending on the severity, symptoms may appear in infancy (often together with other congenital anomalies) or, in the event of less pronounced isolated coarctation, in adulthood (up to 20%). Symptoms include headache, dizziness, pressure sensation, nose bleeds, rapid fatigability of the legs, and cold feet. The time of diagnosis has a significant impact on the prognosis and is therefore aeromedically relevant.

Typically, the blood pressure and pulse are different between upper and lower body parts, identifiable by pressure measurements in the arms and legs at rest and, if necessary, after exercise. On auscultation, a mid-systolic murmur is typically heard left of the spinal column between the shoulder blades. In children, the diagnosis is confirmed by echocardiography in the suprasternal region, and in adults by trans-esophageal echocardiography. Severe grade and extent of the lesion in adults can best be determined by spiral CT or MRA. Accompanying congenital anomalies include bicuspid aortic valves (30%) and cerebral aneurysms.

Therapy consists of the established techniques of surgical elimination of the stenotic isthmus with end-to-end anastamosis as soon as possible at a young age, as well as balloon dilatation. The surgical choice is more traumatic and can result in injury to the spinal cord arteries, resulting in paraplegia. Intervention is fraught with the problem of the appearance of aneurysms in the dilated segment even long after intervention. In case of re-stenosis following surgery (>30 mmHg pressure gradient), intervention together with a stent is the method of choice.

For long-term survivability, the deciding factor is age at therapy. If corrected before 14 years of age, the 20-year survival rate is about 91%. The best survival rates occur in patients who are operated on prior to age nine.[8] In another study, the 30-year survival rate was 92% when surgery was performed between four and 20 years of age.[9] The rate of post-operative persistence or partial appearance of arterial hypertension at rest or after exercise increases with age at surgery (and is 40% if surgery occurs after age 16).

Due to the early onset of arterial hypertension of the upper body, a premature and accelerated process of atherosclerosis develops, with the consequences of CAD, sudden cardiac death, cardiac insufficiency, cerebral vascular events, and aortic aneurysms (dissection and rupture). These aeromedically significant risks should be considered when post-surgery/intervention of coarctation of the aorta is being evaluated.

Applicants who have had therapy prior to the age of 14, have no restenosis, are normotensive at rest and during exercise, and have no associated congenital heart anomalies, may obtain unrestricted certification. With delayed correction, limited certification OML Class I and OSL Class II can be offered. Closely spaced blood pressure, echocardiography, and screening examinations looking for significant CAD are necessary.

PULMONARY STENOSIS (PS)

Depending on the location of the obstruction in the right ventricular outflow tract, the most common valvular pulmonic stenosis can be distinguished from that of subvalvular (infundibular) and supravalvular PS, the latter of which is most often combined with other congenital anomalies, such as VSD, tetralogy of Fallot, or pulmonary atresia. In the case of valvular and infundibular PS (fibromuscular ring of myocardial hypertrophy), one finds a defect in the atrium in 75% of cases as a patent foramen ovale (PFO) or ASD II, often incorrectly depicted as tetralogy of Fallot. By auscultation, a loud 2/3 systolic ejection murmur can be heard. PMI is audible parasternally. At elevated pressures, the ECG shows P pulmonale in the RV, extreme right axis deviation, and signs of RV hypertrophy, which correlates with degree of severity (Fig. 1).

At the initial examination for medical certification, trans-esophageal echocardiography is the examination of choice.

Isolated valvular PS with a maximal systolic pressure gradient <50 mmHg most commonly remains minimally symptomatic or asymptomatic without therapy into adulthood, and does not tend to progress after the age of 20. The prognosis is very good.[10] At a maximal gradient of <20 mmHg, unlimited certification for all classes is possible, as long as no RV hypertrophy exists on echocardiography. At a pressure gradient of 20–30 mmHg, limited certification OML Class I is possible. At a gradient <25, 96% remain free of intervention. Annual 2D-Doppler echocardiography with evidence of stability

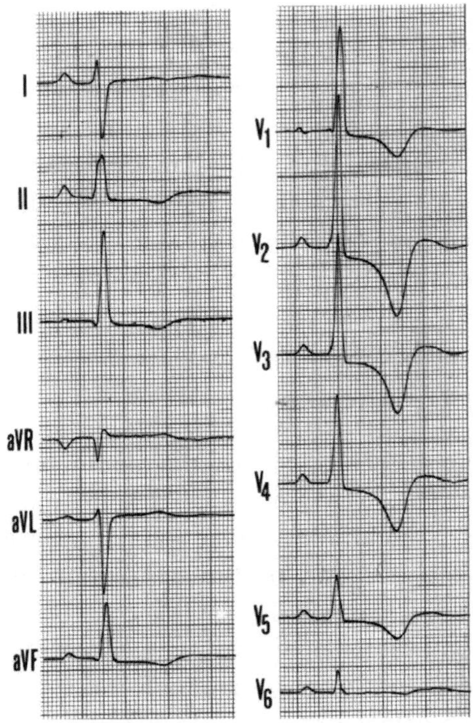

Figure 1. ECG in severe pulmonary stenosis or primary pulmonary hypertension with right ventricular hypertrophy.

is required (only 25% progression). In the case of limited echocardiography, another imaging technique such as cardiac MRI or spiral CT should be utilized.

Valvulotomy[11] is indicated with higher grade symptomatic pulmonary stenosis (pressure gradient >30 mmHg). Intervention with pure valvular PS or surgery with accompanying defect is best performed prior to school age. The long-term course with regard to re-stenosis or sudden cardiac death is very good. In the case when the post procedural maximal gradient is <30 mmHg, unrestricted certification can be obtained. Following valvulotomy, 50% of cases develop significant pulmonary valve insufficiency with chronic volume overload of the RV. So far as this is not determined by echocardiography, such a pilot can, for example, first be identified by ventricular extrasystoles and salvos, which develop due to chronic right heart damage. Therapy in the asymptomatic stage is unclear. Medical certification should then be determined on an individual basis, as long-term data are absent. Although endocarditis is uncommon, lifelong prophylaxis is usually recommended.

Supraventricular PS as a rule leads to disqualification, whereas a corrected infundibular stenosis may be compatible with certification.

AORTIC AND SUBAORTIC STENOSIS

Bicuspid aortic valves and their consequences have been discussed previously. Regarding mild congenital aortic stenosis (often abnormally developed fibrosed or fused valves) with maximal systolic gradient <30 mmHg, absent LV hypertrophy, and good systolic function corresponding to performance of the acquired AS, unlimited certification is possible.

Pediatric non-calcified, high-grade AS is treated with balloon valvuloplasty. It is not unusual for re-stenosis to occur later in life, and aortic insufficiency may result as a consequence of valvuloplasty. Further interventions are necessary in 10–18% until age 15. This problem entails disqualification.

Isolated subaortic stenosis, which is caused by a circular or semi-circular membrane beneath the valve, is conspicuous by its typical murmur. This stenosis can be rapidly progressive in children and young adults. As long as no significant gradient exists, the aortic valve is morphologically normal, and left ventricular wall thickness and function are normal, certification is possible. Frequent echocardiographic examinations are necessary. Significant obstruction in the left ventricular outflow tract must be treated surgically. An extensive excision can lead to conduction disturbances, aortic insufficiency, or LV dysfunction; even VSD can develop. Such cases are incompatible with medical certification. In cases with minor intervention and a good postoperative result, where good long-term results can be expected, certification may be possible.

TETRALOGY OF FALLOT (Fig. 2)

The most common cyanotic congenital heart defect, the tetralogy of Fallot, consists of a combination of pulmonary stenosis (usually infundibular), high riding VSD, and over-riding aorta as a consequence of the dextroposition of the aorta. The degree of severity of the tetralogy is determined by the obstruction in the right ventricular outflow tract. Survival into young adulthood without corrective surgery is possible, but due to the high mortality rate, it rules out any possibility of certification.

The goal of therapy today is primary surgical correction as early as possible with a patch of the VSD, resection of the hypertrophic infandibular musculature, and commissurotomy of a possible PS. In the absence of residual defects following long-term evaluations, the statistical survival rate over 30 years is very good, albeit somewhat less (86%) in comparison to healthy individuals (96%).[12] After surgical correction and valvuloplasty, many patients have significant pulmonary valve insufficiency, which is generally well tolerated over years or decades, even if the spirometric cardiopulmonary performance is reduced and the increase in heart rate with exertion

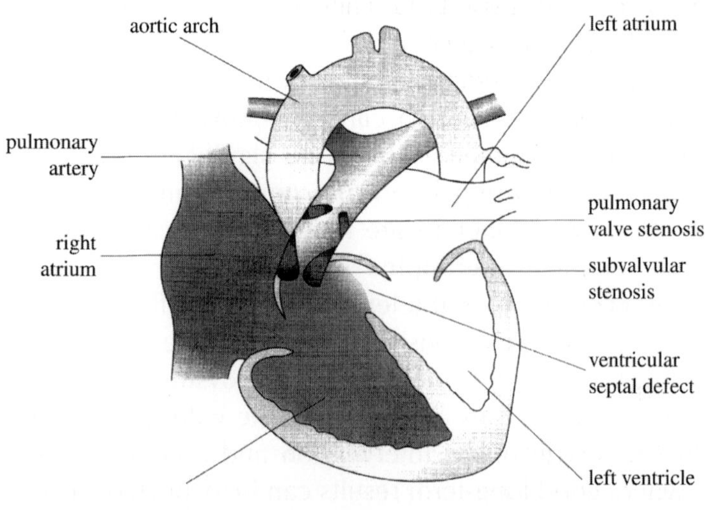

Figure 2. Schematic diagram of Tetralogy of Fallot.

is inadequate. With worsening symptoms, RV dilatation and RV dysfunction eventually necessitates a pulmonic valve replacement via a homograft.

Incidence of sudden cardiac death is as high as 0.46% per year. On the basis of renewed evaluations of 490 long-term patients, the main cause of sudden cardiac death is VT or ventricular fibrillation.[13] Predictors for death and VT are surgery prior to 1970, high preoperative hematocrit, a patch in the right ventricular outflow tract, QRS length >180 ms, chronic RV enlargement, non-sustained VT, late potentials, RV dysfunction, RVOT obstruction, pulmonary insufficiency, and the choice of surgical timing. The incidence of sudden cardiac death increases postoperatively (after 25 years it is 0.94% per year); frequent evaluation is therefore recommended.

On this background, the risk of late sudden cardiac death in asymptomatic, fully active individuals who were operated prior to the age of 12 and who have no hemodynamic problems, is acceptable under the 1% rule, so that limited certification OML Class I and OSL Class II is possible. Frequent cardiology examinations are indicated. With the appearance of risk factors for VT/sudden cardiac death during, certification must be revoked.

Many cardiac examinations are necessary during follow-up after complex cardiac surgery: ECG, chest X-ray, echocardiography, MRI (RV-Volume size and degree of pulmonary insufficiency), as well as electrophysiological studies and spiro-ergometry.[14]

On the basis of the current increases in longevity and improvements in surgical techniques, restricted medical certification may be possible in rare individual circumstances following correction of complex congenital heart anomalies; this requires that the anatomical, functional, and electrophysiological status be determined in specialty centers in order to assess individual risk.

REFERENCES

1. Deanfield JE. (2003) The task force on the management of grown up congenital heart disease (GUCH) of the European Society of Cardiology. *Eur Heart J* **24**: 1035–1084.

2. Murphy JG, *et al.* (1989) The late survival after surgical repair of isolated ventricular septal defect (VSD). *Circulation* **80**(Suppl II): II-490 (abstr.).
3. Allen HD, *et al.* (1974) Postoperative follow-up of patients with ventricular septal defect. *Circulation* **50**: 465–471.
4. Blake RS, *et al.* (1982) Conduction defects, ventricular arrhythmias, and late death after surgical closure of ventricular septal defect. *Br Heart J* **64**: IV–227.
5. Nicholas A, *et al.* (2001) How should patients with patent foramen ovale be managed? *Heart* **85**: 242–244.
6. Meier B. (2005) Closure of patent foramen ovale: Technique, pitfalls, complications, and follow-up. *Heart* **91**: 444–448.
7. Magilligan DJ Jr, *et al.* (1978) Late results of atrial septal defect repair in adults. *Arch Surg* **113**: 1245–1247.
8. Cohen M, *et al.* (1989) Coarctation of the aorta: Long-term follow-up and prediction of outcome after surgical correction. *Circulation* **80**: 840–845.
9. Presbitero P, *et al.* (1987) Long-term results (15–30 years) of surgical repair of aortic coarctation. *Br Heart J* **57**: 462–467.
10. Nugent EW, *et al.* (1977) Clinical course in pulmonary stenosis. *Circulation* **56**: I-38–47.
11. Kann JS, *et al.* (1982) Percutaneous balloon valvuloplasty: A new method for treating congenital pulmonary valve stenosis. *N Engl J Med* **307**: 540–542.
12. Murphy JG, *et al.* (1993) Long-term outcome in patients undergoing surgical repair of Tetralogy of Fallot. *N Engl J Med* **329**: 593–599.
13. Nollert G, *et al.* (1997) Long-term survival in patients with repair of Tetralogy of Fallot: 36-year follow-up of 490 survivors of the first year after surgical repair. *J Am Coll Cardiol* **30**: 1374–1383.
14. 32nd Bethesda-Conference: "Care of the Adult with Congenital Heart Disease." *J Am Coll Cardiol* **37**: 1162–1198.

Chapter 16

Vascular Diseases and Disorders

Ilse Janicke*

AORTIC ANEURYSMS, MARFAN SYNDROME, AND RELATED DISORDERS

Medical provisions (ICAO Standards and Recommended Practices, Annex 1): *There shall be no significant functional nor structural abnormality of the circulatory system.*

Medical Requirements (JAR-FCL 3): *Applicants with aneurysm of the thoracic or abdominal aorta, before or after surgery, shall be assessed as unfit. Applicants with aneurysm of the infra-renal abdominal aorta may be considered by the AMS. Unoperated infra-renal abdominal aortic aneurysms may be considered for restricted Class I or Class II certification by the AMS if followed by six monthly ultrasound scans. After surgery for infra-renal abdominal aortic aneurysm without complications, and after cardiovascular assessment, restricted Class I or Class II certification may be considered by the AMS, with follow-up approved by the AMS.*

In the realm of aeromedical qualification, particular attention should be paid toward true aneurysms, which can appear in sacciform or fusiform versions. The main etiology of aortic aneurysms (70–90% of cases) is arteriosclerosis, followed by idiopathic median

* Herzzentrum, Kaiser-Wilhelm-Krankenhaus, Gerrickstraße 21, D-47137 Duisburg, Germany.

necrosis in 8–10% of cases. Inflammatory (such as syphilitic) aneurysms are rare. The most common location is in the abdominal aorta (68%, in which 95% are infrarenal), followed by the ascending aorta and the arch (22%).

THORACIC AORTIC ANEURYSM INCLUDING MARFAN SYNDROME

The ascending aorta has a diameter of 3–3.5 cm and is visible by echocardiography to within 2 cm of the base of the heart. An increase in the aortic root to 4.0–4.5 cm heightens the risk of dissection, rupture and peripheral embolism and is therefore disqualifying for all classes of medical certification. Surgery is indicated when the condition is symptomatic or when the diameter is > 5 cm (mortality to 13%) or when an increase in diameter of > 0.5 cm per year can be demonstrated. Most aneurysms related to atherosclerosis appear later in life in association with the risk factors of arterial hypertension, diabetes, and smoking. The five year mortality is about 35% of all operated patients and is caused by accompanying CAD or rupture of the aneurysm.[1] Younger pilots with normal blood pressure and who do not smoke are usually not affected by this disease.

At younger ages, cystic medial necrosis Erdheim-Gsell (focal degeneration of smooth muscle/disintegration of the elastic fibers through gene mutation) is typical for the aneurysms associated with the congenital connective tissue disorders of Marfan and Ehlers-Danlos syndromes (autosomal dominant with variable expression). A variety of distinctive features are evident (aortic disease, intraocular lens dislocation, arachnodactyly, and familial or sporadic occurence of the disorder). Prevalence is 1.5/100000, and males are more affected than females (2:1). Because of the risk of progression to aortic/mitral insufficiency, acute aortic dissection or aortic rupture, this is permanently disqualifying for all classes of medical certification. Despite successful surgery, the long term prognosis is not favorable, therefore permanent disqualification is the rule: Marfan syndrome carries a five year survival rate of 75%, and the ten year survival rate is only 56%.[2] On the basis of variable expression, Marfan syndrome includes the so-called *forme fruste,* in which case the diameter of the vessel remains within normal range, but eventually significant aortic or mitral insufficiency develops. In as much as the great vessels and those of the heart remain within normal range, both Classes I and II certification are possible if annual cardiology examinations demonstrate stability (echocardiography, X-rays, MRI).

Abdominal Aortic Aneurysm (AAA)

Abdominal aortic aneurysm is defined as a maximal cross sectional diameter of > 2.5–3.0 cm, or associated with a ratio of dilated segment to normal aorta > 1.5. It is usually an incidental finding in asymptomatic individuals, such as in the case of a sonographic evaluation of elevated liver enzymes. In 30–50% of cases, the aneurysm extends into the pelvic arteries. The etiology in > 90% of cases is generalized atherosclerosis. In the last 30 years, the incidence has increased 10–20 times, the prevalence lies between 2.5 and 5%, and is > 8% in men over 50 years of age. Men are affected four times more often than women. The following risk factors entail a likelihood of a silent aneurysm which is significantly greater than in the normal population:

- First-degree relative with aneurysm
- Pre-existing peripheral arterial vascular disease (~14%)
- Arterial hypertension (~11%)
- Age > 60 and with prior vascular risk factors.

Most aneurysms become larger with time, on the average 0.2–0.3 cm per year. The rate of growth depends, among other things, on the initial diameter. Complications are fatal rupture, embolism and thrombotic aortic occlusion. The average rupture rate is cited as 6–8% every 5–10 years, and is dependent on size. At > 6.0 cm diameter, the rupture rate is about 50% per year. There is no indication for surgery if the diameter is < 5 cm, due to the low complication rate (< 6.0 cm or about 15% per year).

Aeromedical Considerations

Aeromedical significance and the overwhelmingly asymptomatic presentation of AAA indicates that male pilots > 50 years of age with arterial vascular disease should undergo screening examinations by sonography, CT, or MRI. Identified aneurysms entails disqualification. Limited certification may be possible for Classes I and II under the following conditions:

- If < 5.0 cm, semi-annual sonographic examinations.
- Treatment of hypertension, particularly with β-blockers.
- Due to the high correlation with CAD (about 40–50%), noninvasive and, if necessary, invasive coronary artery diagnostic examinations.
- In cases of rapid growth > 0. 5 cm in 6 months or diameter > 5 cm, surgical intervention and renewed disqualification.

Concerning therapy, the pilot's cooperation is important: conventional Y-prosthesis has shown good long term results based on >30 years experience whereas transfemoral stent graft implantation has been marred by not insignificant complications, such as wire fractures, secondary leakage, etc., and the experience with long term results is limited. After successful surgery, medical certification can be renewed with limitations. Blood pressure should be normal at rest and during exercise, and stress ECG testing should be normal. Following Y-prosthesis implantation, regular ultrasound examinations of the abdominal aorta is required. After transfemoral stent graft implantation, frequent X-ray examinations (X ray of the vertebral column, spiral or helical CT with contrast in 5 mm sections, peripheral Doppler pressure testing, etc.) is necessary.

PERIPHERAL ARTERIAL (OCCLUSIVE) DISEASE (PA(O)D)

ICAO Standards and Recommendations: *There shall be no significant functional nor structural abnormality of the circulatory system.*

Medical Requirements (JAR-FCL 3): *Applicants with peripheral arterial disease before or after surgery shall be assessed as unfit. Provided* *there is no significant functional impairment, a fit assessment may be considered by the AMS (following noninvasive, and if necessary, invasive clarification of CAD).*

Arterial occlusive disease encompasses stenotic and occlusive changes of the aorta, extremities, and cerebral vessels. Asymptomatic PAD is three times more common than symptomatic disease. This is aeromedically relevant, in that PAD is an indicator for atherosclerotic changes in the coronary and cerebral arterial vasculature. Patients with symptomatic or asymptomatic PAD (between 55 and 74 years of age, prevalence is 5–10%) have an increased risk of experiencing stroke, heart attack, or sudden cardiac death (incidence 1–3% per year). Atherosclerosis causing PAD is positively correlated with the male gender, age, diabetes, smoking, hypertension, hyperlipoproteinemia, and hyperfibrinogenemia. Smoking is the determining risk factor. Male patients with PAD have a reduced life expectancy of 10 years and usually die of cardiovascular events.

Arterial Occlusive Disease: Screening and Secondary Examinations

In addition to a history of claudication, which pilots often withhold, corresponding risk factors obligate an evaluation of the status of the peripheral pulses (particularly in the feet) and auscultation of vascular sounds in the typical locations. Cessation of stress testing due to leg pain should lead to suspicion of PAD. The simplest instrument for evaluating concerns regarding PAD is *Doppler pressure measurement* (*ABI = Ankle Brachial Index*), such as with a pocket Doppler: after 15 minutes of rest, a supine patient has blood pressure cuffs placed on both arms and both legs (supramalleolar), and the systolic occlusive pressure is measured with a Doppler probe at the brachialis artery, tibialis posterior, and anterior arteries. Proof of PAD lies in the ratio of ankle arterial pressure/arm arterial pressure, which should be < 0.9. This ABI is a very good predictor for mortality. Stress testing and imaging examinations necessarily follow. Initial diagnosis of PAD requires the following **laboratory tests**: complete blood count (polycythemia, thrombocytosis, blood sugar, both fasting and postprandial, HbA1c, urinanalysis, and lipid profile.

If PAD is discovered, a complete **cardiovascular status report** with stress ECG testing/scintigraphy and/or stress echocardiography is necessary. Coronary artery changes are found by angiography in about 70% of patients with PAD.[3] If claudication pain limits stress ECG testing, other methods of evaluation, such as pharmacological scintigraphy/stress echocardiography, or one of the new imaging techniques (multi-slice CT, Cardiac MRI) should be undertaken. The decision to perform a coronary angiogram should be made early.

Due to the high co-morbidity with cerebral arterial vascular disease (30–40%), a **color duplex sonogram of the carotids** should be undertaken. Of significance is the sonographically measured intima-media thickness at the maximal wall thickness (normal < 0.9 mm) due to the association with stroke and heart attack.[4] Significant cerebral arterial vascular disease is disqualifying for all classes.

THROMBOSIS, PULMONARY EMBOLISM AND ANTICOAGULATION

Medical Requirements (JAR-FCL 3): *Systemic anticoagulation therapy is disqualifying. Applicants following anticoagulant therapy require review by the AMS. Venous thrombosis or pulmonary embolism is disqualifying until anticoagulation has been discontinued. Pulmonary embolus requires full evaluation. Anticoagulation for possible arterial thromboembolism is disqualifying.*

Thrombosis (DVT), Pulmonary Embolism, and Flight Fitness

The incidence of acute deep leg or pelvic venous thrombosis is 6/100 000. The absolute risk of thrombosis in individuals under 40 years of age amounts to 1:10 000, and for those over 75 years, 1:100. The mortality rate is 0.6%. 90% of thrombotic events are asymptomatic. Asymptomatic pulmonary emboli and thrombosis extension appear in about 1% of cases, and is the main complication. **Predisposing factors** are trauma, surgery, malignancy, thrombophilic diseases, pregnancy, hormone therapy, varicosities, obesity, and prior history of thrombosis.

Diagnosis: Symptomatic and clinical signs of thrombosis are relatively sensitive, but quite unspecific. The determination of the D-dimer concentration (normal < 500 mcg/l, rapid test simliRED®[5]) rules out the presence of thromboembolism with a high probability. In positive cases (limited specificity), a duplex scan in experienced hands or the gold standard of phlebography is helpful. In the case of suspected pulmonary embolism, the method of choice is the spiral CT. Ventilation-perfusion scans or pulmonary angiography are necessary only in individual cases.

Consequences for pilots: Venous thrombosis followed by pulmonary embolism is rare in young healthy pilots. Regarding recurrence, the etiology of the DVT should be sought for aeromedical considerations. A positive diagnosis requires anticoagulation with warfarin, phenprocoumon, or similar medications. Prior to therapy, laboratory evidence for the not uncommon thrombophilic diseases should be undertaken, upon which the length of therapy depends. All classes are disqualified during therapeutic anticoagulation.

In the case of a suspected or proven **pulmonary embolism**, a 2D Doppler-echocardiogram, or if necessary, a right heart catheterization should be performed in order to determine that there is no evidence of pulmonary artery hypertension (systolic < 30 mmHg). Pulmonary hypertension, whether primary or secondary, with an average pressure > 40 mmHg, is permanently disqualifying for all classes.

Due to a recurrence rate up to 8% in the first year (2% after the third year), recertification may be limited to OML or OSL restrictions in the first two years on the discretion of the AMS. Regular cardiovascular evaluations including echocardiography, initially every six months, followed by annually, is required.

Traveler's Thrombosis

Reports about spectacular fatalities during or after long haul flights in the last few years has lead to a renewed, lively, and partially exaggerated discussion in the lay press, resulting in confusion among passengers and physicians. What the actual data looks like with regard to this so-called **economy class syndrome,** more accurately called **Traveler's Thrombosis**, and the recommendations that can be given at this time, is described as follows.

Definition: Traveler's Thrombosis arises from a deep vein thrombosis (DVT), which can occur up to four weeks after traveling in a primarily seated position (airplane, train, automobile), with or without pulmonary embolism. If the travel occurs after several hours on an airplane, it is called air traveler thrombosis. Currently, there are several studies regarding this topic.

Pathophysiology: Regarding causes for this air and travel thrombosis, the following items are discussed:

- Kinking of the popliteal vein in the popliteal fossa with lengthy seated position (venous stasis).
- Dehydration through significantly low humidity in the cabin (8–12%), fostered by alcohol and caffeine, through which more fluid is lost by way of diuresis.
- Decreased partial pressure of oxygen in the cabin (2000–2500 m in elevation) may reduce fibrinolytic activity, and by the release of EDRF/NO, facilitate vasodilatation and stasis,[6,7] while other studies show no significant effect of hypoxia on the coagulation parameters in the general population.[8]

Data: In 1954, two thrombosis cases following long flights of over eight hours were first reported. Until 1999, the only reports were exclusively case reports or retrospective studies concerning about 200 cases of flight-associated thrombosis.[9] More studies since 1999 have investigated the relative risk of long flights and the value of compression stockings. The LONFLIT 1 and 2 studies merely showed an incidence of 4–6% for DVT in high-risk groups (with predisposing factors, see below) after over 10 hours flight.[10] A few studies showed no association between flight and thrombosis, while others showed a strong association.[11] The LONFLIT 4 study demonstrated a significant reduction of edema and DVT in the low and moderate risk factor group for DVT, and in those individuals with edema, a lower rate of microangiopathy.[12]

Current consensus: At a WHO conference, it was determined that an association between long haul flights and thrombosis is possible according to the current data, but that it is a weak correlation. This association particularly concerns people with predisposing factors (see above). Further prospective studies to determine the thrombosis risk associated with flight involving satisfactory numbers of passengers are currently underway. For passengers and airline companies, important consequences may be determined, such as the distance between seat rows and liability issues.

Current Recommendations

(1) For trips less than three hours duration or under 2500 km, no intervention is necessary.
(2) Without additional risk of thrombosis, the following is recommended for longer trips: foot and ankle circles, isometric exercises, frequent standing, drinking 150 ml fluids/hour (no alcohol or coffee), and avoid taking sedatives.
(3) With one or more additional risk factors for thrombosis, depending on the risk profile: additional to (2), compression stockings Classes I–II.
(4) High-risk individuals (prior thrombosis, malignancy, thrombophilic diseases, major surgery in the preceding six weeks), low molecular weight heparin in higher dose subcutaneously two hours prior to departure. On the basis of the current studies, there is no indication to use Aspirin® for the prevention of venous thromboembolism. Many airline companies are passing out related information with their tickets, or providing further information on their web sites.

REFERENCES

1 Crawford EF, *et al.* (1989) Surgical treatment of aneurysm and/or dissection of the ascending aorta and transverse aortic arch: Factors influencing survival in 717 patients. *J Thorac Cardiovasc Surg* **98**: 659–674.
2 Svennson LG, *et al.* (1989) Impact of cardiovascular operation on survival in the Marfan patient. *Circulation* **80**: 1233–1242.

3. Darbar D, *et al.* (1996) Prediction of late cardiac events by dipyridamole thallium szintigraphy in patient with intermittent claudication and occult coronary artery disease. *Am J Cardiol* **78**: 736–740.
4. O'Leary DH, *et al.* (1999) Carotid-artery intima and media thickness as a risk factor for myocardial infarction and stroke in older adults. *N Engl J Med* **340**: 12–22.
5. Wells PS, *et al.* (1995) A novel and rapid whole blood assay for d-dimer in patients with clinical suspected deep vein thrombosis. *Cirulation* **91**: 2184–2187.
6. Gertler JP, *et al.* (1993) Ambient oxygen tension modulates endothelial fibrinolysis. *J Vasc Surg* **18**: 939–946.
7. Bendz B, *et al.* (2000) Association between acute hypobaric hypoxia and activation of coagulation in human beings. *Lancet* **356**: 1657–1658.
8. Crosby A, *et al.* (2003) Relation between acute hypoxia and activation of coagulation in human beings. *Lancet* **361**: 2207–2208.
9. Landgraf H, *et al.* (1994) Economy class syndrome: Rheology fluid balance and lower leg oedema during a simulated 12-hour long-distance flight. *Aviat Space Envir Med* **65**: 930–935.
10. Belcaro G, *et al.* (2001) Venous thromboembolism from air travel: The LONFLiT study. *Angiology* **52**: 369–374.
11. Mendis S, *et al.* (2002) Air travel and venous thromboembolism. (Review). *Bulletin of the World Heath Organization* **80**: 403–406.
12. Cesarone Mr, *et al.* (2003) The LONFLIT4-Concorde Deep Venous Thrombosis and Edema Study: Prevention with travel stockings. *Angiology* **54**: 143–154.

Chapter 17

Ophthalmology for the Medical Examiner

Rüdiger Schwartz*,† and Jörg Draeger†

INTRODUCTION

Over 90% of flight-relevant information comes to the pilot through the eye, making it the most important sensory input system for aviators. Despite technological advances in aircraft engineering and information technology, nothing has changed in that regard. On the contrary, research is being undertaken to transfer even more flight-relevant information from the aural into the visual realm. With the introduction of "fly-by-wire" technology, even residual mechanical input is slipping away; neither stick pressure nor power setting changes are noticeable by feel or hearing when the Flight Management System (FMS) activates its programmed settings, whereas a glance at the primary FMS display provides the pilot with decisive information regarding the functional conditions and flight profile of the aircraft.[1] Developments in recreational flying are heading in the same direction, with display panels becoming similar to those of corporate aircraft. Even high performance airplanes, although not flown by an FMS, nonetheless have relatively large instruments displays that are not only designed for navigational purposes but are also linked to flight data recorder information. The pilot can only utilize the displayed information if he can discern the information precisely.

* Corresponding author.
† Department of Ophthalmology, Hamburg University, Hamburg, Germany, E-mail: r.schwartz@yke.uni-hamburg.de.

This chapter does not deal with the cognitive side of signal processing, but rather with the optical. The eyes produce an unambiguous signal image, which is transmitted to the optical cortex for interpretation and reaction. As in all of our sensory systems, a certain stimulus size must be exceeded in order to be perceived. In physiology, this is termed "threshold." This does not necessarily have to do with energy levels, such as the quantum amount required to sense light, but rather with the resolution limits for distinguishing geometric patterns. On the one hand, the cockpit signals must be designed such that they exceed the threshold for perception, and on the other hand, the receptor (the eye) and its performance must meet regulatory standards.

The concept of visual acuity encompasses many aspects and must therefore be narrowed down.

"Point visual acuity" is defined as the ability to discriminate a single point. This can be important in aviation, such as when a distant aircraft can be discerned as only a point. In clinical practice, however, point visual acuity is not measured quantitatively.

"Visual acuity of separation," or minimum angle of resolution, describes the ability to discriminate two closely neighboring points as separate. This is the conclusive criterion for signal perception.

"Visual acuity of localization" is defined as the smallest recognizable change in spatial relationships between two objects. An example is the so-called "nonius" visual acuity, demonstrated by the ability to place one vertical line precisely on top of another line, such as is used in calipers with a vernier scale. It is possible to determine inaccurate positions at less than 10 seconds of arc.

"Visual acuity of recognition" (minimum legible acuity): the point at which an object can be perceived as such. This is within the realm of cognition.

The resolution of the eye is the visual acuity of separation as given by the smallest angle subtended by two points still visible as separate. This angle is called the "minimum angle of resolution" (MAR) and is measured in minutes of arc. The visus is defined as the reciprocal of this threshold angle, measured in minutes of arc. Visus 1 means the MAR is one minute, visus 0.5 means the MAR is two minutes, etc. Sometimes, the $\log_{10}$ form of MAR is used.

Relationship between Snellen notation, MAR, logMAR, and decimal notation:

Snellen Notation				
Metric	**Imperial**	**MAR**	**logMAR**	**Decimal**
6/60	20/200	10	1.0	0.10
6/48	20/160	8.0	0.9	0.13
6/38	20/125	6.3	0.8	0.16
6/30	20/100	5.0	0.7	0.20
6/24	20/80	4.0	0.6	0.25
6/19	20/60	3.2	0.5	0.32
6/15	20/50	2.5	0.4	0.40
6/12	20/40	2.0	0.3	0.50
6/9.5	20/30	1.6	0.2	0.63
6/7.5	20/25	1.25	0.1	0.80
6/6	20/20	1.00	0.0	1.00
6/4.8	20/16	0.80	–0.1	1.25
6/3.8	20/12.5	0.63	–0.2	1.58
6/3.0	20/10	0.50	–0.3	2.00

Many individuals, especially young people, possess a visus of >1. In other words, the MAR is significantly smaller than one minute. Examination is usually performed using test letters with defined identifiable angles in the shape of physically defined figures, either Landolt coptotypes or numbers with defined angular relationships. For maximal resolution, only an area of about 1° of the fovea centralis is needed. If the image drifts onto the retinal periphery, the resolution will deteriorate exponentially. At a distance of 20 cm from the eye, the area of clarity has a diameter of about 3.5 mm, while at a distance of a meter, this area enlarges to 17 mm. It is therefore not possible to visualize two flight deck instruments simultaneously with full resolution, whether they are next to each other or at different distances. To achieve this, eye movements are needed. These are very fast and are directed with considerable accuracy, but this requires a distinctly structured space, in which particular features provide an optical orientation. A display built from completely equal units will more likely lead to search errors than one where the units are marked unequally. This is particularly important for rapid reading of charts and checklists.

The MAR changes not only with the position of the image on the retina, but also with the lighting, due to the adaptability of the eye. The eye adapts its sensitivity to changes in lighting conditions. This occurs partly via regulation of the pupillary diameter and partly by adaptation of the sensitivity of the photoreceptors. When it is bright, this occurs very rapidly by photoadaptation; this takes much longer in darkness when only the parafovea rods are being utilized scotoptically. A quick glance from a bright instrument panel to a dimly lit region is not possible; dark adaptation takes much more time. This is important at twilight or at night. A similar situation exists when dealing with contrast, such as a figure on a display, when rapid and precise recognition is critical.

Precise object recognition is predicated upon optimal geometric optics projecting the corresponding image of the object onto the eye. In this endeavor, accommodation is utilized when an image is made of differing points along the optical axis. This process is slow and the time required increases with a person's age; the ability to accommodate begins to wane after a particular age, to the point where accommodation is no longer feasible. For this reason, all the visual surfaces in the cockpit should require as little accommodation as possible, in order to appear on virtually the same point along the optical axis. As this is not usually the case in practice (between the primary flight display, glare shield fixture, center console, and heads-up display), the workload of the visual system is increased significantly. In addition, normal binocular vision is coupled with accommodation-related convergence movements of the eyes: If a close object is to be visualized clearly, both vision axes must be brought together. This drive for convergence and accommodation are coupled.

This means that every time accommodation occurs, convergence is evoked. If the image on the retina is not sharp, the eye begins to initiate accommodation and, therefore, also convergence. This leads to further problems of image recognition. The ability to accommodate declines with age, as the near point moves further away (presbyopia). The near point of a 20 year old is about 10 cm, whereas it is about half a meter for a 50 year old. Corrective lenses are particularly important for a presbyopic pilot as they must allow the pilot to meet the regulatory standards for distant vision, and at the same time provide a clear picture of a number of objects inside the cockpit at varying distances from the pilot's eyes. It is not physically-technically possible to produce lenses that allow the presbyopic pilot to focus immediately on any object regardless of distance. Because cockpit geometry is complex, the pilot may have to search for that segment in the glasses where the image is seen most clearly. In addition to this problem, lateral distortion also leads to further, unavoidable visual deterioration.

The additional effect that chromatic aberrations have on accommodation is only briefly mentioned, but this is an issue that is becoming increasingly important as modern flight decks employ an increasing number of color applications. Colored indicators, located at equal visual distance, require changes in accommodation with visualization of each chosen color.

With regards to the refractive errors, myopia, hyperopia, and astigmatism, more will be detailed in relation to the regulatory standards and examination techniques, as well as refractive methods of eyeglasses and contact lenses.

In the past few years, refractive corneal surgery has become widely used to correct the refractive errors that occur due to variations in bulbar length. This is done by reshaping the corneal surface and flattening it. One method is to make radial cuts into the corneal surface, leading to scarring in the periphery that in turn leads to a bowing-up of tissue there, which then leads to a flattening of the central area. The same goal is achieved by using excimer-laser-ablation of the central area of the cornea. The removal of tissue flattens the corneal curve, reduces the refractive power, and allows a sharp image on the retina despite the long bulbar length. This excimer-laser-ablation can also be performed in the intrastromal tissue. To this end, the anterior corneal lamella is excised (Lasik), central corneal material is removed, and the lamella is reinserted. Common for these procedures is an increased risk for scar formation and subsequent structural changes within the cornea. The first case of keratoconus after such surgeries has been reported.

It is obvious that, besides questions of optical imaging such as resolution, color vision, contrast, and dark adaptations, other flight-specific issues can influence visual performance. The relative drying of the corneal surface due to low air humidity in most commercial aircraft is well known, and can be particularly bothersome to older pilots. However, the effect of acceleration as having hydrostatic effects on the eyes can be disregarded in commercial aviation but not always in private flying.

The duty of the aeromedical ophthalmologist is to utilize particular knowledge regarding the actual performance requirements in the cockpit, the work environment of air traffic controllers, the regulatory standards, and to perform accurate examinations.

ANATOMY AND PHYSIOLOGY OF THE EYE

Introduction

The human eye (Fig. 1) is one of the most complex organs of the body. Next to the kidney, it has the highest metabolic rate. Hypoxia impairs all visual functions. Besides the parasympathetic and sympathetic nervous system, half of all brain neurons participate in the innervation of the eye.

Visual performance encompasses many different qualities, such as visual acuity, contrast, dark adaptation, glare sensitivity, spatial vision, color vision, and peripheral vision. Only with regular and diligent examinations can vision problems that may endanger aviation safety be recognized early.

Eye Lids and Tear Ducts

The eyelids are muscular soft tissue with extensive safety functions. Form and function are such that the eye can be covered entirely by closure of the lids. Lid closure occurs reflexly by way of mechanical, optical, and acoustic stimulation. An even distribution of tear

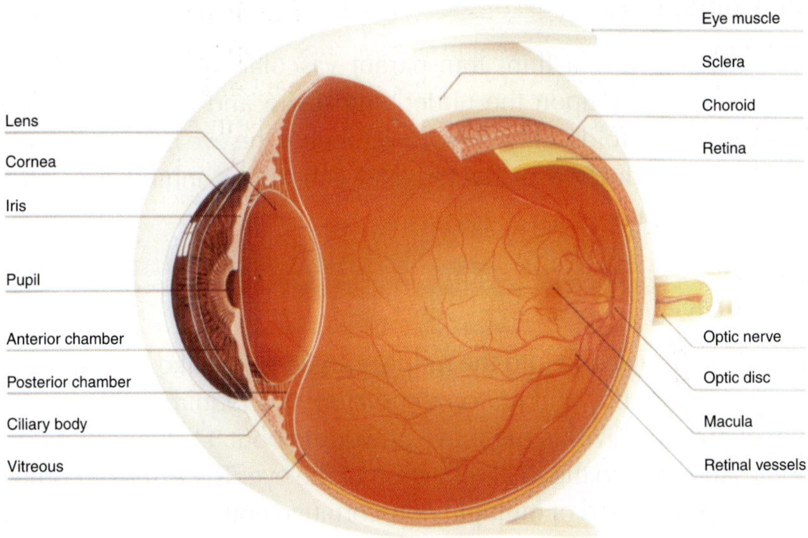

Figure 1. Cross-section of the human eye.

secretion occurs through regular blinking about 20–30 times per minute, preventing drying of conjunctival and corneal tissues. The edges of the lids contain countless sweat and sebum secreting glands, which have the effect of lubricating the lid margins in order to prevent overflow of tear fluid. The inner aspect of the lids is lined with conjunctiva. Accessory tear glands reside in the upper and lower folds; they produce serous tear fluid along with that from the main ducts, which are located under the temporal area of the upper eyelid. Tear film has three layers. The outer lipid layers consist of secretions from the sebum and tear glands; they prevent too rapid evaporation of the tear film. The middle watery layer's function is primarily to cleanse the cornea surface and to facilitate a high quality image. The inner mucinous layer comes from the goblet cells of the conjunctiva and the main tear gland; it serves as a stabilizer of the tear film upon the otherwise hydrophilic corneal surface. Tear fluid discharges by way of the upper and lower tear ducts. From there, the tears flow via the upper and lower duct canals into the lacrimal sac and through the nasal tear duct into the nasal cavity.

The Conjunctiva

The conjunctiva is a thin, transparent vascular mucous membrane layer. Its mobility upon the underlying sclera and the tissue redundancy in the lid folds allow free movement of the eye ball in all visual directions. Production of bactericidal substances inhibit eye infections significantly.

The Cornea

The cornea is inserted into the mildly curved sclera like a watch crystal. Its transparency and uniform curvature is a requirement for good optical imaging. With a refractive power of about 43 diopters, it contributes the most to the total refraction of the eye. The external corneal surface is composed of multiple non-cornified epithelial layers, which can rapidly regenerate when injured. The basal cell layers are joined to the very tough Bowman's membrane by a thin mucosal membrane. An injury to this layer does not regenerate tissue, but forms a scar.

The corneal stroma, which regenerates slowly owing to lack of vasculature, is made of collagen lamellae. The stroma is bound in the anterior chamber by the durable Descemete's membrane. This serves as the basal membrane of the single layered corneal epithelium. The pumping action of this non-regenerative endothelium maintains the transparency of the cornea. The average diameter of the adult cornea is about 11 mm, and the axial thickness about 500 μm. The cornea is sensitive to touch via innervation from the trigeminal nerve; injuries are very painful.

The Sclera

Together with the cornea, the sclera forms the protective, outer layer of the eye, onto which six external eye muscles are attached. The sclera is white, opaque, and fibrous, and contains *collagen* and *elastic fibers* with a high water content.

The Lens

The lens of the eye focuses the incoming light onto the retina. Allowing for accommodation, the portion of refraction attributed to the lens is in the order of 10–20 diopters. The lens is clear and biconvex, with a greater curvature on the posterior surface. It lies in the back of the anterior chamber between the posterior aspect of the iris and the vitreum, and is therefore a component of the iris–lens–diaphragm system, which separates the anterior chamber from the posterior. Zonular fibers are attached to the equator of the lens and connected to the ciliary body (Fig. 2).

When the ciliary muscle contracts, the tension on the lens, maintained by the zonular fibers, is reduced, and its intrinsic elasticity brings it to a rounder shape. This is called accommodation (Fig. 3).

Since the elasticity of the lens continuously decreases after birth, there is a continued deterioration of the lens' power of accommodation.

Accommodation

Normal vision (emmetropia) exists when parallel light rays enter the eye and are focused onto the retina (Fig. 4). This is the rule when the axial length of the eye is 24 mm. The refractive power increases through accommodation, whereby near objects can be seen clearly (Fig. 5). The unit of measurement is a diopter (D), which is the reciprocal of the focal length measured in metres (i.e., 1/m). In the case of emmetropia, an accommodation of 5 D will bring an object at a distance of 20 cm $\left(\frac{1\text{m}}{5}\right)$ sharply into focus on the retina (Figs. 2, 3 and 5).

Refraction

Refraction is determined primarily by the axial length of the eye.

If the eye is one mm too long or too short, a 3D-discrepancy exists. The eye axis generally lengthens until puberty, increasing

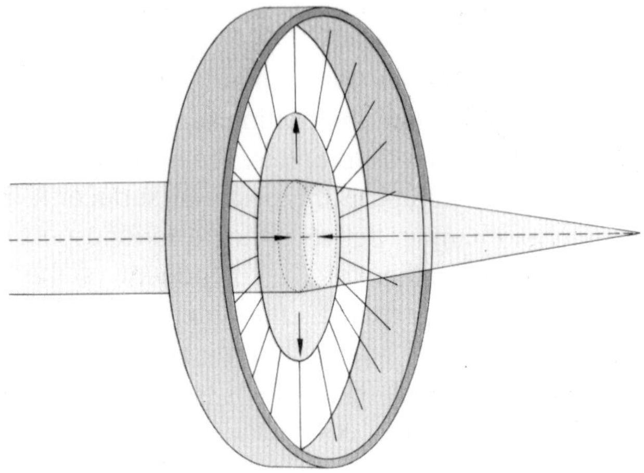

Figure 2. Relaxed ciliary muscle.

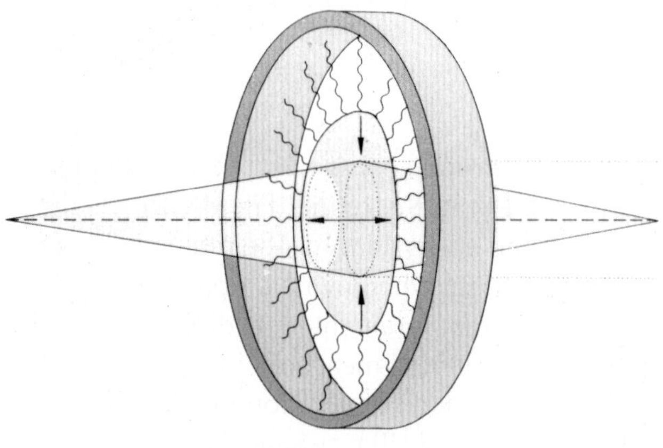

Figure 3. Contracted ciliary muscle.

nearsightedness and decreasing farsightedness. Loss of lens elasticity results in a loss of accommodation, as does an increase in lens density. This creates a higher optical density and refractive index with age, and therefore increases nearsightedness, which is additional to the axial ametropia.

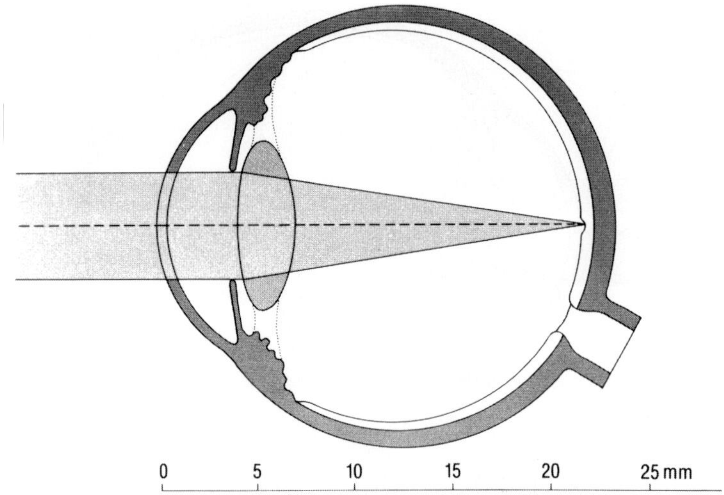

Figure 4. Emmetropia.

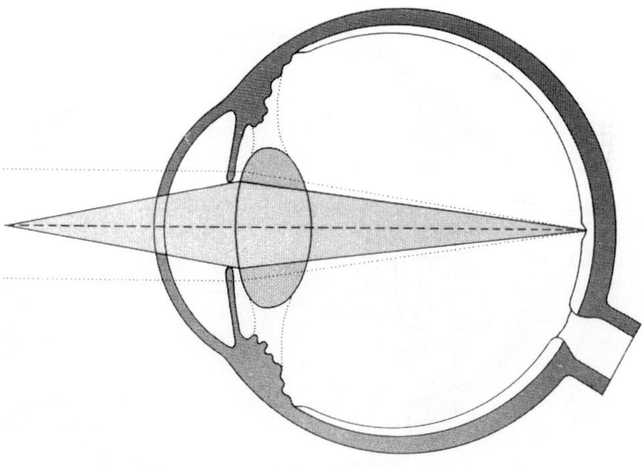

Figure 5. Accommodation with emmetropia.

Nearsightedness (myopia)

In an elongated eye, the focal point (without accommodation) lies in front of the retina (Fig. 6). This is nearsightedness or axial myopia. Placement of a concave lens before the eye displaces the focal point posteriorly and thus corrects the myopia (Fig. 7).

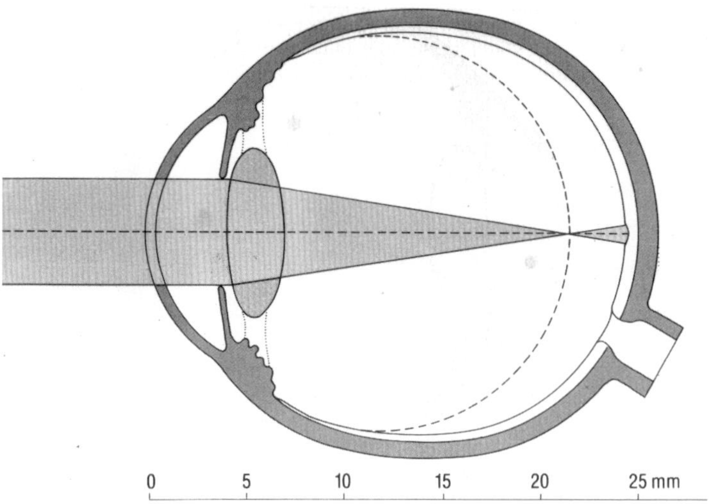

Figure 6. Myopia.

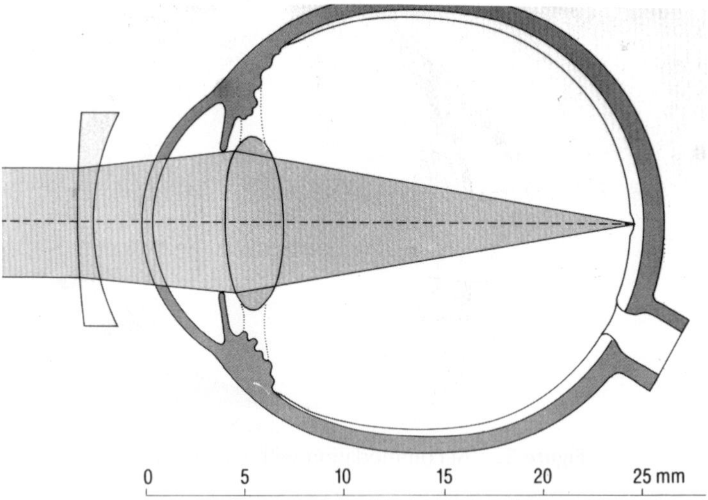

Figure 7. Myopic eye with corrective lens.

Farsightedness (hyperopia)

If the eyeball is too short, the focal point lies behind the retina (Fig. 8). This is called farsightedness or axial hyperopia.

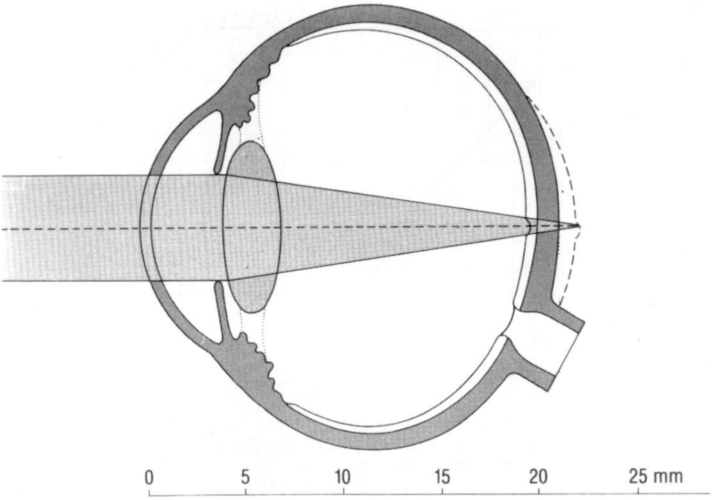

Figure 8. Hyperopia.

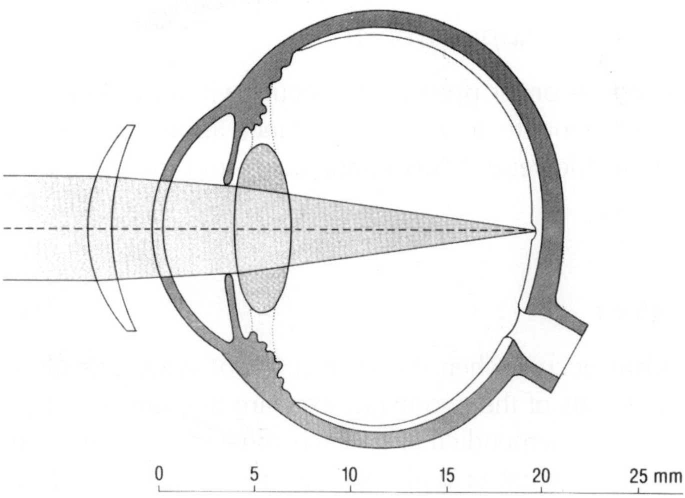

Figure 9. Hyperopic eye with corrective lens.

Through accommodation or placement of a convex lens before the eye, the focal point can be transferred to the retinal plane (Fig. 9).

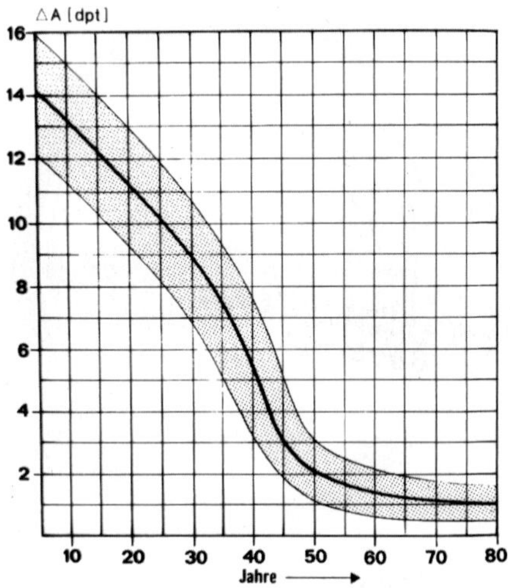

Figure 10. Accommodation and age.

Age related vision (presbyopia)

Age related vision or presbyopia occurs when accommodation is no longer adequate to focus an object about 30–40 cm away clearly onto the retina. This happens around the age of 45 years (Fig. 10).

Astigmatism

Astigmatism occurs when the cornea is not symmetrically curved. The focal points of the two major axes are not identical (Fig. 11). If these axes are perpendicular to each other, a cylindrical lens can bring the focal point of both axes together (Fig. 12) and project a sharp image onto the retina.

The Iris, Ciliary Body, and Chorioid

These structures form the uvea. The iris is opaque and shields the eye from overly intense light exposure. The variably sized pupillary diameter

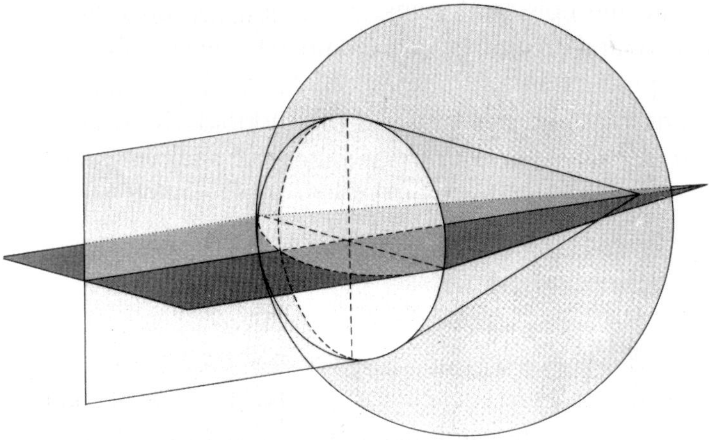

Figure 11. Differing axes with differing focal points.

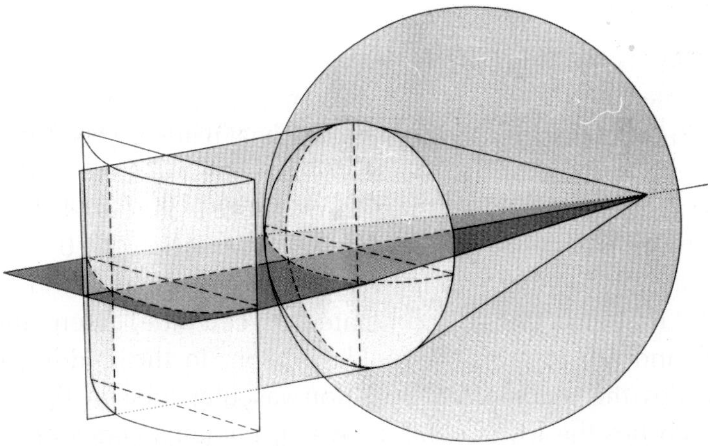

Figure 12. Correction of astigmatism with a plus-cylindrical lens.

serves as an optical aperture. The root of the iris transitions to the ciliary body, the muscles of which are responsible for accommodation and whose epithelium regulates the aqueous humor. This traverses from the posterior chamber through the pupil into the anterior chamber and drains from there, via the trabeculae in the iridocorneal angle, into the episcleral veins. A uniform eye pressure, generally between 10 and 20 mmHg, is maintained by an equilibrium between aqueous production and absorption. At the ora serrata, the ciliary body transitions into arterial tissue, the chorioid. This structure is very vascular and serves to nourish the outer retina and regulates the eye temperature. The interior retinal layers are supplied by the central retinal arteries.

The Vitreum

The vitreum is a clear, gelatinous structure, which becomes somewhat more fluid with age. It functions as a bulbar stabilizer and fills about three-quarters of the total eye volume.

The Retina

The retina is the "film" in the eye. Here, all the optical stimuli are transformed into electrical impulses by photoreceptors, and transferred to the optic nerve through the neuronal retinal layers. The retina contains two types of light sensitive cells, the rods and the cones. Although the two are mixed, the rods dominate in the periphery of the retina and the cones in the central part. About 120 millions rods transmit twilight and are responsible for night vision, while about 7 millions cones discriminate between blue, green, and red colors and are responsible for day vision. In the middle of the retina lies the macula, an oval non-vascular area in the center of which lies the fovea centralis which contains cones only. It is here the sharpest image is projected. This layout explains why there is no color perception in the peripheral vision, and why visual acuity declines from the central to the peripheral parts of the retina.

Adaptation to varying light intensities occurs not only by pupillary action, but also by way of transition from rod to cone vision. Adaptation to light occurs substantially faster (in seconds) than adaptation to darkness (~30 minutes).

The Optic Nerve (n. opticus)

The retinal nerve fibers in the optic nerve merge together in the papilla. There are no photoreceptors in this area, thereby creating the "blind spot." The optic nerve stretches from the posterior aspect of the eye to the optic chiasm, where the nasal fibers cross over to the opposing side and, together with the temporal fibers of the optical tract, arrive at the corpus geniculatum. The optic nerve as such is not a real cranial nerve but rather an advanced brainstem, and it is therefore encased by dura and pia mater as well as arachnoid tissue. Consequently, a blurred or elevated optic disc can indicate an increased intracranial pressure.

Ocular Muscles and Binocular Function

The large mobility of the eyeball increases the visual field greatly, and thus makes head movements less necessary. The normal human visual field extends to approximately 60 degrees nasally in each eye, to 100 degrees temporally, and approximately 60 degrees above and 75 degrees the horizontal meridian. This mobility is produced by the action of four straight and two diagonal muscles. Through the cooperation of sensory and motor systems, binocular vision is produced.

Slightly different images are projected onto the retinas, but perceived simultaneously. If the two images can be melted together in the brain, fusion is created and the object is seen as one. In addition, the brain's analysis of the double images provides depth perception. Man's highly developed binocular vision is the basis of spatial or stereoscopic vision.

If the eye muscles are unbalanced and there is no parallel position of the eyes, strabismus is present; if the strabismus angle is the same in all directions, then a concomitant strabismus is present. Concomitant strabismus most often appears in early childhood. Usually the brain favors visual perception in one of the eyes and sight is suppressed in the other (amblyopia). Due to this unilateral suppression of visual perception, double vision is avoided, but binocular function is lost. Eye injuries or diseases of the nerve or nuclei may lead to incomitant or paralytic strabismus with double vision and compensatory head positioning. The strabismus angle occurs only in the direction of the paralyzed muscle.

Phoria has to do with latent strabismus, which is only revealed when decompensation occurs, usually because of fatigue of the ocular muscles. Decompensation can lead to outright strabismus with double vision.

DISEASES OF THE EYE

Diseases of the Tear Duct System and Lids

Dry eye (keratoconjunctivitis sicca, xerophthalmia)

This condition is caused by decreased tear production or increased tear film evaporation. Symptoms consist of reddened, burning eyes and a foreign body sensation. Although it may seem strange, the dry eye condition can cause the eyes to water. By way of a reflex, excessive tearing is initiated but tearing time is usually shortened (less than five seconds), and the mucinous component so minimal that a good contact between the hydrophobic corneal surface and the watery phase of the tear film cannot be sustained.

The air in modern commercial airliners is quite dry, with a relative humidity of 4–14%; this can substantially worsen symptoms. Tear supplementation (artificial tears) or punctum plugs can be helpful.

High viscosity tear supplements or eye ointments can temporarily interfere with visual acuity and should be avoided during flight.

Excessive tearing (epiphora)

Overproduction of tears frequently occurs in the setting of inflammation or external irritation. Often there is an interference within the drainage system causing recurrent conjunctivitis. Lid anomalies can also cause tearing, especially when the lower lid curls outward, whereby the lower punctum no longer lies in the tear pool. Since epiphora often leads to a reduction in visual acuity, the cause should be investigated.

Drooping upper eyelid (ptosis)

Ptosis can be congenital or acquired. A prominent ptosis can indicate myotonia, sympathetic damage, or a disorder of the oculomotor nerve. Trauma or instillation of a local anesthetic can also induce ptosis. Whether or not flight fitness is impaired depends on the visual field evaluation. It is particularly important to monitor this when dealing with myotonic ptosis, as the degree of lid narrowing can be variable.

Incomplete lid closure (lagophthalmos)

The inability to close the eye is usually caused by a facial nerve paresis. Bell's palsy, which induces the eye to turn upwards when the patient attempts to close the eye, can lead to insufficient protection of the corneal surface. Often a surface disorder with irritation of the corneal surface develops. To what extent flight fitness is affected must be determined on a case by case basis, using aeromedical judgment.

Misalignment of the lids

As mentioned above, an outward curl of the lower lid (ectropion) can result in increased tearing, in that the lower punctum no longer lies within the tear pool. An inward curling of the lower lid leads to a scouring of the eyelashes on the cornea, giving rise to a foreign body sensation. A primary malformation of the lids can result in similar symptoms. In general, corrective surgery can eliminate the misalignment and the functional impairment.

Inflammatory changes and tumors of the eyelid

Meibomian cysts (chalazion) and styes (hordeolum) are relatively common disorders of the eyelid. They are secondary to inflammation or infection of gland ducts, in most cases caused by Staphylococcus aureus. In general, they do not have any functional significance. Hordeola are often painful and should be treated locally with antibiotics, and sometimes even systemically. Chalazion, in contrast, are minimally painful and encapsulated, and should be removed surgically. In that all chronic inflammations of the lids can progress to a functional impairment, any effect on flight performance should be determined. In general, all tumors in the area of the eyelids should be treated surgically.

Disorders of the Conjunctiva

Conjunctivitis

Conjunctival inflammation is a relatively common disorder. It can appear in response to bacteria, viruses, Chlamydia, or be a topical allergic reaction. Allergic conjunctivitis from pollen is often improved during flight, as there are few or no allergens in the filtered cabin air. Viral conjunctivitis not uncommonly leads to corneal involvement in which case visual acuity can be affected due to glare and reduced corneal transparency. Keratoconjunctivitis epidemica can lead to temporary unfitness for flight, such as in the case of lymphocytic infiltration of the cornea, or to permanent disqualification, such as in the case of corneal damage from a herpes infection.

Pterygium

A pterygium is a duplication of the conjunctiva; it generally grows into the cornea from the nasal side. Vision could be impaired if it reaches the optical zone. Surgical removal can be performed, but recurrences are not uncommon.

Symblepharon

Through a fusion of the conjunctivae of the bulbus and the inner eyelid, ocular motility can be impaired. Symblepharon usually arises due to infections or an ocular pemphigoid. If the restriction of eye movement causes double vision, flight fitness could be affected.

Cornea

A uniformly curved and transparent cornea is a prerequisite for projecting optimal quality images onto the retina. Cloudiness of the cornea leads to significant glare, especially when it affects the optic center. Edema can develop when the endothelium loses cells, leading to deterioration of vision, especially in the morning hours. With irregular corneal curvature, visual acuity can usually be significantly improved with a shape-stabilizing contact lens. Flight fitness is determined by the corrected vision. If there is an increasing corneal irregularity, keratoconus must be suspected and corneal topography studies are required. If there is a known family history of corneal dystrophy, it is important to remember that these often do not manifest themselves until middle age, and then may be incompatible with continued medical certification.

The Uveal Tract: Iris, Ciliary Body, and the Choroid

Iris and pupil

Iritis is the most common form of uveitis, and is most often combined with an inflammation of the ciliary body (cyclitis). Recurrence is frequent and often associated with rheumatoid diseases. Iritis is marked by pain, photophobia, and excessive tearing. Visual acuity can be reduced by inflammatory cells from exudates or from protein deposits, such as fibrin, in the anterior chamber.

The most serious consequence occurs when the posterior aspect of the iris and the anterior aspect of the lens stick together. In order to avoid this complication, the pupil is kept dilated during the acute phase. During this time of induced mydriasis, the loss of accommodation and the increased sensitivity to light are a bar to medical certification. If synechia develops, which interferes with pupillary light reaction, future flight fitness must be evaluated on an individual basis. The applicant with a history of uveitis must be informed that medical certification might be in jeopardy.

Non-inflammatory pupillary disorders should be evaluated neuro-ophthalmologically. Pronounced iris colobomas or pupilloplegia are often compatible with flying duties after determination that it is an isolated situation. Medications affecting the pupil will be discussed in the section on eye medications and their effects on flight fitness.

Inflammation of the ciliary body (cyclitis)

Isolated cyclitis is rare, but appears more commonly together with iritis as iridocyclitis. With involvement of the ciliary body, the posterior chamber can become involved and intersperse the vitreous with inflammatory mediators and cells. This can additionally impair vision.

Inflammation of the chorioid (chorioiditis)

Due to the lack of sensory innervation of the chorioid, inflammation to this part of the uvea is not painful. Inflammatory foci of the chorioid usually heal within a few weeks. Depending on their localization and size, they can lead to circumscribed scotomas in the peripheral field, or macular involvement and therefore a reduction in visus. If the retina is involved as an inflammatory component, the condition is called retinochorioiditis. Here, the inflammatory cells are also found in the vitreous. The most common disorder of this type is the congenital or developed manifestations of toxoplasmosis. This leads to retinal scarring with corresponding scotomas and loss of nerve fibers. Recurrences are not uncommon.

Tumors of the uvea

Malignant melanoma is the most common tumor of the chorioid. Diagnosed early, it responds well to brachytherapy (sealed source radiotherapy), albeit creating a corresponding scotoma.

Disorders of the Vitreous Humor

Opacities of the vitreous humor can lead to a reduction in vision. Opacities can develop from inflammation of the uvea and are often not reversible. Floaters are deposits of various size, shape, consistency, refractive index, and motility. They may be of embryonic origin or acquired due to degenerative changes of the vitreous humor or retina. The perception of floaters is known as *myodesopsia.* Floaters appear as shadow-like shapes, either alone or together with several others in the field of vision. They may be seen as spots, threads, or fragments of cobwebs which float slowly before the eyes. Since these objects exist within the eye itself, they are not optical illusions but entoptic phenomena. One specific type of floater is called m*uscae volitantes* or *mouches volantes* and consists of small spots. These are present in most people's eyes and are attributed to minute remnants of embryonic structures in the vitreous humor. Rarely are they precursors or consequences of a retinal disorder. Nearsightedness and advanced age favor the development of *mouches volantes.*

The extent to which vision is impaired by opacities depends on the size and number of the cloudy areas as well as their locations. Only in unusual cases do opacities develop into a significant functional impairment. This is also true for the so-called asteroid hyalosis, a primarily unilateral degenerative disorder involving small white opacities in the vitreous humor.

Disorders of the Lens

As the lens ages, its elasticity changes and so does its refractive index. Cataracts develop when there is an interference with light transmission. If the refractive index increases, the eye can become myopic, yet fully correctable. Subluxation of the lens can lead to similar symptoms. A discontinuous refractive index can result in double or multiple refractions, so that monocular double vision can occur. A cataract can influence near and distant vision acuity differently. Cataracts have a tendency to increase glare sensitivity.

Medical certification after intraocular lens implant depends not only on the resulting refraction and the visual acuity, but also on the degree of pre-operative refraction.

Disorders of the Retina

Introduction

Hereditary retinal degenerative disorders, such as retinitis pigmentosa, are usually disqualifying for aviation duties due to their progressive nature. If function is not yet significantly impaired, the applicant should be informed that this condition might in the future deteriorate visual acuity to below the requirements.

Retinal disorders with macular involvement usually lead to decline in function. With regard to medical certification, the progressive nature of these disorders dictates frequent testing of vision.

Retinal detachments (amotio retinae)

Retinal detachments cause a peripheral field defect corresponding to the site of the detachment. Even after successful intervention, peripheral field defects can persist. In order to re-attach the retina, a plomb is often sewn onto the posterior part of the eyeball. This can lead to a restriction of ocular motility and consequential double vision. Even the axial length of the eyeball can be altered by such surgical intervention, resulting in a change in refraction. Replacement substances that are imported into the vitreous can cause a change in refraction; if it is gaseous, a rapid decompression can create a serious rise in intraocular pressure. In the event of a very small, circumscribed retinal detachment, laser coagulation is indicated and may be adequate to encase it. In general, this entails no functional impairment; with the onset of retinal healing at about 10–14 days, further retinal detachment is not likely. Areas of degeneration, which can further deteriorate into retinal detachments, should be prophylactically treated with laser coagulation. In general, there is no flight restriction necessary after a coagulation of a peripheral retinal area. The existence of peripheral retinal degeneration should always initiate a complete eye examination by an ophthalmologist, including a detailed visual field test.

Central serous retinopathy

This disorder, which mostly affects active men in their middle years, is caused by a serous effusion into the retina. If the macula is involved, patients usually complain of distortion of vision or micropsia (the perception of objects as being much smaller than they actually are). In many cases, the warping of the retina leads to hyperopia. This disorder has a good prognosis and spontaneous healing is common. In some cases, the source points can be visualized with fluorography and coagulated by laser. Often, this results in a minimal decrease in function and diminished contrast sensitivity. Medical certification may be considered when there is no further evidence of leakage as shown by fluorography. Persistent serous leaks can result in unpredictable vacillations in visual acuity.

Vascular diseases of the retina

Tissue changes resulting in functional losses due to underlying internal diseases, such as diabetes mellitus or arterial hypertension, are generally not compatible with aviation duties as the underlying disease process may be disqualifying. Retinal artery occlusion can lead to an irreversible loss in the supply area of the affected branch of the artery. Occlusion of the central retinal artery leads to complete blindness. When a smaller branch artery is blocked, only the part of the retina supplied by that branch is affected and vision is not as severely affected. Arterial retinal occlusions are therefore not compatible with aviation duties. Occlusion or stenosis of retinal veins can lead to a stasis with disseminated bleeding.

The course of a vascular occlusion is thereby quite variable. Extensive retinal ischemia can lead to the development of neovascularization, resulting in many types of late complications, such as secondary glaucoma. Even laser treatment cannot always prevent blindness and the need of eventual enucleation. On the other hand, cases occur where there is total regress and new collateral vessels develop in the area of the papilla. Such cases may be entirely compatible with aviation duties. In all other cases, medical certification is not possible due to the unpredictable course of this disease. As retinal vascular occlusions usually are caused by an embolus, a full work-up is required to look for possible embolic sources. A pilot who has had a retinal artery occlusion is at increased risk for a stroke or myocardial infarction.

Diseases of the Optic Nerve

Inflammation of the optic nerve (neuritis nervi optici, retrobulbar neuritis)

Optic neuritis typically affects young adults ranging from 18 to 45 years of age, with a mean age of 30–35 years. There is a strong female predominance. The main symptoms of optic neuritis are a decrease in visual acuity, a change in color vision, and pain on eye movements. Younger patients often develop multiple sclerosis later on, resulting in recurrent optic neuritis. Vision can recover completely between episodes, yet a relatively central defect of the visual field usually remains. Due to the high rate of recurrence and the danger of progressive functional deterioration, medical certification can only be considered under certain conditions, viz. that the time of presentation is after the age of 45, when multiple sclerosis is not likely to develop, and that no indication of localized defects is found on retinal imaging.

Ischemic optic neuropathy

Whether inflamed or not, ischemic optical neuropathy usually leads to visual loss below the standards for aviation duties, and is only relatively reversible. An indication of ischemia is a swelling of the optic nerve followed by atrophy.

Glaucoma

Worldwide, glaucoma is the most common cause of permanent blindness. The incidence is estimated to be approximately 2% in the

Caucasian population, substantially increasing after the 45–50th year of life.[5,6] The damage to the neuronal structures of the visual axis, especially of the optic nerve fibers, along with ascending atrophy of the optic nerve is caused by a decrease in the so-called perfusion pressure. This is the pressure gradient between the retinal capillaries, the chorioid, and the anterior uvea. The intraocular pressure, which is the pressure of the circulating aqueous humor, is necessary for the optical function of the eye, as the shape of the globe determines the proper imaging of the object onto the retina. In order to ensure the geometric configuration of the eyeball against the soft tissue counter pressure of the orbit, the tension of the eyelid, and the pull of the extraocular muscles, an intraocular pressure of at least 10 mmHg is required. The average intraocular pressure of a healthy adult is approximately 15 mmHg (in the newborn it is about only 8–9 mmHg). Empirically, a slow and steady rise in pressure occurs with increasing age, so that average pressures found in youths are about 12 mmHg rising to about 16–18 mmHg in the elderly. As arterial blood pressure also increases slightly with aging, the ocular perfusion pressure is adequately supported throughout life.

Nutritional support of the eye is very sensitive and immediately suffers with continued changes in perfusion pressure, whether due to a reduction of circulatory pressure or an elevation of anterior chamber pressure from a pathologic hindrance of chamber fluid drainage. It is inexpensive to measure the intraocular pressure. The tonometer (a word coined by Albrecht von Graefe in 1865) provides a non-invasive estimate of intraocular pressure. In order to physically ascertain the true intraocular pressure, one would have to puncture the eyeball with a needle and attach the needle to a manometer, which is not possible in routine clinical circumstances. An elevated intraocular pressure is in general the decisive cause for the development of glaucoma. Aqueous humor is continually produced by the ciliary processes. It is important that this production is balanced by an equal rate of drainage. Small variations in production or outflow of aqueous humor will have a large influence on the intraocular pressure. Figure 13 shows the irido-corneal angle. The primary route for aqueous humor flow is first through the posterior chamber, then via

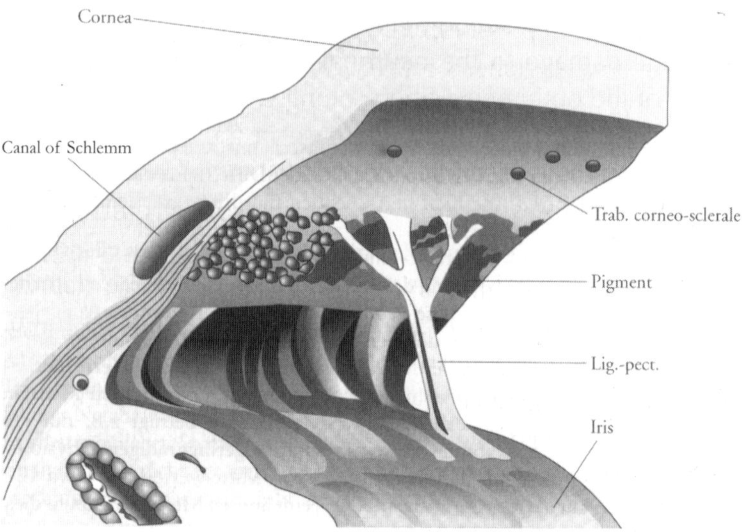

Figure 13. The irido-corneal angle.

the iridocorneal angle (the narrow space between the posterior iris and the anterior lens) through the pupil into the anterior chamber.

The influx of fluid to the anterior chamber is stable at about 1 mm^3/min, resulting in an astonishingly well-equilibrated pressure.

Drainage occurs through a circumferential split in the sclera, called the canals of Schlemm, into the extraocular venous plexus. Apart from rare cases of elevated extraocular venous pressure, a reduction in drainage into the outflow tract is usually caused by an increased resistance in the canals of Schlemm. This can be caused by deposition of cellular detritus and inflammatory proteins (secondary glaucoma), by deposition of pigmented cells (pigmentary glaucoma) and, most important clinically, by age-related structural changes in the outflow tract.

Particularly in hyperopia, due to a short eyeball, a flattening of the anterior chamber with narrowing of the chamber angle can exist, so that with a widened pupil, the root of the iris can close the iridocorneal angle, resulting in an acute angle-closure glaucoma. Pressure then rises abruptly and dramatically, leading to malaise and vomiting. The pupil is fixed in mid-position, the cornea becomes edematous with surface dullness, and the conjunctivae are red. Release of the angle closure results in a slow drop in eye pressure. In order to prevent another acute angle-closure glaucoma, peripheral iridectomy is performed, so that a direct connection between the anterior and posterior chamber is created. With this procedure, the danger of another angle closure is eliminated.

Because acute angle-closure glaucoma causes pain, the diagnosis is generally made before the optic nerve is damaged.

Since glaucoma is eminently treatable, initially with medications and later with surgical intervention, it is obvious that early detection is critical in order to protect the eye from damage. For the aviation medicine practitioner, glaucoma is particularly important from the perspective of functional consequences: initially the visual field is pared down in the outer or middle peripheral regions, eventually also involving central vision, and finally leading to blindness (Fig. 14).[7]

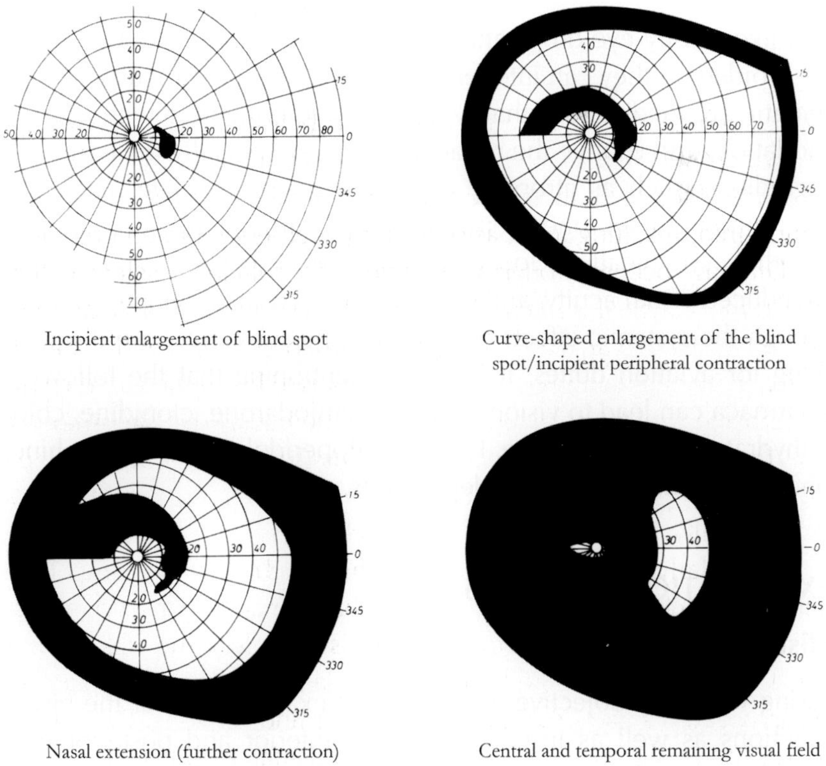

Incipient enlargement of blind spot

Curve-shaped enlargement of the blind spot/incipient peripheral contraction

Nasal extension (further contraction)

Central and temporal remaining visual field

Figure 14. Perimetry visual field changes caused by glaucoma.

Such a development is obviously disqualifying for medical certification. However, cases without gross morphologic changes and without functional damage, usually where glaucoma has been detected early, may be compatible with aviation duties. The prerequisite is, of course, adequate management of the intraocular pressure through appropriate therapy of a kind that does not cause a secondary disqualifying condition. In the past, therapy was limited to the miotic agent pilocarpine, which interferes with adaptation and accommodation and often results in refractive changes. Today, treatment consists primarily of beta blockade, which may cause side effects in the circulatory system, especially hypotension. Careful monitoring of such patients is required.

Effects of Medication on Visual Acuity

Gel-like or oily eye drops and eye ointment should, when possible, be avoided, as they can interfere with visual acuity. Particularly problematic are medications that widen the pupil, interfere with accommodation, and change the refraction. This is especially the case with ingredients such as atropine, carbachol, cyclopentolate, naphazoline, neostigmine, phenylephrine, pilocarpine, and scopolamine, whether systemically or locally applied. Beta blockade can also lead to reduced visual acuity, and can often worsen sicca symptoms. Even though the systemic effects of the following substances are disqualifying for aviation duties, it is worth mentioning that the following pharmaca can lead to vision disorders: amiodarone, clonidine, chloralhydrate, chlorpromazine, L-dopa, haloperidol, lithium, morphine, phenytoin, and tricyclic antidepressants.

EXAMINATION METHODS

History

Along with the subjective and objective examinations of the visual functions as well as inspection of the anterior and posterior eye, the history is of particular importance. Questions regarding family history should not only include inherited diseases such as corneal dystrophy or pigmentosa retinopathy, but also diseases that are not directly hereditary but often occur in familial patterns, such as glaucoma. The strength of the parents' eyeglasses can also be helpful, when future progression of a refractive error is of concern. Frequent headaches can indicate a non-corrected hyperopia or a high-grade phoria. Further questions should include:

- Strabismus in childhood
- Injuries, infections, or surgeries of the eye
- Regular application of eye drops or ointment
- Light sensitivity or photophobia
- Poor twilight vision
- Temporary blurriness
- Eye pain and double vision.

One should emphasize to the applicant that withholding information, for example about having undergone refractive surgery, can later lead to the loss of medical certification.

In spite of the fact that refractive corneal surgery is an efficient method to correct refractive errors, one must keep in mind that in some cases the applicant will still not meet the requirements for medical certification. Postoperative refractive instability, increased glare sensitivity, or other pathological findings may entail unfitness for aviation duties. Furthermore, "iatrogenic keratectasy" is a long-term complication, which in an increasing number of cases leads to serious complications, threatening the function of the eye.

Eye Examination

When examining the external eye, one should be particularly mindful of asymmetry, such as unequal lid opening or a unilateral exophthalmus, which can be quantified with an exophthalmometer according to Hertel's method. Additionally, unequal pupils should be looked for. All asymmetry requires a careful search for the etiology.

Pupillary Movement

Light reaction

The reaction of the eye to direct light is evaluated by illumination in a semi-darkened room. Normally, the illuminated pupil constricts after about 0.2 seconds. Consensual light reaction is observed in the other eye, but one must avoid shining light on the other eye. The pupils normally constrict simultaneously without delay. The swinging flashlight test lends itself to the diagnosis of afferent pupillary disturbance. The patient is asked to look into the distance, as accommodation should be avoided. The eyes are illuminated alternatively, at the same distance and for the same length of time, whereby the initial constriction and the subsequent dilatation of the pupils can be evaluated. If one pupil constricts and dilates more slowly than the other, the affected eye has a relative afferent pupillary disorder. This evaluation may be difficult, so this is the remit of examiners with experience. The test is particularly helpful in the diagnosis of retrobulbar neuritis.

Examination of near vision alignment

The subject looks into the distance and then at a near object (such as a pencil), which is slowly brought close to the eye. This causes a convergence of the optical axes, brought about by a near vision alignment miosis. If the object is brought even closer to the eye, convergence often cannot be maintained and the eye diverges. Depending on the age, convergence is coupled to accommodation. Insufficiency of convergence is a common cause of asthenopic complaints, such as cephalgia.

Slit Lamp Biomicroscopy

Anterior chamber

With slit lamp biomicroscopy, the anterior as well as the posterior chambers of the eye can be examined. The examination of the anterior chamber includes the position of the lids, changes in the conjunctivae and cornea. By means of fluorescein dye and illumination with blue light, defects of the cornea can be determined, as defects stain greenish-yellow. It is also possible to evaluate the tear film break-up time (in seconds) with fluorescein: a drop of 2% fluorescein solution is placed in the lower lid and the patient is asked to blink three times. The interval between the last blink and the appearance of the first precorneal hypofluorescent spot, streak, or other irregularity interrupting the normal homogenous fluorescein pattern is the tear film break-up time.

The transparency of the aqueous humor and the existence of cells or protein in the anterior chamber must be noted. The depth of the anterior chamber must be evaluated and the iris and lens examined for pathological changes.

Posterior chamber

In order to evaluate the iridocorneal angle and the posterior eye, a fundus contact lens is placed on the anesthetized eye. By way of the central portion of the contact lens, the vitreum and the posterior pole can be evaluated (Fig. 15). The optic nerve papilla can be evaluated and described with respect to sharpness of the disc edge, coloration, notching, and swelling. The vessels, the macula, and the fovea are examined. With a mirror system, the retina can be examined well into the outer circular periphery. This is particularly important in nearsightedness as degenerative areas often lie in the periphery. Whenever possible, the examination should be performed during maximal mydriasis, which suppresses accommodation and therefore facilitates refraction. Appropriate medications include tropicamide and cyclopentolate, which are applied twice over 10 minutes into the conjunctival sac. The evaluation of the anterior chamber is similarly performed utilizing a mirror in the contact lens whereby the anterior chamber angle can be examined and possible structural abnormalities can be noted.

The fundus examination with the direct ophthalmoscope (eye mirror) covers only the posterior pole, but is not adequate to evaluate the peripheral retina. With indirect methods, a virtual, upside-down mirror image is created. Either a biconvex magnifier is

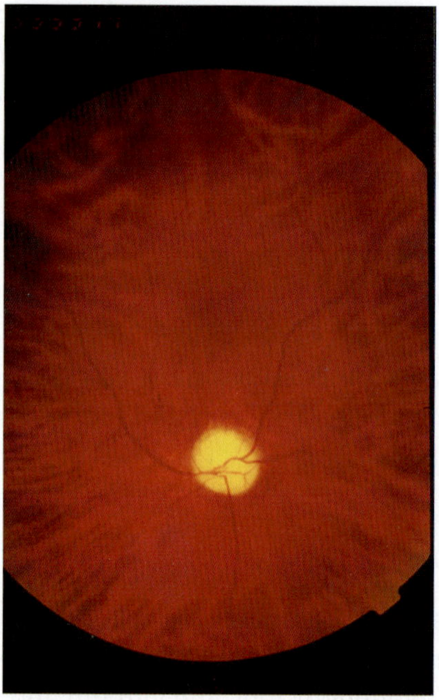

Figure 15. Normal fundus, optic disc with small physiological cupping.

placed on the slit lamp in front of the eye, or an indirect ophthalmoscope is used for the examination. This technique requires much experience, but allows examination of the peripheral retina. It has the advantage that the eye is not touched and therefore no local anesthetic is necessary.

Pressure Measurement

In the course of time, a variety of principles has been applied to assess the intraocular pressure. Very early on "applanation tonometry" (Fick, 1888) was recommended, and it is still the most commonly utilized method: it is based on the concept that internal eye pressure can be determined by distortion or oblation of a small central area of the cornea. The first truly clinically useful eye tonometer using this principle was proposed in 1954 by Hans Goldman in Bern (Fig. 16).

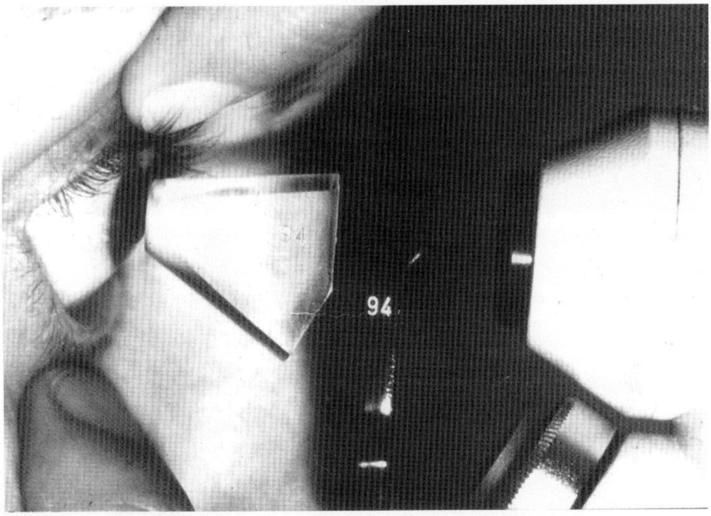

Figure 16. Applanation tonometer after Goldman.

This tonometer utilizes the conventional slit lamp microscope for evaluation of the anterior chamber and also for visualization of the corneal surface and the applanation produced by the tonometer. The force required to flatten a defined surface of 3.06 mm in diameter can then be read from a dial. This device today belongs to the standard equipment in most eye practices, but is somewhat cumbersome for the medical examiner as a non-ophthalmologist, apart from its substantial cost. Not only for these reasons, but also in order to improve handling and operation of such a tonometer, the so-called hand applanation tonometer (Draeger, 1965) was developed. In addition to being very simple to use, this device is completely independent of position and gravity; it can be used on supine patients or also in weightlessness during space missions. More recently, the advances in microelectronics have allowed a fully automatic hand applanation tonometer to be developed.[9–14] It requires use of local anesthetic, but can measure the intraocular pressure with precision in a few seconds. A coaxial optic allows observation of the applanation surface, and measurement is fast and automatic (Fig. 17).

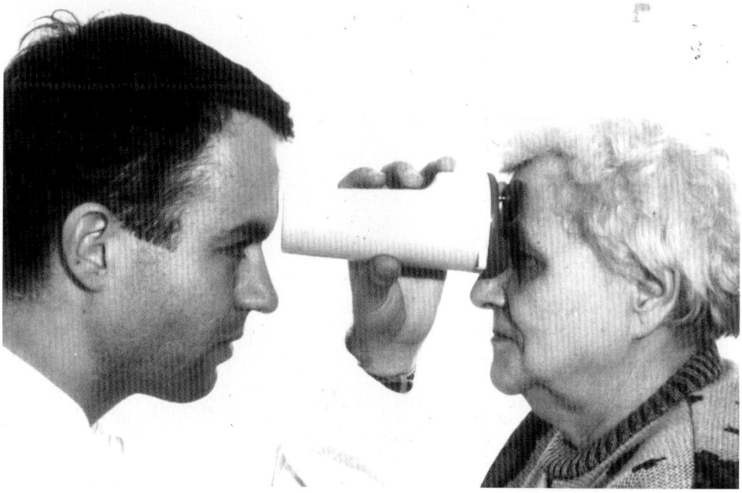

Figure 17. Fully automatic hand applantion tonometer.

A single discretionary measurement of elevated eye pressure is not necessarily valid evidence for the existence of glaucoma. Sampaolesi (1964) demonstrated that the amplitude of daily pressure changes is a more important diagnostic feature (Fig. 18).

It is entirely possible that an afternoon reading in the eye clinic is inconspicuous, while the pressure is 10 to 15 mmHg higher during the critical hours of early morning. In doubtful cases, it is therefore recommended to take several measurements.

Especially in the USA and with opticians, the so-called air-puff tonometer is in general use. It can, if necessary, be used without local anesthesia (although this is very unpleasant for the patient). Measurements with this device become increasingly inaccurate with increasing eye pressure.

The so-called "impression tonometry" (Hjalmar Schiötz, 1905), which was earlier a routine method, is no longer in common use because of its relative inaccuracy. It is, however, a comparatively easy method for non-ophthalmologists.

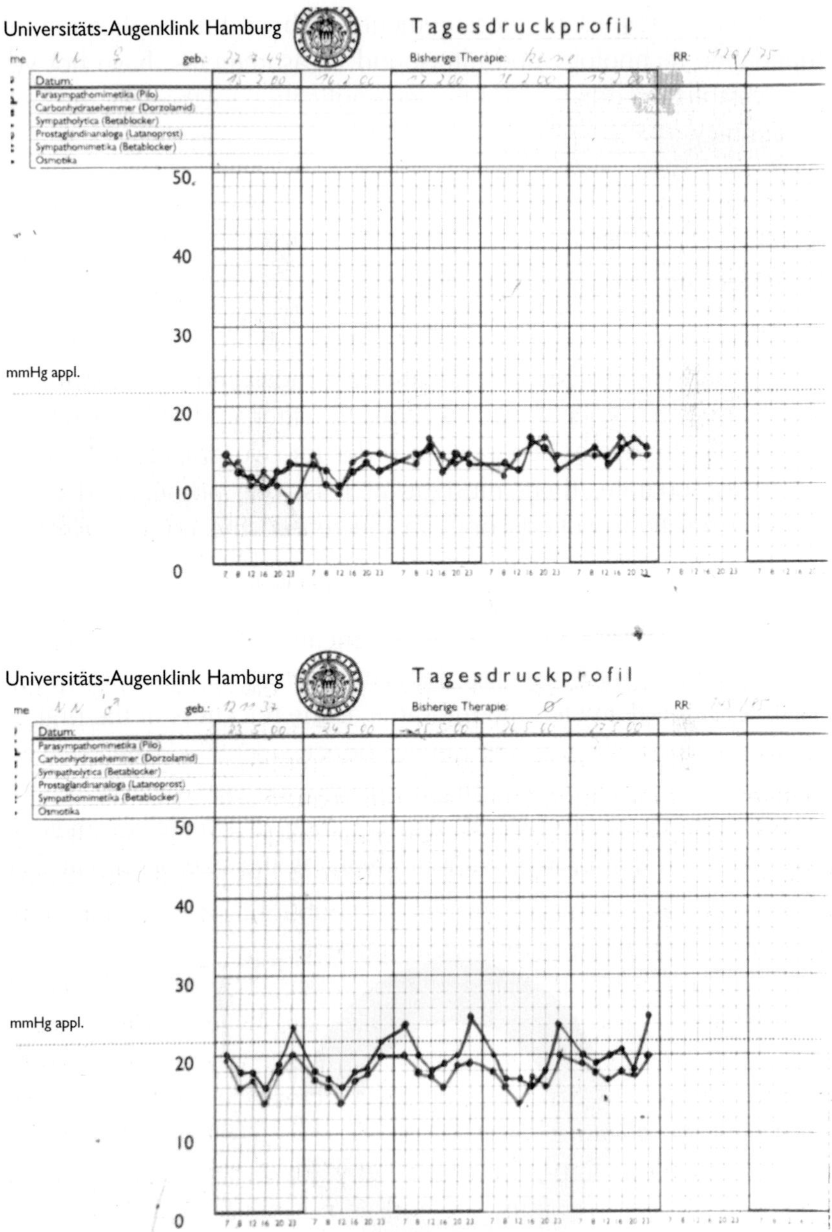

Figure 18. Circadian pressure curve.

Other principles of measurement, such as the application of impedance technology and ultrasound measurements, have not yet been established due to complicated application methods or the lack of accuracy.

Visual Acuity (Visus)

Visus testing

Visual acuity is defined as optimal resolution ability, if necessary with correction by optical aids. Visual acuity is measured by determining how close two objects can be to each other and still be distinguished by the eye as separate. In order for two objects to be perceived as separate, there must be at least one non-excited cone between the two excited cones in the retina. The normal eye has the ability to resolve a spatial pattern separated by a visual angle of one minute of arc.

Visual acuity can be evaluated by means of the Landolt broken ring (Landolt C optotype) (Fig. 19). The opening of this optotype is one-fifth of the diameter and the same as the thickness of the ring. If the localization of the opening can be correctly identified when viewed under a visual angle of one minute of arc, the visual acuity is 1.0. The chart is generally placed at a distance of five to six meters. A doubling of the distance without changing the size of the Landolt

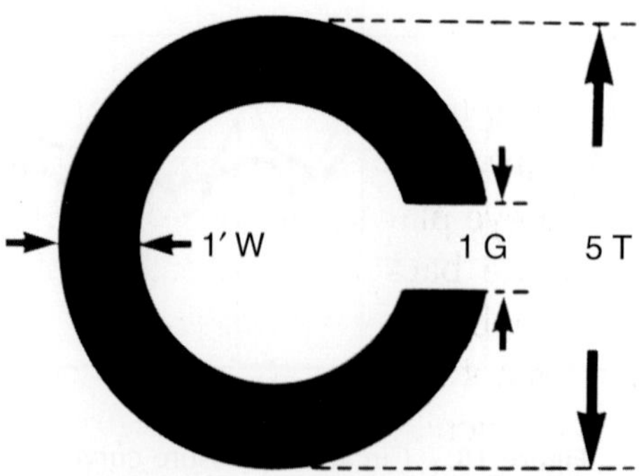

Figure 19. Landolt-Ring (T = total size, G = space, W = ring thickness).

rings requires a resolution ability of 0.5 minute of arc, which corresponds to a visual acuity of 2.0. Similarly, a visual acuity of 0.5 is adequate to properly localize the opening at half the distance with the same size Landolt rings.

Although a visual acuity of 1.0 defines "normal vision" (normal visual acuity), young people in general possess a visual acuity ranging between 1.2 and 1.6. For visus testing, the Landolt rings should be positioned with the opening in the four straight axes and also in the four diagonal axes. With a visual acuity of at least 0.4, a visus level is recognized when six out of 10 Landolt rings are identified without hesitation. With lower visual acuity, at least three out of five must be correctly identified without hesitation. Additional visual acuity results, such as "partially recognized" should be avoided. In some countries, the visus levels are reported as quotients. The quotient is the ratio between the examination distance and the distance at which a test letter of equal size corresponds to a visus of 1.0. The visus levels commonly used in Germany are 6/6 = 1.0, 6/9 = 0.7, 6/12 = 0.5, 6/18 = 0.3, and 6/60 = 0.1. In practice, visual acuity examinations are often made by using Snellen test charts with numerals or letters. The disadvantage of such test letters is that they are not equally legible. Round numbers, such as 8, 9, 6, 3, and 0 are more easily confused than straight numbers such as 4 and 7. Some alphabetic letters are easily recognizable, such as L, I, and T, while others, such as G, R, and B can easily be confused.

Static visus testing

Not only the type of test letter, but also its color, the contrast to its environment, presentation length, peripheral illumination, and the adaptive ability of the eye play significant roles. Test letters are generally black on a white background. Visual acuity declines with reduced object contrast, but very high contrast can also impair visual acuity. If contrast does not go below 85%, no effect on visual acuity is to be expected. Visual acuity rises with background illumination up to a maximum, and then falls off when the illumination is so strong that glare develops. Commercially available test letter displays that are illuminated from behind usually fulfil the requirements, as long as the ambient illumination does not fall below 20% of the display illumination. Near vision testing takes place at 30–50 cm and 100 cm. Also here, sufficient illumination of the test letters is necessary. The test letter display should be clean and exhibit high contrast, while the surface should be non-reflective and dull. When illumination has been optimized, it should no longer be changed. Daylight tends to vary and is therefore unsuitable for vision testing. Because not everyone is in the position to ascertain contrast and light intensity, it may be necessary to utilize the services of a professional optometrist prior to starting vision testing and refraction.

Dynamic visus testing

In addition to the described static visus testing, it is also possible to test dynamic visual acuity by utilizing moving optotypes. Although the dynamic visual function is very important for pilots, neither standardized test procedures nor requirement limits have been established. Dynamic visual acuity does not directly correlate with static visual acuity.

Pinhole test

To differentiate refraction errors from organic disease, a pinhole test can be used. If vision improves with pinhole, the reduced visual acuity is due to refractive error.

Contrast sensitivity

In order to evaluate contrast sensitivity, stripe patterns with sinusoidal contrast dispersion and a variety of frequencies are presented. The stripe pattern is presented in the vertical as well as inclined to the left and right positions, in order to better determine recognition.

Contrast sensitivity and visual acuity are two different functions that are not correlated. In many cases, it makes sense to determine contrast sensitivity in addition to visual acuity. Because requirement limitations do not exist, this examination has not yet found its way into aeromedical certification evaluations.

Refraction

Normal vision (emmetropia) exists when parallel light rays are sharply focused onto the retina without accommodation. In many cases, this can only be achieved by way of corrective lenses. If the focal point is shifted away from the incoming light, a convex lens (spherical plus lens) is necessary. If the focal point is shifted toward the incoming light, a concave corrective lens (spherical minus lens) is required.

Often, there is an additional corneal curvature (astigmatism) that must be offset with a cylindrical lens. A cylindrical lens breaks light most strongly perpendicular to its axis. In a plus-cylindrical lens, one surface is flat, the other convex; in a minus-cylindrical lens, one is flat and the other concave. When both radii of curvatures are perpendicular to each other, a regular astigmatism exists, which can be equalized with a cylindrical lens. If the axes are not perpendicular to each other, then the focal point cannot be optimally corrected with glasses. Most common is regular astigmatism, which is curved steeper in the vertical (tangential) meridian than in the horizontal (sagittal) meridian — so-called with-the-rule astigmatism. In the reverse case, one speaks of an astigmatism against-the-rule. Because the total astigmatism of the eye is the combined astigmatism of the lens and the cornea, a determination of the corneal curvature with an ophthalmometer may not be adequate.

Above all, it is important to deactivate accommodation in order to perform an objective refraction examination in those younger than 20 years and in adult hyperopes. Paralysis of the ciliary body (cycloplegia) can be accomplished by instilling cycloplegic drops (tropicamide, cyclopentolate) in the eyes. The examination is then carried out with an autorefractor, which is quick, simple, and painless, or by skiascopy (shadow test), which is a task for a specialist. However, when performed by an experienced clinician, skiascopy has been found to provide a more accurate estimation of refractive error than refraction done with an autorefractor. In order to avoid influencing the test results, the pupil size must not be decreased by squinting, which increases depth perception. The distance between the corrective lens and corneal crown should always be 12 mm. One should be mindful of this when using phoroptor and trial lenses. Even though the aeromedically recommended limitations for spherical and cylindrical correction may be subject to criticism, there are good reasons for these limitations, not only regarding visual acuity but also regarding correction requirements. The stronger the correction, the poorer the uncorrected visual acuity in the event of lost glasses. As a security measure, substitute glasses should be immediately accessible in flight. Retinal detachment is more common in individuals with severe myopia, as the retina becomes thinner and overly stretched with increasing size of the eye, and the risk of angle closure glaucoma is higher in individuals with high-grade hyperopia. But these are not the salient reasons for the stipulated limitations. The real reason lies much more with the corrective lenses themselves. Increasing refractive power leads to optical aberrations in the periphery of the lenses, which are particularly troublesome when the pupils are dilated. High plus-lenses additionally lead to a reduction in peripheral vision. Corrective lenses are allowed in the cockpit provided they are suitable for distant, near, and intermediate vision, so that the pilot will not need to change glasses in flight. This creates an additional problem for early presbyopic individuals. Although they can read charts with the near vision portion of their glasses, see the instrument panel with the intermediate portion and outside of the cockpit with the distant vision portion, they can only read the relatively close overhead panel by extreme extension of the neck in order to look through the lower segment of their glasses.

Placing relevant flight information onto the instrument panel at an intermediate distance would alleviate much of this problem. An alternative to bifocal or trifocal lenses are the so-called progressive lenses or Varilux lenses, where the distant vision area transitions smoothly into the near vision area. Some pilots find it difficult to get used to progressive lenses and may need a familiarization period of one to two weeks on the ground before they can comfortably and safely use such lenses in the cockpit.

Visual Field Examination (Perimetry)

The visual field is the area that can be perceived by the non-moving, forward-looking eye. It encompasses all the points in space that can be seen simultaneously while the eye is fixating on a point. The visual field examination is performed one eye at a time. The subject fixates on a central point inside a hemisphere under defined adaptation conditions and certain peripheral illumination.

Kinetic visual field testing is performed by moving light sources from the periphery into the hemisphere. Light sources of equal size and intensity provide a concentric circle of equal perception (isopter). When the subject perceives the light source, he activates an acoustic signal, and the location of the perception is recorded by the examiner. As the test markers become smaller and less intense, the distance of the isopters from the center become smaller.

Static perimetry is often preferred, as it can be done automatically and independent of an examiner; this, however, can in certain cases be a disadvantage. In static perimetry, the intensity of a non-moving light source increases until it is perceived. The position of the presented light source occurs randomly. The testing grid becomes coarser toward the periphery. During the test, light sources appear in the area of the anatomic blind spot in order to verify fixation. Relative or absolute visual field defects always require additional diagnostic evaluation. The outer limit of a normal visual field for high stimuli lies approximately 90° temporally, 60° nasally, 50° above, and 80° below. Scotomas that lie far outside the usable visual field or scotomas in the nasal area, which is covered by the other eye, are not necessarily disqualifying, but must not be of a progressive nature.

Color Vision

Disorders of color perception can be inherited or acquired. Most common are disorders of red-green vision, which occurs primarily in males, as it is inherited as a recessive x-chromosome. Green weakness (deuteranomoly) is the most common, followed by red weakness (protanomaly), followed by green blindness (deuteranopia) and red blindness (protanopia). Disorders of blue-yellow vision are very rare. There is no area where aeromedical ophthalmologists are in more disagreement than in the selection of appropriate color vision examinations and the standardization of regulatory limitations. Certainly, the evolution of multicolor displays increases the need for reliable color vision ability.

Pseudoisochromic color plates

In Germany, the Ishihara and Velhagen tests (Fig. 20) are prevalent. The instructions accompanying these tests are to be followed closely, particularly regarding illumination (daylight or artificial daylight) as

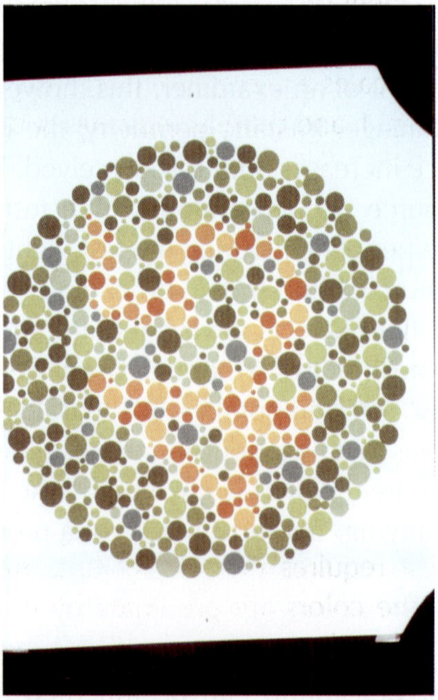

Figure 20. Pseudoisochromatic plate.

this can profoundly affect the outcome. Presentation time of each plate is also stipulated and should not exceed three seconds. The order of the plates should be random and unknown to the examinee. If all plates are correctly identified without hesitation, a normal trichromatic vision can be assumed.

Anomaloscope

A quantitative assessment of color perception is possible by using Nagel's anomaloscope or other similar devices. The test method is based on Raleigh's color matching equation: red + green = yellow. The test ocular consists of two halves; a lower yellow half which can change in intensity, and a red–green upper half which the patient adjusts by turning a knob, thus mixing red and green until the color of the upper half corresponds to the yellow color of the lower half. The anomaly quotient can be determined by the amount of adjustment used. A normal trichromatic person sets a medium setting and has an anomaly quotient of 1.0, but values between 0.7 and 1.4 are generally considered within normal limits. An anomaly quotient between 0 and 1 indicates a defect in the red range, while an anomaly quotient between 1 and infinity indicates a defect in the green range.

Simulator test

Currently, there is no suitable test, so this option is not yet available. The author is currently working on the development of a simulator test, in which perception of colors used in aviation can be tested.

Signal light test

The signal light test requires the subject to correctly identify red, green, and white. The colors are presented by way of lightbulbs or light signals in an irregular and previously unknown series, which must be recognized without hesitation. Test results are unreliable and the method cannot be recommended.

Lantern test

Just as the anomaloscope is not widely used outside Gemany, so is the lantern test not common in Germany. For the purpose of testing for medical certification, the Holmes Wright and the Beyne's lanterns play a particularly important role, but other lanterns are in use around the world. Basically, they are all acceptable for aeromedical color vision testing as they are used under controllable clinical conditions and provide reliable and reproducible results. Further information can be obtained from their operation manuals.

Evaluation of Binocular Function

Stereopsis

Stereopsis means spatial depth perception. Useful tests are the Titmus test or the random-dot test. These tests rely in part on the polarization process, whereby each eye looks at a slightly displaced image. Through sensorial fusion, an impression of spatial perception occurs. To what extent and to what degree intact stereopsis is necessary for safe flight has not been established and the issue is not entirely without controversy. Stereopsis is only possible up to a distance of about 30 meters. In the flight standards of ICAO and JAA there are no requirements for stereopsis for any class of medical certification.

Heterophoria

Phoria is the relative directions assumed by the eyes during binocular fixation of a given object in the absence of an adequate fusion stimulus. Heterophoria (latent strabismus) is a reaction to an interruption of the sensory-motor feedback control system. The need to compensate for heterophoria by sensory-motor fusion can cause asthenopic complaints, such as headaches. Fatigue can lead to decompensation and double vision. If visual perception is uncoupled between the right and left eye, each eye will take a resting position. If the relative directions assumed by the eyes are parallel to each other, orthophoria is present. Commonly, there is a deviation toward the midline (esophoria) or laterally (exophoria), or less commonly vertically (hyper- or hypophoria). The quantitative testing of phorias is best accomplished at five meters with a Maddox rod and rotating prisms, and close up with the Maddox wing.

Eye position and motility

It is easy to test eye position by illumination with a flashlight and determine the corneal reflex. Testing of eye motility is performed in both horizontal axes (abduction and adduction) as well as the oblique axes (upward in abduction and adduction, downward in abduction and adduction). Evaluation of eye motility disorders requires considerable experience and the AME should not hesitate to refer doubtful cases to an ophthalmologist.

Convergence

Convergence is the simultaneous inward movement of the eyes toward each other, necessary to maintain single binocular vision when an object is viewed at close distance. The near-point of convergence is generally determined by asking the examinee to focus on an object (e.g., the top of a pencil), which is then slowly moved closer and closer to the eye until one eye diverges. In the healthy subject, this point is less than 10 cm.

REFERENCES

1. Stern C, Schwartz R, Groenhoff S, Draeger J, Uettig G, Bernhard H. (1998) Clarity of flight information in the cockpit of the new aircraft generation. *Ophthalmologe* **91**(4): 548–550.
2. Draeger J, Schwartz R, Stern C, Wurster J. (1994) Evaluation of current guidelines for flying capacity and internationally proposed revisions. *Ophthalmologe* **91**(4): 543–547.
3. Draeger J, Schwartz R, Kohlhaas M, Boehm A, Lombardi M, Goerne M. (1993) Pressure-induced change in corneal curvature in patients with

refractive surgery and unoperated probands. *Ophthalmologe* **90**(6): 711–715.

4. Draeger J. (1999) Glaukom. Entstehung Diagnostik, Therapie und Prophylaxe. Deutsche. *Aphakiezeitung*: 1–8.
5. Draeger J, Jessin K, Rumberger E. (1993) *Tonometrie*. Thieme.
6. Draeger J, Schwartz R, Deutsch, Groenhoff S. (1991) Clinical and experimental results with a fully automatic self-tonometer. *Fortschritte der Ophthalmologie* **88**(3): 304–307.
7. Draeger J, Wirth H, Schwartz R. (1986) "TPMEX," monitoring of intraocular pressure under micro G conditions. *Naturwissenschaften* **73**(7): 450–452.
8. Draeger J, Schwartz R, Groenhoff S, Stern C. (1995) Self-tonometry under microgravity conditions. *Aviat Space Env Med* **66**(6): 568–570.
9. Draeger J, Schwartz R, Groenhoff S, Stern C. Self-tonometry during the German 1993 Spacelab D2 mission. *Ophthalmologe* **91**(5): 697–699.
10. Schwartz R, Draeger J, Groenhoff S, Flade KD. (1993) Results of self-tonometry during the first German-Russian MIR mission 1992. *Ophthalmologe* **90**(6): 640–642.
11. Draeger J, Schwartz R, Wiezorrek R. (1996) Ophthalmological experiments and results in Space Flight — MIR 1992 — Mission and Spacelab D2-Mission 1993. *An Inst Barraquer (BARC)* **25**: 767–770.
12. Draeger J, Michelson G, Rumberger E. (2000) Continuous Assessment of intraocular Pressure — Telematic Transmission, even under Flight — or Space Mission Conditions. *Eur J Med Res* **5**: 2–4.
14. Draeger J, Rumberger E. (2000) Automatische ophthalmolodynamometrie — ein neuer weg zur direkten messung des aktuellen perfusionsdrucks. *Search on Glaucoma* **8**(1): 3–7.

Chapter 18

Ear, Nose and Throat (ENT) Medicine and Dentistry for Aeromedical Examiners[a]

Jürgen Kressin[‡] and Reinhard G. Matschke[*,†]

INTRODUCTION

Although practically all relevant sensory modes are grouped together or at least closely associated within the specialty of otorhinolaryngology, ENT medicine is accorded comparatively little attention in aviation medicine. Yet it is precisely this discipline that has the most specific involvement with the standards for medical fitness, and we intend therefore to deal with it accordingly in the following.

By prevention and therapy, dentistry contributes to aviation medicine with a reduction in the risk of aerodontalgia, which may occur during flight, caused by pressure changes in the aircraft cabin.

THE EAR

The ear is the unit of organs and body parts that facilitate hearing and balance. The auditory system is divided into the outer ear, the middle

[a] An outline of ear, nose and throat diseases and dysfunctions, including their anatomical and physiological bases, of relevance for the assessment of medical fitness.

* Corresponding author.
[†] Lister Krankenhaus, Lister Kirchweg 43, D-30163 Hanover, Germany.
[‡] Dortplatz 9, D-12526 Berlin-Bohnsdorf, Germany.

ear, and the inner ear. The outer ear consists of the auricle, the external auditory canal, and the external surface of the eardrum. The middle ear is situated in the pars petrosa of the temporal bone and is surrounded by air-filled cavities lined with mucosa, the mastoid cells, which are ventilated via the tympanic tube (tuba Eustachii) from the nasopharynx. The most important auditory structure of the middle ear is the ossicular chain, comprising hammer, anvil, and stirrup. These transmit sound from the eardrum to the inner ear. This is likewise located in the petrosal pyramid and consists of a system of cavities filled with lymph fluid in a particularly dense bone capsule. In its anatomy and evolution, the inner ear is one unit, which, however, contains organs with two different functions, namely organs for hearing and balance[1] (Fig. 1).

External Ear

The external ear includes the auricle, the external ear canal, and the outer surface of the eardrum. The soft skin of the auricle (auricula) is

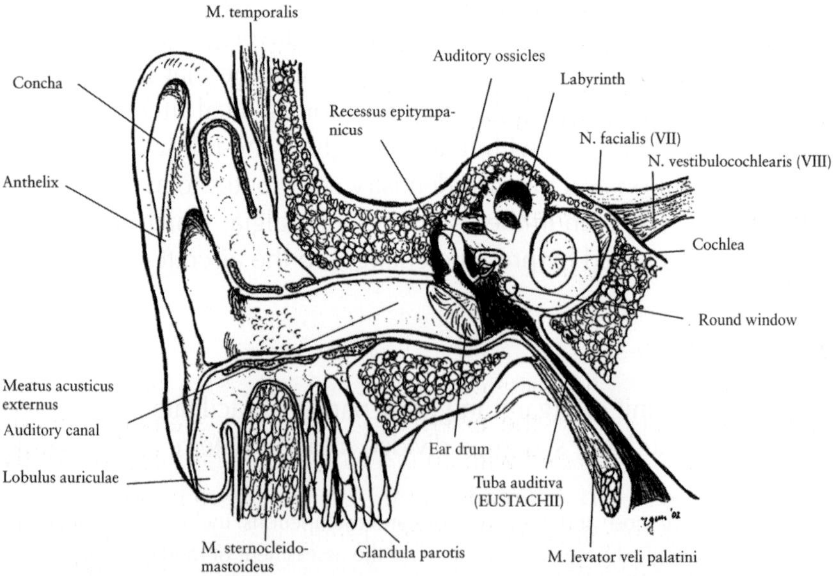

Figure 1. Diagram of the external ear, the middle ear (in color), and the inner ear (hearing and balance organ); drawing by author.

supported by elastic cartilage; the only part without cartilage is the earlobe (lobulus), which consists only of fatty tissue. Every normal auricle has certain folds, divided into the helix, the antihelix, the cavum conchae, the porus acusticus externus, and the tragus. There is a great range of variation between individual forms. The cartilage structure of the auricle is linked to several small muscles, which are very rudimentary in humans and are no longer relevant for their original task of changing the position of the auricle to improve directional hearing.

The external ear canal is approximately 3.5 cm long and contains several bends. It is lined with epidermis, extends to the eardrum; the outer third consists of cartilage and the inner two-thirds consist of bone. Here, the skin lies directly on the wall of the bony canal, which is formed from the pars tympanica, the pars petrosa, and the pars squamosa of the temporal bone. The front wall of the osseous ear canal helps form the temporomandibular joint, while the posterior wall and the roof border on the air-filled cavities of the middle ear, in particular, the mastoid.

Hairs are present only in the external part of the ear canal. They become sparser towards the bony part and are completely absent in the interior. Ceruminous glands produce cerumen, emerging next to the hair follicles in the external ear canal.

Disease of the external ear

Diseases of the external ear include deformations, consequences of trauma, infectious and non-infectious processes, and tumors. Since unobstructed sound conduction to the middle ear is necessary for normal hearing, all dysfunctions can be relevant for the AME. Infectious processes in the external ear can be extremely painful. Complications associated with an initially superficial infection (otitis externa) occur when it spreads to the cartilage (perichondritis) or to the bone (osteomyelitis) in the surrounding area. Foreign bodies in the ear canal normally result in diminished hearing and numbness. They should be removed by flushing with water at body temperature but only if the eardrum (anamnesis) is intact. Otherwise, foreign bodies are removed with instruments, best under a microscope. In the event of a lesion of the ear canal, pain, bleeding, and purulent secretion may occur.

Post-traumatic or surgical loss of the auricle, if not resulting in loss of hearing, does not in general reduce medical fitness; neither does reconstructive surgery or bone-anchored epithesis.

The Middle Ear and the Barofunction

The middle ear consists of the eardrum (membrana tympani) and the tympanic cavity (cavum tympani). The eardrum is a three-layered membrane separating the ear canal from the middle ear. It is approximately 0.3 mm thick and has an area of about 0.55 cm^2. The pars tensa is a thin epidermal layer of skin from the ear canal covering a mesodermal, elastic layer of connective tissue which allows the eardrum to oscillate. The connective tissue layer is missing only in the area of the pars flaccida, which is located to the upper rear, where the eardrum is double-layered. The surface of the eardrum facing the tympanum is covered by mucosa.

The tympanic cavity is the largest and most important cavity in the middle ear. To the front it borders on the canal of the internal carotid artery, and to the rear on the processus mastoideus, below on the bulbus of the jugular vein, and its medial wall is next to the labyrinth. Above the roof of the tympanic cavity is the medial cranial fossa. The tympanic cavity provides air to the mastoid. It contains the ossicular chain, consisting of the hammer (malleus), anvil (incus), and stirrup (stapes), the middle ear muscles (m. stapedius and m. tensor tympani) and the chorda tympani, the fibers of which are integrated into the facial nerve (n. facialis). The canal of the facial nerve passes the stirrup and forms with the promontorium the oval niche. The oval window contains the stapes footplate, while the round window by means of a membrane separates off the scala tympani of the inner ear. The oval and round windows are movable in the direction of the inner ear. A functionally important connection from the tympanic cavity to the nasopharynx at the back of the nose is the tuba auditiva Eustachii, a cartilagenous tube that ensures the supply of air to the middle ear cavities and is controlled by m. tensor and m. levator veli palatini. The mucosa in the tympanic cavity is supplied with sensory nerve fibers from the plexus tympanicus and, to a lesser degree, from the sympathetic plexus of the internal carotid artery. M. stapedius is supplied by the facial nerve, and m. tensor tympani by the trigeminal nerve. The lymph canals in the middle ear are connected with those in the external ear and the eardrum.

In line with the requirements set forth in the Medical Provisions of Annex 1 to the International Convention on Civil Aviation and detailed in various medical standards[2–4] for examinations of medical fitness for Class 1 and 2, we intend to set out the main dysfunctions of aeromedical relevance.

According to Boyle-Mariotte's Law, the volume of a gas behaves at constant temperature proportionately to its pressure. The most frequent pressure-related dysfunction of the ears and sinuses occurs during descent due to the increased air pressure in the cabin. This happens both in private aeroplanes and in simple business planes without pressurized cabins and in larger passenger aircraft. In airliners at normal cruising altitudes of 33 000 to 41 000 ft above sea-level, a cabin altitude of maximum 8000 ft is ensured and the cabin pressure adjusted to the cruising altitude by means of a pressure-regulating air conditioning system. During normal flight conditions, computerized regulators ensure a rate of climb, tolerable for ears and sinuses, of 500 ft/min and a rate of descent of 300 ft/min (Fig. 2).

Particular circumstances may, however, demand a rapid descent and thus cause a rapid rise in ambient pressure, and the ear will then have to equalize the air pressures on either side of the drumhead very quickly. Regular aeration of the middle ear by trouble-free ventilation of the Eustachian tube is a prerequisite for safe flying. Tube ventilation is partly an active, partly a secondary process. In its normal condition, the tube is closed by virtue of the tension of the elastic tube cartilage and the surface tension of the membrane from the tube ostium in the epipharynx to the middle ear cavity. By means of

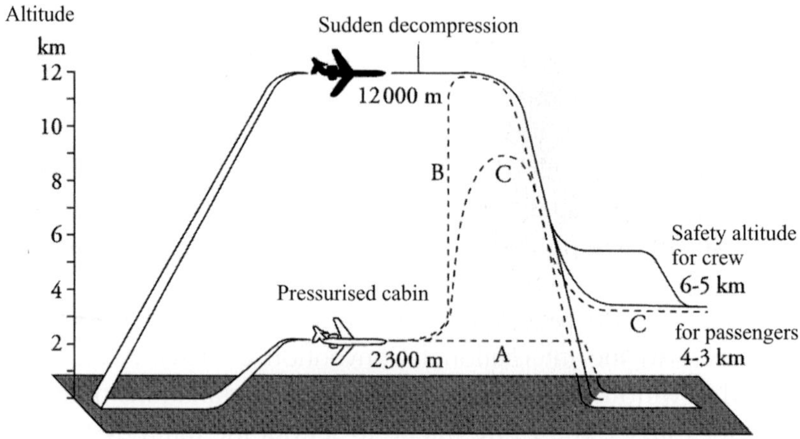

Figure 2. Diagram of flight profile at altitude (cruising) and emergency descent with rapid decompression of the pressurized fuselage to ensure capability of the crew to work and act and avoids health risks to passengers. If the automatically lowered oxygen masks are used properly, risks are reduced. The emergency descent maneuver varies from aircraft type to aircraft type. The interior altitude of the cabin (------) to a maximum of 3000 m (A) in cruising flight ensures a lower pressure difference in the event of rapid decompression to 1200 m, in the event of a large hole of the size of a door (B), or lower altitude in the event of a smaller hole (e.g. a burst window (C)).

techniques such as swallowing, yawning, jaw movements, speaking or singing, the tube is opened by synergetic contraction of the mm. tensor et levator veli palatini[5] (Fig. 3).

Spontaneous opening of the tube, even without any auxiliary action such as yawning or similar, has been observed regularly during decompression chamber tests with simulated rate of descent of 15 m/s (2700 ft/m). Opening of the tube, which takes about 0.2 seconds, occurs regularly throughout the day provided the tube mucosa, the middle ear cavities, and the tube ostium in the nasopharynx are normal and not pathologically swollen as during a common cold. During ascent, a passive equalization of pressure in the middle ear to the nasopharynx takes place when a pressure difference of 1.5–1.8 kPa is reached. The pressure difference can also be equalized by swallowing or pinching the nose. During descent with increased ambient

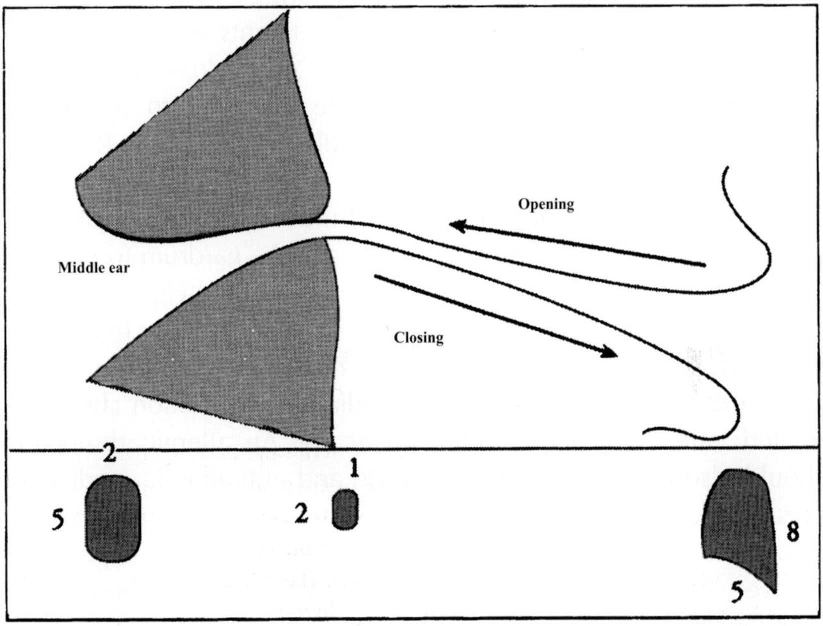

Figure 3. Opening and closing process of the 3.5 cm long Eustachian tube during pressure equalization of the middle ear. Normal widths of the tube lumina in millimeters.

air pressure in the cabin, tube opening is facilitated by speaking, yawning, or by Valsalva manoeuvre, but this is possible only up to a pressure difference of 0.8–1.2 kPa; beyond this level, it is no longer possible to force open the tube and barotrauma of the middle ear occurs. This is known as aerootitis or aviator's ear.[6]

Aerootitis

In the event of acute symptoms occurring after landing, painkillers and decongesting nose drops are indicated. Individuals who frequently experience mild aerootitis when traveling by air may be helped by a special kind of ear plugs known as ear planes which have proved to be useful in ensuring long and continuous equalization of the rapid change of pressure in the cabin during take-off and landing. They can be used also by those cabin attendants who are prone to barofunctional disturbances. In the case of eardrum secretion or haemotympanum, myringotomy may be indicated to relieve the symptoms and prevent subsequent middle ear problems. Recurring aerootitis should be treated by an ENT specialist. Treatment modalities include corticoid preparations and mucolytics and, if tube dysfunction persists, insertion of small tubes in the eardrum to equalize the pressure and facilitate the drainage of secretion (Figs. 4A and B). The tubes must be left in place until trouble-free function of the Eustachian tube is restored. If aerootitis recurs, the cause may be one of various forms of chronic otitis media. This condition should be treated with medication and/or surgically. An allergic rhinopathy should also be considered as a cause and anti-allergic medication prescribed. Although tube closure is found less frequently than obstructed breathing through the nose. Return to flying depends on recovery of hearing (audiogram) and proof of normal tube function (tympanogram). The AME should always inspect the ear canals and the eardrum, if necessary after cleaning of the ear canal. Changes in the eardrum (scarring or perforation) and eardrum movement (test of the patency of the tube) can only be clearly seen when a pneumatic otoscope is used.

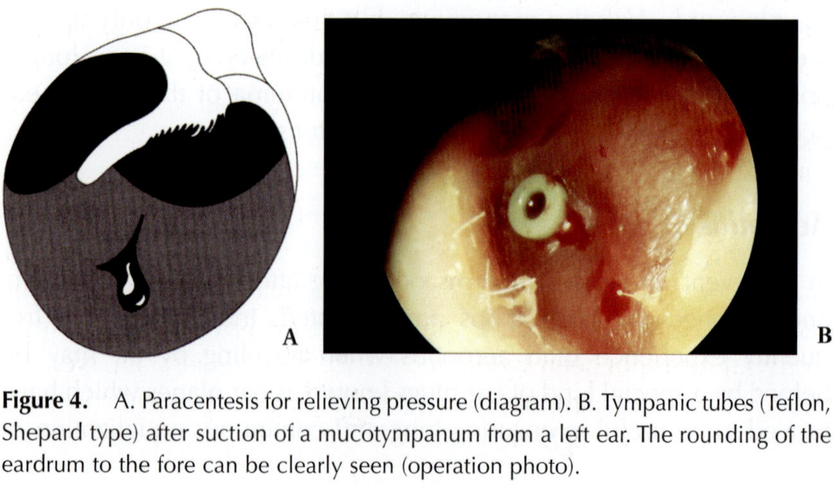

Figure 4. A. Paracentesis for relieving pressure (diagram). B. Tympanic tubes (Teflon, Shepard type) after suction of a mucotympanum from a left ear. The rounding of the eardrum to the fore can be clearly seen (operation photo).

Diseases of the middle ear, reconstructive surgery

Depending upon course and degree of seriousness, three different middle ear pathologies are distinguished: tube and middle ear catarrh, acute otitis media, and chronic otitis media. Each of these pathologies occurs in different forms, which vary diagnostically and with regard to treatment, possible complications, and long-term effects on hearing.

The mucosa in the tuba auditiva and middle ear is affected to a greater or lesser degree by any inflammation in the nose and nasopharynx. This results in swelling of the mucosa with increased secretion. Acute middle ear catarrh leads to reddening of the eardrum and hearing loss due to secrete collecting in the tympanum. If the secrete does not drain into the nasopharynx within a few hours, the secondary mucosal reaction results in additional swelling which causes the secrete to remain in the tympanic cavity (otitis media serosa acuta). Chronic middle ear catarrh (otitis media serosa chronica), characterized by mucotympanum, is the result of a particular disposition of the mucosa (allergy), recurring middle ear infections, insufficient medication or anatomical obstructions (tumors, scars, or adenoids). The main symptom is conductive hearing loss, combined with a feeling of numbness in the affected ear. Treatment consists of myringotomy and the incision may have to be held open with an aeration tube (tympanic tube) for several weeks depending on the viscosity of the secretion. If a middle ear catarrh is left untreated, there is a risk of irreparable changes in the middle ear with sclerosis of the ossicular chain (tympanosclerosis) and permanent hearing loss. Long-lasting under-pressure in the middle ear then results in an adhesion process or tearing of the eardrum and a permanent perforation. A cholesteatoma can also develop from an adhesion process.[1]

A tympanic tube correctly fitted removes pressure equalization problems and restores normal hearing straightaway but is not compatible with safe flying. The tube should be removed after three months if it has not been spontaneously rejected before then. Normal tube function and eardrum should be demonstrated by tympanometry before return to flight duty.

Acute middle ear infection (otitis media acuta) is caused by bacterial infection supervening a middle ear catarrh; primary symptoms are serious earache and fever. At the height of the infection, myringotomy is indicated. If not undertaken, a spontaneous eardrum perforation often occurs, which brings significant relief to the patient. The eardrum perforation normally closes spontaneously as the infection clears up, within two to three weeks. During this period, hearing becomes normal again. Infectious diseases, particularly virus infections, may follow an atypical course.

Chronic middle ear infection (otitis media chronica) is generally not caused by insufficient treatment of the acute form of the disease, but rather by recurring infections in patients with reduced mucosal resistance of the upper respiratory system and the middle ear, either constitutional or acquired in childhood. The chronic infection has essentially two forms, either a relatively harmless chronic suppuration from a large eardrum defect in the area of the pars tensa (mesotympanal otitis media chronica), or a more dangerous bone suppuration with a defect in the area of the pars flaccida (epitympanal otitis media chronica).[7]

Hearing is in most cases restricted, but the extent of the eardrum defect bears no relation to the loss of hearing. Scarring of the middle ear structures and damage or interruption of the ossicular chain may result in conductive hearing loss of 30 to 50 dB, while inner ear performance may remain unaffected. Over time, however, recurring infections and toxic influence also lead to diminution of the inner ear function.

When bone suppuration with epitympanal defect occurs, the epithelium in the ear canal grows into the middle ear and forms a gathering of epidermal scales, which are unable to flow out of the close confines of the middle ear. The chronic infection and the build-up of detached skin scales provide a good breeding ground for a cholesteatoma. Depending on the state of the infection and the extent of the cholesteatoma, the neighboring middle ear structures are destroyed. If a cholesteatoma grows, all otogenic complications such as mastoiditis, labyrinthitis, facialis paresis, sinus thrombosis, meningitis, epidural abscess, and brain abscess may occur. If untreated, a cholosteatoma can, in spite of slow growth, cause death via one of the complications mentioned above. This distinguishes it fundamentally from chronic mesotympanal otitis media. A cholesteatoma must always be surgically treated.

The aim of the operation is complete removal of the cholesteatoma without damage to functionally important structures to the extent they have not already been destroyed by the cholesteatoma. In the same session, if possible, tympanic reconstruction is carried out with closure of the eardrum perforation and reconstruction of the ossicular chain (to improve hearing). Improved hearing should, however, be regarded as being of secondary importance to complete sanitation. Large and recurring cholesteatomas are treated with a radical operation, which leaves behind a radical cavity that needs constant care. Smaller cholesteatomas may be operated on endaurally, retaining the posterior wall of the ear canal. To prevent recurrence, it has proved useful to carry out a follow-up operation to check that all is well. Even after a successful middle ear operation with a reconstruction of the sound conduction chain with bone, cartilage, ceramic, plastic, or precious metal implants, more or less heavy sound conduction dysfunction is to be expected from scarring. Aeration of the middle ear cavities via the Eustachian tube is an indispensable prerequisite for the long-term success of surgical sanitation of the middle ear.[7]

Medical certification after reconstructive and prophylactic ear surgery may be considered in consultation with an ENT specialist.

Inner Ear (Vestibulo-Cochlear System)

The hearing organ (cochlea) and balance organ (vestibular system) together form the "inner ear" in the petrosal pyramid. The sensory apparatuses are located in the membraneous labyrinth, which is filled with endolymph. The membraneous labyrinth is located in the bony labyrinth where it is surrounded by perilymph. The skin-lined labyrinth includes the three semicircular canals, the vestibulum, and the cochlea.

The cochlea contains the sensory cells of the hearing organ. The cochlear canal in the adult has two-and-a-half bends and a total length of 32 mm. It winds about a cylindrical axis and is subdivided into three chambers: the scala vestibuli and the scala tympani, which are filled with perilymph and are connected at the tip of the cochlea via the helicotrema, and the scala media (ductus cochlearis), which is filled with endolymph. The ductus cochlearis is separated from the scala vestibuli by Reissner's membrane (the vestibular membrane) and from the scala tympani by the basilar membrane, on which Corti's organ, the actual hearing organ, is located. It reaches from the basal bend to the apex and consists of sensory cells (hair cells) and supporting cells. The approximately 17 000 sensory cells of Corti's organ are distributed into one row of inner hair cells and three rows of outer hair cells. 95% of the nerve fibers of the n. cochlearis are connected with the inner hair cells, and only 5% of the fibers are connected with the outer hair cells. In the inner ear canal is the VIIIth cranial nerve (n. vestibulocochlearis), which contains the nerve fibers from the sensory organs of both the hearing and the balance systems (Fig. 5).

The central auditory pathway includes the afferent hearing system with its peripheral part, pars cochlearis of n. vestibulocochlearis, and a central part, which contains the central auditory pathway as well as sub-cortical and cortical hearing centers. The section of the auditory nerve above the cochlea is also described as retrocochlear, which is why hearing dysfunctions originating there are also so designated. The ascending nerve fibers run to the nucleus cochlearis dorsalis and the descending ones to the nucleus cochlearis ventralis. From the dorsal core, the fibers cross over to the contralateral olivary nucleus. Other interfaces for the central auditory pathway are the lemniscus lateralis, the colliculus inferior, the corpus geniculatum mediale, and the primary hearing cortex[8] (Fig. 6).

Hearing is tested at several different levels. In the whisper test, understanding of conversational speech and whispered speech is tested.[9]

It should be noted that this test is purely for screening, as it is not standardized and the results are not reproducible. Nevertheless,

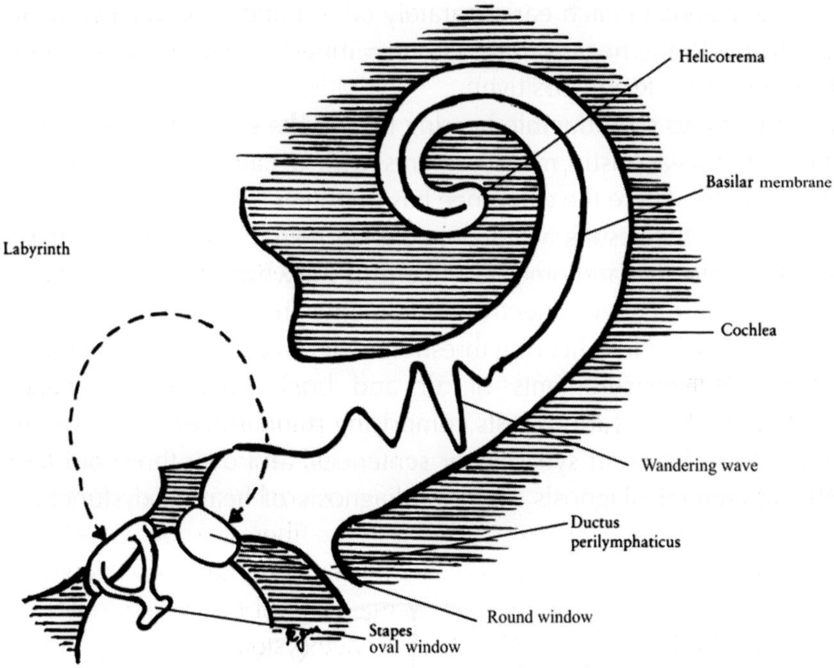

Figure 5. Diagram of the pressure transfer between the oval and round windows with creation of a wandering wave on the basilar membrane (modified after Plath[9]).

whisper tests are widely used for renewal examinations for the medical certificate. Schöder, in his paper presented at the Medicine and Mobility Conference in Berlin in September 2000, has convincingly shown the difficulties of testing hearing without an audiometric test,[10] as the degree of noise-induced hearing impairment that restricts speech comprehension is significantly less than the degree of hearing loss accepted for medical certification (Fig. 7).

Tuning fork tests provide valuable diagnostic information. In Weber's test, the sound from the tuning fork placed on the center of the cranium is lateralized to the affected ear in the case of conductive hearing loss and to the better ear in the case of inner ear (sensorineural) hearing loss. In Rinne's test, air and bone conduction are compared in each ear separately (air < bone = conductive hearing loss = Rinne negative; air > bone = inner ear hearing loss or normal hearing = Rinne positive).

Exact and reproducible hearing test results can only be obtained from electro-acoustic measurements with a calibrated audiometer. Audiometry where the examinee has to state what he or she can hear and where the results are dependent on his or her cooperation are called subjective audiometry, while tests for which no cooperation is necessary are called objective audiometry. The subjective test methods are divided into hearing threshold determination (sound audiometry) with measurements of air and bone conduction, speech audiometry with various tests comprising standardized words of one syllable and several syllables or sentences, and over-threshold tests for differential diagnosis and topodiagnosis of hearing dysfunction.

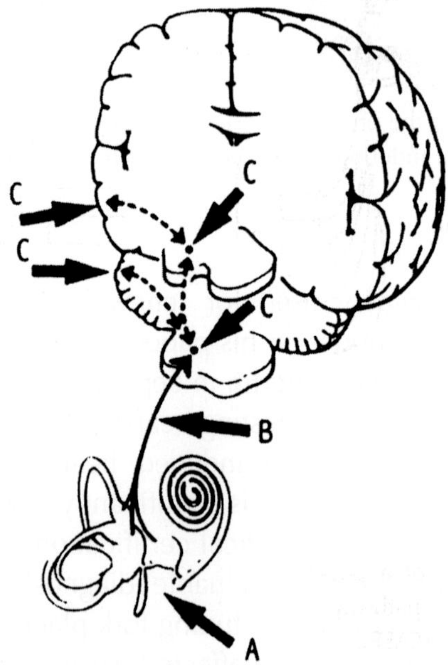

Figure 6a. Possible localizations of damage that can result in peripheral (vestibular) (A) intermediary (along the course of the VIIIth cranial nerve) (B), and central vertigo (C).

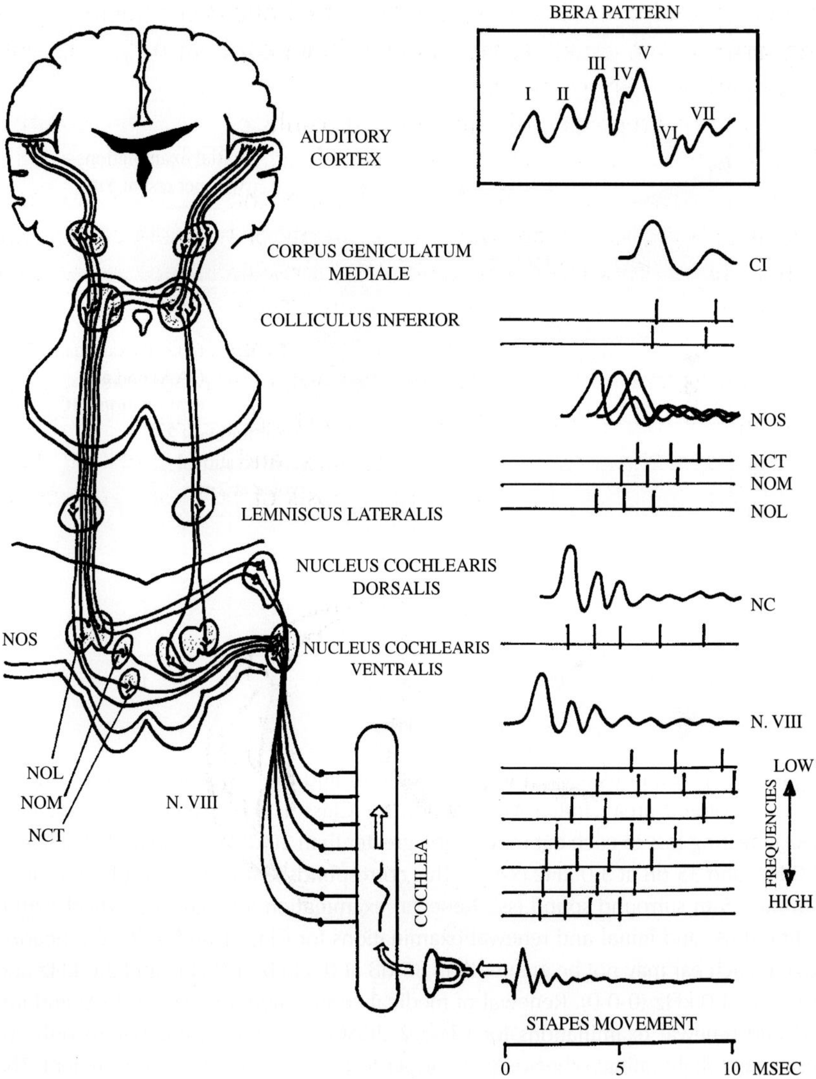

Figure 6b. Diagram of a possible overlaying of action potentials from various regions of the auditory pathway to the characteristic potential pattern of early auditory evoked potentials (EAEP).

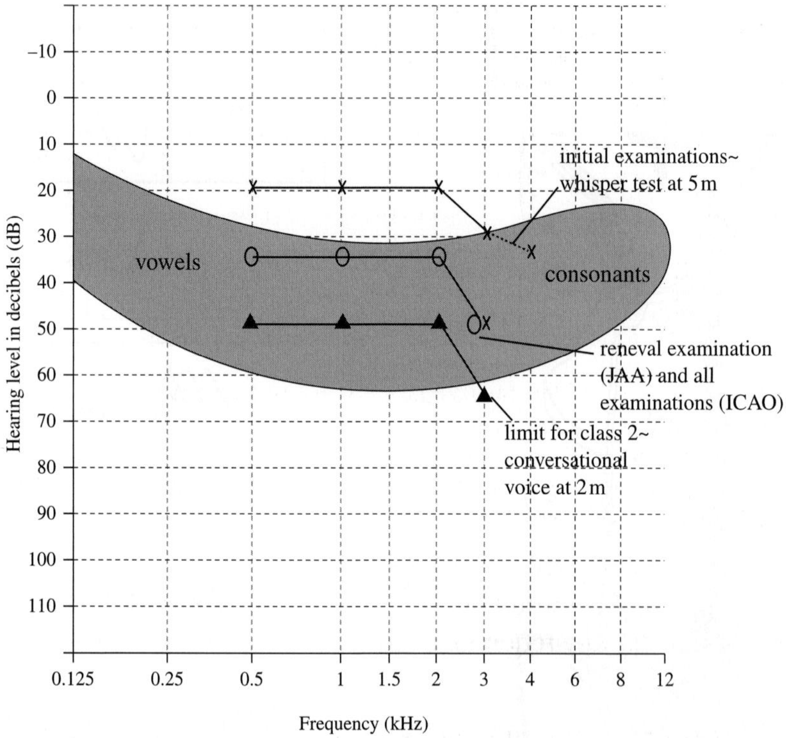

Figure 7. JAA and ICAO hearing requirements and the frequency range of human speech (colored area). Initial examination for Class 1 and 2 medical certification (JAA): hearing loss in each ear may not be greater than 20 dB at 0.5 kHz, 1.0 kHz and 2.0 Hz, and 35 dB at 3.0 kHz (x-x-x). This corresponds to a whisper test from around 5 m and 5 m surround sound (ss). Renewal examination for Class 1 medical certification (JAA) and initial and renewal examinations for Class 1 and 3 (ICAO): hearing loss in each ear may not be greater than 35 dB at 0.5 kHz, 1.0 kHz and 2.0 kHz and 50 dB at 3.0 kHz (0-0-0). Renewal of medical certification for Class 2 (JAA) and initial and renewal examinations for Class 2 (ICAO) requires an audiogram only for instrument flight rating; otherwise, a whisper test at 2 m is considered sufficient. The minimum hearing in both ears for Class 2 is conversational voice at 2 m (▲-▲-▲). Except in the latter case, the other ear must be masked during testing.

The results are noted in internationally standardized forms and are reproducible. The most important objective hearing test methods are the measurement of otoacoustic emissions (OAE) and tympanometry with stapedius reflex measurement and the derivation of auditory

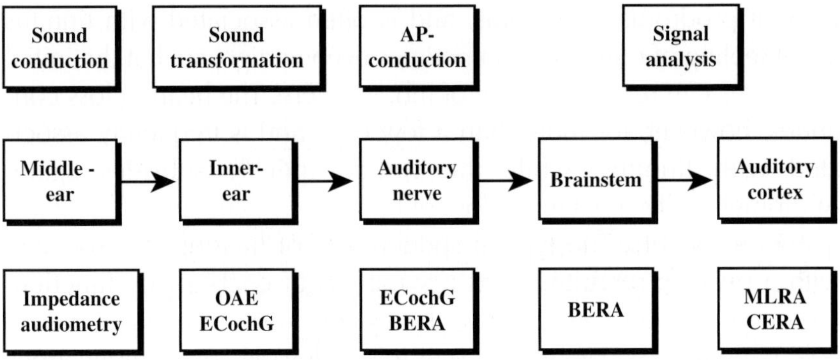

Figure 8. Summary of the "audiological test battery" for differential diagnostic examination of the auditory system from the middle ear to the auditory cortex (OAE = otoacoustic emissions; BERA = brainstem evoked response audiometry; EcochG = electrocochleography; MLR = middle latency response; CERA = cortical evoked response audiometry.

evoked potentials. These have today largely superseded the simulation tests, previously required[9] (Fig. 8).

Sudden hearing loss, mb. menière, acoustic trauma, tinnitus

Cochlear inner ear infections are always accompanied by a degree of hearing loss. The etiological factors resulting in the symptoms are, however, not always the same. The long-held view that sudden hearing loss, mb. Menière and Menière-like symptoms with and without noise in the ears (tinnitus) are consequences of circulatory disorders in the inner ear can no longer be upheld. While circulatory disorders can play a part in the etiology of these complex pathologies, they are, however, not obligatory but rather co-factors. The pathogenic and etiological problems of this pathological complex, which is not clear even today, can only be dealt with in a cursory manner here. Since these pathologies are always accompanied by sensorineural hearing loss and frequently by vertigo, they are of essential significance for fitness to fly. Sudden hearing loss is a pathology that has developed into a therapeutic problem in the recent past due to its frequency.[11] Deterioration of hearing in one ear occurs quite suddenly, mostly without prodromal symptoms, and is often associated with tinnitus and a feeling of numbness, sometimes even vertigo, so that the initial symptoms can resemble those of mb. Menière. The hearing loss continues, however, for more than a few days and is frequently associated with tinnitus, while the vertigo quickly subsides again. Audiometrically speaking, a loss of hearing, which can affect all frequencies, occurs. The typical sudden loss of hearing is associated with a positive recruitment as a symptom of cochlear dysfunction. For every sudden hearing loss, the existence of an acoustic neurinoma, an apoplectic insult, multiple sclerosis, or complications triggered by cerebral processes must be eliminated by careful audiometric and vestibular differential diagnosis. Immediate treatment of hypotensive regulatory disorders and psycho-vegetative dysregulation usually results in rapid remission. Spontaneous remissions are common during the first few days but therapy may still be indicated.

Morbus Menière is a paroxysmal disease of the inner ear, always accompanied by the triad of rotational vertigo attacks, hearing impairment, and tinnitus. Etiologically, it is a hydrops of the membraneous labyrinth. The vertigo attacks last from a few minutes to several hours and recur within days or weeks and may be accompanied by nausea and even vomiting. During the attack, for a short time, an irritation nystagmus can be observed on the affected side, while a loss nystagmus can be observed later on the healthy side.[11] Hearing impairment is mostly associated with a diplacusis (double disharmonic hearing), where the sound is perceived as higher in the affected ear. The tinnitus, accompanied by a feeling of pressure and bloatedness in the affected ear, is a particular nuisance. Therapeutic measures during the attack are symptomatic, and no causal therapy is known. To begin with, hearing loss is reduced during the attack-free interval, but later it becomes deeper from attack to attack and the affected ear may become completely deaf. In the vestibularis test, normal functions are likewise found during the initial intervals, but later, and after repeated attacks, under-excitability occurs on the affected side. If the frequency of attacks cannot be controlled, destructive surgery may be used, the usefulness of which, however, is disputed. In any case, in the event of recurring attacks, the subject is not fit to drive or fly. The acoustic trauma is also part of the complex of inner ear affections, but unlike sudden hearing loss, it is triggered by an identifiable factor. Bangs, explosions, noise, dull cranial traumas, and sudden changes of pressure can result in degeneration of the hair cells in the organ of Corti. Mostly, permanent hearing loss results, which is associated with a tinnitus of the same frequency as the damaged hair cells. But tinnitus has many causes. Since the characteristics of tinnitus involve subjective auditive perception without a corresponding sound event, it can occur as an accompaniment to all kinds of hearing impairment. The current view is that tinnitus is generated by a disorder of the spontaneous activities in the auditory passage with the effect of creating the apparent existence of a sound that does not, in fact, exist. By definition, tinnitus cannot be objectified; it is an individual perception without correlation to anything outside the body. It is, however, possible for the patient to classify it; this may be done in order to assess the extent to which the patient is subjectively affected. Tinnitus is not a disease but a symptom, which can occur as a warning signal for several organic and psychological disorders.

Otosclerosis and implantable hearing aids

Otosclerosis occupies a special place between the diseases of the middle ear and those of the inner ear. It is a disease of the bony labyrinth, the cause of which is unknown; it results in bone transformation from spongy to sclerotic bone. Changes in the composition of the perilymph and endolymph cause degeneration of the sensory cells and inner ear loss of hearing. Otosclerosis most frequently begins in the area of the oval window niche, causing ankylosis of the stirrup, and thus resulting in progredient conductive hearing loss. Affected persons occasionally complain of tinnitus whereas vertigo occurs only in exceptional cases. Small deformations in the middle ear, post-traumatic chain interruptions, scarring residues following middle ear infections and tympanosclerosis should be eliminated by differential diagnosis. A tympanoscopy is necessary for final diagnosis.

Otosclerosis is treated surgically with a stapes prosthesis and/or stapedectomy, in which the immobilized stirrup is removed and replaced with a prosthesis that is attached to the long arm of the anvil and transmits sound vibrations through the perforated footplate to the inner ear (vestibulum). Regardless of the technique and the prosthetic material used, hearing is restored in 90% of cases by this operation. If left untreated, otosclerosis progresses and can result in almost complete deafness (Fig. 9).

The patient will be unfit for flying for at least three months after an operation involving a temporary opening of the inner ear. Provided the vestibular function is normal, medical certification may be considered in consultation with an ENT specialist.

Implants are being used less and less in reconstructive middle ear surgery, more and more giving way for complete hearing prostheses. Technologies and methods in this area vary from osseo-integrated

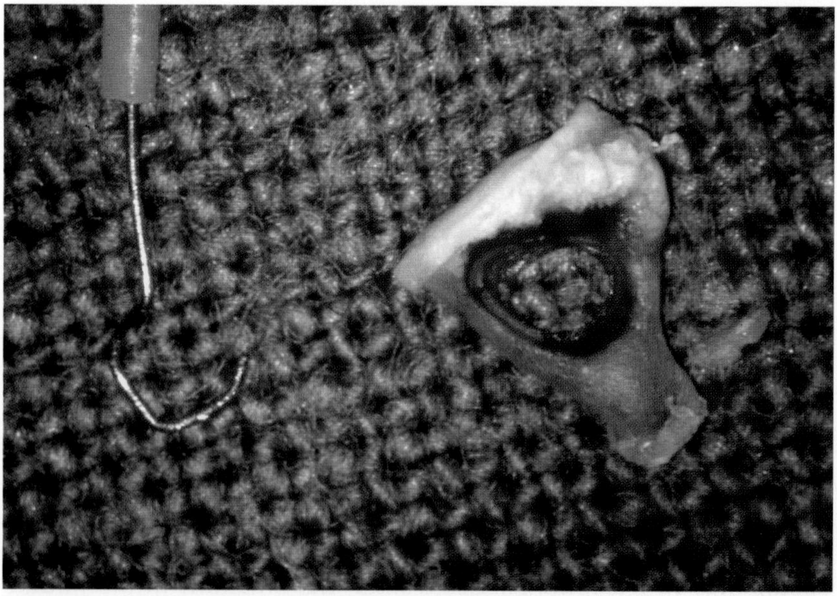

Figure 9. Surgically removed stapes with advanced otosclerosis of the footplate and stapes replacement prosthesis made of platinum wire with a teflon piston.

titanium anchors (BAHA™) to implanted electronic inner ear prostheses (Cochlear Implants). Indication for implantation of a hearing system vary from problems with wearing a hearing aid due to skin infections with chronic inflammation and suppuration, ear canal stenosis, cranial and mandibular fractures, allergies and deformations, to acoustic and cosmetic problems. A distinction is drawn between vibratory amplifier implants, partially implantable ossicle-coupled implants, fully implantable ossicle-coupled implants, and endocochlear implants.

Not all implantable hearing systems assume the destruction of middle ear and inner ear structures. Passengers can be assumed fit to fly with authorized systems after successful implantation, provided structures have healed without irritation. There is still insufficient experience to permit any assessment of pilots and flight crews.

Hearing protection

The inner ear is damaged in typical ways by sound of high intensity. Noise-induced hearing loss always occurs if there is exposure to an unphysiologically high sound stress over a period of years. To begin with, there is a temporary threshold shift (TTS), which can be reversed after a sufficient recovery phase, but on further exposure and a lack of rest phases, there is high frequency hearing loss with a typical dip at 4000 Hz, which represents a permanent threshold shift (PTS). Noise protection measures are prescribed by law for all workers exposed to damaging noise in the workplace. This does not, however, apply to people in the private sphere, where noise-induced damage caused by recreational noise is increasingly common. In particular, listening to loud music through headphones, in discotheques and at concerts but also being exposed to noise from artillery, firearms, fireworks, and engine noise of all kinds result over time in excess strain on the organ of Corti. It is not possible to distinguish between chronic noise damage acquired in the workplace and that acquired elsewhere. There is no treatment for noise-induced hearing loss, so prophylaxis is of utmost importance. Both avoidance of unnecessary noise and personal ear protection such as ear plugs, protective ear muffs, and ear protection helmets are necessary.

Problems emerge, however, if spoken communication is absolutely necessary and is obstructed because of ear protection.[12] Earlier studies of speech intelligibility in flight noise have failed to take into consideration the fact that coherent speech structures can, according to the listener's level of knowledge and experience, be perceived, even if heavily masked by disruptive noise. A realistic assessment of speech intelligibility in the cockpit can only be made by using simple non-aviation sentences and test words such as two-digit numbers, phonetically balanced words (PBW) and spondee words, and by recording sound reception in the pilot's ear canal (MIRE = measure in real ear) (Fig. 10).

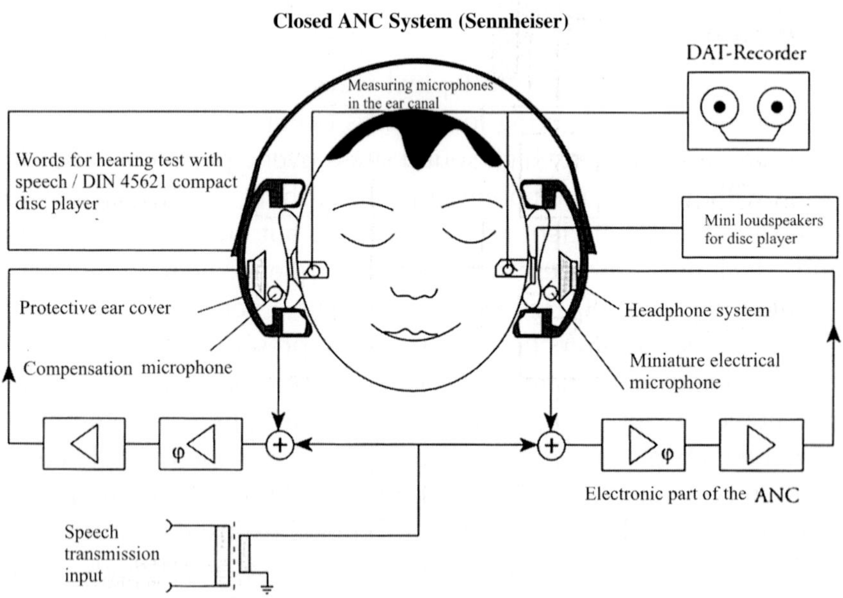

Figure 10. Measuring system for speech audiometry with the pilot in the cockpit during flight with active noise compensation.

It is possible to reduce noise intensity and at the same time improve speech intelligibility with active compensatory systems (ANC = active noise compensation) based on the principle of "anti-noise." It is anticipated that more electronic communication aids will be developed in the future to avoid undesired disruptive noise[13,14] (Fig. 11).

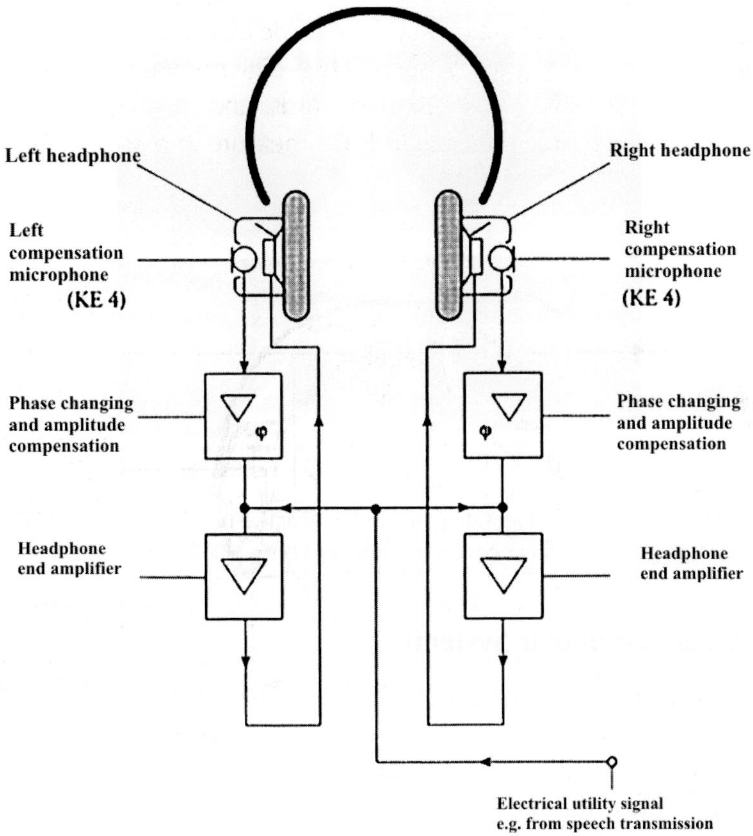

Figure 11a. Block circuit diagram of active noise compensation in conjunction with an open headphone.

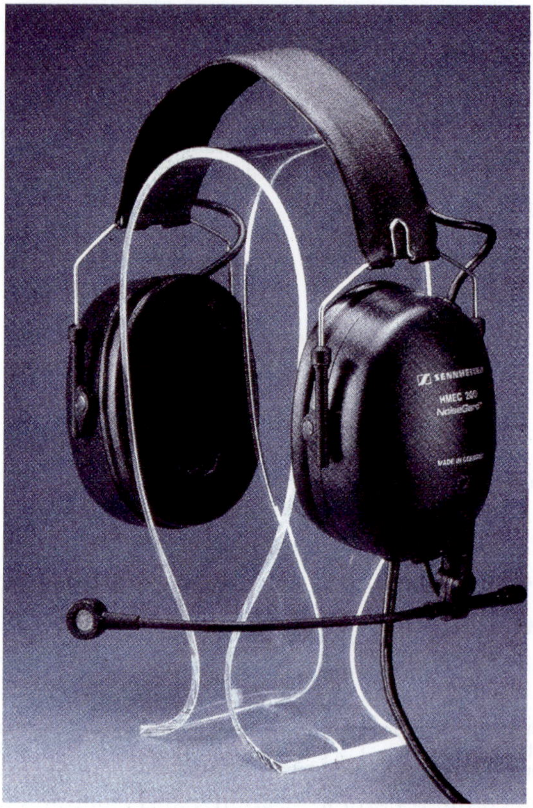

Figure 11b. Actively compensating headset with active noise compensation in passively damping protective ear covers (Sennheiser HMEC 2000).

Inner Ear (Vestibular System)

Pursuant to the medical provisions for licensing, pilots and other applicants for a career in aviation are obliged to give details of previous or current illnesses or health disorders. In addition to the medical history, the AME must eliminate balance function disorders by examining the subject. Assessment of medical fitness requires a thorough examination by an otorhinolaryngologist as part of the initial examination for Class 1 medical certification. These otorhinolaryngological examinations must be repeated at five-year intervals until the age of 40 and every two years thereafter. Otorhinolarygological specialist examinations are not required for Class 2 medical certificates. At renewal examinations, the same dysfunctions and illnesses must be eliminated as for the initial examination, therefore the AME must eliminate with a high degree of probability dysfunctions of the balance system when carrying out renewal examinations for Class 1 and Class 2 medical certification.

During flight, eyesight and the vestibular system provide the main sensory information for balance. Acceleration, hypoxia, and reduced barometric pressure, as typical in-flight stress factors, influence the pilot's ability to maintain body balance.[15]

The balance organ, arranged in pairs and located in the pyramids of the petrosal bones, consists of a membraneous, liquid-filled canal system with three semi-circular canals and two sac-like extensions (saccule and utricle). The three semi-circular canals (ductus semicirculares) are positioned at right angles to each other, beginning at the vestibular aqueduct (vestibulum) with an extended part, the ampule, in which the sensory cells are located. In the vestibular aqueduct, there are also two sensory cell centers, the utricle and saccule, each with a small sac of about 3 mm in length for the sensory cells (macula), which are embedded in a colloidal mass and contain on the surface crystalline particles (otoliths and calcium carbonate particles) that react to horizontal and vertical stimuli of linear acceleration. The utricle and the saccule are placed at 90° to each other. When the head is inclined, the effect of gravity on the otolith membrane is changed and triggers a feeling of inclination, comparable with the feeling caused by forward acceleration of an airplane with the head held straight.

The sensory cells in the semi-circular canals transmit the changes from head-turning movements by means of the movement of liquid, which results in distortions of the cupula. The otolith organs have for some time now been accorded much more significance for the vestibular system than the semi-circular canals[16] (Fig. 12).

Balance stimuli are conducted via the vestibular part of the VIIIth cranial nerve and processed with the acoustic part of the nerve

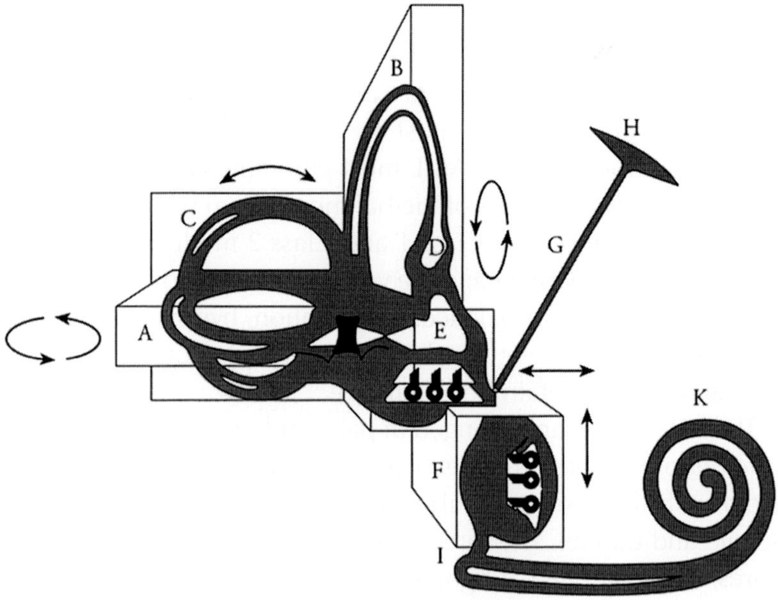

Figure 12. Diagram of acceleration forces acting on the vestibular apparatus. A: lateral semi-circular canal; B: upper semi-circular canal; C: posterior semi-circular canal; D: cupula; E: utricle; F: saccule; G: ductus endolymphaticus; H: sacculus endolymphaticus; J: ductus reuniens; K: cochlea.

(important for directional hearing) and via the various switching points and control circuits with the optic system. The proprioceptive system, the "measuring sensors" in the skin, muscles, and joints, also helps maintain the sense of balance of the body. Finally, the intellectual performance (such as reading and believing flight display information) plays an important role for spatial orientation (Figs. 13 and 14).

The particular importance of this combined function of the three most important systems for balance is shown in Fig. 15. Many different dysfunctions of the sense of balance can be derived from this. The forces and axis equivalents affecting the entire person on take-off and landing are shown in Fig. 16.

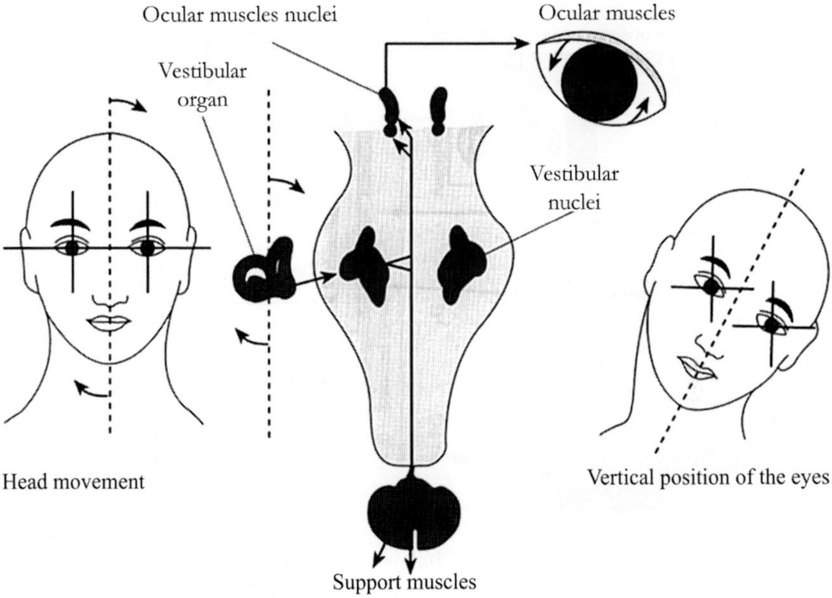

Figure 13. Vestibular effect on visual motor performance (after Ref. 26).

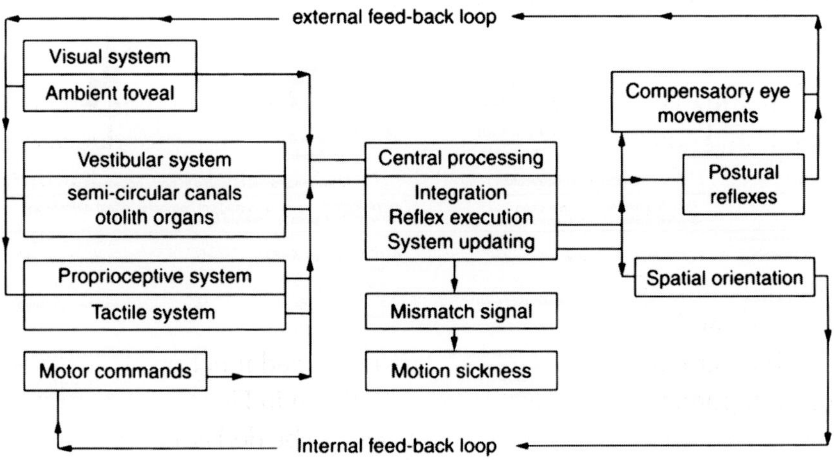

Figure 14. Diagram of the control circuits of the optic and balance systems.

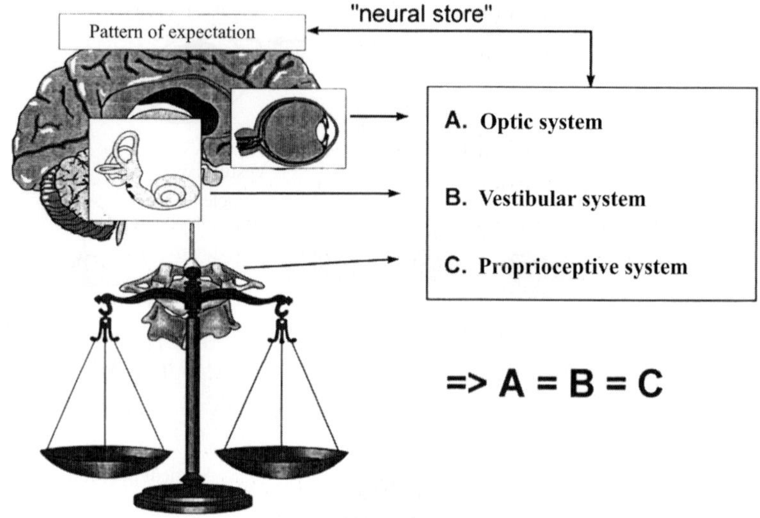

Figure 15. Illustration of the complex balance state (after Ref. 21). Balance is established when information from A, B, and C is identical. Kinetosis can result from mismatch of single bits of information.

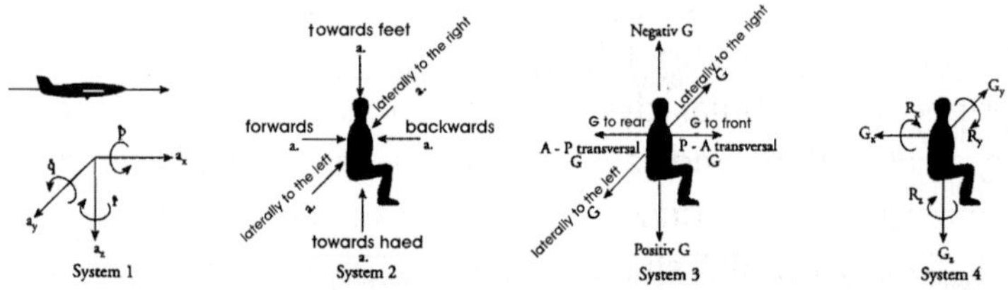

Direction of acceleration			resulting forces of inertia in body acceleration		
	Aircraft, Computer Standard (System 1)	Acceleration description (System 2)	physiological description (System 3)	physiological computer Standard (System 4)	effect description
linear movement					
forwards	$+a_x$	acceleration forwards	(1, 2) transverse A - PG leaning back chest to back G	$+G_x$	eyeball looking inwards
backwards	$-a_x$	acceleration backwards	transverse P - AG leaning forward back to chest G	$-G_x$	eyeball looking outwards
upwards	$-a_z$	acceleration in head direction	positive G	$+G_z$	eyeball looking down
downwards	$+a_x$	acceleration in foot direction	negative G	$-G_z$	eyeball looking upwards
to the right	$+a_y$	sideways acceleration to the right	left lateral G	$+G_y$	eyeball looking to the left
to the left	$-a_y$	sideways acceleration to the left	right lateral G	$-G_y$	eyeball looking to the right
angular movement					
roll to the right	$+p$		roll	$-R_x$	
roll to the left	$-p$		porpoise	$+R_x$	
porpoise up	$+q$		yaw	$-R_y$	
porpoise down	$-q$			$+R_y$	
yaw to the right	$+r$			$+R_z$	
yaw to the left	$-r$			$-R_z$	

Figure 16. Body accelerations, axis equivalents modified during take-off, flight and landing (after Ref. 31).

Dysfunctions of the opto-vestibular-proprioceptive system, vertigo, kinetosis, whiplash injury, positional vertigo, canalolithiasis

The medical history of the examinee is especially important for cranial and brain traumas, metabolic dysfunctions, reduced blood supply (hypotension, badly adjusted hypertension, reduced perfusion of the a. labyrinthi and the inner ear capillaries), brain tumors, arachnoidal cysts, middle ear dysfunctions, disorders of the baro-function of the Eustachian tube and inner ear function (morbus Menière, chronic tinnitus, sensorineural hearing loss different on either side, acute unilateral vestibular dysfunction), and any kind of "vertigo."

Vertigo is the second most frequent symptom encountered in general practice. Possible causes are numerous, so it is important to trace a past history of vertigo. If it is assumed that around 10% of patients complaining of vertigo offer an unusable, uninterpretable anamnesis, and 50% of vertigo symptoms are caused by psychogenic factors, then a great number of symptoms with neurological, internal medical, and otological causes remain, which can be identified by means of thorough history taking.[17]

Peripheral vestibular dysfunctions include rotational vertigo, a feeling of elevation, and lateropulsion. Central vestibular disorders include unsteady legs, dizziness, general uncertainty when walking, "feeling slightly drunk," stupefaction or gaps in consciousness.

Non-vestibular vertigo has many symptoms, including an empty feeling in the head, blackouts, seeing stars, unsteady vision, sudden stupefaction, an empty feeling in the stomach, nausea, salivation, breathlessness, weakness in the legs, quick or irregular pulse rate, stabbing pains in the heart, collapse or loss of consciousness, blurred vision or diplopia.

Two diagnoses should be given special attention, since they occur more frequently than is usually supposed. These are "centrifugal trauma" (whiplash injury)[18] and "benign positional vertigo."[19] In Germany, a figure of around 400 000 compensation claim cases per year has been given for whiplash injury (i.e. damage to the cervical vertebrae caused by an accident). The figure for annual accidents with centrifugal traumas with "slight" head acceleration of under 4 G to 15 G can be assumed to be far greater, since there is a great degree of equalization in the region of the cervical vertebrae. Late consequences with positional vertigo or spontaneous nystagmus must also be allowed for. The connection between deforming velocity, head acceleration, and degree of severity of the whiplash injury is shown in the following table:

Velocity	<5 km/h	8–30 km/h	30–80 km/h	>80 km/h
Car damage	slight	slight-moderate	moderate-severe	severe
Head acceleration	<4 G	4–15 G	16–40 G	>40 G
Severity of whiplash injury	nil	slight-moderate	severe	fatal

Different relative acceleration rates between head and body in car collisions can result in severe damage to the cervical vertebrae and cranio-vertebral joints, even at velocities of less than 10 km/h. The most frequent injury is in the C1/C2 region, followed by the second most frequent injury in the C4/C5 region.

Benign positional paroxysmal vertigo (BPPV) is one of the most frequent forms of vertigo. Rotational vertigo attacks of very short duration are always caused by head movements. Otoliths or otolith parts are loosened from the mucopolysaccharid membrane via the macula organ in the saccule/utricle and repositioned in the posterior vertical semi-circular canal, rarely in the lateral horizontal semi-circular canal. They float free in the semi-circular canals, thus irritating the cupula and causing benign positional paroxysmal vertigo.[19]

The otolith fragments are washed back again by means of deliberate or unconscious counter-positioning maneuvers (freeing maneuvers). This is why BPPV is now also known as "canalolithiasis." Canalolithiasis can be cured in 70% of cases by a single "freeing manoeuvre," and in nearly 30% of cases by the use of several "freeing maneuvers."[20] Otoneurological evaluation is crucial in order for any decision about medical fitness to be made.

Kinetosis, also known as motion sickness, can happen to any person with an intact balance apparatus.[21] For trainee pilots, it is usually of significance in the training period, and over 50% of pilots ditched and rescued at sea become "seasick."

It is, however, rare for pilots to give up their careers because of recurring kinetosis. This occurs much more frequently among cabin staff, and "air-sickness" in passengers is an important aspect of air travel.

Common for all illusions associated with vertigo are a linear or angular acceleration. Particular intensive is the Coriolis cross-coupling illusion, which can occur in all kinds of flying, especially in aerobatics or in crash situations. Also turbulence can result in balance disturbance, caused by a mismatch of optical, vestibular and proprioceptive information. The safe conduct of the flight may thus be endangered.

For evaluation of a pilot's fitness, a small set of examination instruments is useful to rule out dysfunctions in the opto-vestibular-spinal system and to examine the balance function.[22]

A few brief ENT examination procedures should be part of all routine aeromedical examinations. If anything noticeable is found, an otorhinolarygological explanation is necessary.

Every head movement triggers a contrary eye movement to stabilize the field of vision. A fast reflex return movement of the eyes then takes place. This vestibular-ocular reflex, determined by the position of the head and the position of the eyes, ensures a sharp optical image by adaptation of the velocity of the reflex eye movement to the head movement. Nystagmus is coordinated eye movements in certain directions with rhythmic fast and slow phases. Vestibular nystagmus is eye movements triggered by vestibular stimuli or diseases of the balance system or by head movements. Nystagmus is an important indication of vestibular dysfunction.

It is only possible to evaluate nystagmus behind Frenzel glasses,[23] which eliminate the examinee's ability to fixate (Fig. 17). The occurrence of spontaneous nystagmus, provocation nystagmus, and positional nystagmus should be examined.

Spontaneous nystagmus is always pathological. Provocation nystagmus is tested by shaking the examinee's head with Frenzel glasses on. The examiner takes the head of the seated subject in both hands and moves it 10 times quickly to and fro, horizontally at an angle of around 120°. In this way a latent nystagmus can be detected and a provocation/stimulus nystagmus accentuated.

A positional nystagmus (reproducible rotational vertigo) is tested with Frenzel glasses using the positioning maneuver according to Hallpike.[24] It is a provocation test for positional nystagmus through change in position (benign positional paroxysmal vertigo) (Fig. 18).

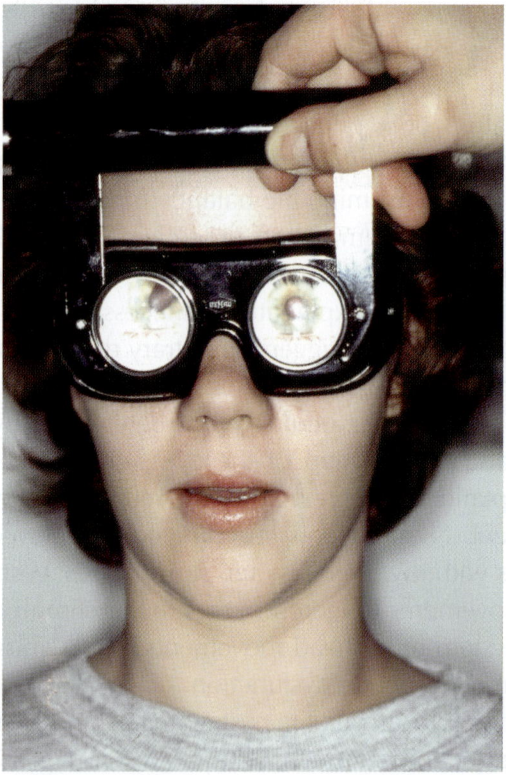

Figure 17a. Examination of spontaneous nystagmus allows detailed evaluation in the slow direction of the beat: Looking to the right, straight ahead, to the left, up, and down behind Frenzel's glasses. The magnification effect of the magnifying lenses largely prevents fixation, while the internal illumination makes the pupils contract and prevents optical input from the surroundings.

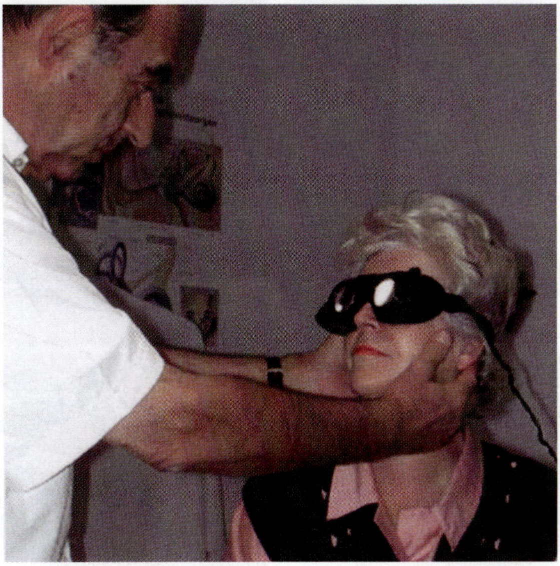

Figure 17b. Testing provocation nystagmus in seated person after several rapid left-right turning movements of the head.

Static and dynamic balance should be assessed by testing the vestibule-spinal reaction. Following an extensive aeromedical examination, two balance tests are sufficient[25,26]:

The "intensified" Romberg test: the examinee places the feet firmly, one in front of the other, crosses the arms loosely across the chest, stands for at least 15 seconds with the eyes closed; equilibration is allowed. Walking blind: blindfolded or with eyes closed and with arms loosely crossed over the chest, the examinee walks straight ahead, placing the feet heel to toe. After ten steps, the deviation should not be more than a foot's width from the straight line that has been drawn or imagined. Larger deviations must be clarified by further examination.

As mentioned before, all dysfunctions of the balance system, which occur spontaneously or are found by provocation, should be further examined and treated by an otoneurologist.

The prognosis is always individual and depends upon the cause, treatment and subsequent re-training of the balance function. This is

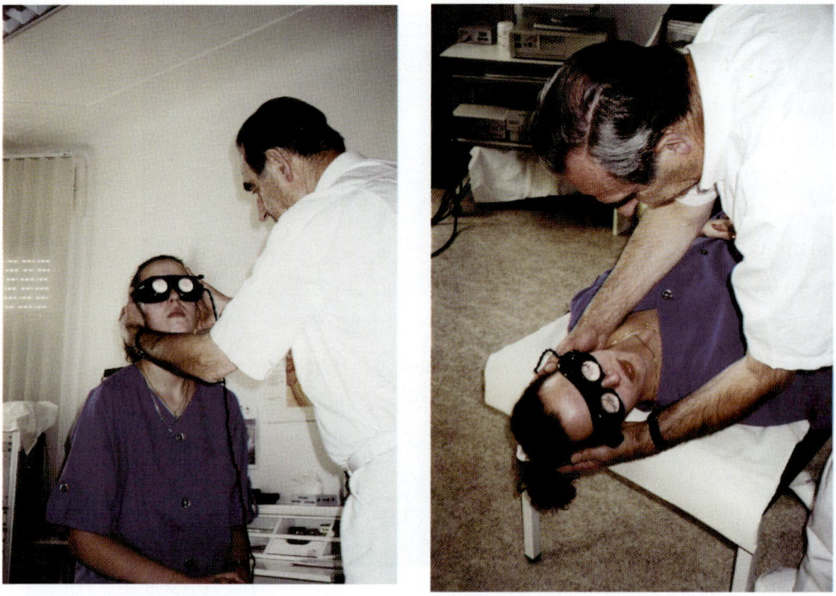

Figure 18. Hallpike's positional maneuver: test of nystagmus while examinee is sitting, then lying-down, and then sitting up again. Clockwise nystagmus shows affection of the left labyrinth, while anti-clockwise nystagmus shows affection of the right labyrinth. A rotating nystagmus can occur after sitting upright. The duration of the nystagmus is usually less than 30 seconds.

so in many cases following ear operations with short-term vestibular irritation, after acute unilateral vestibular dysfunction, and following a benign positional paroxysmal vertigo or after a slight whiplash injury.

SINUSES/BAROFUNCTION

The air-filled sinuses (frontal sinus, ethmoidal cells, maxillary sinuses, and sphenoidal sinus) have a 1 to 2% share in barotraumatic dysfunctions. If the nasal mucosa and the mucosal lining of the sinuses are in normal condition, there is open access between the nose and the sinuses and no difference in pressure will occur during climb and descent. Air exchange takes place by breathing through the nose with a slight difference in pressure of +/– 10–17 Pa; if breathing through the nose is heavier, if the nose is blown, or if a Valsalva manoeuvre is carried out, a value of 1.3 kPa can be reached.

If the mucosa in the nose, the ostia or the sinuses are swollen, or if there is blockage due to secretion or polyps, the air in the affected sinus is largely resorbed or evacuated through the nose during ascent due to the relative over-pressure compared to the cabin pressure. During descent, severe pain can occur in the affected sinus in the upper jaw, retrobular, or in the temple, often combined with streaming eyes and, more rarely, epistaxis. It is not possible to equalize the pressure, apart from attempting to relieve it with decongestant nose drops or by direct puncture of the temple or maxillary sinus. Because of the often very severe pain experienced, with all consequences, including collapse, aerosinusitis is a serious risk to the pilot's capacity to act, and its cause must be clarified. Certain diseases are incompatible with medical certification if they cause or merely facilitate the occurrence of aerosinusitis (Fig. 19).

The AME should focus on any pressure problems in the ears and sinuses revealed by anamnesis. If breathing through the nose is obstructed (ascertained by attempting to blow through the left and right nostrils), if the patient has a cold with heavy swelling of the mucosa, or if there is chronic infection of the nasopharynx or allergic rhinitis of permanent or seasonal type, or if there are polyps in the nose or hyperplasia of the nasal conchae, these conditions should be clarified and treated by an otorhinolaryngologist or allergologist.[27] Aeration of the nasal cavities can be inspected by looking into the right and left main sinuses with a lit nasal speculum.

Aerosinusitis, Disorders in the Barofunction

Once aerosinusitis has occurred, the aim of any treatment must be to restore the aeration of the affected sinuses. Acute aerosinusitis is treated with decongestant nose drops, painkillers, and application of moist heat to the face. Allergic diseases are usually seasonal and

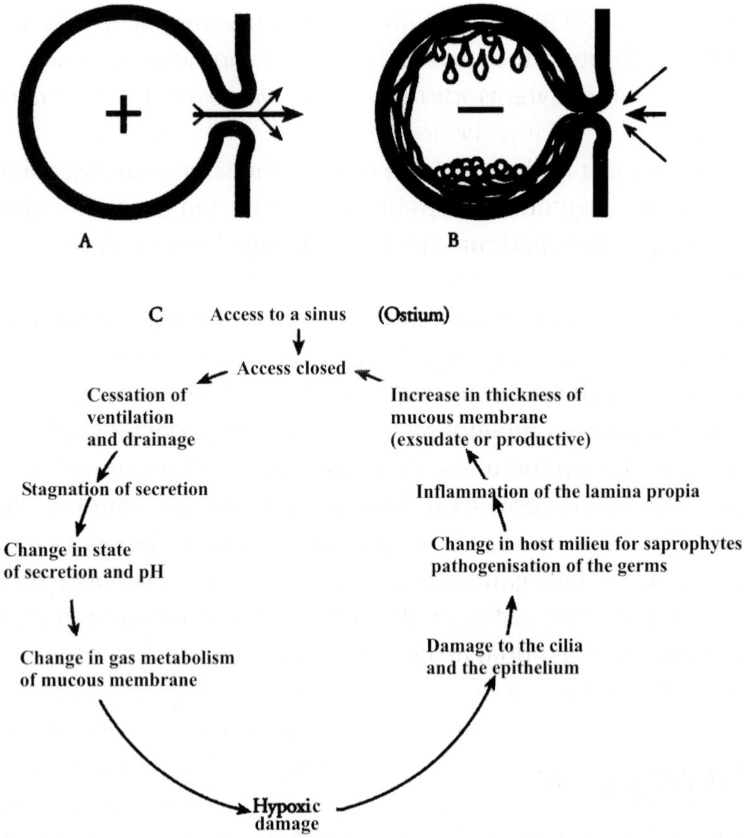

Figure 19. A. Pressure equalization between a sinus and the surrounding air (nose) during ascent. B. Diagram of barofunction disorder of the sinus caused by infectious swelling of mucous membranes. C. Cycle of formation of aero-sinusitus or aerootitis.

may restrict fitness for flying; to avoid unfitness for flying, the results of treatment by hyposensitization as a special immunity therapy over two to three years must be confirmed by an allergologist or other doctor working with allergies.

Where seasonal therapy with non-calming second generation antihistamines (e.g. loratadin) is used, the effect must be tested and proven in each single case while the pilot is on the ground.[27] Chronic obstruction to breathing through the nose and inflammations of the mucosa in the sinuses (purulent sinusitis or proliferative changes in the mucosa or naso-sinusoidal polyps) are the most common causes of aerosinusitis, mostly due to acute exacerbation. The aim must therefore be to achieve free breathing through the nose. The therapy comprises a septum operation if there is septum deviation, and cauterization of the nasal conchae if there is hyperplasia, when necessary combined with fenestration of the maxillary sinus.

Following surgery, unfitness for flying is likely to last for at least six weeks, depending on the healing process and how well free breathing through the nose has been restored as shown by rhinomanometry. Chronic polypous infections of the sinuses and tumors ought to be discovered at an early stage if the AME is careful when conducting aeromedical examinations. For chronic sinusitis, often polypous, a long healing phase with intensive aftercare is necessary. Medical certification is usually possible, even after endonasal sinus surgery, but requires a thorough otorhinolaryngological evaluation. Tumors require individual assessment by the medical assessor of the licensing authority.

SMELL AND TASTE

When we sniff, eddies of air with water-soluble olfactory substances in a gaseous or dusty form are inhaled through the nostrils. When we swallow or exhale via the nasopharynx, these substances reach the regio olfactoria. We smell in fact much of what we believe we are tasting. Only the five qualities, sweet, sour, salty, bitter, and umami (fresh flavor) are detected with the sense of taste. If the concentration of olfactory substances remains constant, the sense of smell adapts, and our sensitivity to smell diminishes quickly.

The olfactory epithelium is a multi-layered vacillating epithelium which contains Bowman's glands. The olfactory pathway begins with the olfactory cells in the regio olfactoria. Its neurites are gathered together into about 20 fila olfactoria and run through the lamina cribrosa of the base of the skull and form the primary olfactory center in the bulbus olfactorius. From there, the nerves run via the tractus olfactorius to the secondary and tertiary olfactory centers. Connections from the olfactory pathway to the vegetative and extrapyramidal system trigger reflexes such as the secretion of saliva and stomach juices in the case of appetite-stimulating smells, or nausea, vomiting and refusal movements in the case of foul smells. The organ is very sensitive and can sense more than 10 000 different qualities of smell and distinguish more than 200. It is also involved in the subjective sense of taste ('gustatory smell'); this olfactory perception is unconsciously processed together with the gustatory sensation to form an overall impression of taste.

Olfactory Dysfunctions

When examining the sense of smell, a distinction must be drawn between a subjective smell test and an objective olfactometry. The threshold for smell stimuli can be determined subjectively and semi-quantitatively by means of various olfactory stimulants (aromatic substances, coffee, lavender, terpentine, vanilla, cinnamon, and benzaldehyde) in increasing concentrations. This enables a distinction between a perception threshold and a recognition threshold; in additional testing with a trigeminal stimulant (acetic acid) and a hypoglossus stimulant (pyridine), distinctions can also be drawn for aggravations and simulations. However, more precise information is provided by objective olfactometry, in which olfactorily evoked potentials are measured. The laborious procedure permits a distinction between olfactory and trigeminal dysfunctions and a topodiagnosis of central dysfunction of the sense of smell.

Dysfunctions of the sense of smell are divided into quantitative dysfunctions (hyposmia or anosmia) and qualitative dysfunctions (parosmia or cacosmia). They can occur peripherally through the blocking of the olfactory cleft when the mucosa is swollen or by polyps or tumors (respiratory anosmia), or be caused by injury to the specific sensory epithelium from viral or neurotoxic factors or the effects of biting smoke, solvents, and medications (essential anosmia). Dysfunctions of varying severity of the sense of smell can be expected from neurosurgical operations to the base of the nose or following accidents with traumatic tearing of the fila olfactoria in fractures of the base of the skull (post-traumatic anosmia) and injuries to the bulbus olfactorius and the olfactory pathway in space-occupying intracranial processes. Anosmia is incompatible with fitness for flying because of inability to detect smoke or leaking solvents in flight.

Dysfunctions of the Sense of Taste

Taste or taste components can be tested with sugar, citric acid, common salt, and quinine solutions in various concentrations. Sweetness is primarily perceived at the tip of the tongue, sourness at the edge of the tongue, and saltiness and bitterness at the base of the tongue. Taste perceptions can also be triggered by electrical stimuli (electrogustometry).

A dysfunction of the sense of taste (dysgeusia, ageusia) can be triggered by peripheral or central lesions. Damage to the taste buds can be caused by smoking, heavy alcohol use, acid or alkali burns, stomatitis, or atrophy of the mucosa. It occurs with dryness of the mouth (xerostomy) as a consequence of radiogenic mucositis after treatment of a tumor with radiation. Scarring in the posterior part of the oropharynx after tumor operations or enucleation of the tonsils can result in dysfunctions of the sense of taste in the posterior third of the tongue. Injury to the chorda tympani after middle ear operations also causes a unilateral peripheral dysgeusia.

STOMATOGNATHIC SYSTEM, BAROFUNCTION DISORDER/AERODONTALGIA

In some medical standards,[2–4] it is emphasized that dysfunctions or pathological conditions of the buccal cavity, teeth, and larynx are incompatible with medical certification.

The AME should, when examining the buccal cavity, pay attention to the condition of the teeth, the parodontium (tooth retention apparatus), and the prosthetic situation; even retinated teeth present a risk. Aerodontalgia is a barofunction disorder with the same frequency as aerosinutisitis of around 2%. We found in a long-term aeromedical study over 20 years a frequency of 7%.

Aerodontalgia is characterized by its sudden appearance and intense pain. In a pilot, aerodontalgia is likely to lead to a considerable reduction of performance.

Only healthy teeth, or teeth that have been repaired *lege artis*, can be assumed not to present any risk. In vital teeth aerodontalgia may be caused by caries, acutely and chronically inflammatory processes of the pulp, and loss of hard substance after crown preparations. In teeth with dead pulp causes are trapped gas in the case of gangrene or incomplete root fillings. During ascent, trapped gas expands via the root canal into the apical tissue and causes pain; the symptoms usually diminish during descent. Dental repair must in all cases be carried out following episodes of aerodontalgia. Depending on the extent of the surgery, the pilot should refrain from flying for two to ten days following extractions and oral surgery. Regular dental examinations and prompt repair with required prophylactic programmes ensure aesthetic appearance, normal chewing and speaking function, and retention of own teeth into old age.[28,29]

Provision of a firmly fitting dental prosthesis should be aimed for after tooth loss. Missing natural teeth may, depending on anatomical conditions, be replaced by artificial tooth roots (implants) to avoid removable dentures (Fig. 20).

LARYNX AND SPEECH

The skeleton of the larynx consists of the thyroid cartilage, the signet-ring-shaped cricoid cartilage (Adam's apple), the two pyramid-shaped arytenoid cartilages, the epiglottis, and a few unimportant smaller cartilages. The inferior horn of the thyroid cartilage articulates on each side with the cricoid cartilage. The cricoid cartilage also has other important articulations with the arytenoid cartilage. The base of the arytenoid cartilage rests on the upper edge of the cricoid cartilage and runs laterally into a processus muscularis for the posterior and

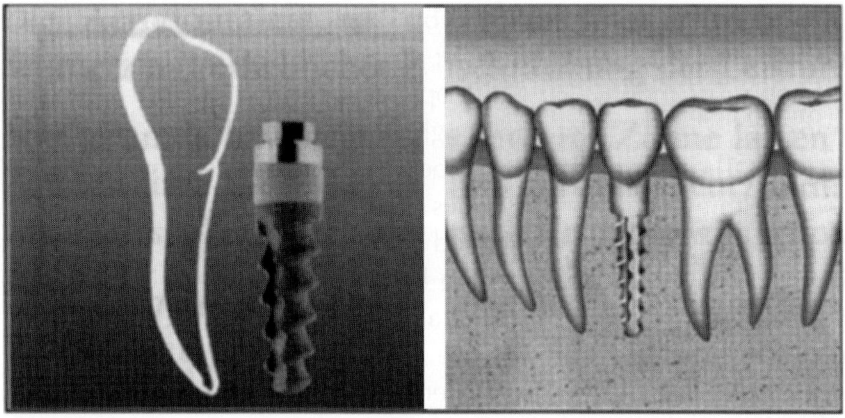

Figure 20. Titanium tooth implant modeled on natural tooth root (Dentaurum-Implants™).

lateral cricoarytaenoid muscles. In a ventral direction, they form a processus vocalis for the beginning of the vocal cord. The epiglottis is leaf-shaped and consists of elastic cartilage. It has a stem inclining in a caudal direction and is here fixed with ligamentum thyreoepiglotticum to the posterior side of the thyroid cartilage. With its free, moveable part, the epiglottis can close the larynx during the act of swallowing.

The most important functions of the larynx are respiration and phonation. The larynx also helps prevent aspiration by facilitating complete closure of the trachea during swallowing. Stabilization of the thorax, vital for the application of abdominal muscular pressure, is furthermore facilitated by closure of the glottis.

Nerve supply in the larynx takes place via n. laryngeus superior from the vagus nerve with sensitive fibers supplying the mucosa and the front part of the vocal cord. M. cricothyreoideus (internus) is motorically innervated via the ramus externus. N. laryngeus inferior (recurrens), which likewise originates from the vagus nerve supplies all other laryngeal muscles and the mucosa below the glottis. It winds to the right around arteria subclavia and to the left around the aorta.

Examination of the larynx is by inspection and palpitation from outside (tumors, perichondritis); internal inspection is by laryngoscopy. For indirect laryngoscopy, a light source and a laryngeal mirror or a magnifying wide-angle lens (magnifying endoscope) is needed. The larynx and the upper trachea may also be inspected through thin, flexible endoscopes inserted through the mouth or the nose. Rigid tubes or illuminated hollow tubes are used for direct laryngoscopy, as a rule with the help of the operation microscope and with the patient under general anaesthesia. With six to 40 times magnification, not only precise diagnosis but also microsurgery is possible. The use of a CO_2 laser further makes it possible, in case of malignant laryngeal diseases, to preserve organs and functions while ensuring the complete removal of the tumor. Image-forming procedures (X-ray tomography, laryngography, core spin tomography, and echolaryngography) are also used for examination of the larynx.

Diseases of the Larynx

Diseases of the larynx, in particular hoarseness, coughing, breathing difficulties, soreness and swallowing disorders (dysphagia/globus) are frequently occurring. Hoarseness is the most common early symptom of diseases of the larynx and is caused by a dysfunction in the movement of the vocal cords. This can be caused by inflammation, deformation, vocal cord paralysis or injuries, or it can be the consequence of surgery, tumors, and voice dysfunctions.

Any hoarseness of more than three weeks duration must without fail be referred to an ENT specialist.

Hoarseness should be differentiated from the feeling of having a lump in the throat when speaking, which is usually caused by infections and tumors of the throat and the hypopharynx. Dry laryngeal coughing (the constant need to clear the throat) is a reaction of the sensitive mucosa to various irritations. Breathing difficulty is caused by a stenotic formation process and results, if the upper respiratory passages are blocked, in a typical inspiratory stridor. It occurs in the presence of inflammations, injuries, foreign bodies, synechia, and benign or malignant tumors. Pain from the ear on the affected side may be misinterpreted as an ear infection. In the case of tumors and acute infections of the larynx, dysphagia may occur, while globus (the lump-in-the-throat feeling) frequently accompanies various functional and organic disorders.

Voice and Speech

Speech dysfunctions may have a central nervous cause or arise as a result of faulty articulation, while voice dysfunctions are caused by faulty phonation. In addition to anamnesis and inspection of the larynx, examinations of timbre, vocal range, note-holding duration as well as voice strain tests, vocal field measurements, and stroboscopy are required to evaluate a voice disorder.

Speech is based on articulation and phonation. Many speech disorders are caused by the wrong use of the respiratory musculature when speaking and the wrong breathing technique that results from this. Articulation is the presice movements of the organs that form speech. The various speech sounds are formed by changes in the supraglottic air passages (resonance cavity), which include the supraglottic cavity, the throat, the buccal cavity, and the main nasal cavities and sinuses. The form of this resonance cavity can be changed by movements of the lips, tongue, jaw, and the soft palate. A person who is unable to hear cannot develop speech (deaf-muteness).

Intact speech tools are absolutely vital for the pilot in order to communicate by speech. Good vocal abilities are required in the cockpit, as drying-out of the mucosas due to the low air humidity in flight is a great strain and also carries a high risk of infection. Unless an intercom system is used, noise in the aircraft also forces the pilot to speak very loud to be understood.[12] For untrained speakers, uneconomical use of the voice can result in frequent problems, even temporary loss of voice (aphonia) (Fig. 21).

A disorder of the speech function can be caused on all levels of the resonance cavity and must always be examined phoniatrically by an ENT specialist in order to evaluate fitness for flying. This is

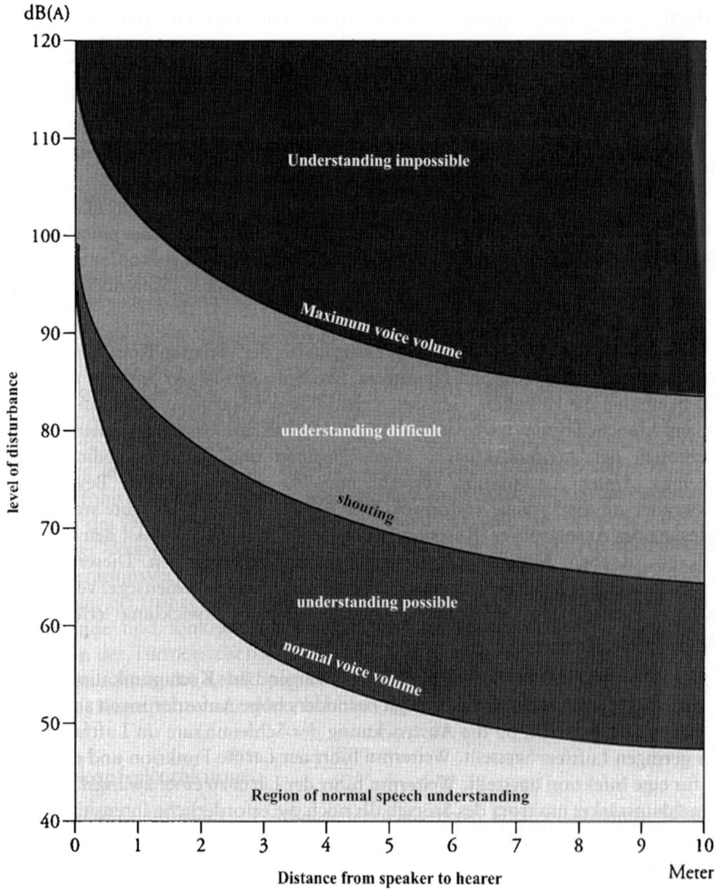

Figure 21. Diagram of the effect of surrounding noise on intelligibility of speech, allowing for speech volume and distance from speaker to hearer.

also necessary following surgery in the otorhinolaryngological area if impairment of vocal and/or speech functions have occurred. The loss of parts of the larynx or the whole larynx usually entails unfitness for medical certification. Speech dysfunctions following central nervous diseases (aphasia) require additional evaluation by a neurologist.

REFERENCES

1. Berghaus A, Rettinger G, Böhme G. (1996) *Hals-Nasen-Ohren-Heilkunde (Ear, Nose and Throat Medicine).* Hippokrates Verlag, Stuttgart.
2. *U.S. Naval Flight Surgeon's Manual, Otorhinolaryngology, Second edition.* (1978) US Government Printing Office, Washington, D.C. 20402.
3. Publication of the regulations amending rules concerning medical provisions for licensing aircrew. *Bundesanzeiger (Federal Gazette)* **No. 94a**: 1–37 (2007) (JAR-FCL3-German). *Bundesanzeiger (Federal Gazette)* **No. 82a**: 1–35 (2008) (1st DV Luft VZO-German).
4. Joint-aviation requirements, flight crew medical requirements. *JAR-FCL Part 3 (Medical),* Subpart, B, C, Section 3.230/3.350, Section 2, pp. 425. Joint Aviation Authorities (1997).
5. Kressin J. (1999) Flugreisemedizinische Probleme des Hals-, Nasen- und Ohrenfachgebietes (*Aeromedical Problems of Otorhinolaryngology*). Urban und Fischer-Verlag, Z.ärztl.Fortbildung.Qual.sich. (ZaeFQ), pp. 509–510; München.
6. Kressin J. (1990) Die flugmedizinische Bedeutung von Luftdruckveränderungen für den menschlichen Organismus in der Luftfahrt (The importance in flight medicine of air pressure changes for the human organism in air travel). In: Heinig R (ed) *Luftfahrt-Handbücher, Flugmedizin,* pp. 121–183, Schulze E, Schöder H-J, Lehwess-Litzmann I, Kressin J. Transpress Berlin.
7. Matschke RG. (1996) *Mittelohrchirurgie bei chronischer Otitis media und Cholesteatom (Middle ear surgery for chronic otitis media and cholesteatoma)* Part 1 and 2 — HNO aktuell, pp. 4, 127–131, and 163–169.
8. Matschke RG. (1993) *Untersuchungen zur Reifung der menschlichen Hörbahn (Investigating the Maturing of the Human Auditory Pathway).* Georg Thieme Verlag, Stuttgart, New York.
9. Plath P. (1992) *Das Hörorgan und seine Funktion. Einführung in die Audiometrie (The Auditory Organ and its Function. An Introduction to Audiometry), 5th ed.* Edition Marhold Spiess, Berlin.
10. Schöder H-J. (2000) "Medizin und Mobilität": Untersuchungstechniken der fliegerärztlichen Untersuchung — Ohren (Vortrag) ("Medicine and

mobility": Techniques for examination by the AME — ears (lecture). *38. Jahrestagung der Deutschen Gesellschaft für Luft- und Raumfahrtmedizin (38th Annual Conference of the German Aerospace Medicine Society).* Berlin.

11. Michel O. (1998) *Morbus Menière und verwandte Gleichgewichtsstörungen (Morbus Menière and Related Balance Disorders).* Georg Thieme Verlag, Stuttgart, New York.
12. Matschke RG. (1987) Lärmschwerhörigkeitsrisiko durch Sprechfunkverkehr? Audiologische Befunde bei Hubschrauberbesatzungen und Piloten von Propellerflugzeugen (Risk of hearing loss induced by noise from voice radio traffic? Audiological findings in helicopter crews and pilots of propeller aircraft). *HNO* **35**: 496–502.
13. Matschke RG. (1994) Speech intelligibility of aircraft pilots with and without electronic noise compensation. In: Draeger J, Schwartz R. *Proceedings of the 41st International Congress of Aviation and Space Medicine, Hamburg 12–16 September 1993.* Monduzzi Editore, Bologna, Italy.
14. Matschke RG. (1994) Kommunikation und Lärm, Sprachverständnis bei Luftfahrzeugführern mit und ohne aktive Lärmkompensation (Communication and noise, speech intelligibility with and without active noise compensation). — *HNO* **42**: 499–504.
15. Schöder H-J. (1990) Das Gleichgewichtssystem — Funktion und Funktionsstörung unter luftfahrtspezifischen Bedingungen (Function and dysfunction under air travel-specific conditions). In: Heiniig R (ed), *Luftfahrt-Handbücher, Flugmedizin,* pp. 58–80, Schulze E, Schöder H-J, Lehwess-Litzmann I, Kressin J, Transpress Berlin.
16. Scherer H. (2000) Otolithenerkrankungen: Diagnostik und Therapie. Vortrag Dezemberfortbildung HNO-Klinik des Unfallkrankenhauses Berlin (Otolith diseases: Diagnosis and treatment. December training course lecture in the Ear, Nose and Throat Clinic of the Berlin Accidents Hospital).
17. Stoll W. (1994) Schwindel und schwindelbegleitende Symptome (Vertigo and its Accompanying Symptoms) Springer-Verlag, Vienna, New York.
18. Ulrich D. (2000) Das HWS-Distorsionssyndrom aus HNO-ärztlicher Sicht: Aspekte zur Dokumentation und Klinik. (The whiplash trauma

from the ENT doctor's perspective: Aspects for documentation and clinic, Norddeutsche Gesellschaft für Otorhinolaryngologie und zervikale Chirurgie, Mitteilungen (Communications of the North German Society for Otorhinolaryngology and Cervical Surgery), pp. 91–96.
19. Hamann KF. (2000) Der gutartige Lagerungsschwindel (Benign Rotational Vertigo), *HNO* aktuell **8**: 311–316.
20. Hamann KF. (2000) Therapie des benignen paroxysmalen Lagerungsschwindel (Treatment of benign paroxysmal rotational vertigo). *Laryngo-Rhino-Otol* **79**: 625–626.
21. Thümler R. (1996) Kinetose. In: Landgraf H, Rose DM, Aust PE, *Flugreisemedizin (Air Travel Medicine)*, pp. 169–189. Blackwell Wissenschaftsverlag, Berlin, Vienna.
22. Stoll W, Matz DR, Most E. (1992) *Schwindel und Gleichgewichtsstörungen (Vertigo and Balance Dysfunctions).* Thieme-Verlag, Stuttgart, New York.
23. Scherer H. (1992) Das Gleichgewicht, Band 2 — (Balance, Vol. 2), Springer, Berlin, Heidelberg, New York, Tokyo.
24. Hallpike CS. (1995) Die kalorische Prüfung (Calorific testing), *Pract. oto-rhino-laryngol* **17**: 173–178.
25. Graybiel A, Fregly AR. (1965) A new quantitative atoxia test battery. *Acta Oto-Laryng* **61**: 292–312.
26. Graybiel A, Fregly AR. (1965) NASA — Order No. R-93, US Government Printing Office, Washington D.C. 20402.
27. Heppt W, Bachert C. (1998) *Praktische Allergologie, Schwerpunkt HNO-Heilkunde (Practical Allergology, focussing on ear, nose and throat medicine),* Georg Thieme Verlag, Stuttgart, New York.
28. Kressin ST. (1991) Zahnmedizinische Probleme beim Fliegen (Dentistry Problems in Flying). *Quintessenz* **28**: 1311–1315.
29. Kressin ST. (1990) Ergebnisse 20-jähriger präventiv orientierter Betreuung am Beispiel des Personals der zivilen Luftfahrt, Inauguraldissertation (Results of 20 years of prevention-oriented caretaking of civil aircrew as an example, Inaugural Dissertation), Berlin.
30. Silbernagl S, Dospopoulos A. (1983) Taschenatlas der Physiologie (Pocket Atlas of Physiology). G. Thieme Verlag, Stuttgart, New York.
31. Gell CF. (1961) Table of equivalents for acceleration terminology. *Aerospace Med* **32**: 1109–1111.

Chapter 19

Neurology for the Aeromedical Examiner

Jürgen Kriebel*,† and Frank Weber‡

INTRODUCTION

Area of Responsibility/Relationship between Structure and Function

Neurology deals with prevention, diagnosis, therapy, rehabilitation, and specialist evaluations of diseases of the central (brain and spinal cord), of the peripheral, and of the autonomic nervous system, and with myopathies. Basic functions of the CNS are perception and processing of information from the interior and exterior world. The information from different perceptive modalities is analyzed, validated, and compared with experience, i.e. with items learned before (memory). Against the background of their individual, situational, and general sense, they receive affective tinting, and, if necessary, are put into appropriate action. This sequence of perception, multisensory convergence, and purposeful action is of particular importance in the man-machine-interface of the cockpit. Thinking, feeling, willing, action, and consciousness are brain functions. This might seem trivial, although according to our experience in aviation medicine,

* Corresponding author.

† Facharzt für Neurologie und Psychiatrie-Psychotherapie-Flugmedizin, Scultetusweg 8, D-98075 Ulm, Germany.

‡ Flugmedizinisches Institut der Luftwatte, Postfache 1264 KFL, D-82242 Fürstenfeldbruck, Germany.

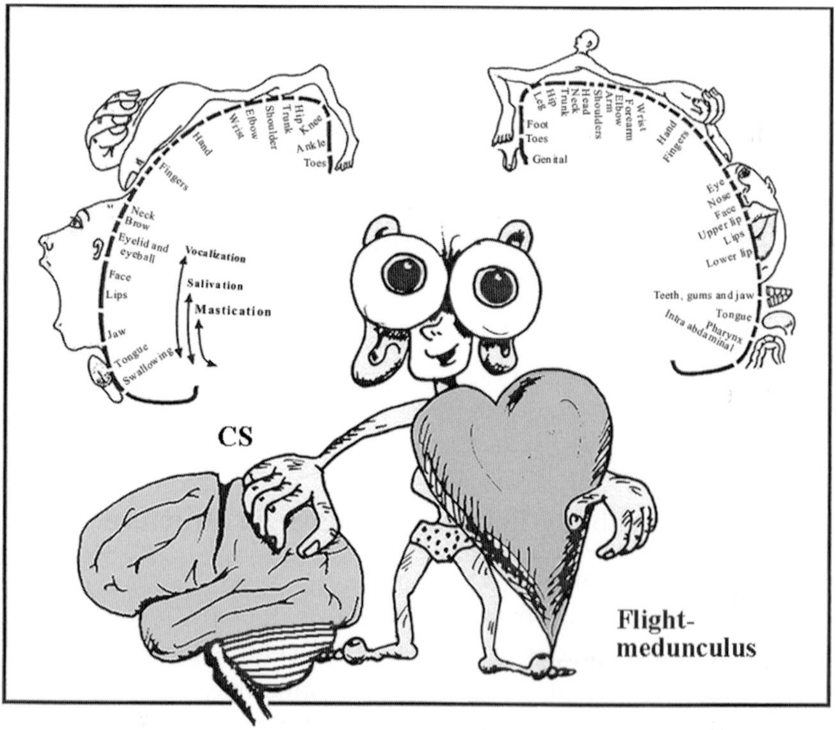

Figure 1. Homunculus and aeromedical homunculus. The motor (upper left) and sensor (upper right) homunculus are somatotopically organized. The more complex the function, the greater the cerebral representation. Similarly the aeromedical homunculus symbolically represents the aeromedical significance of various medical specialities CS: Central Sulcus between motor and sensory strips. For the liver gap see Chapter 20 on "Psychiatry for the Aeromedical Examiner."

there is a strong need for promotion of neuroscience among aeromedical examiners.

Aeromedical Homunculus

Figure 1 presents the basic neurological informaton in aviation medicine. Large parts of the CNS are somatotopically organized. Afferent and efferent projections, the nuclei, the basal ganglia, and the different cerebral and cerebellar cortical regions are arranged in a topical and functional way.

The areas in medicine that are particularly important in aviation medicine are presented symbolically (SC: sulcus centralis). The somatotopical organization of the cortical sensorimotor homunculus is well known. In front of the central sulcus, Fig. 1 shows in the upper left corner the motor homunculus and in the upper right corner the sensory homunculus. The more complex the motor or sensory function, e.g., for speaking or for fine-tuned three-dimensional coordination tasks, the larger the cortical representation area and the greater the number of efferent and afferent projections. In analogy to the sensorimotor homunculus, the impact of the different organ systems for aviation medicine is encoded by their size. Cardiology is so dominant that the heart has to be drawn outside the body. The "liver gap" is reviewed in the psychiatric chapter. Eye and ear symbolize the significance of ophthalmology and otorhinolaryngology. The cranium is invisible. In a symbolic and cartooning way, this represents the previous neglect of neurology and psychiatry in aviation medicine.

Cordially or Cerebrally

On this occasion we would like to eliminate a misunderstanding which is deeply rooted and detrimental to neuroscience. The poet and pilot Antoine de Saint Exupéry once wrote: "Only the heart can see well — the essentials are invisible for the eyes." Why do we welcome each other cordially? We describe others as kind-hearted, warm-hearted, heartless, etc. Thus, we describe character traits and ascribe them to the heart. Colloquially, we assign emotions to the heart and intellect to the brain. But the muscle of the heart is incapable of such complex tasks. Fear, shock, and pleasure lead to significant changes of the cardiac rhythm, which we realize. Human behavior, the individual meaning of an event, and the affective coloring of it are brain functions. The confusion between cause and effect has a long tradition in literature, religion, journalism, and everyday life. Having clarified that point — which is important for psychiatry, too — we stay in the cardiocentric tradition and continue to welcome each other cordially and not cerebrally. We do not touch the heart-breaking in romanticism and do not rename the church of Sacre Coeur to Sacre Cerveau (i.e., holy brain). Saint Exupéry would turn in his grave if we did that. One further remark to the functional cerebral organization of teleception is that it is true we see through the eyes and hear with the ears, but this sensory performance is limited to the mediating of the visual and acoustic stimuli. Vision and hearing in the sense of an understanding and judging perception is made possible only by the brain. Free from these misunderstandings, we can now focus on practically relevant neurological topics. We will deal only with frequent diseases and refer to the textbooks for a comprehensive review.[1]

NEUROLOGICAL TOPICS IN AVIATION MEDICINE

Database

The diagnostic entities reviewed in this chapter are taken from our database. Up to 2007, we gave specialist evaluations (or so-called 'expert opinions') on 626 neurological cases. Approximately 70% were professional cockpit crews, about 25% military pilots, about 1% air traffic controllers (ATCs), and the last 4% cabin attendants.

VERTEBRAL COLUMN

Degenerative Joint Disease

Degenerative joint disease of the spine was the third largest group we had to investigate. They occur as a result of changes in the intervertebral disks (spondylosis) with aging. Spondylosis leads to osteophyte formation, meningeal fibrosis, and disk herniation. Spondylosis in the cervical spine can cause progressive myelopathy, radiculopathy, or both. Thoracic lesions become evident mainly as paraparesis. Lumbar lesions cause radiculopathies, neurogenic claudication, or acute back syndromes. One has to keep in mind that neuro-imaging shows degenerative changes, especially in the cervical and lumbar spine, even at the age of 30. These changes might reach an alarming size, but clinical symptoms and signs remain critical for clinical and aeromedical decision-making. In about 1%, considerable disk herniations are found incidentally and asymptomatically without significant clinical symptoms. It is not neuro-imaging that needs to be treated, but the patient. Indication for surgery in disk herniations is crucial. Usually the treatment of disc disease is conservative with initial bed rest (later physiotherapeutic training) and non-steroidal anti-inflammatory agents. The majority of patients improve with time regardless of the type of intervention. Surgical decompression is indicated only when symptoms are unresponsive to conservative therapy, if there is progressive weakness, or when central herniation results in myelopathy or cauda equina syndrome. Radiculopathy is usually manifested by radiating pain, weakness, loss of deep tendon reflexes, and sensory changes in a segmental distribution. Neck or lower back pain and stiffness are common in cervical and lumbar radiculopathies, respectively. Symptoms may be aggravated by sneezing, coughing, straining with defecation, or neck or trunk movement. Bed rest usually offers relief. On examination, Lasègue's sign (the straight leg raising sign) may be present in cases of lumbar radiculopathy. Crossed straight leg raising usually indicates a larger lesion. An isolated root lesion may result in a smaller area of sensory disturbance than expected by standard dermatomal maps due to cutaneous nerve overlap. Hyporeflexia is restricted to the involved root level. Weakness may occur in the appropriate myotomal distribution and may indicate a larger lesion with greater anterior root involvement. Central lumbar lesions may result in a cauda equina syndrome. Although herniated intervertebral disc material is the most common cause of radiculopathy, other mass lesions and structural abnormalities should be excluded. These may include tumors, epidural abscesses and spondylosis. Nowadays, this exclusion is usually made by MRI. The other diagnostic studies include nerve conduction studies and EMG. The latter serve to exclude brachial or plexus neuropathy and peripheral neuropathy. Furthermore, EMG may identify evidence of denervation in a root distribution before clinical weakness develops. Neurogenic claudication is usually due to spondylotic narrowing of a lumbar spinal canal. Like vascular claudication, it causes exertional pain, but differs from vascular claudication: the pain may be felt in the buttock or thigh with prolonged standing or walking, the pulses are normal, reflexes may decrease while at peak pain, and the pain is relieved with waist flexion or rest but usually takes several minutes or more to resolve.

Herniated Discs

In our airmen, herniated discs ($N = 65$) and degenerative or traumatic lesions, the latter due to helicopter crashes or ejection seat escapes, were distributed in 75% in the lumbar spinal column, in 20% in the cervical region, and in 5% in the thoracic region. Aeromedical disposition is easy. Return to cockpit after full recovery is the rule. This applies even to military pilots of fast jets with ejection seats after cervical spinal surgery if the surgical procedure applied does not lead to osseous instability.[2] A problem is the subgroup of pilots who do not become pain free even after full resolution of all neurological symptoms. In these cases, a consequent long-term rehabilitation is necessary, which sometimes collides with the needs of the employer, creating a compliance problem for the pilot. If long-term rehabilitation is unsucessful, one should look for non-neuro-orthopedic problems, i.e., psychosomatic disorders, loss of motivation to fly, or fear of flying. Many insurance companies do not cover occupational disabilities based on psychiatric or affective disorders. This may lead to a situation where the pilot accepts untreated low back pain as an "acceptable alternative."

EPILEPSY AND NON-EPILEPTIC PAROXYSMAL SYNDROMES

Diagnostic Group

The epilepies are a group of conditions marked by recurrent seizures that are the clinical manifestation of abnormal electrical discharges in the brain. Here, the diagnostic group "cerebral seizures/EEG-abnormalities" is the most frequent in our areomedical specialist evaluations, and primarily includes non-epileptic paroxysmal syndromes. There were confirmed idiopathic epilepsies in 18 cases, and in the same number of cases the suspected seizure or syncope could not be confirmed. In 17 cases, a non-epileptic cause was probable, and these cases were referred to the internist (cardiologist). Interictal epileptiform activity (spikes, sharp waves, spike-wave complexes) was found in 18 cases. Interictal epileptiform activity is strongly but not absolutely correlated with epilepsy. Thus, its presence does not unequivocally indicate a diagnosis of epilepsy nor does its absence exclude it. Evidence of interictal epileptiform activity in an otherwise healthy pilot is a bar to medical certification. In about 2000 healthy male applicants for military aviation, the prevalence of interictal epileptiform activity was 1.48% (95% confidence interval 0.92% to 2.35%).[3] Symptomatic seizures and single non-provoked seizures are not included in this diagnostic group. They are assigned to the causal diagnoses and will be reviewed there. For didactic reasons they are mentioned here, in the case reports, to sensitize the aeromedical examiner to become attentive in suspicious cases and to look for symptomatic seizures.

Free Interval

Both cerebral fits and faints can last for seconds or minutes, or even longer. There are free intervals lasting days, weeks, months or years, so the person's competitiveness or ability to endure stress is usually not affected. Consequently, it is a common fallacy by affected persons, jurists, and even some physicians that free intervals must entail medical fitness for flying, especially in the case of long free intervals as one finds them in oligo-epilepsia and in patients who comply well with antiepileptic treatment. The aeromedical examiner rarely witnesses epileptic paroxysms. He sees the pilot in the free interval and relies crucially on history. As in other neurological disorders with a time-limited course, a careful history taking, including interview with family members and colleagues, is here usually far more informative than the physical examination.

Case 1: At the airfield, a private pilot had a convulsive, generalized seizure with unresponsiveness for several minutes. The aeromedical examiner was informed by a third person and learned of some additional seizures in the past. The pilot was confronted with his uninformative history and answered that he had not been asked about seizures during the periodic medical examinations and had misunderstood the questions on the examination sheet.

Doctor-hopping and fragmentary statements are a problem with relevance to flight safety not only in this diagnostic group. Epilepsy is a frequent disorder of the central nervous system with a prevalence of 0.5% (0.2% to 0.8%) in the general population. A single provoked seizure is thought to have a lifetime prevalence of 5%. Every brain is able to respond with a seizure to appropriate stimulation. Fever, sleep deprivation, hyperventilation, photic stimulation, certain drugs, and alcohol can provoke seizures or contribute to them. The diagnosis of epilepsy is usually made after two spontaneous seizures. There are certain exceptions to this rule, e.g., patients referred for evaluation of a first seizure often report previous episodes that are highly likely to be earlier, undiagnosed seizures. These can include events that are similar to the one that has led to the current consultation (e.g., a patient consulting for a generalized tonic clonic seizure reports a history of awakening with a bitten tongue, fatigue, and myalgia) or other types of seizures (e.g., absences or myoclonic seizures in a patient with a first generalized tonic clonic seizure). The diagnosis of epilepsy does not apply in the case of only one seizure, especially if the seizure is provoked by certain conditions such as alcohol or drug over-consumption or when related to severe sleep deprivation (provoked seizures).

In aviation medicine, not only epileptic syndromes during adolescence and adulthood, but also epileptic fits in childhood, especially after age 5, may be relevant. Complicated or prolonged febrile seizures may lead to a chronic epilepsy syndrome after puberty.

Symptomatic Seizures and Standards in EEG

Epileptic fits are often part of a symptomatic syndrome, i.e., they are caused by a neoplasm, especially low-grade gliomas, cortical dysplasia, and vascular malformations, or are of ischemic, inflammatory, toxic, or post-traumatic origin. In some intracranial tumors or vascular malformations, focal or generalized seizures are the presenting symptom. Therefore, in seizures of unknown origin, as well as in seizures with a well-founded suspicion of cause, there should be a throrough diagnostic work-up including MRI (magnetic resonance imaging) with contrast enhancement and MRA (magnetic resonance angiography). In certain cases we reviewed, the neuro-imaging was insufficient. Similar critical remarks must be made about the quality of some EEG-recordings. JAR requires clear quality standards (20 electrodes placed according to the 10/20-system, information regarding the duration of the recording, the placing of the electrodes and the calibration). The aeromedical examiner is obliged to do the EEG-recordings in institutions that fulfill these requirements. In some countries, an EEG is required at the initial medical examination for commercial pilots; in other countries, however, EEG is considered necessary only on clinical indication.

Case 2: A high school graduate with a glider pilot's licence applied for certification as a professional pilot. The EEG at the initial medical examination showed interictal epileptic activity. Since there was no family history of epilepsy, the parents and the general physician did not accept this EEG-reading. ("There is no such thing as epilepsy in our family.") The interictal epileptic activity could be reproduced in subsequent EEGs, but further diagnostic work-up was rejected. Two years later, a series of generalized, convulsive seizures developed without aura. Adequate work-up at this time showed no causation, and successful antiepileptic treatment was established. Only now could the medical rejection be accepted subjectively.

This case report contains some important aspects. In the author's opinion, initial aeromedical examinations should include an EEG. This recommendation is not shared by ICAO, FAA, and JAR-FCL 3, primarily because there is wide interreader variation in sensitivity and specificity of EEG interpretations and this variation influences the ability of EEG to discriminate between those who will and those who will not have seizures in the future. In practice, interpreting the degree to which a positive EEG result predicts increased seizure risk in an individual patient is difficult. However, interpreting EEG with higher specificity yields more accurate predictions. Given a prevalence of epilepsy in the general population of 0.5%, a sensitivity of the EEG of 0.52, and a specifity of the EEG of 0.97, the conditional probability of an otherwise healthy applicant with interictal epileptic activity in his EEG-recording to develop epilepsy in the future is 8%.[3,4] The conditional probability of a person with a negative EEG to develop epilepsy in the future is 0.25%. Thus, a negative EEG halves the predictive risk. Since there are no better predictors for risk stratification, the occasional unfairness to the individual applicant should be accepted as preferable to endangering aviation safety by epileptic fits. In pilots, the diagnosis of epilepsy is felt as shameful and degrading. Thus, the aeromedical examiner must not take for granted that the pilot will be responsible and inform him of previous fits. Some pilots offer an insignificant history in spite of seizures because they fear to lose their licence, especially if the seizures are alcohol or drug related. The next case report shows an example.

Case 3: While flying as pilot-in-command, a professional pilot experienced a generalized tonic-clonic convulsive seizure with initial cry, unresponsiveness for 15 minutes and postictal drowsiness and amnesia for one hour. In the tonic phase, the rudders were blocked and the stick was fixed in a downward position. In a huge effort, the co-pilot succeeded to just barely scrape past a high-tension line and land in a nearby airfield. It was an epileptic fit due to alcohol withdrawal. For years the pilot had been alcohol addicted. The meaning of the chronically elevated γ-GT had been minimized by his aeromedical examiner. He had forced his wife to silence about earlier fits by severe threats.

We can learn from this case not to ignore elevated liver enzymes. Significant information from history might be unavailable. In fits with amnesia, the affected persons themselves often cannot give reliable information.

Diagnosis

Important diagnostic hints are tongue bites or wounds from bites in the cheeks, micturition during the fit, postictal aching muscles, and elevated CK or prolactin. Wounds due to falling are usually at the back of the head ("faints fall forward, fits fall backward"). EEG-recordings can be unproductive. Provocation during the EEG (hyperventilation, photic stimulation) may be helpful and is standard in aviation medicine. Most importantly, after one abnormal EEG, normal recordings lose their meaning. Another well-founded provocation is the sleep-deprived EEG. We were the first to show the value of sleep-deprived EEGs in the diagnosis of epilepsy.[5] It is particularly important in these EEGs to look for the phases of drowsiness, falling asleep and wake-up, which are diagnostically productive. Sometimes this extended EEG work-up provides indication for simultaneous EEG and video-recording, which can yield additional diagnostic information.

Classification of Epileptic Seizures

Epilepsies provide a wide variety of clinical phenotypes. Epileptic seizures are classified as focal (partial, local), beginning in a part of one hemisphere, generalized, beginning bilaterally, or unclassified as to focal or generalized. Focal seizures that subsequently evolve to generalized seizures are said to exhibit secondary generalization.

Even simple partial seizures without compromise of consciousness rule out medical certification for flying. The international guidelines leave no room for personal judgement if epilepsy is confirmed. If the aeromedical examiner is aware of petits maux in childhood, he should seek neurological advice. Most of these cases stop in puberty, but some can persist into adulthood. In our experience, most of the epilepsy cases in pilots are primarily or secondarily generalized seizures. Sometimes they may lead to traffic accidents. So-called "simple febrile seizures" that occur after the age of five need a thorough work-up. Seizures with a special connection to the time of day (on awakening or when falling asleep) are not compatible with flying. It is a sign of progression when formerly focal seizures change to generalized ones, or when formerly focal seizures become complex-partial ones. The latter might be a sign of mesial temporal sclerosis. It belongs to the tasks of the aeromedical examiner to initiate a thorough work-up if there is any doubt whether a pilot could suffer from epileptic seizures.

Case 4: A young man, achievement-orientated and successful in his profession, paid for the ATPL out of his own pocket. After a phase of strong workload and sleep deprivation he suffered from a disturbance of consciousness for several seconds after drinking a small amount of alcohol. While sitting on a bar stool, he sank slowly to the ground, with prompt re-orientation. Some weeks later, his spouse reported some spasms during sleep that occurred at least once. Anxious and responsible, the pilot contacted his aeromedical examiner who consulted a neurologist. History revealed an unequivocal description of a tonic-clonic convulsive generalized seizure with bluish discoloration and foaming at the mouth during sleep. Physical examination, EEG, and neuro-imaging were not informative. Medical certification was rejected in spite of the fact that the first event could not with certainty be classified as an epileptic seizure. International guidelines justify this for the individual pilot severe decision.

Aeromedical Disposition

Patients who experience a single unprovoked seizure have a significant chance of recurrence over the next five years, varying from 23% to 71% depending on the study.[6] Those with an underlying cerebral lesion and an abnormal electroencephalogram or who have a high-risk epilepsy syndrome, such as juvenile myoclonic epilepsy, have the greatest likelihood of recurrence and probably should be treated after their first seizure. The risk of recurrence after two seizures is higher than 80%.[7] If the EEG is normal on several occasions, the risk of recurrence declines to 12% within two years.[8] These numbers are definitively higher than the incidence limit of 1% per year that is internationally accepted. There is little room for flexibility. Restricted recertification, however, may be considered after an appropriate observation time without seizures and free of medication. A time period of 10 years has been suggested.[9]

Non-epileptic Fits

Conditions producing symptoms and signs that may be mistaken for epileptic seizures include the following: syncope, transient ischemic attacks, migraine, metabolic derangements (e.g., hypoglycemia), parasomnias, transient global amnesia, paroxysmal movement disorders (e.g., paroxysmal kinesiogenic choreo-athetosis), and non-epileptic psychogenic pseudoseizures. The differential diagnosis is particularly important if the non-epileptic fits share phenotypic features of the epileptic seizures. In 10% of the affected persons, epileptic and non-epileptic fits are confused. Evaluation of a first seizure-like event is usually most difficult, especially if there is no sufficient history.

The most frequent differential diagnosis affects syncopes. Convulsive syncopes can be confused with generalized, convulsive seizures. Convulsion in syncopes is brief, about 10 seconds, and starts after, not before, the fall; there is no disturbance of breathing, the face is pale, eyes are closed, and re-orientation is prompt. In generalized seizures, the eyes are open, pupils are wide, and re-orientation is slow. Regrettably, a normal EEG-recording does not support the diagnostic decision. A sleep-deprived EEG and sometimes long-term observation may be necessary.

Transient Global Amnesia (TGA)

The syndrome occurs in middle-aged or elderly individuals and recurs in about 3%.[10] An individual behaves in an apparently automatic fashion for minutes to hours (<24 hours) without recollection of those events and has retrograde amnesia that may be spotty. During the ictus, the patient repetitively asks questions about his or her plight, identity, or location in ways that indicate an acute awareness of the amnesia. Although the patient recovers, a permanent island of memory loss for the period encompassed by the TGA may remain. TGA attack can follow a wide variety of stresses, including strenuous exertion, sexual intercourse, immersion in water, pain, or emotional stress. The pathogenesis of TGA is unknown but may be a manifestation of migraine, transient vascular insufficiency, either arterial or by venous ingestion due to insufficiency of the venous valves in the internal jugular venes, or complex partial seizure. MRI revealed cellular edema in the anterior part of the temporal lobe in TGA. Delayed cell destruction in the CA1-region of the hippocampus, however, is possible, leading to hippocampal cavities, detectable by MRI.[11]

Aeromedical disposition: An epileptic or an arterial cause (transient ischemic attack) should be ruled out. Since the recurrence rate decreases exponentially over time, unrestricted certification may be considered after an appropriate observation time, usually a year or two.

OTHER NEUROLOGICAL DISEASES

This relatively large group is a colorful collection of different neurological disorders. In addition to the different diagnostic bars in Fig. 2, these diagnoses with less than 10 cases cover the whole field of neurology. This group contains paraneoplastic syndromes, syringomyelia, porphyria, degenerative disorders, hereditary polyneuropathies, several other disorders of the peripheral nervous systems, and myopathies. These are case-by-case decisions, some may require accredited medical conclusion.

TRAUMATIC BRAIN INJURY (TBI)

Case Definition

The diagnosis of brain injury would seem to be relatively straightforward, based on the history of exposure to a blunt or penetrating injury of the head followed by a temporary or persisting neurological deficit. However, wording in the guidelines, e.g., in JAR FCL 3, FAA- and ICAO-regulations do not distinguish injuries of the head that do not affect the brain itself from injuries of the brain *per se*. "Head trauma" is a collective name for any kind of injury to the head, with or without involvement of the brain.

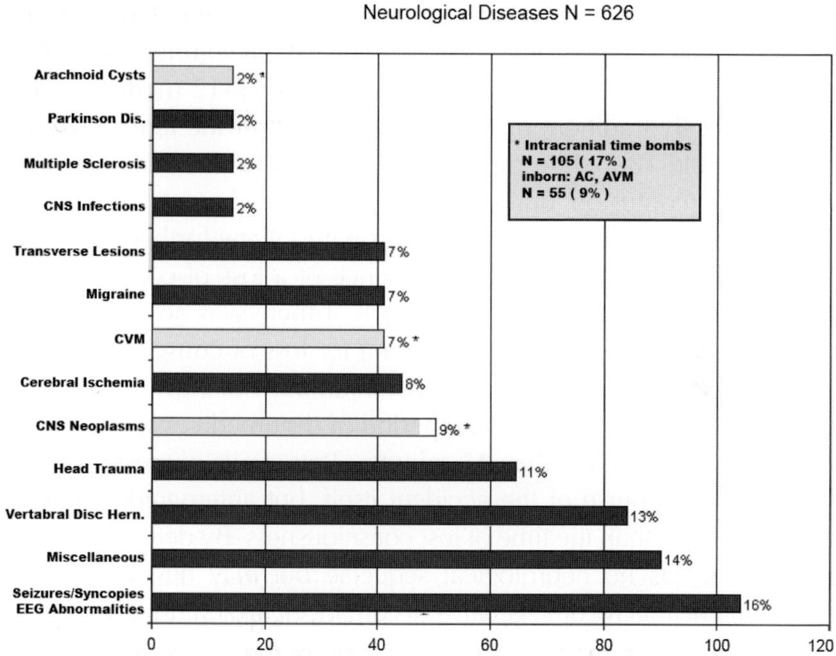

Figure 2. Distribution of aeromedical neurologic diagnoses. Abscissa: absolute numbers. Diagnoses with the less than 10 cases are in the miscellaneous bar. Asterix indicates diagnoses with high risk of sudden incapacitation (intracranical time bombs). This also accounts for the idiopathic epileptic seizures hidden in the "Seiz./Sync./EEG" bar.

Evidence for the involvement of the brain includes disturbance of consciousness, retrograde or anterograde amnesia, and neurological deficits with or without associated abnormalities in neuro-imaging or in electrophysiological tests. These criteria can be used for differential diagnosis and for grading the severity of the TBI. Vegetative symptoms, nausea, and vomiting are frequent in TBI. They do not *per se* provide evidence for involvement of the brain but can be explained by concussion of the labyrinth. There are several different scales with different criteria for grading the severity of brain injuries. In clinical studies, the severity of brain injuries is usually graded using the Glasgow Coma Scale (GCS). The scale has three components based on eye movement, motor, and verbal responses. It can be reported by a single score that ranges from 3 to 15 points. Brain injuries associated with GCS scores of 13–15 are considered mild, 9–12 moderate, and 3–8 severe. By tradition, many neurologists prefer the term "concussion" for mild TBI, while moderate and/or severe TBI traditionally is called brain contusion. Brain concussion is defined as a traumatic loss of consciousness for less than 24 hours without any further neurological deficits. Retrospectively, the presence of a loss of consciousness might be difficult to decide, particularly if there was an overlapping drug effect for narcosis, etc. The criteria for loss of consciousness are antero- or retrograde amnesia or post-traumatic dozing.

In mild TBI (concussion), the period of disturbed consciousness is usually brief, often less than 15 minutes. Retrograde amnesia is often limited to the course of the accident itself, but anterograde amnesia may last longer than the time of lost consciousness. By definition, brain concussion has no neurological sequelae but may be followed by unspecific headache or vegetative disturbances, which usually subside within weeks. In cases of simple brain concussion, pilots can routinely return to flying within a few weeks, in individual cases within a few days. These intervals are usually extended in cases of more severe TBI.

Moderate and Severe TBI

In moderate and severe TBI, morphological lesions and/or focal neurological deficits as aphasia or paresis are often found in addition to the disturbance of consciousness. Furthermore, one can find neuropsychological deficits with impairment of several aspects of cognition, such as thought content and judgement, impaired attention and altered mood, and even post-traumatic personality disorders. These deficits are often diffucult to recognize and require specialized neuropsychological assessment (for details, see the neuropsychology chapter in this book). Morphological basis for these deficits is diffuse axonal injury (DAI), most often demonstrable with MRI. Subjective complaints correspond to brain concussion and are not necessarily more severe. There are also moderate and severe TBIs without a concussion syndrome.[12] In this group of TBI ($N = 68$), we assessed

36 concussions and 32 moderate/severe TBIs. Most of them were returned to flying duties.

Post-traumatic Intracranial Hematoma

Close observation of the patient is essential in any kind of TBI. A particular problem is the so-called lucid interval. The initial loss of consciousness with regaining of consciousness is followed hours later by progressive headache and deterioration of the mental status; lateralizing signs may be present. The reason is acute subdural hematoma, acute epidural hematoma, or any other kind of intracranial hematoma with mass effect. Acute subdural hematoma is usually caused by traumatic tearing of bridging veins, and acute epidural hemorrhage results from skull fracture with laceration of the middle meningeal artery and vein. The clinical course is similar to acute subdural hematoma but more rapidly progressive. Rapid herniation, respiratory depression, and death may ensue. The diagnosis is established with CT scan. An acute subdural hematoma appears as hyperdensity over the cortex, an acute epidural hematoma is a lens-shaped hyperdensity. The prognosis for survival and recovery of patients that are neurosurgically treated immediately is generally good. This also applied in our case series. In two cases, we found coincidental traumatic subarachnoid hemorrhage and traumatic intracerebral hemorrhage. These pilots did not regain their medical certification due to persisting neuropsychological deficits.

Case 5: A captain was found unconscious, lying on the sidewalk in a Middle-Eastern country. After hospital admission, his mental status deteriorated with lateralizing signs. An acute epidural hematoma was suspected and was immediately evacuated. His condition improved fast, and after the third day he was free of complaints. There were signs of skin lacerations and skin contusions in the parietal region of the skull. The captain had retrograde amnesia, there was no history of an accident, and neuro-imaging and EEG were unremarkable. Thus, the cause of the trauma was unclear. A first-time manifestation of a generalized convulsive epilepsy could not be ruled out, and the pilot was classified as unfit. An additional expert evaluation by a specialist in forensic medicine concluded that the skin lacerations were the result of criminal violence. In the case of simple falling, skin contusions are not found above the brim of the hat. After the cause of the incident was thus identified, the pilot was permitted to return to the cockpit.

Long-term Outcome, Blunt or Open Head Trauma

Case 6: A professional pilot suffered a severe open traumatic brain injury after a motorcycle accident. He had an impression fracture in the fronto-lateral region, tearing of the dura, focal frontal brain contusions, and a countre-coup contusion contralaterally in the parieto-occipital region. Management included neurosurgical evacuation and intensive care. The patient remained unconscious for one week, and then improved gradually. After two years of intensive rehabilitation, there was a post-traumatic personality disorder with prevailing altered mood status with euphoria, uncriticality, and severe over-estimation of his own abilities. EEG-recordings showed no epileptic acitivity, and there were no infectious complications. With this argument, he insisted on regaining his medical certification. He was even able to procure legal support for this request.

This case report highlights the difference between open and blunt head injuries. The criterion for an open (penetrating) head injury is the opening of the dura, e.g., in basal skull fractures with cerebrospinal fluid fistulae. This can cause infectious complications, even brain abscesses, sometimes month or years after the acute event.

From a retrospective point of view, diagnosis and documentation of traumatic brain injuries are sometimes insufficient, especially in cases of polytraumas, where life-saving surgical procedures dominate the initial care. In these cases, TBIs simply can be overlooked and neurological and neuropsychological treatment can be missed. We saw several of these cases, where family, friends, and company realized the possibility of TBI late, and then only when the pilot failed his simulator checks for relicensing. Close observation of the clinical course, combined with EEG-recordings, is of particular importance in aviation medicine. The time period for observation follows the risk for post-traumatic epilepsy, which typically begins six months to two years after the head trauma, but the risk persists for 10 to 20 years. Risk factors for post-traumatic epilepsy include intracranial hemorrhage, depressed skull fracture, early seizures, and duration of post-traumatic amnesia greater than 24 hours. According to cited literature,[13] mild head injuries (including brief unconsciousness or amnesia) have a slightly elevated risk for post-traumatic epilepsy within five years after the injury (with SIR, standardized incidence ratio, of 1.5). Patients with severe injuries (with contusion, focal neurological deficits, intracranial hematomas, or more than 24 hours of unconsciousness or post-traumatic amnesia) have an SIR of 17.0, while those with moderate injury (skull fractures or at least 30 minutes of unconsciousness or post-traumatic amnesia) have a SIR of 2.9.[13] These numbers point the way for the aeromedical disposition.

CEREBRO-VASCULAR MALFORMATIONS

Intracranial Time Bombs

The cases of cerebro-vascular malformations in our series are of congenital origin. They can remain clinically silent for a long time or even lifelong, as can be shown by autopsy series or by incidental findings in neuro-imaging.[14] The majority of them can lead to serious neurological complications without prodromal symptoms or triggers. These complications include subarachnoid hemorrhages, intracerebral hematomas, epileptic fits, and other neurological deficits. We know of several such complications that have occurred in flight and were survived only because of the other pilot in the cockpit. It is difficult to estimate how many crashes of military single-seated fast jets, often attributed to spatial disorientation, are due to such intracranial catastrophies. Post-mortem examinations of the brain are often impossible or at least seriously limited, e.g., in crashes on the high seas or in crashes with impact explosions. Epidemiological data support such considerations, because the prevalence of intracranial vascular malformations or of aneurysms in the general population is reported to be between 1% and 3%.[14–17] The experience from our specialist evaluations confirms the areomedical relevance of this topic. From the aeromedical point of view we call them intracranial time bombs. There are no existing predictors other than the size of the aneurysms, which could indicate which malformation will remain clinically silent and which will not. For military pilots we therefore consider preventive screening with MRI a necessity. The present group of cerebrovascular malformations consists of 18 aneurysms, 20 arteriovenous malformations (AVM), and six cavernomas.

Aneurysms

Epidemiology and clinical signs

Recent studies argue that 3.6% to 6% of the population aged over 30 years harbor an unruptured aneurysm, that these are more common in females than males, and increase in frequency with age; they are associated with smoking and alcohol consumption, possibly with hypertension, and with hypercholesterolemia.[18] There is no evidence that aneuryms occur — at least in significant numbers — in younger age groups.[19] Rupture with subarachnoid hemorrhage (SAH) is the primary manifestation. Overall incidence of SAH is six to eight per 100000 person-years, with a case fatality rate between 25% and 50%; one-third of survivors remain disabled. Ruptured saccular aneurysms account for 80% of non-traumatic SAH. A severe headache of sudden onset is characteristic. The size and location of the hemorrhage and the presence of intraparenchymal and ventricular extension affect the level of consciousness (lethargy to coma). Sudden loss of consciousness is the presenting feature in 20% of the cases. Meningeal signs, papilledema, retinal hemorrhage, and seizures are common. Diagnostic evaluation includes CT (results are negative in about 15% of the cases) and lumbar puncture, if the CT finding is negative. MRI with FLAIR (fluid attenuated inversion recovery) technique demonstrates SAH in the acute stage as reliably as CT. Angiography may locate and define the cause of SAH.

The Hunt and Hess grading scale is commonly used for the prognosis and timing of aneurysm surgery: 0 — unruptured aneurysm (symptomatic or incidental discovery); I — asymptomatic rupture or minimal headache and nuchal rigidity; Ia — no meningeal or brain reaction, but fixed neurologic deficit; II — moderate to severe headache, nuchal rigidity, no neurological deficit other than cranial nerve palsy; III — drowsiness, confusion, or mild focal neurological deficit; IV — stupor, moderate to severe hemiparesis, possibly early decerebrate rigidity and vegetative disturbances; V — deep coma, decerebrate rigidity and moribund appereance. Complications and sequelae of SAH result from systemic dysfunction (syndrome of inadequate antidiuretic hormone, cardiac arrhythmias, diabetes insipidus, pulmonary embolism, gastrointestinal bleeding, respiratory depression, and cardiac arrest), vasospasm, rebleeding, seizures, herniation, and hydrocephalus. Cerebral ischemia or infarction is frequent in the first four to 14 days after the initial hemorrhage because of arterial vasospasm. The amount of subarachnoid blood correlates positively with the rate of occurrence of vasospasm. Lysis of the clot surrounding the aneurysm after the initial bleed results in rebleeding, which may become evident as new focal signs develop or the clinical status worsens. Slightly more than 20% of patients rebleed in the first two weeks, and more than 30% rebleed in the first month. The mortality rate with rebleeding is up to 40% and higher than with the initial bleeding. After the first six months, the annual rebleeding rate is about 5%, with an annual mortality rate of 1% to 3%. Treating hypertension and maintaining the blood pressure within the normal range helps prevent rebleeding.

Surgical clipping of the aneurysm is the definitive therapy. Endovascular treatment by platinum coils has a lower morbidity and mortality than surgical clipping, but achieves complete aneurysm occlusion in only 52% to 78% of the cases. Both should be performed as soon as possible, especially in stable patients (Hunt and Hess grades I to III) to avoid the risk of rebleeding. Late occurrence of hydrocephalus may require shunting. The incidence of recurrent subarachnoid hemorrhage after clipping for ruptured intracranial aneurysms is less than 1% per year (286 of 100 000 patient-years, 95% CI 160 to 472 per 100 000).[20]

Case 7: During check-out after an intercontinental flight, a captain experienced an unusually severe headache that started suddenly. His FO found him in the toilet in a somnolent state. A prompt diagnostic procedure, successful surgical clipping of an aneurysm of the posterior communicating artery, an uneventful postsurgical course, and successful rehabilitation enabled medical recertification after one year.

Case 8: While acting as pilot-in-command during a night flight, an FO suddenly began to moan due to a severe headache; he developed nausea, vomitus, meningism, and a third nerve palsy. He remained incapacitated for the rest of the flight. After landing, the SAH was diagnosed and successfully treated. Course and long-term outcome correspond to the previous example. These case reports can be classified as Hunt and Hess grade III.

Figure 3 shows the most common sites for aneurysms in adults. A higher frequency of aneurysms has been reported in some familial cases and in patients with polycystic kidneys, coarctation of the aorta, and fibromuscular dysplasia. Most aneurysms are in the anterior circulation: approximately 40% in the anterior cerebral artery, about 30% in the internal carotid artery, about 13% in the middle cerebral artery. About 13% occur in the posterior circulation (basilar or vertebral artery). Nowadays, these proximal aneurysms in the circle of Willis can be visualized by MRA (magnetic resonance angiography). Prior to surgery, the conventional angiography, especially digital subtraction angiography, is still used. Figure 4 offers an example and indicates, due to the vasospasm, that the clipping of the aneurysm should be postponed.

Case 9: A 36-year-old private pilot suffered an SAH with acute, very severe headache, nuchal rigidiy, vomitus, and nausea. He had two large aneurysms in the anterior cerebral artery and in the middle cerebral artery. For many years, he had been treated with beta-blockers for his hypertension. Both the ruptured and the unruptured aneurysm

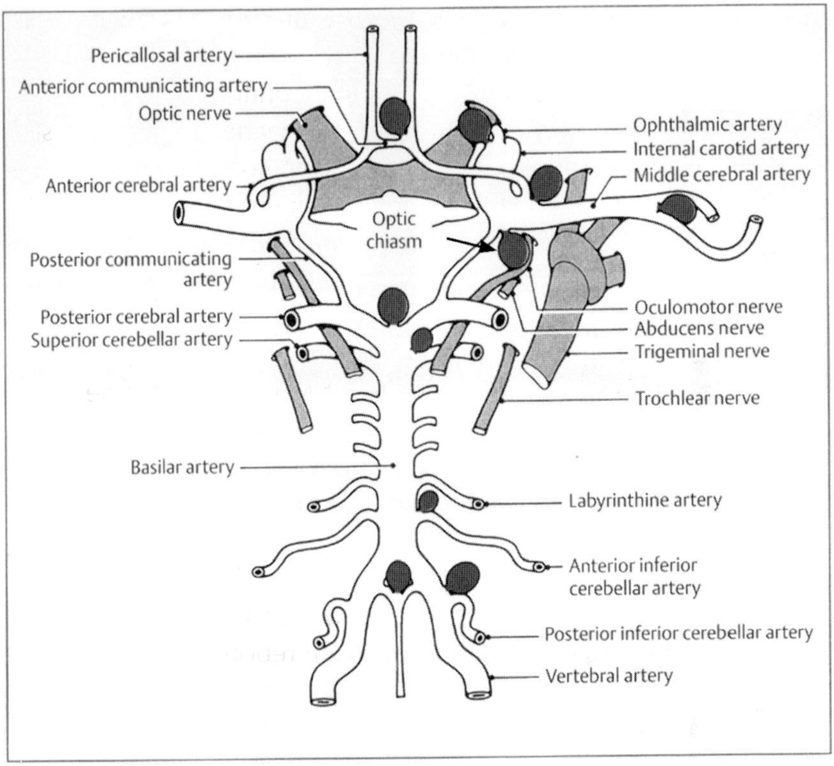

Figure 3. Most common sites of aneurysms. The aneurysm at the branching of the middle cerebral artery and the posterior communicating artery exemplifies (arrow) another clinical representation (besides SAH by rupture): pressure related palsy of the oculomotor nerve, sometimes also involving the abducens nerve.

With kind permission by the authors and the publisher.[1]

were clipped surgically. After successful rehabilitation, neurological and electrophysiological follow-up, and normal neuropsychological testing, he was recertificated for PPL after one year. Four years later the pilot had a new specialist evaluation because he wanted to become a professional pilot. There were new risk factors: he was overweight (BMI 29), had hypercholesterolemia, hypertension (treated with beta-blockers), and a raised γ-GT. Neurological, psychiatric, neuropsychological, and electrophysiological findings were unremarkable. Thus, he got a Class I medical certificate under the

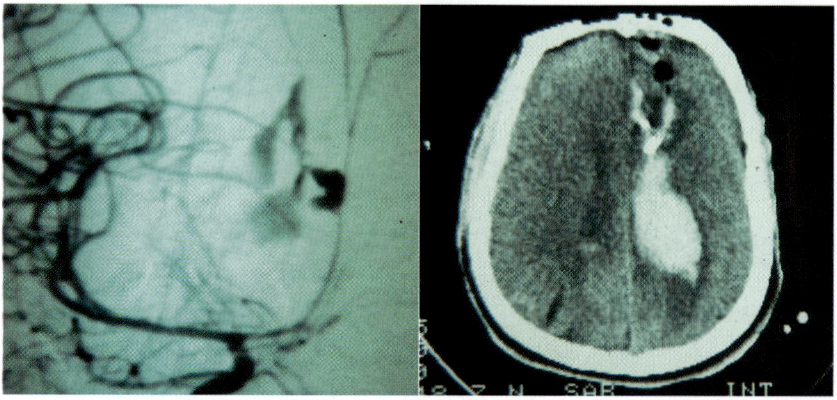

Figure 4. Conventional angiography (left) shows a rupturing bleeding aneurysm and vasospasm (indicating rebleeding) of the anterior cerebral artery. The contrast material/blood in the subarachnoid space surrounds the gyrus. (Right): ruptured giant aneurysm with lethal intracerebral hemorrhage.

condition that he reduce his risk factors. The raised γ-GT as a marker of potential alcohol consumption requires further evaluation. Aerobatics were not allowed.

The previous examples show that the size of the aneurysm is not necessarily associated with the clinical findings in any clear-cut way. As a rule the larger the aneurysm, the higher the risk for bleeding, but also small aneurysms can cause severe hemorrhages. A very serious problem is the misjudgement of the first bleeding in lower graded Hunt and Hess SAH (I, II). In about 30% of SAH, there are so-called "warning leaks," minor bleedings that occur before the first "real" bleeding. In pilots, there is a tendency in those cases to make the diagnosis of migraine, especially if these pilots have a history of migraine, which was usually not revealed to the AME. This constellation applied to 25% of our SAH cases. Even if the initial diagnosis is correct, medical mismanagement in the course of the disease is still possible:

Case 10: A 40-year-old professional pilot was overwhelmed by very severe headache, nausea, vomitus, and slight nuchal rigidity during stressful pre-Christmas activity. Aspirin, which used to help his migraine (never revealed to the AME), did not help in this particular case. MRI and MRA showed an aneurysm of the anterior communicating artery. His condition temporarily improved and he was allowed by his physician to travel abroad to visit his parents. On Boxing-day, his mental status deteriorated and a positive lumbar puncture with bloody and xanthochromatic cerebrospinal fluid confirmed both initial bleeding and rebleeding. Rather late, surgical clipping was performed; fortunately there were no vasospasms. Also in this case the Class I medical certificate could be reactivated after one year. The migraine, by the way, did not reoccur postoperatively.

The next case exemplifies that aeromedical recertification is possible not only after the definitive treatment of surgical clipping of the aneurysm but also after endovascular treatment:

Case 13: A 41-year-old private pilot, with a history of new-onset migraine that had not been evaluated, suffered a SAH level IV/V according to Hunt and Hess by a fusiform aneurysm of the vertebral artery on the right side. Clinical manifestation was sudden loss of consciousness that required intubation and artificial ventilation. The aneurysm was located shortly after the branching of the inferior posterior cerebellar artery (PICA) and was obliterated by coils. There was enough collateral supply via the opposite side. An accompanying hydrocephalus had to be shunted for a short time only. Clinical symptoms resolved quickly, and full recovery was regained after one year. Flexibility was applied and he was recertificated.

In the past, each individual aneurysm was discussed between neurointerventionalists and the vascular neurosurgeons. Now there are many institutions that prefer the endovascular route if technically possible, e.g., if the geometry and anatomy of the aneurysm makes it suitable for embolization. Nowadays, most of the aneurysms are treated by an endovascular technique (up to 75%). Whilst the management of ruptured aneuryms is pretty clear, it is rather unclear what to do with unruptured aneurysms, because there are no clear predictors for bleeding. Unruptured aneurysms are a heterogeneous entity, both in terms of morphology and behavior, e.g., tendency of rupture.

This is in part reflected in the extreme variation in reported risk of rupture in the literature, between 0.05% and 5% a year. Both size and location are influential. Traditionally, 10 mm was thought to be a critical size. However, some authors report a five-year cumulative rupture rate of aneurysms <7 mm in the anterior circulation of 0% (!) and 2.5% in the posterior circulation: the corresponding numbers for aneurysms >25 mm are 40% or 50% respectively.[21]

Aeromedical disposition

Although the actual rupture risk of aneurysms is rather variable (<5 %), it is evident that the rupture risk lies in the magnitude of or above the critical 1% incidence rate. Thus, a person carrying an incidental aneurysm must be classified as unfit. Flexibility should be dependent on a detailed specialist evaluation of the individual case, which should include a statement about possible neurosurgical or endovascular treatment. Due to the high prevalence of aneurysms in the general population, we advocate the screening of military pilots and military applicants by MRI and MRA. We currently perform this policy in German military pilots. This is justified because we use the 1%-rule in aviation medicine. However, the efficacy of the screening is difficult to decide for the general population, because there is a *de novo* rate of aneurysma formation in the range of 1% to 2% per year, with a rupture rate of <5 %, while non-invasive imaging tests are not yet accurate enough to detect small aneurysms, and the morbidity and mortality for elective surgical treatment of unruptured aneurysms is not low. 15% of SAHs are not attributable to saccular aneurysms. Two thirds (10% of the total) are caused by non-aneurysmal SAH and the remaining 5% by a variety of rare conditions. Perimesencephalic hemorrhage constitutes about 10% of all episodes of SAH, and two-thirds of those with a normal angiogram. In this radiologically distinct and strinkingly harmless variety of SAH, the extravasated blood is confined to the cisterns around the midbrain. This disease is defined only by the characteristic distribution of the extravasated blood in combination with the absence of an aneurysm. Clinically, there is little to distinguish idiopathic perimsesencephalic SAH from aneurysmal SAH. On admission, all patients are in perfect clinical condition apart from their headache. The clinical course is uneventful, rebleeding and delayed cerebral ischemia do not occur. The period of convalescence is short, and the quality of life in the long-term is excellent.[22] This is the only condition among the SAHs, where recertification after nine months is reasonable.

Arterial Dissection

Arterial dissection in the carotid or vertebral artery deserves separate consideration. Subadventitial dissection leads to bleeding into the different layers of the arterial wall; this narrows the volume of the vessel, thus reducing arterial supply to the brain. This may be asymptomatic if there is sufficient collateral supply, but a dissection is a good source for local thrombosis with consecutive arterio-arterial emboli. About 25% of all ischemic strokes in young patients are said to be caused by arterial dissection of the carotid artery. Local trauma may be contributive, but often the origin is unclear. We saw one case where a dissection of the vertebral artery led to brainstem infarction; it was possibly caused by chiropractic manipulation of the cervical spinal column. Recertification was not possible.

Case 12: A 43-year-old captain collapsed while jogging in a park. A long-distance dissecting aneurysm of the internal carotid artery on the right side with an embolic infarction of the middle cerebral artery was found; thrombolytic therapy was successful. Neuro-imaging showed a large area of infarcted brain tissue, extending to the temporal lobe, the basal ganglia, and the insular cortex. Left-sided hemiplegia and supranuclear ophthalmoplegia resolved slowly. A hemiparesis with special involvement of the arm and consecutive impairment of fine finger movements remained in combination with a temporary homonymous hemianopia. These focal deficits and bad scoring in neuropsychological tests made the pilot unfit in a first specialist evaluation two years after the stroke. However, the pilot remained highly motivated, worked in a ground job for his company, and continued to pass neuropsychological training. After four years, he mastered all simulator checks and regained medical certification. This case is a nice example of the functional plasticity of the brain, even in an "older" person, something which should not be underestimated.

Arteriovenous Malformations (AVM)

AVMs are another intracranial vascular topic of aeromedical relevance. AVMs are the most common symptomatic vascular malformation with a prevalence in population-based studies of 0.18%. Prevalence in hospital-based post-mortem studies extends up to 6%; our own data show a prevalence of 0.2%.[19] AVMs represent a disordered regulation of angiogenesis and are a result of continuous vascular modelling. In contrast to hemangiomas, they have normal endothelial tissue and turnover. They can be located anywhere in the brain tissue, with about 80% located supratentorially. The vessels involved arise anywhere out of the spectrum of arteries and veins (therefore arteriovenous). Most often, AVMs become symptomatic between the ages of 20 to 40 and account for one-third of all intracranial hemorrhages in the young adult and up to 9% of all SAHs. Clinical manifestations include (with overlapping) hemorrhage (67%), seizures (20%), migraine-like headache (20%), and gradually progressive focal neurological deficits (10%). Only 15% remain long-term free of symptoms. Overall lethality is 1% to 1.5% per year, and the cumulative bleeding rate is between 2% to 4% per year; the case-fatality-rate is up to 20% the first 30 days after bleeding. The rate of rebleeding is 18% in the first year. Angiography detects most AVMs, and MRI is the preferred noninvasive neuroimaging modality. Therapeutic modalities include surgical excision, embolization, and radiotherapy.[23]

AVMs are another example, where an (unrevealed) history of migraine may lead to the diagnosis. In contrast to migraine, which always alternates between the right and left side, a migrainous hemicrania that continually stays on the same side is suspicious of an underlying vascular malformation. If the hemicrania is joined by a seizure, an AVM is highly probable.

Aeromedical disposition

If surgical excision is complete and postoperative recovery is unremarkable without complications, medical recertification is possible. This applied to nine of our 16 cases. In incidental unruptured AVMs, we face the same problem as in unruptured aneurysms: The risk of rupture lies in the magnitude of or above the critical 1% annual incidence rate. Thus, a person carrying an incidental AVM should be classified as unfit. Flexibility should be dependent on a detailed specialist evaluation of the individual case, including a statement about recommended future treatment.

Case 14: A first officer, while acting as pilot-in-command, suddenly stopped radio transmission and developed a generalized convulsive seizure. He lost consciousness for several minutes and needed 20 minutes for reorientation. A physician among the passangers injected diazepam. After landing, a large AVM on the right hemisphere with feeding from the middle cerebral artery was found; complete surgical removal was successful. EEG-recordings showed interictal epileptic activity, and phenytoin was prescribed. The patient did not adhere to the medication, which provoked additional seizures. Carbamazepin was then prescribed and adhered to; it could be discontinued after the third year. Neuroimaging showed an ischemic area in the temporal pole, while further EEG-recordings confirmed interictal epileptic activity. Therefore medical recertification was not possible. There had been a history of migraine (unrevealed to the AME) before the bleeding; it subsided after surgery.

Case 15: A 19-year-old glider pilot suddenly lost consciousness after an extraordinarily severe headache. There was an intracranial hemorrhage at the right hemisphere with expansion in the ventricle from an AVM in the temporal region. It was fed by the posterior cerebral artery and the inferior temporal artery. After partial endovascular embolization, it could be successfully surgically removed. The postsurgical course was uneventful with regular neurological and EEG controls. Restricted recertification was possible after the second postsurgical year.

Our experience from specialist evaluations in aviation medicine tells us that some hemorrhages could have been prevented if pilots would not offer "empty" histories so often. In most of our cases, we found some complaints, often migraine, in the time period before the incident. Such complaints offer the opportunity for diagnostic work-up, thus including an important preventive potential.

Cavernomas (CAV)

After AVMs, cavernomas or cavernous angiomas — sinusoidal vessels without intervening neural tissue — are the second largest group of angiomas that become symptomatic. Surprisingly, cavernomas are angiographically "occult", i.e., they cannot be visualized in angiography, and CT fails to detect them in 30% to 50% of cases. The preferred method of neuro-imaging is again MRI which shows cavernomas with a characteristic "popcorn"-like appearance due to different stages of minor bleeding, which are often clinically silent. Cavernomas are dynamic in behavior, they can arise *de novo*, can enlarge, and can reduce their size. Prevalence is 0.5% in the general population, with 75% of the cavernomas solitaire, and 10% to 30% familial. Clinical relevant symptoms usually present between the ages of 40 to 60 and consist of seizures (50%) and progressive neurological deficits (25%). About 20% are asymptomatic. Sporadic cavernomas carry a risk of bleeding in the range of 0.25% to 0.7% per year, familial cavernomas one of 1% per lesion per year. Therapy is surgical excision after bleeding.[23] In five of the six pilots in our series, seizures were the presenting symptom, which persisted after surgical therapy of the underlying cavernoma. Although each of these cavernomas could be successfully removed by surgery, the pilots remained permanently unfit. Because the spontaneous bleeding rate is less than 1% per year, carriers of incidental cavernomas may be considered fit for restricted certification. However, they should be kept under close observation with MRI monitoring, because of the tendency of cavernomas to grow and bleed. Therefore, a restriction to multicrew operations is appropriate.

Finally, to conclude the chapter on vascular malformations, it is of special aeromedical importance that any cerebral vascular malformation may be multiple or accompanied by other vascular malformation. Therefore, the diagnostic procedures recommended are four-vessel-angiograhies.

TUMORS OF THE CENTRAL NERVOUS SYSTEM

The presence of tumors within the nervous system is often suspected when subacute or acute focal symptoms develop. Some tumors, particularly metastases or carcinomatous meningitis, can give rise to multifocal signs. The combination of location, patient demographics, and neuro-imaging often suggests the most likely histopathology. Metastases account for the majority of CNS tumors in adults; approximately 20% of all patients with systemic cancer have CNS involvement at some time during their illness. Symptoms and signs of CNS neoplasms may be generalized and non-localizing, usually as a result of diffuse edema, hydrocephalus, or increased intracranial pressure. Headaches are variable and may resemble tension or migraine headaches. Most headaches are ipsilateral to the tumor. With increased intracranial pressure, a bifrontal or bi-occipital headache is common, regardless of tumor location. Seizures occur more often with slow-growing tumors and with tumors in the frontal and parietal lobes. Vomiting occurs most consistently with posterior fossa masses. Localizing symptoms and signs depend on the location of the tumor. Frontal lobe masses may be silent or, if anterior or midline, may produce changes in personality and memory. Third ventricle and pineal region tumors often produce ventricular and aqueductal obstruction leading to hydrocephalus. Brainstem tumors produce cranial neuropathies, long-tract signs, and hydrocephalus resulting from compression of the aqueduct. The diagnosis of a brain tumor is usually confirmed by neuro-imaging, either through CT scan or MRI. Hemorrhage occurs most often with glioblastoma multiforme and metastatic tumors. Calcification occurs more commonly with oligodendrogliomas and meningiomas. Available treatment modalities include debulking surgery, radiation therapy, chemotherapy, and a combination of the three.

In our series, the group of tumors consisted of 50 tumors (46 intracranial tumors, and four spinal cord tumors), representing 9% of the neurological diagnoses. In two of the four spinal cord tumors (one lipoma, one astrocytoma WHO grade 1), complete postsurgical recovery made recertification for PPL possible. Two pilots, one with a spinal ependymoma and the other with a higher grade astrocytoma, were assessed as unfit.[24]

Table 1 summarizes the brain tumors according to histopathological classification and aeromedical disposition. The next case vignette exemplifies the uncharacteristic appearance of malignant

Table 1. Intracranial Neoplasms

Histological Classification		**N**	**WAIV**	**PEND**	**UNFIT**
Neuroepithelial tumors	Glioblastoma	3			3
	Astrocytoma	8		4	4
	Oligodendroglioma	3	1	1	1
Meningeal tumors	Meningeoma	15	12	1	2
Germ cell tumors	Teratoma/ Germinoma	4	1		3
Malformative tumors	Craniopharyngeoma	1	1		
Hypophyseal tumors	Adenoma	5	5		
Nerve sheath tumors	Schwannoma	7	4	1	2
Neuroectodermal tumors	Neuroblastoma	2	1		1
Misc	Cerebellar, unclassified	1		1	
Metastastatic tumors	Bronchial carcinoma	1			1
		50	**25**	**8**	**17**

Histopathological classification and areomedical disposition of intracranial neoplams, N = 50. Abbreviations: Waiv: a waiver was granted; Pend: temporarily unfit, decision still pending, Unfit: permanently unfit.

brain tumors. These tumors carry a poor prognosis with short survival time. Most often they are diagnosed late in the course of the disease. For this reason, the affected pilots may still be flying while unaware of their progressive malignant brain tumors.

Case 16: Over a period of several months, a 32-year-old helicopter pilot, a good sportsman and dedicated to many social activities, became socially isolated and gave up one kind of sport after the other. He went to his aeromedical examiner, complaining of headaches, fatigue, and impairment of concentration and initiative "for some time." The aeromedical examiner noticed a ptosis, and the pilot was referred to our hospital. One day before admission, the pilot had flown passenger flights. We diagnosed a large glioblastoma in the right frontal lobe with surrounding edema and mass effect with ventricular obstruction. The pilot died four months later in spite of all available therapies.

Benign Tumors

Among the benign tumors, meningeomas and acoustic neuromas deserve some special remarks. Meningeomas usually present with seizures (in about 80% of cases); they can often be removed completely without neurological deficits, and seizures cease after removal. Thus, pilots with meningeomas can often be recertificated (in our series, 12 out of 15 cases). This does not apply to the rare cases where, due to personal indolence, the tumors reach the size of an orange and cause pressure-related deficits. Acoustic neuromas (vestibular schwannomas) represent about 6% of all intracranial tumors. They are benign, slow-growing tumors, which arise from cells in the sheaths that surround the vestibulocochlear nerve. The neuromas usually manifest themselves as one-sided hearing impairment, which may go ignored by the patient or be dismissed by the doctor. Continued growth of these neuromas ultimately results in compression of the brainstem due to raised intracranial pressure. About 90% of patients experience gradual, progressive hearing loss in one ear. However, about 5% experience a sudden hearing loss.

Many (about 70%) experience tinnitus in one ear. However, about 3% of patients with acoustic neuromas will have normal hearing at presentation. The incidence of acoustic neuromas is around 13 cases/million/year, and a recent radiological study found seven unsuspected acoustic neuromas per 10 000 brain MRI studies — equivalent to 700 cases in a population of one million.[25] There are three management options: interval scanning, surgical removal, or radiotherapy. Interval scanning with no intervention (watchful waiting) may be considered, at least in the short term, for patients with a small neuroma and good hearing. For intracanalicular neuromas, an observation period between scans of approximately one year may be appropriate as there is evidence that some of these neuromas cease to grow, at least in the short term.[26] Growth in the first year following diagnosis is predictive of later neuroma enlargement.[27] All patients being managed conservatively should be reviewed by annual imaging, to look for neuroma growth. It should be kept in mind that interval scanning bears the risk of complications like facial palsy or hearing loss. Therefore, in our opinion, early surgical removal — especially by an experienced neurosurgeon — is the treatment of choice and should be offered to the majority of patients with acoustic neuromas. Complete neuroma removal is achievable in over 95% of cases. Operative mortality in experienced centers is less than 1%, the risk being slightly greater with larger neuromas. Permanent facial paralysis, either partial or complete, remains the greatest single source of disability following neuroma removal; those patients with large neuromas are at greatest risk of this complication.

If there are contraindications against surgery, stereotactic radio-surgery and fractionated stereotactic radiotherapy may be considered: Small and medium-sized neuromas up to 3.0 cm in diameter are considered potential candidates for radiotherapy. All patients who undergo radiotherapy must submit to serial scanning for the rest of their lives or until neuroma growth ceases. No controlled studies exist to show that radiotherapy is better than no treatment. Concern exists about treating benign lesions, such as acoustic neuromas, with radiation, especially in the absence of tissue diagnosis. The long-term risks of such complications as brainstem ischemia and injury to cranial nerves (such as the facial nerve) are uncertain. Aeromedical disposition: Recertification is possible if there are no or acceptable neurological deficits. In our experience, most pilots prefer watchful waiting or radiotherapy, because these treatment options do not affect the fitness to fly in the short term. We have no experience with long-term results of radiotherapy in pilots.

PARAPLEGIC PILOTS

Paraplegia

In industrialized nations, the incidence of acute traumatic paraplegia is estimated at 20 to 50 per 1 000 000 and year. Some of these handicapped persons may have an astonishing performance ability, which can be seen at the paralympics.

In recent years we have been asked for specialist evaluation of 41 paraplegic patients applying for PPL. 36 were of traumatic origin, and five cases were neurodegenerative or tumorous. Until 1988, these pilots would have been considered unfit in Germany (and still are in many other countries today), even to fly without passengers. The reason was that a handicapped person might be unable to save himself in case of an accident. In 1972, the "International Wheelchair Aviators" (IWA), the first association of handicapped pilots, was founded in the USA. It was followed by the "Delta Foxtrot" (Disabled Flyers) in the United Kingdom and by the "Interessengemeinschaft luftsporttreibender Behinderter e.V." (Rolliflieger) in 1993 in Germany. These associations are devoted to helping persons with physical handicaps obtain a pilot's licence. They also mediate an exchange of experience between handicapped and non-handicapped pilots, give advice on the development of technical means to compensate for various handicaps, and provide assistance to applicants in aeromedical cases.

In the community of aeromedical examiners, it is still disputed whether paraplegic pilots can be certificated to fly. However, our experience with steadily increasing accumulated flight time by handicapped pilots is positive. Up to now, there has been no serious incident or accident attributed to a pilot's handicap. Of course, our specialist evaluations represent a selected group of paraplegic persons. All were socially integrated, most of them working full-time and holding a driver's licence. The average age was 38 years, and the time between the onset of the disease and application for medical certification was 11 years on average. Most of them had pretraumatic flying experience, and they all applied for PPL only. Most lesions were in the thoracic spinal cord and in five cases in the cervical cord. 22 handicapped applicants suffered from neurogenic bladder dysfunction, but they were able to carry out intermittent self-catheterization without complications. Besides the absence of secondary complications, another important criterion was stability in the sitting position and a sufficient function of the muscles of shoulder, arm, and hand to operate aircraft in which also rudder and brakes were converted to manual control. In seven out of 41 pilots (17%), a restricted medical certification could not be recommended. The reasons for not recommending certification were: weakness in muscles of the hand and arm due to high cervical lesions in two cases, additional traumatic brain injury with neuropsychological deficits in two cases, additional functional monocularity in one case, and in two cases, infiltrating growth of a partially resected astrocytoma. Myelopathies, relapsing or progressive demyelinating lesions, or progressive neoplastic growth of extramedullary or intramedullary tumors are conditions for which certification usually cannot be recommended. Sometimes, the recommendation not to issue a certificate leads to legal actions. The applicant then learns the rationale for the specialist's recommendation and, although formerly positive-minded, self-confident and motivated, now develops anxious self-observation and fear of the future. This is an aspect of the appeal's procedure of which all aeromedical examiners should be aware. Furthermore, we assessed eight pilots with amputations. We recommended certification in cases where the functional deficit was adequately compensated with a prosthetic device.

Manual Control

In accordance with ICAO Standards and Recommended Practices in Annex 1 — Personnel Licensing, JAR-FCL 3 has made it easy to assess the medical fitness of handicapped applicants. The applicant should not have any abnormality within the musculosceletal system that might affect flight safety. A new development is that the applicant has the opportunity to prove by a practical test that he is able to compensate safely for his handicap. Technical aids, such as certified manual controls, are expressively permitted. There is certified equipment that can be retrofitted in some gliders and some types of flying vehicles in the E- and K-Class. Conversion is rather fast, so these types can be flown with normal controls, too. During conversion, landing flaps can be fixed stepwise, and the movements of the rudder with pedals are replaced by a forward and backward movement of a hand-held lever. Regrettably this kind of equipment does not work in the same way in gliders and motor planes, so there can be adjustment problems for pilots who fly both gliders and motor planes. In the cases we describe, receiving certification and the joy of flying contributed to the self-esteem and social integration of these persons. From our experience, and international experience, this kind of "therapeutic flying" should be advocated whenever compatible with flight safety.

STROKE

Incidence

As cerebrovascular and cardiovascular pathology is often interrelated (see the Cardiology chapters), 80% of strokes are ischemic, while 20% are due to intracerebral hemorrhage. Of the latter, about a quarter is due to subarachnoid haemorrhage, with the other 75% being due to primary intracerebral hemorrhage. Hemorrhages due to vascular malformations and aneurysms have already been reviewed. We now focus on cerebral ischemia, represented by 44 cases, i.e., 8% of our case series. We had only one intracranial hemorrhage due to hypertension. In industrialized nations, after coronary artery disease and cancer, stroke is the third leading cause of death and the leading cause of premature disability.[1] Incidence depends on age, gender, and race-ethnicity, and was estimated at 200–350/100 000 in industrialized countries, with a prevalence of approximately 600/100 000.[1] Cerebral ischemic events are classified by anatomic location, size of blood vessels (small and large vessel disease), duration of deficit, and mechanism (cardioembolic, atherosclerotic, lacunar). The recognition and reduction of risk factors is the most effective method to prevent stroke. Risk factors may be modifiable or non-modifiable and vary with age and race. In young adults trauma, drugs, oral contraceptives, migraine, and spontaneous arterial dissection are the most common cause of ischemic stroke. In older patients (>55 years) hypertension, prior stroke or TIAs, coronary artery disease, congestive heart failure, and diabetes are important risk factors. Smoking, obesity, increased fibrinogen level, family history of premature death from stroke, and excessive alcohol use are also recognized as risk factors. Studies show that atrial fibrillation is associated with a six-fold increased risk for stroke. In our experiene, the influence of chronic alcohol intake in socially accepted dosages on hypertension is underestimated.[28–31]

In aviators, the incidence and prevalence of stroke in the older age groups is lower than in the general population. This might be due to a preventive effect of the periodical medical examinations ('healthy worker effect').

Aeromedical Disposition

Stroke is a disqualifying condition. Certification may be possible, if the outcome is good (without any or with very minor neurological and neuropsychological deficits), and if the recurrence rate in the individual case is low. In our case series, we could recommend a restricted certification only in eight cases. In what follows, we focus on a discussion of the recurrence rate and on measures of secondary prevention, which should be included in the review process. Recurrent stroke is not infrequent. In ischemic stroke, the risk of recurrence may be as high as 10–12% in the first year and 5–8%

yearly thereafter, with a cumulative risk of up to 30–40% in five years. 15% of these patients will have a myocardial infarction and a similar proportion will die as a consequence of vascular disease.[31,32] More than 75% of secondary ischemic events (such as myocardial infarction, ischemic stroke, or vascular death) are strokes.[33] In non-aneurysmal brain hemorrhage, the risk of recurrence following the initial hemorrhage is 3–7% after one year and 19% after five years.[34] The immediate post-stroke period carries the greater risk of early recurrence. In the Stroke Data Bank 3.3% patients with infarcts had an early recurrence within 30, accounting for 30% of recurrent strokes in the following two years.[35] The rate of stroke recurrence varies for stroke subtypes, being higher in patients with cardio-embolic stroke and those with stroke due to high-grade carotid stenosis than in patients with lacunar stroke or moderate to minimal carotid stenosis (Fig. 5).

Whilst a second stroke is most often caused by the same mechanism as the first stroke, some patients will have strokes of a different etiology.[34] Patients with cardio-embolic stroke are most likely to have recurrent stroke from the heart; there is a lower frequency of same etiology recurrence in those in whom the initial stroke was due to arterial emboli, hemorrhage or lacunar infarction. In patients with cerebral infarction, 5% of recurrent strokes will be hemorrhagic, whilst in those with intracebral hemorrhage, 42% of recurrences will be ischemic. Also the territory of the recurrent stroke is not always the same.[34] The mechanism of recurrent ischemic events may well be different from the index event, because the risk factors that predispose to different subtypes of cerebral ischemia are largely similar. Transient cerebral or ocular ischemic attacks (TIA) are a strong predictor of subsequent stroke.[36] The risk of stroke is highest during the first few days after a TIA. The 90-day risk of ipsilateral stroke is 20.1%, while the two-day risk is 5.5%. Most ischemic strokes, regardless of duration, are athero-embolic in origin and a manifestation of more widespread vascular disease, which might comprise large-artery occlusive disease, including the aorta and the coronary arteries, with resulting atrial fibrillation. About half of all patients are hypertensive. Recurrent stroke may therefore be caused by coexistent

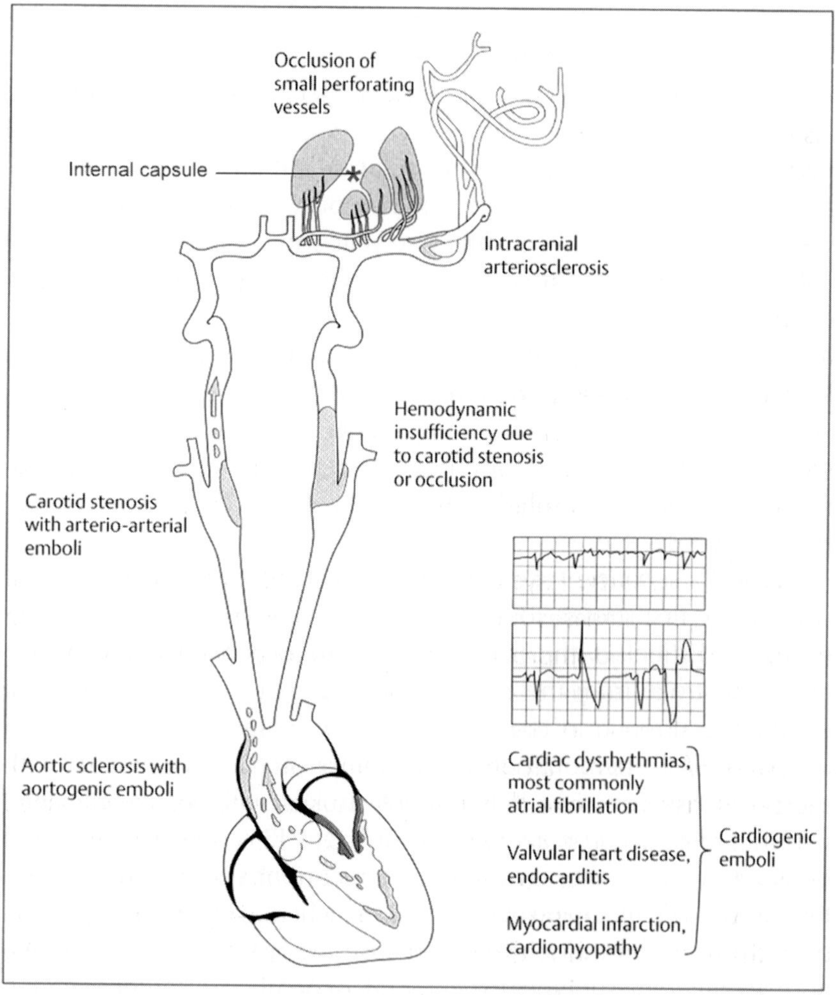

Figure 5. The most important etiologies of cerebral infarction: cardiovascular emboli; arterio-arterial emboli; atherosclerosis; stenosis and occlusion; vasculopathies and dysrhythmias. Modified after Ref.1 with kind permission of the authors and the publisher.

pathology present at the time of the index event but not etiologically related to that event.

Thus, certification should be dependent on a detailed specialist evaluation of the individual case after an appropriate observation time (usually in the magnitude of one year) that should include a statement about stroke classification and recurrence rate. Certification should not be unconditional, but bound to lifestyle and risk factor modification. In practice there is a continuum between primary and secondary prevention, but it should be pointed out clearly to the pilots that the absolute benefit of lifestyle and risk factor modification is likely to be much larger in those who are at high risk after having had a stroke than in those without symptomatic vascular disease.

Tobacco smoking: Smoking increases the risk of stroke by a factor of 1.5 to three. In people who smoke less than 20 cigarettes a day, cessation decreases the risk of stroke to the level of non-smokers. Cessation by those who smoke more than this also reduces the risk of stroke, though their risk remains higher than that of non-smokers.[37]

Physical activity: Physical activity favorably influences vascular risk factors: it decreases blood pressure, helps patients to maintain normal weight, and improves glucose tolerance. Moderate exercise, at least 30 minutes per day, decreases the risk of a first stroke, but there is no evidence of the effect on recurrent stroke.

Alcohol: Heavy alcohol consumption is associated with increased risk of stroke.[38] It is controversial whether middle-aged people, drinking one or two drinks (i.e., between 10 and 30 g ethanol) daily have a lower risk of stroke than non-drinkers.[39,40] People who do not drink should not be encouraged to do so; however, those who do should be encouraged to drink no more than the appropriate amount, i.e., as little as possible.[41]

Diet: High dietary salt intake contributes to blood pressure elevation and hypertension. Increasing the dietary intake of potassium containing food such as fruits and vegetables potentiate the effect of lowering dietary salt intake. Limitation of saturated fatty acids in the diet may also lower blood pressure and be of benefit to the lipid profile.[38] Whilst evidence would suggest that elevated blood homocysteine increases the risk of stroke,[42] there is no evidence available as to whether dietary supplementation with vitamins B6, B12, and folic acid might prevent stroke.[43]

Blood pressure: Elevated blood pressure increases the relative risk of stroke by four to five times. Systolic hypertension (>140 mmHg) and diastolic hypertension (>95 mmHg) are independent risk factors for stroke.[38,44,45] In 17 world-wide trials of blood pressure reduction involving nearly 50000 patients, a 38% reduction in risk of all strokes and a 40% reduction in fatal strokes followed antihypertensive treatment.[46] The target of antihypertensive treatment is to achieve normal levels of systolic and diastolic blood pressure, i.e., systolic blood pressure <140 mmHg and diastolic blood pressure <90 mmHg; the recommended maximum level is <150/90 mmHg.[47–49] There have been fewer data confirming the role of blood pressure lowering treatment in secondary stroke prevention.[50] However, the recent PROGRESS trial demonstrated that against a background of standard treatment blood pressure reduction, a flexible regime with an ACE inhibitor (perindopril) and a diuretic (indapamide) was beneficial and reduced the risk of stroke by 28% over four years.[51] The target level of blood pressure control in the secondary stroke prevention has not been precisely defined by PROGRESS, though benefit was present even in patients who at baseline were not hypertensive (as defined in the study) or had blood pressure less than 140/85 mmHg. It appears that the lower the pressure, the lower the risk of stroke.

Dyslipidemia: High levels of cholesterol, LDL cholesterol, triglycerides, and low concentration of HDL cholesterol are independent risk factors of coronary artery disease. Meta-analysis of clinical trials of reductase HMG-CoA inhibitors (statins) has shown that their use in people with unstable coronary artery disease and a history of myocardial infarction is associated with a 30% reduction in stroke incidence.[52,53] The largest studies have been done with the use of simvastatin and pravastatin, but other statins may have a similar effect. Dietary modification or the use of fibrates has not proved to be effective. As yet specific data on the secondary preventive effect of statins in patients with stroke or TIA are available mainly from the stroke subgroup of a large, randomized, placebo-controlled study (Heart Protection Study, HPS) of high-risk patients.[54] The result in the stroke subgroup is similar to the overall result of the trial: about one-quarter reduction of a combined end-point of serious vascular events (including stroke) and revascularization.[55] The benefits were additional to those of existing treatments, and there were no substantial safety concerns. Statins are now widely used in patients with stroke. Their use should be considered mainly in patients with coronary heart disease, atherosclerotic changes in carotid or peripheral arteries, high level of cholesterol, and diabetes.

Antiplatelet drugs: Acetylsalicylic acid (Aspirin7) or another oral antiplatelet drug is protective in most types of patients at increased risk of occlusive vascular events, including those with stroke. Late stroke prevention: Antiplatelet drugs reduce the risk of late stroke recurrence and other vascular events. Treatment of 1000 patients for three years after stroke resulted in 36 fewer serious vascular events per 1000 patients. This benefit reflects a significant reduction in non-fatal stroke (25 fewer/1000), non-fatal myocardial infarction (six fewer/1000), vascular mortality (seven fewer/1000), and the reduction in mortality (15 fewer deaths/1000).[56] As it is the most cost-effective antiplatelet drug, acetylsalicylic acid is most widely used. Gastro-intestinal side effects are dose related, whereas bleeding complications are not related to dose. Acetylsalicylic acid in doses of 75–150 mg daily is an effective antiplatelet regimen for long-term use.[56] Other antiplatelet drugs available include ticlopidine, clopidogrel, and dipyridamole.

Carotid surgery: The efficacy of endarterectomy of the carotid artery in secondary stroke prevention was demonstrated in two large, randomized trials: ECST and NASCET for patients with carotid territory TIA or non-disabling stroke during the last six months and a severe stenosis of the ipsilateral carotid artery.[57–61] The pooled analysis confirmed that the benefit was substantial in 70–99% of symptomatic stenosis of the carotid artery, with an absolute risk reduction of 16.0%, corresponding to a number needed to treat (NNT) of six to prevent one ipsilateral stroke or any stroke or surgical death.[58] The benefit of surgery was modest in patients with 50–69% stenosis, with an NNT of 24 to prevent one ipsilateral stroke, or 14 to prevent one stroke of any origin or death. There was no benefit for patients with 30–49% stenosis, and surgery was harmful for patients with <30%

stenosis. Carotid angioplasty with stenting has up to now not convincingly been proven to be an alternative to the use of carotid endarterectomy. Carotid surgery in primary prevention is indicated only for 70–99% stenosis and provides only a small beneficial effect compared with best medical treatment. Oral anticoagulants have not been reviewed here because they cause medical unfitness *per se*.

INFLAMMATORY DISORDERS OF THE CENTRAL NERVOUS SYSTEM

Multiple Sclerosis

Our case series contains 14 cases of multiple sclerosis (MS). MS is best understood as an immune-mediated disease that affects the central nervous system's white matter and is the leading cause of neurological disability in the western hemisphere. Onset of the disease peaks between the ages of 20 and 30. The incidence of MS increases with latitude in moderate climates. The risk of developing the disease correlates with the latitude at which one lived before the age of 15 years. There is a familial predisposition for its development; women are more affected than men and whites more than blacks or Asians. Approximately 80% of patients will have relapsing-remitting MS, while 20% follow a primary progressive course. Of the patients with relapsing-remitting disease, 50% will develop secondary progressive MS. Clinical features cover a broad spectrum and include fatigue, limb weakness, spasticity, hyperreflexia, paresthesias, Lhermitte's sign (barber's chair phenomenon), ataxia, tremor, nystagmus, vertigo, optic neuritis, internuclear ophthalmoplegia, bowel or bladder dysfunction, depression, emotional lability, and cognitive abnormalities. The diagnosis is made on clinical grounds and is supported by radiological (MRI) and laboratory studies (CSF analysis). Treatment options include methylprednisolon for acute relapses and beta interferon or glatiramer acetate or intravenously applied gamma-globulins to reduce the frequency of relapses and the formation of new lesions. Favorable prognostic factors include relapsing-remitting disease at onset, younger age of onset, opticus neuritis or sensory symptoms at onset, high degree of remission, and few functional systems involved. In long-term studies of MRI as a predictor of outcome, the extent of imaging abnormalities detected at initial presentation of an isolated clinical syndrome suggestive of MS (such as opticus neuritis) provided information regarding the potential development of MS. There is a significant and positive correlation between the number of new or enlarging lesions on MRI and clinical disability over two to three years.[62,63]

Aeromedical Disposition

Restricted medical certification is possible early in the course of the disease, after complete recovery of the first or second relapse. Close observation at short intervals is necessary, and a multi-crew restriction is indicated. New relapses may be incapacitating, but almost never evolve paroxysmally. After complete remission, a new attack usually takes at least 24 to 48 hours to develop. In view of the usual course of the disease, it should be pointed out to the pilot that certification cannot be guaranteed in the long-term. However, we have seen some cases with a minor deficit stable for many years, which was compatible with certification, including airline pilots. Given the fact that the cause of MS remains unknown, there has been an extensive search for risk factors for the development of the disease. These suspected "risk factors" include trauma, stress, specific environmental exposures such as cold temperature, infections, diet, pregnancy, and breast-feeding. Up to now, there is no conclusive result, but it is possible, that a number of unspecific agents could trigger MS in genetically susceptible individuals. We have no reasons to believe that flying *per se* could be such a trigger.

Infections

Here, we focus on meningitis, brain abscesses, and encephalitis. These conditions deal with inflammation of the brain related to infectious, post-infectious, or demyelinating states. Encephalitis can occur as an acute febrile illness associated with headache, seizures, lethargy, confusion, coma, ocular motor palsies, ataxia, abnormal movements, and myoclonus. Alternatively, it may present as a slowly progressive, afebrile disease. Prognosis depends on the causative agent and the use of antiviral agents. Variable degrees of residua include impaired cognition and memory, behavioral changes, hemiparesis, and seizures.

The most common cause of fatal viral encephalitis in the western world is herpes simplex encephalitis (HSV type I), but there are also arthropod-transmitted epidemic encephalitis, immune-deficient related encephalitis, and non-viral causes as prion infections, rickettsia, bacteria, etc., and post-infectious encephalomyelitis. We present a case of herpes simplex encephalitis.

Case 17: After a flight, a 50-year-old captain with more than 12 600 flying hours experienced a slight illness with headache, dizziness, lethargy and fever. Symptoms improved, and he decided to drive home from the airport. Although he obviously knew the way well, he could not find his home. He phoned his spouse who gave him directions, and he tried to follow her instructions. Shortly after, he was found sitting in his car, confused and restless. He was admitted to a near-by neurological clinic with memory deficits and sensory aphasia. CSF-analysis and MRI were performed. MRI showed increased signal intensity in the medial and inferior temporal lobe, particularly on the left side. A diagnosis of herpes simplex encephalitis (HSV type 1) was made and treatment with aciclovir was started immediately. Diagnosis was confirmed by lymphocytic pleocytosis and positive PCR. Acute treatment and rehabilitation led to complete recovery of the sensory aphasia and improvement of the cognitive deficits, but problems with learning new information remained. EEG recordings showed no focal slowing or interictal epileptic activity. After an observation period of two years there were still memory deficits, and therefore recertification could not be recommended.

HIV and AIDS

AIDS is caused by the retrovirus HIV (human immunodeficiency virus). Neurological manifestations at any level of the neuraxis at any stage of infection are seen and can be a result of direct HIV infection, HIV-induced immune dysregulation, or opportunistic infections. In early HIV infection, HIV meningoencephalitis can accompany the syndrome of viral infection, resulting in self-limited encephalopathy. In midstage HIV-infection, HIV meningitis can recur at any point and may remain asymptomatic. In late HIV infection (CD4 count <200/μL), neurological complications include focal brain lesions caused by cerebral toxoplasmosis, primary CNS lymphoma, progressive multifocal encephalopathy, fungal abscesses, tumors, and stroke, in addition to cryptoccocal meningitis, syphilitic meningitis, tuberculous meningitis, and HIV encephalopathy. Neurological manifestations of late HIV infection are always a bar to medical certification. In early HIV infection without any kind of neurological deficit, close observation is necessary. It is often a problem that the time of infection cannot be determined, thus the length of the time interval up to clinical manifestations is difficult to estimate. On the basis of case-by-case decisions, some pilots may be given restricted certification but close follow-ups are mandatory.

HEADACHE AND MIGRAINE

Unrecorded Cases, Symptomatology

Headache is extremely common. The lifetime prevalence of headache (any kind), migraine, and tension-type headache has been estimated as 93%, 8%, and 69% respectively for men, and 99%, 25%, and 88% respectively for women. The prevalence of tension-type headache decreases with increasing age, whereas migraine shows no correlation to age. The brain itself is not sensitive to pain. Headache develops with irritation of pain sensitive structures, i.e., the large vessels of the brain, the basal dura and pia, the sinus, and the cranial nerves. A current hypothesis claims that the pulsating headache during a migraine attack originates from the inflamed and dilated walls of dural vessels.

Epidemiological and twin studies indicate that migraine, in particular migraine with aura, is an inherited disease. Multiple genes, however, must be involved. Migraine is characterized by unilateral, pulsating, moderate to severe headache, often increasing with physical acitivity and helped by sleep. Migraine may be preceded or accompanied by auras, most commonly visual fortification spectra, scintillating scotomas, or flashes of light (photopsias). Migraine subtypes include those with aura (classic, complicated, opthalmic, hemiparesthetic, hemiplegic, or aphasic) and without aura (common migraine), ophthalmoplegic migraine (most commonly complete oculomotor palsy), retinal migraine, and basilar migraine. Aura symptoms develop within minutes and last usually less than one hour. Occasionally, migraines may be pure acephalalgic auras (migraine sine hemicrania), but these may require investigation to rule out other intracranial processes.

Migraine is a highly prevalent illness that remains substantially under-diagnosed, both in primary care and in aviation medicine. Diagnosis is made exclusively by history. For this reason, migraine is probably the diagnosis with the highest number of unrecorded cases in aviation medicine. Additional investigations (EEG, neuro-imaging, etc.) only serve to rule out other intracranial processes. We have already pointed out that a strictly unilateral migraine that does not change side within the time course of the disease, should be carefully investigated to rule out vascular malformations. Complicated migraines, like ophthalmoplegic ones or those with focal neurological syndromes are often symptomatic, i.e., caused by vascular malformation, etc.

Treatment of Migraine

Headache therapy involves three components: Psychological (reassurance and counseling, stress management, relaxation therapy), physical (identifying headache triggers such as diet, hormone variations, stress), and pharmacotherapy. A headache calendar documenting the occurrence, severity and duration of headaches, the type and efficacy of medication taken, and triggering factors should be recorded by the patient. Pharmacotherapy can be divided in two approaches, symptomatic and prophylactic. Treating the migraine attack: Mild to moderate migraine attacks should be treated by analgesics or non-steroidal anti-inflammatory drugs (NSAIDs), either alone or in combination with an anti-emetic drug. The new class of COX-2 inhibitors is not superior to non-steroidal anti-inflammatory drugs in the treatment of migraine attacks. Acetylsalicylic acid (Aspirin) should be taken in doses between 500 and 1000 mg. Paracetamol (acetaminophen) is available as tablets, suppositories and drops. The usual dose is 1000 mg. Ibuprofen, naproxen, or diclofenac can be used for the treatment of a migraine attack. Other frequently used NSAIDs are indomethacin, flubiprofen, ketoprofen, and tolfenamic acid. Metamizol is effective in doses between 500 and 1000 mg and has a good tolerability. Many patients are nauseated during a migraine attack. Therefore, the use of antiemetics (metoclopramide or domperidone) is indicated. In addition, these drugs speed up the gastrointestinal absorption of many analgesics and ergots. Antiemetics can either be taken some time before analgesics or at the same time. Moderate or severe migraine attacks should be treated with specific migraine drugs.[64] These include ergot alkaloids (also called ergots), and triptans. Migraine "specific" means that these drugs only work in migraine (and in cluster headache), but not in tension type headache or other pains like tooth pain or general pain. Ergotamine and dihydroergotamine (DHE) have been available for a long time. Ergots are less effective than most of the triptans and can cause nausea and vomiting as a side effect.[65] They have vasoconstrictive properties and are therefore contraindicated in uncontrolled hypertension, coronary heart disease, peripheral vascular disease, cerebro-vascular disease (stroke and TIA), hepatic or renal disease, and during pregnancy.

Severe migraine attacks that disable the patient should be treated with a triptan (sumatriptan, zolmitriptan, naratriptan, rizatriptan etc). About 20–30% of patients are non-responders to triptans. Triptans may have a peripheral mode of action and will not be effective once central sensitization has taken place, i.e., they should be administered before allodynia of the head or face develops. Prevention of migraine: Established drugs for the prevention of migraine include betablockers (e.g., propranolol, metoprolol), flunarizine, valproic acid, and tricyclic antidepressants. The variety of effective drugs indicates that the mode of action of drugs used for migraine prophylaxis is unknown.

Case 18: During a holiday period, a 32-year-old FO with a positive family history for migraine developed an attack with aura. A sudden speech arrest was followed by repetition of syllables. Language understanding and perception was not impaired. After 30 minutes, a severe pulsating headache in the fronto-temporal region with nausea, photophobia, and phonophobia developed, lasting for several hours. The attacks recurred three to four times a week, aphasia became weaker, but paresthesia developed in the right arm. Neuro-imaging (MRI, MRA) and EEG were normal. Preventive treatment with propanolol was stopped by the patient after four months. Stress management and muscle relaxation were supportive. A continuous therapy with acetylsalicylic acid was finally sucessful. Recertification was recommended.

Aeromedical Disposition

In five Class 1 pilots, we did not recommend recertification due to hemianopia during the aura and inadequate effect of pharmacotherapy. In one case, a binocular central scotoma developed in flight during the final approach. In general, we recommend recertification if the frequency of the attacks is low and if the attacks (inlcuding the aura) can safely be controlled by pharmacotherapy without significant side effects. A multi-crew restriction is necessary. We are very reluctant to recommend certification for single-pilot operations. This reduces the room for certification of general aviation pilots. Furthermore, migraine patients often do not habituate on repeating sensory stimuli, making them prone to airsickness.

PARKINSON'S DISEASE

Diagnosis and Clinical Course

Parkinson's disease (paralysis agitans) is a progressive movement disorder resulting from defective neurotransmission of dopamine in the basal ganglia. The neurodegenerative process is characterized by a triad of symptoms: Tremor at rest, rigidity (cogwheel rigidity), and bradykinesia (slowness of movements).

Frequently the onset is unilateral but the course is variable. In some cases, resting tremor ("pill-rolling tremor", 4–7 Hz) as hemitremor may be the first and only symptom for some time.

The symptoms of the triad may start in different combinations and sequences. Relatively modest limitations may progress to complete invalidism.

The diagnosis is clinical. Cases with slow and modest symptomatology need time and follow-ups to ensure the diagnosis.

Case 19: A 50-year-old captain underwent orthopedic treatment for about two years. First then his back pain, related to the vertebral column, could be diagnosed as Parkinson's disease with pronounced axial rigidity.

In most cases rigidity is pronounced in arms and hands due to increased muscle tone simultaneously in the extensor and flexor muscles. Besides rigidity, the motor system is affected by bradykinesia, especially by reduced self-initiation of movements as indicated by passive behavior. The clinical presentation may also show reduced mimic movements progressing to mask-like face, slow and hypophonic speech, reduced size of fine motor activities leading to micrography, forward flexed posture, walking with reduced arm swing, shuffling gait, and, in the later course, postural instability.

Rather often, the patients develop autonomic dysfunctions, e.g., orthostatic hypotension or impaired thermoregulation, with sometimes pronounced sweating, especially at night.

From an aeromedical point of view, attention should be paid to cognitive impairment, in some cases with later manifestation of dementia. Depressive and anxious symptomatology is likely to get worse. Cognitive dysfunctions and depression may even precede the neurological diagnosis.

The onset of Parkinson's disease peaks in the sixth decade, but much earlier onset is possible. The colorful bundle of symptoms, in varying interacting combinations, and the need for treatment make close cooperation between the aeromedical examiner and a neurologist necessary.

Differential Diagnoses and Treatment

Impaired eye movements, severe dysautonomic features, cerebellar symptoms, ataxia, dyskinesia, etc., make a precise differential diagnosis necessary. Before medical treatment is commenced, Parkinson's-plus syndrome and other neurodegenerative diseases should be excluded.

Treatment remains symptomatic and combines physiotherapy and medication. The individual medication is age-related and depends on the clinical picture and the progression of the disease. All medications used (levodopa, dopamine agonists, anticholinergic drugs, COMT inhibitors, MAO B inhibitors, etc.) bear the risk of side effects, such as drowsiness, unexpectedly falling asleep during daytime activities, confusion, blurred vision, dyskinesia, and even psychotic reactions with visual hallucinations.

For detailed information and staging and rating scales, see neurology textbooks.

Aeromedical Disposition

Only cases with little impairment and slowly progressive symptoms without side effects of treatment may be considered for medical certification and only on a case-to-case basis. Re-examinations and follow-ups are mandatory to assure that flight safety is not endangered.

ARACHNOID CYSTS

Risks of Arachnoid Cysts in Aviation Medicine

Arachnoid cysts are cavities within the subarachnoid space, filled with cerebrospinal fluid. They can be diagnosed radiologically as cystic expansions of the subarachnoid space with a smooth, sharp demarcation. The content of the cyst is homogeneous with the same signal intensity as cerebrospinal fluid. Our series contains 13 pilots with arachnoid cysts, corresponding to 2% of our neurological diagnoses in aviation medicine. However, these cases are significant, because they represent intracranial time bombs just like the aforementioned vascular malformations. Ten of these cases had cysts in the medial cranial fossa, while two cysts were infratentorial and led to aplasia of the ipsilateral cerebellar hemisphere and to displacement of the brain stem. The affected pilot suffered from vertigo and ataxia, which subsided after surgery; recertification was recommended. The residual 11 cases, presenting predominantly with complex focal seizures, remained permanently disqualified.

Prevalence, Clinical Symptoms and Signs

We conducted a large ($N = 1772$) prospective MRI trial in healthy young applicants for military flying in the German Air Force and found a prevalence of arachnoid cysts of 1.5% (= 27/1772, 95% confidence interval 1.0% to 2.2%).[14] This was confirmed by a later study in the same population, which showed a prevalence of 1.7%.[19] As described in the literature, arachnoid cysts were usually found in the temporal fossa (22/27) and more on the left than on the right side (14/8). All were unilateral. The prevalence was confirmed by an even larger retrospective study on MRIs and CTs of neurological and psychiatric patients. Here, we found a prevalence of 1.8% (= 142/7705; 95% CI 1.5% to 2.2%).

Arachnoid cysts are considered a disorder of leptomeningeal development; the arachnoid top layers of the temporal and parietal lobe do not merge and form a non-communicating liquid compartment that is entirely surrounded by arachnoid membrane. Depending on the size of the cyst, it is associated with a more or less expressed hypoplasia or aplasia of the ipsilateral temporal lobe. Arachnoid cysts are usually described as purely incidental findings without any pathological significance and that may be correct for the majority of the findings. On the other hand, there are many case reports arguing in favor of a pathogenic potential of these cysts, but there is always a discussion about whether pathological findings in carriers of arachnoid cysts are purely coincidental. There is no classic symptomatology besides the tendency to provoke seizures. Symptoms can be related to the cysts themselves (tendency to subdural hematoma in minor traumatic head injury, epileptic fits through pressure on adjacent brain substance, grouped rhythmic discharges in the EEG, headache) or to the maldeveloped temporal lobe. Cognitive deficits include impaired learning and memory, attention deficits, and personality disorders. Also psychiatric disorders, including paranoid psychosis, can be seen. However, there are no known predictors for the development of a neuropsychiatric problem in a carrier of an asymptomatic arachnoid cyst. We present the case of a 45-year-old captain with a longstanding asymptomatic cyst.

Case 20: A 45-year-old pilot with more than 12000 flying hours developed affective lability, increased irritability, and aggressiveness on trivial occasions that could be compensated in the professional, but not in familial environment. The familial conflict was amplified by imperative, often incomprehensible orders to the family. The pilot, however, often did not even remember these orders. After a dispute with his wife, a divorce was initiated. Due to his strange behavior, a psychiatric investigation was carried out on the lawyer's advice. A large temporal arachnoid cyst with aplasia of the anterior aspects of the temporal lobe was found, additional to memory disorder and frequent psychomotor attacks with consecutive amnesia. Spikes and sharp waves in the temporal region of the EEG-recording confirmed interictal epileptiform activity. Neuropsychological assessment showed slow cerebration with impaired learning, attentiveness, and information processing. Retrospectively, it was astonishing that all these impairments could be compensated for such a long time in the professional environment. Recertification was not recommended.

Intracranial Hemorrhage

Another major problem in arachnoid cysts is their proneness to develop intracranial, in particular subdural, hemorrhages after minor head injury.

In Fig. 6, the upper row illustrates this with an impressive example. In this case, the pilot hit his head against the edge of a door while playing with his daughter. He had only brief pain, no skin contusion and no impairment of consciousness; he continued playing.

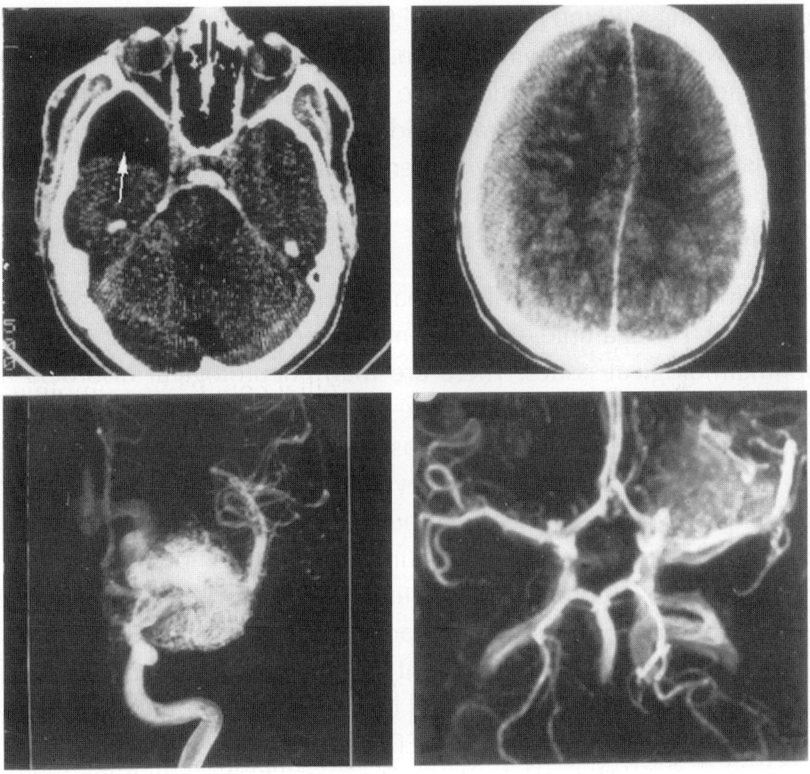

Figure 6. Upper left: Arachnoid cyst (arrow) loco typico with hypoplasia of the temporal lobe pole. Upper right: Subdural hematoma following minor head injury of the same patient. Notice increased intracranial pressure with midline shift. Lower row: Arteriovenous angioma (AVA — Case 14). Left: Angiography. Right: Magnetic Resonance Angiography (MRA): Feeding of AVA by the middle cerebral artery.

Aeromedical Disposition

Pilots with symptomatic arachnoid cysts are unfit. In our case series, one case presented with recurring nystagmus and double vision. Another two showed marked impairment of learning and concentration and general slowing with a drop in efficiency as the presenting symptom. Eight pilots were Class 1. In pilots with incidental asymptomatic arachnoid cysts, our current aeromedical policy is to consider recertification of those pilots who have no additional abnormal findings in monitoring-MRI (no progress), EEG and neuropsychological testing, usually with a multicrew restriction. If we obtain an abnormal finding in the additional investigations, we classify the pilot as unfit. The relative large prevalence of arachnoid cysts (>1%) is another argument for MRI screening of military fighter pilots and astronauts.

CONCLUSIONS

Neurology has an interdisciplinary orientation towards aviation medicine. For example, there are many neuro-otological and neuro-ophthalmological issues. There are many neurological disorders in the daily work of the internist. The neurologist often sees manifestations or sequelae of internal diseases. In the brevity of this chapter, we cannot offer a complete survey of neurology. We have followed the frequency of the disorders in our daily neurological aeromedical practice. A special problem in neurology is the "empty history." This can only be overcome by a "trusting" attitude of the pilots/patients towards neurology. Our aim is to preserve the pilots' medical fitness. Another issue we wanted to point out is that certain conditions in neurology can only be diagnosed by additional technical investigations such as electrophysiology (EEG, evoked potentials, EMG) and neuro-imaging. The relatively high frequency of hitherto silent intracranial abnormalities (aneurysms, arachnoid cysts) justifies MRI screening in military pilots and astronauts. In addition to internal medicine, ENT, and ophthalmology, there is a considerable overlapping to psychiatry. Some of our case reports could have been presented just as well in the psychiatric chapter, which follows next.

REFERENCES

1. Mumenthaler M, Mattle H. (2004) *Neurology, 4th ed.* Thieme. Stuttgart, New York.
2. Pippig T, Kriebel J. (2000) Prevalence of cervical and lumbar disc disorders in pilots of the German Armed Forces. *Eur J Research* **26**(5): 8.
3. Weber F. (2005) Value of the EEG in the medical selection of military pilots. In: Rödig E (ed), *German Flight Surgeons Conference.* Königsbrück: Surgeon General of the German Air Force.

4. Hendriksen IJ, Elderson A. (2001) The use of EEG in aircrew selection. *Aviat Space Env Med* **72**: 1025–1033.
5. Bechinger D, Kriebel J, Schlager M. (1973) EEG following sleep deprivation — an important tool for diagnosis of epileptic seizures. *J Neurol* **20**: S193–S206.
6. Berg AT, Shinnar S. (1991) The risk of seizure recurrence following a first unprovoked seizure: A quantitative review. *Neurology* **41**: 965–972.
7. Hauser WA, Rich SS, Lee JR, Annegers JF, Anderson VE. (1998) Risk of recurrent seizures after two unprovoked seizures. *N Engl J Med* **338**(7): 429–434.
8. van Donselaar CA, Schimsheimer RJ, Geerts AT, Declerck AC. (1992) Value of the EEG in adult patients with untreated first seizures. *Arch Neurol* **49**: 231–237.
9. Merry RTG. (1999) Neurological diseases. In: Ernsting J, Nicholson AN, Rainford DJ (eds), *Aviation Medicine, 3rd ed.*, pp. 312–318. Oxford: Butterworth-Heinemann.
10. Hodkes JR. (1991) *Transient Global Amnesia: Clinical and Neuropsychological Aspects*. Saunders, London.
11. Nakada T, Kwee IL, Fujii Y, Knight RT. (2005) T2 reversed MRI of the hippocampus in transient global amnesia. *Neurology* **64**: 1170–1174.
12. Kornhuber AW, Bischoff W, Kriebel J. (1994) Frequent problems of neurologic and psychiatric assessment of flying personnel. In: Daeger J, Schwarz R (eds), *International Congress of Aviation and Space Medicine*. Bologna: Monduzzi Editore.
13. Annegers JF, Hauser WA, Sharon PC, Rocca WA. (1998) A population based study of seizures after traumatic brain injuries. *N Engl J Med* **338**: 20–24.
14. Weber F, Knopf H. (2004) Cranial MRI as a screening tool: Findings in 1772 military pilot applicants. *Aviat Space Env Med* **75**: 158–161.
15. Winn HR, Almaani WS, Berga SL, Jane JA, Richardson AE. (1983) The long-term outcome in patients with multiple aneurysms. Incidence of late hemorrhage and implications for treatment of incidental aneurysms. *J Neurosurg* **59**: 642–651.
16. Yasui N, Suzuki A, Nishimura H, Suzuki K, Abe T. (1997) Long-term follow-up study of unruptured intracranial aneurysms. *Neurosurgery* **40**: 1155–1159.

17. Rinkel GJ, Djibuti M, Algra A, van Gijn J. (1998) Prevalence and risk of rupture of intracranial aneurysms: A systematic review. *Stroke* **29**: 251–256.
18. Wardlaw JM, M WP. (2000) The detection and management of unruptured intracranial aneurysms. *Brain* **123**: 205–221.
19. Weber F, Knopf H. (2006) Incidental findings in magnetic resonance imaging of the brains of healthy young men. *J Neurol Sci* **240**: 81–84.
20. Wermer MJH, Greebe P, Algra A, Rinkel GJ. (2005) Incidence of recurrent subarachnoid hemorrhage after clipping for ruptured intracranial aneurysms. *Stroke* 362–394.
21. Wiebers DO, Whisnant JP, Huston Jr, Meissner I, Brown JDj, Piepgras DG, Forbes GS, Thielen K, Nichols D, O'Fallon WM, Peacok J, Jaeger L, Kassell NF, Kongable-Beckman GL, Torner JC. (2003) Unruptured intracranial aneurysms: Natural history, clinical outcome, and risks of surgical and endovascular treatment. *Lancet* **362**: 103–110.
22. van Gijn J, Rinkel GJ. (2001) Subarachnoid hemorrhage: Diagnosis, causes and management. *Brain* **124**: 249–278.
23. Osborn A. (2004) *Diagnostic Imaging: Brain Amirsys.* Salt Lake City.
24. Kriebel J, Mühlsiepen F, Kornhuber AW. (1998) Neoplasms of the central nervous system: Risk of incapacitation, diagnosis and treatment. *Aviat Space Env Med* **69**(3): 249.
25. Anderson TD, Loevner LA, Bigelow DC, Mirza N. (2000) Prevalence of unsuspected acoustic neuroma found by magnetic resonance imaging. *Otolaryngol Head and Neck Surgery* **122**: 643–646.
26. O'Reilly B, Murray CD, Hadley DM. (2000) The conservative management of acoustic neuroma: A review of 44 patients with magnetic resonance imaging. *Clin Otolaryngol* **25**: 93–97.
27. Tschudi DC, Linder T, Fisch U. (2000) Conservative management of unilateral acoustic neuromas. *American J Otology* **21**: 722–728.
28. Kornhuber HH. (1984) Bluthochdruck und alkoholkonsum. In: Rosenthal J (ed), *Arterielle Hypertonie*, pp. 149–162. Springer.
29. Kornhuber HH. (1993) Risikofaktoren und prävention des schlaganfalls. In: Hijfemann G, Braune HJ, Grieving B (eds), *Durchblutungsstörungen im Bereich des Nervensystems*, pp. 18–36. Einhorn-Presse Verlag.
30. Aschoff JC, Knaps A. (1990) "Normal" alcohol consumption and well-being: Relationship between reduction of alcohol consumption and

changes in well-being. In: Deecke L, Eccles JC, Mountcastle VB (eds), *From Neuron to Action*, pp. S31–S37. Springer.
31. Sacco RL, Wolf PA, Kannel WB, McNamara PM. (1982) Survival and recurrence — The Framingham Study. *Stroke* **13**: 290–295.
32. Wilterdink JL, Easton JD. (1992) Vascular event rates in patients with atherosclerotic cerebrovascular disease. *Arch Neurol* **49**: 857–863.
33. Vickrey BG, Rector TS, Wickstrom SL, *et al.* (2002) Occurrence of secondary ischemic events among persons with atherosclerotic vascular disease. *Stroke* **33**: 901–906.
34. Yamamoto H, Bogousslavsky J. (1998) Mechanisms of second and further strokes. *J Neurol Neurosurg Psychiat* **64**: 771–776.
35. Sacco RL, Foulkes MA, Mohr JP, *et al.* (1989) Determination of early recurrence of cerebral infarction. Stroke Data Bank. *Stroke* **20**: 983–989.
36. Eliasziw M, Kennedy J, Hill MD, *et al.* (2004) For the North American Symptomatic Carotid Endarterectomy Trial (NASCET) Group. *Canad Med Ass* **170**: 1105–1114.
37. Feinberg WM. (1996) Primary and secondary stroke prevention. *Current Opin Neurol* **9**: 46–52.
38. Gorelick PB, Sacco RL, Smith DB, *et al.* (1999) Prevention of a first stroke. A review of guidelines and multidisciplinary consensus statement from the National Stroke Association. *JAMA* **281**: 1112–1120.
39. Sacco RL, Elkind M, Boden-Albala B, *et al.* (1999) The protective effect of moderate alcohol consumption on ischemic stroke. *JAMA* **281**: 53–60.
40. Malarcher AM, Giles WH, Croft JB, *et al.* (2001) Alcohol intake, type of beverage, and the risk of cerebral infarction in young women. *Stroke* **32**: 77–83.
41. Sacco RL. (2001) Newer risk factors for stroke. *Neurology* **57**(Suppl 2): S31–S34.
42. Collaboration HLT. (1998) Lowering blood homocysteine with folic acid based supplements: Meta-analysis of randomized trials. *BMJ* **316**: 894–898.
43. Toole JF, Malinow MR, Chambless LE. (2004) Lowering homocysteine in patients with ischemic stroke to prevent recurrent stroke, myocardial infarction, and death: The Vitamin Intervention for the Stroke Prevention (VISP) randomized controlled trial. *JAMA* **291**: 565–575.
44. Sacco RL, Benjamin EJ, Broderick JP, *et al.* (1997) Conference proceedings. Risk factors. *Stroke* **281**: 507–1517.

45. Fotherby MD, Panayiotou B. (1999) Antihypertensive therapy in prevention of stroke. What, when and for whom. *Drugs* **58**: 663–674.
46. MacMahon S. (1996) Blood pressure and the prevention of stroke. *J Hypertens* **14**(Suppl): 636–646.
47. Hansson L, Zanchetti A, Carruthers S, *et al.* (1998) Effects of intensive blood pressure lowering and low dose aspirin in patients with hypertension: Principal results of the Hypertension Optimal Therapy (HOT) randomized trial. *Lancet* **351**: 755–762.
48. Organization WH. (1999) International Society of Hypertension Guidelines for the Management of Hypertension. *J Hypertens* **17**: 151–183.
49. Staessen J, Wang J, Bianchi G, Birkenhäger WH. (2003) Essential hypertension. *Lancet* **361**: 1629–1641.
50. Association AD. (1998) Clinical practice recommendation. *Diabetes Care* **21**(Suppl 1): S1–S89.
51. Group PC. (2001) Randomized trial of perindopril-based blood pressure lowering regimen among 6105 individuals with previous stroke or transient ischemic attack. *Lancet* **358**: 1033–1041.
52. Bucher HC, Griffith LE, Guyatt GH. (1998) Effect of HMG CoA reductase inhibitors on stroke: A meta-analysis of randomized, controlled trials. *Ann Intern Med* **128**: 89–95.
53. Corvol JC, Bouzamondo A, Sirol M, Hulot JS, Sanchez P, Lechat P. (2003) Differential effects of lipid-lowering therapies on stroke prevention: A meta-analysis of randomized trials. *Arch Intern Med* **163**: 669–676.
54. Group HPSC. (2002) MRC/BHF Heart protection study of cholesterol lowering with simwastatin in 20536 high-risk individuals: A randomized placebo-controlled trial. *Lancet* **360**: 7–21.
55. Group HPSC. (2004) Effects of cholesterol lowering with simvastatine on stroke and other major vascular events in 20536 peoples with cerebrovascular disease or other high-risk conditions. *Lancet* **263**: 221–227.
56. Collaboration AT. (2002) Collaborative metaanalysis of randomised trials of antiplatelet therapy for prevention of death, myocardial infarction, and stroke in high-risk patients. *BMJ* **321**: 71–86.
57. Group ECSTC. (1991) MRC European Carotid Surgery Trial: Interim results for symptomatic patients with severe (70–99%) or mild (0–29%) carotid stenosis. *Lancet* **337**: 1235–1243.

58. Group ECSTC. (1998) Randomized trial of endarterectomy for recently symptomatic carotid stenosis: Final results of the MRC European Carotid Surgery Trial (ECST). *Lancet* **351**: 1378–1387.
59. Collaboration NASCET. (1991) Beneficial effect of carotid endarterectomy in symptomatic patients with high-grade carotid stenosis. *N Engl J Med* **325**: 445–453.
60. Barnett HJM, Taylor DW, Eliasziw M, *et al.* (1998) Benefit at carotid endarterectomy in patients with symptomatic moderate and severe stenosis. *N Engl J Med* **339**: 1415–1425.
61. Cina CS, Clase CM, Haynes RB. (2003) Carotid endarterectomy for symptomatic carotid stenosis (Cochrane Review). *The Cochrane Library 3*.
62. Runmaker B, Anderson O. (1993) Prognostic factors in a multiple sclerosis incidence cohort with 25 years of follow-up. *Brain* 110–117.
63. Achiron A, Barak Y. (2000) Multiple sclerosis — From probable to definite diagnosis. A seven-year prospective study. *Arch Neurol* **57**: 974–979.
64. Ferrari MD, Roon KI, Lipton RB, Goadsby PJ. (2001) Oral triptans (serotonin 5-HT1B/1D agonists) in acute migraine treatment: A metaanalysis of 53 trials. *Lancet* **358**: 1668–1675.
65. Diener HC RA, Pascual J, Jansen J-P, Pitei D, Steiner T, on behalf of the Eletriptan and Cafergot Comparative Study Group. (2002) Efficacy, tolerability and safety of oral eletriptan and ergotamine plus caffeine (Cafergot) in the acute treatment of migraine: A multicenter, randomized, double.

Chapter 20

Psychiatry

Jürgen Kriebel*,† and Matthias M. Weber‡

INTRODUCTION

Epidemiology of Psychiatric Disorders

Internationally, psychiatric and/or neuropsychiatric disorders follow internal somatic diseases as the second most frequent cause of unfitness for medical certification. Psychiatric disorders are relatively common and are a greater cost to society than cardiovascular diseases. Epidemiological research has proven that mental disorders are highly relevant to general medical, internal medical, orthopedic, and other medical practices, but are sometimes not identified or misdiagnosed and incorrectly treated.

Competency of Psychologists and Psychiatrists

Mentally conspicuous behaviors are extremely diverse and lie within the competencies of many fields of specialization. The tasks of the psychiatrist, and partly also those of the neurologist, are not easily distinguished from those of the psychologist, especially within clinical psychology and neuropsychology. The lack of etiological specificity in

*Corresponding author.

† Facharzt für Neurologie und Psychiatrie-Psychotherapie-Flugmedizin, Scultetusweg 8, D-98075 Ulm, Germany.

‡Max-Planck Institute for Psychiatry, Munich, Germany.

psychopathological syndromes is mentioned in the chapter devoted to neurology. Mentally conspicuous behaviors may be triggered by toxins, inflammations, cerebral trauma, and other diseases and disorders. The primary responsibility for their diagnosis and treatment rests with psychiatrists or neurologists. Contrary to the opinions of some AMEs, the treatment of psychotic (e.g. schizophrenic) pilots is not the responsibility of aviation psychologists, whose primary competence involves the testing of pilots' aptitude and practical capabilities. Such tests may indicate that an applicant is unsuitable for training as a pilot but are not sufficient to confirm the existence of a psychopathological condition. Simply put, a psychologist's remit is the testing of flight aptitude which is comparable to the remit of a clinical physiologist. In the event of a somatic disease such as a heart attack, it goes without saying that the patient would be referred to a cardiologist rather than to a cardiac physiologist. Similarly, flight personnel who exhibit mentally conspicuous behavior should initially be referred to a psychiatrist, not to a psychologist. However, after having recuperated from a psychiatric disorder, an aviator should perhaps be required to repeat certain parts of a flight-aptitude examination. The undoubtedly complex overlapping of clinical psychology and psychiatry demands information and cooperation rather than unproductive competition.

Subsequent chapters in this book discuss various psychological task fields, especially psychological testing and neuropsychological examination to determine whether a perceived abnormality might have a somatic cause, e.g., brain damage resulting from a trauma. Such examinations may also disclose problems that might otherwise elude detection by AMEs, many of whom tend toward a one-sided somatic view and who may therefore overlook general symptoms of organic brain disease, e.g., cognitive functional deficiency, reduction of cognitive adaptability, abnormally early onset of fatigue, reduction in retentiveness and comprehension, difficulties with concentration, increased irritability, affective instability, etc. The phrasing of the requirements in JAR-FCL3 should contribute toward reducing the number of misdiagnoses. The medical provisions and guidelines of FAA and ICAO are clearer.

CLASSIFICATION AND DIAGNOSIS OF MENTAL DISORDERS

The ICD-10 and the DSM-IV

Let us now return to psychiatry and the scope of its responsibilities. Psychiatry uses somatotherapeutic, psychotherapeutic, and sociotherapeutic methods, and it concerns itself with the diagnosis of mental disorders, their non-surgical therapy, prevention, rehabilitation and evaluation, as well as their social components and psychosomatic aspects.

The preceding definition has created a problem with regard to nomenclature and classifications. Unlike the traditional diagnostic concept (which was strongly oriented toward etiological notions), current diagnostic practice primarily relies on descriptive, phenomenological, and operational criteria. The DSM-IV, i.e., the "Diagnostic and Statistic Manual of Mental Disorders, 4th Edition" of the American Psychiatric Association, precisely defines these criteria for each nosological entity.[1] Whereas the DSM-IV is the preferred basis for practitioners in English-speaking countries in particular and for international neurobiological research in general, the psychiatric chapter in ICD-10 (the World Health Organization's "International Statistical Classification of Diseases and Related Health Problems 10th Revision), chapter F[2] is the authoritative reference to assure international uniformity of diagnostic terminology. Although the codes in WHO's ICD-10 are commonly used in international aviation medicine and are the basis for ICAO's medical provisions, psychiatrists who treat outpatients or inpatients and who examine pilots often also use terminological codes specified in the DSM-IV, so AMEs should be familiar with both terminologies. Although the DSM-IV and the ICD-10 F differ in many details, these divergences are negligible from an aeromedical perspective because both taxonomic systems rely on the same basic principles and use nearly identical terminologies and criteria for the majority of disorders. Of practical importance is the fact that the DSM-IV has retained the numerical codes from the obsolete ICD-9, whereas the ICD-10 uses an alphanumeric code. The letter "F" is assigned to psychiatric disorders and the letter "G" is used for neurological disorders. In accord with standard international practice, the ICD-10's codes will be used on the following pages, and reference will be made to DSM-IV codes only in cases where this seems more suitable to the matter at hand.

One consequence of this operationally and phenomenologically defined diagnostic system is that many terms that formerly played an important role in psychiatry (e.g., "endogenous" or "psychogenic") are no longer used. Furthermore, the DSM-IV and the ICD-10 have largely replaced the concept of "illness" with the concept of "disorder" and have abandoned the traditional "psychosis/neurosis" dichotomy. Another feature shared by both classificatory systems is the principle of co-morbidity in the coding of diagnoses. If the symptomatology satisfies the inclusive and exclusive criteria for several mental disorders, then all of them must be listed side-by-side, even if biological and psychological understanding would suggest the existence of a common etiology.

Among the other important benefits of this international nomenclatural consensus is the fact that terminological concurrence makes it easier for a non-psychiatrist to assign a diagnosis to an empirically observed psychopathological profile. However, unrestricted reliance on the ICD-10 and the DSM-IV remains problematic for aviation medicine and necessitate certain compromises. In particular, the outmoded "psychosis/neurosis" dichotomy and other traditional psychiatric terminologies have not yet entirely disappeared from aeromedical guidelines for the assessment of flight fitness. Such terminologies are also still sometimes encountered in written evaluations of flight personnel. The etiological orientation remains important for the prognosis, so this vocabulary is also used in this and other chapters. In addition to relying on guidelines for the evaluation of flight fitness, many psychiatrists and neurologists who collaborate with flight surgeons still use classical psychiatric terminologies. Comparable compromises persist even in newer editions of authoritative textbooks, to which readers seeking more detailed information are referred.[3–5] Sporadic usage of classical vocabulary will probably persist throughout a lengthy transitional period.

Psychiatric Diagnosis

After this introduction to psychiatric nosology, it seems expedient to briefly describe the psychiatric examination, which should consist of a physical examination, including a complete neurological profile, and if necessary, laboratory testing and examinations with technical methods, including CNS imaging. To increase the accuracy of the diagnosis, structured interviews augment psychological tests designed to evaluate cognitive capacity and personality characteristics. Clinical psychopathology's purely phenomenological orientation, which tends to neglect somatic aspects and the results of psychological tests, is no longer acceptable. The absence of etiological specificity in the syndromes, as well as the interweaving of neurological, psychiatric, and general medical aspects, should always be borne in mind. Personality and affectual disturbances can surely be traced to cerebral-organic factors in the narrower sense of this term.

The chapter on neurology discussed the inadequate therapeutic consequences of a purely phenomenological orientation, e.g., the futile attempt to use psychotherapy to treat a brain tumor. No purely phenomenological, reliably appraisable, etiologically specific, nosological entities exist within psychiatry. The dualistic "somatic versus mental" model is obsolete.[3,4] Somatically oriented examinations also play an important role in psychiatry, but they must be clearly indicated. Dissociative personality disorders without proof of organic cause, or "psychosomatic" disorders with organic manifestations, are presently classified as somatoform disorders, but the minds of patients suffering from such disorders are often strongly fixated on purely somatic symptoms. Because these patients tend to change physicians frequently, the same examinations may be repeatedly many times over.

Flight Fitness

The psychiatric requirements for flight fitness, specified in the JAR-FCL 3 and in the FAA and ICAO regulations, stipulate that a pilot's licence should not be granted to a person suffering from a psychiatric disorder that could conceivably interfere with his or her ability to safely fly an airplane. The disqualifying disorder may be acute or chronic, congenital or acquired, and its existence can be determined either through medical history or clinical diagnosis. Particular attention should be paid to schizophrenic and affective disorders, anxiety and personality disorders, and problems associated with alcohol or the misuse of other psychotropic substances.

PSYCHOTIC DISORDERS

Definition and Etiology

Sporadic psychotic symptoms are not necessarily indicative of a psychosis because they may also occur transiently during the critical phases of other disorders. A genuine psychosis is a pathological condition in which the impairment of mental functions becomes so severe that it significantly interferes with reasonable insight, drastically impairs the ability to cope with the demands of daily life, and/or seriously disrupts contact with objective reality.[3,4] Continuity of perception is disordered and contact with objective reality is lost.

The traditional triadic nosological system distinguishes between organically explicable psychoses in the narrower sense on the one hand, and schizophrenic and affective psychoses on the other hand. Among the organic psychoses, it differentiates between brain-inherent disorders (e.g. encephalitis, vascular processes, and tumors) and disorders in which the brain participates (e.g., intoxications, infections, endocrinopathies). The outcome of an aeromedical examination depends upon the prognosis and the degree of success in the treatment of the underlying disorder.

Affective psychoses may occur as monopolar depression or monopolar mania, as well as in bipolar form, i.e., with alternating depressive and hypomanic or manic episodes. Although genetic components play a significant role in the etiology of schizophrenic and affective psychoses, genetic factors alone cannot fully explain the type of symptoms or the moment in time when they appear. Recently developed examination techniques such as positron-emission tomography (PET) and functional magnetic-resonance imaging (fMRT) combine structural and functional depictions. Advances in the fields of neurotransmission and psychopharmacology are yielding an increasingly large body of evidence that suggests schizophrenic and affective psychoses are accompanied by pathological somatic changes in the central nervous system.

As Fig. 1 shows, our aeromedical results conform to this threefold classificatory scheme and categorize psychiatric disorders *sensu stricto* into organic, schizophrenic, and affective disorders.

The Significance of Epidemiology in the Practice of Aviation Medicine

The above mentioned categories of mental disorders (organic mental/behavioral, schizophrenic delusional and mood-anxiety disorders) account for 38% of the 338 psychiatric diagnoses. About half of the bar with mood and anxiety disorders contains about 16% of major depression of the former "endogenous" type. All patients in this group and those represented by the first two bars were permanently disqualified from flight duties. Patients with organic-psychotic disorders constituted 2% of the group: if they had received sufficient treatment, and if such treatment had been lastingly successful, then these individuals might have been granted waivers, albeit with specified restrictions. However, because of insufficient therapeutic measures (e.g. due to tardy diagnosis of the underlying disorders), and also partly as a result of the patients' lack of insight into their own illnesses, none of them were deemed fit for flight duties.

Case 1: A polytoxicomanic PPL-A holder with more than 500 hours of flight experience who had abused alcohol for many years. He also ingested analgesics, sedatives, amphetamines, and other psychotropic substances. Ignoring his elevated levels of liver enzymes and MCV, AMEs had repeatedly re-issued his medical certificate.

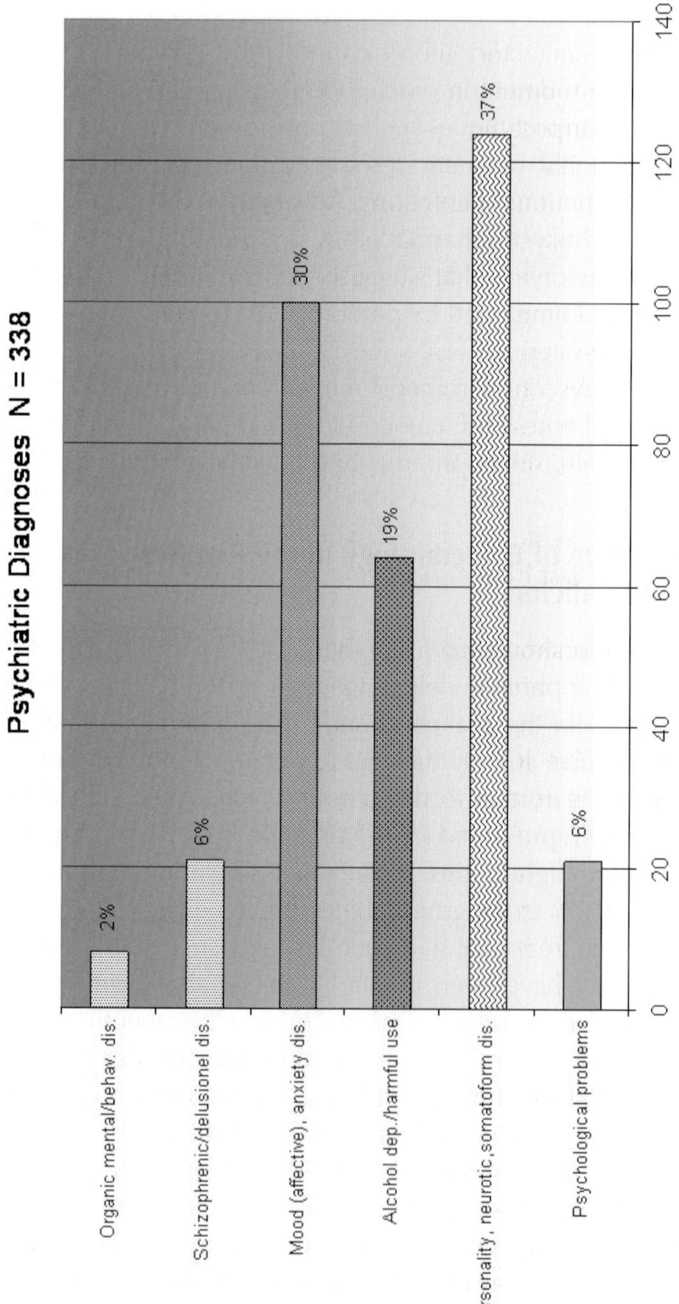

Figure 1. Distribution of psychiatric diagnostic groups ($N = 338$). Abscissa: absolute numbers.

One day, he went to the airfield at which he had chartered airplanes for many years and, without prior authorization, took an airplane out of the hangar, damaging two parked planes in the process. He then flew to an airport he was quite familiar with. The flight seemed to have passed without further mishaps. After landing, he disobeyed orders to switch off the engine, left it idling, and walked into the airport restaurant. When the chief air-traffic controller asked him for an explanation, he seemed disoriented, confused, and agitated. He took off his clothes, ran across the airfield stark naked while gesticulating wildly, thereby disrupting normal flight operations. The police escorted him to the nearest psychiatric ward, where he was admitted against his will as an inpatient and diagnosed as suffering from a substance-induced psychotic disorder (ICD-10: F14.5). After undergoing insufficient therapeutic measures (his detoxification was not followed by treatment for substance abuse), he enlisted the aid of a lawyer to assist him in his struggle to regain a Class 2 medical certificate.

This example shows how a psychiatric disorder can induce its sufferer to violate behavioral norms and regulations, jeopardize his own and others' safety, and fail to appreciate well-founded criticism of his actions. The ICD-10 assigns organic mental disorders and behavioral disorders due to the use of psychotropic substances to Chapters F0 and F1. From a purely phenomenological perspective, it is often difficult or impossible to distinguish the symptoms of these disorders from symptoms associated with disorders in the F2 categories, which include schizophrenia, schizotypal, and delusional disorders.

Case 2: A private pilot with PPL-A and C who toward the end of his academic studies had been diagnosed as suffering from a schizophrenic disorder (ICD-10: F.20) with ego disorders (derealization, thought insertion), formal thought disorders (scattered and incoherent thoughts, flight of ideas, talking past the point), paranoid symptoms (delusions of grandeur), and hallucinatory symptoms (commenting and imperative voices). Subsequent episodes exhibited additional hypomanic aspects (elevated mood, euphoria, feelings of happiness, hyperactivity, hardly any sleep but without an apparent sleep deficit). He was 35 years old at the time of his first aeromedical examination, during which he recounted an inconspicuous medical history while maintaining a regular regimen of neuroleptic medication. He was given a Class 2 medical certificate. He suffered a relapse after discontinuing his antipsychotic medication "with the approval of the family physician." Megalomaniacal symptoms predominated during several weeks of inpatient psychiatric treatment. He felt as though he was a messiah who could save the world, and he was unshakably convinced of his delusion that he could end all wars. He resumed taking antipsychotic medication, and after recounting another inconspicuous medical history at his next medical examination, he was again assessed as fit to fly. After having decided on his own to discontinue taking his medications, he suffered a third psychotic episode. At times he felt a "split of personality" and frequently experienced auditory hallucinations, during which he always heard the same familiar voice. During a flight, this voice ordered him to change his destination and land at an airport with his radio and transponder turned off. If he failed to comply, the voice warned that "something bad would happen." After a bizarre approach to the airport, he landed his plane between the airliners and was subsequently confined for several weeks in a psychiatric hospital, where he felt as though he was "the immortal messiah." Because he was unable to convince others of this belief, he jumped through a windowpane: "I didn't even know what floor I was on." The impact of his plunge was partly absorbed by a sand heap at a construction site, so he suffered only minimal bruises and lacerations. He interpreted this good fortune as further confirmation of his invulnerability to injury, which he used to justify his violent resistance to the police, whom he regarded as "Judases." His symptoms quickly disappeared after resuming taking antipsychotic medications. Because of the risk of relapse, this was now assessed as a permanently disqualifying disorder.

Risk of Relapse

Neurologists and psychiatrists frequently encounter the problem of inconspicuous medical histories. The example above of a paranoid hallucinatory schizophrenia (ICD-10: F20.2) shows the risks that this disorder can pose to flight safety. It also clearly indicates that psychotic episodes can recur without recognizable triggers and that they often go initially unnoticed by people in the individual's social surroundings. The duration of intervals between episodes varies drastically from patient to patient and can be very lengthy. Nonetheless, international rules for fitness of aviation personnel stipulate that a history of a schizophrenic disorder with subsequent confirmation of this diagnosis renders the applicant permanently unfit for all classes of medical certification, despite optimal medical treatment and good compliance.

Rather than citing numerous additional examples from our first-hand experience of such cases, we shall recount the history of a spectacular accident that occurred in 1982 during an approach to Tokyo-Haneda airport in Japan. The accident report revealed that cultural aspects also played a role, especially the extreme inequality in the hierarchal positions of the captain and his first officer. Shortly before his DC-8 with 174 persons on board reached the airport, the captain, who suffered from schizophrenia with florid paranoid symptoms, deliberately crashed the aircraft into the shallow waters of Tokyo Bay. 24 passengers perished in the accident, which would have claimed even more lives were it not for the first officer's energetic counter-steering. Approximately six years before the accident, this experienced captain had repeatedly exhibited conspicuous psychopathological behavior. He was treated several times by his physicians, who suspected that he may have been suffering from depressive and psychosomatic disorders. His sister had long before been diagnosed as suffering from a schizophrenic psychosis. He was disqualified from flight duties for approximately one year. After a check flight with an AME on board, the captain was reconfirmed as fit for flight duty. Two years prior to the accident, copilots reported that the captain behaved in a peculiar way while piloting his aircraft. Among his idiosyncrasies, he would remain silent during a flight, refuse to answer questions posed directly to him or laugh uncontrollably (parathymia). His paranoid psychosis gradually evolved but was ignored for a long time by people in his surroundings. He was absolutely convinced that spies in his homeland were preparing bloody confrontations. He gravely threatened his wife, whom he imagined to be one of the spies. With absolute delusional certainty, and perhaps under the influence of imperative voices, he began to exhibit suicidal symptoms which culminated in an expanded suicide.

This case story shows, *inter alia,* that family medical histories may be of great importance and that check flights during symptom-free intervals, with or without physicians on board and with or without supporting psychological tests, are improper as they may create a false sense of security. Schizophrenic and affective psychoses render those suffering from them permanently unfit for all classes of medical certification.

The crash of a Royal Air Maroc ATR-42 on a domestic flight in 1994 is another case of expanded suicide. The captain, who likewise suffered from a schizophrenic disorder, killed himself and his 43 passengers. Though he had repeatedly been treated as a psychiatric inpatient in the past, the necessary aeromedical consequences were not forthcoming. Though suicidal behavior is not uncommon in psychiatry, it can be difficult to properly assess and can often occur unexpectedly, much to the dismay of even the most experienced clinicians. This fact is impressively confirmed by the numerous international cases of suicides that occur either during psychiatric hospitalization, shortly after patients have been released, or on furloughs from hospitals.[3,4,6]

Though airplanes are seldom flown with suicidal intent, the Internet confirms that they are often discussed as potential "tools" for vehicular suicide.[7–9] The histrionically staged suicide of a private pilot in November 1996, who announced that he was preparing to crash his plane into the Zugspitze (Germany's tallest mountain peak), defies classification in any of the above mentioned diagnostic groups and seems more likely to have resulted from a histrionic personality disorder. We shall return to the topic of suicide later and in another context. As these examples show, even distinctly pathological symptoms sometimes go undetected, not only by people in the patient's social environment, but also by physicians, including neurologists and psychologists.

Case 3: A 32-year-old private pilot (PPL-A and C) with nearly 800 hours of flight experience was hospitalized for four months with what appeared to be the initial manifestations of a paranoid-hallucinatory psychosis. He suffered a relapse after opting to discontinue his regimen of antipsychotic medication. Upon his re-admittance for inpatient treatment for an additional period of more than two months, the diagnosis of a schizophrenic disorder was definitely confirmed. After being informed about the patient's psychiatric treatment, an AME erroneously referred him for a psychological evaluation for flight fitness during a symptom-free interval. Such testing was clearly inappropriate, as he should have been referred to a psychiatrist. The patient's preexistent and clearly psychotic symptoms were now erroneously reinterpreted as psychoreactive conflict constellations in the context of personality disorders. The regimen of antipsychotic medication was discontinued in the wake of this incorrect diagnosis, and as one would expect, he suffered a relapse. His comrades found him engaging in a hunger strike in his room, where he had barricaded himself several days previously because of ideas of persecution. A psychiatric and aeromedical assessment following another interval of inpatient therapy confirmed the patient's permanent unfitness for all classes of medical certification.

Psychopathological symptoms vary from person to person and are frequently associated with the patient's biography. Symptom-free intervals are variable, too: if no residual psychosis persists during these intervals, patients return to normal behavior, perform well in their jobs, and are able to cope with stress. Symptom-free intervals after psychotic episodes may last for weeks, months, years or even decades.

Psychopharmacological treatment, augmented by social-therapeutic measures, often enables post-psychotic patients to recover their ability to work. It would, however, be irresponsible to allow a post-psychotic pilot to return to flying. AMEs also frequently underestimate the significance of uncharacteristic premonitory symptoms, which may appear years before the onset of a full-fledged psychosis and which can be correctly diagnosed only after the appearance of obviously schizophrenic symptomatology.

Typically, schizophrenic and affective symptoms appear simultaneously and with equal severity during a psychotic episode. The ICD-10 and the DSM-IV assign these schizoaffective disorders to the schizophreniform group. The three pilots suffering from schizoaffective disorders are therefore categorized in the corresponding column in Fig. 1. The international classificatory system differentiates among schizodepressive (F25.1), schizomanic (F25.0), and mixed schizoaffective disorders (F25.2).

Case 4: A 30-year-old postgraduate student and glider pilot with about 300 hours of flight experience discontinued his regimen of antipsychotic medication during a sojourn abroad. His concentration and attentiveness became severely disturbed and he developed manifold symptoms, including incoherence, talking past the point, delusional thoughts including fantasies of omnipotence, experiences of depersonalization and derealization, parathymias (affective behavior inappropriate to the situation), agitation, panic attacks, depressive intervals followed by hypomanically euphoric moods, loose associations, and a massively reduced need for sleep without any feeling of sleep deprivation. He believed that cancer had been implanted in him and that he would be able to cure it. He was also unshakably convinced that he had invented a cure for AIDS. Only vague information could be gleaned about his auditory hallucinations. His father suffered from a paranoid disorder. The patient first underwent psychiatric treatment at age 22 and was afterwards repeatedly hospitalized, on one occasion against his will. The diagnosis of a schizoaffective disorder (ICD-10 F25.2) could be confirmed, his regimen of antipsychotic medication was successfully fine-tuned, and his capacity to work was restored. However, his fitness for flying could never be restored.

Although these aeromedical decisions are responsible and appropriate, they are often difficult to accept for the affected individuals, as well as for colleagues who lack aeromedical training. This is one of the reasons why "inconspicuous" medical histories are frequently presented at aeromedical examinations. Important information from the patient's own medical history and/or from his family's medical history usually comes to light only in retrospect.

This is frequently, and unfortunately, the case in aviation medicine, especially in neurology and most particularly in psychiatry, as we can see in the following example, where psychotic disturbances repeatedly recur but are not unambiguously interpreted as indicative of schizophrenia.

Case 5: A high-school graduate who hoped to become a commercial airline pilot twice failed the requisite psychological aptitude tests. Alongside his work in another career, he earned an ATPL and amassed more than 3000 hours of flight experience. For many years, he did not tell his AME about his six inpatient psychiatric treatments of more than five months' duration, nor did he divulge that he had undergone several weeks of inpatient treatment in a closed ward.

Diagnosis: Episodes of acute psychotic disorder without a confirmed diagnosis of schizophrenia (ICD-10 F23.0). This diagnosis belongs to the ICD's Group F2, which includes schizophrenia, schizotypal, and delusional disorders. Various conspicuously pathological behaviors were observed alternately and in different combinations. These included: a delusional system with delusional perceptions, ideas of persecution, loosening of associations, formally accelerated thought processes, persevering, loosening of ego boundaries, thought insertion, obsessive thoughts and impulses, temporary feelings of perplexity and desperation, irritability, aggressiveness alternating with depressive moodiness, suicidal thoughts and ideas, etc. Psychopharmacological treatment and psychotherapy were able to restore productive and work-capable intervals, but relapses occurred whenever the treatments were interrupted or discontinued. After each treatment, the patient staunchly insisted that he had permanently overcome all his former problems and that he would certainly never again suffer a relapse. Despite severe problems with his family and occupation, he failed to achieve sufficient understanding and insight from his experiences. Only in the wake of a court order did he finally accept the fact that he was permanently unfit to pilot an aircraft.

Aeromedical literature has devoted very little attention to the principal negative symptoms of schizophrenic disorders, which can reappear as residua. This negative symptomatology may include leveling of individualistic personality characteristics, affect reduction, diminished motivation to the point of autistic withdrawal, thought disorders, marked decrease in the ability to work, slowing of psychomotor activity, and abrupt decline in overall performance. The presence of such a constellation of negative symptoms is unlikely to trigger a reexamination of an individual's fitness for flight duties. As the above-mentioned case studies show, medical examinations are far more likely to ensue when individuals display positive psychotic paranoid-hallucinatory syndromes. These syndromes may have very lengthy symptom-free intervals, and aeromedical examinations performed during such intervals generally reconfirm flight fitness because of blank medical histories. This constitutes a very rare but nonetheless grave risk to flight safety.

Psychopathologically conspicuous behaviors, and this also applies to the affective disorders ("affective psychoses") that will be discussed below, may develop either gradually or with surprising rapidity and acuteness. Patients suffering from such disorders withdraw from consensus reality and everyday life into a psychopathologically determined constellation of problems that they experience as unquestionably and absolutely real. Persons who are unaffected by such disorders may be unable to comprehend the situation and especially its positive symptoms, whereas the affected individuals become unable to comprehend the "normal situation." In cases of absolute delusional certainty, no amount of rational argumentation can dissuade the patients from believing in even the most improbably bizarre delusional systems; contact with objective reality no longer exists. Auditory hallucinations, especially commanding voices, are experienced as unquestionably real, and the patient is likely to obey their commands without regard for the harm this may cause to himself or others. The majority of similar disorders, however, run their course with far less drama and danger. Though there is no reason to exaggerate the potential dangers, neither should the existing aeromedical risks be minimized. This warning seems worthy of mention here because aeromedical professionals, some of whom are not sufficiently aware of the national and international flight-fitness guidelines and requirements, repeatedly certify pilots as fit for flight duty, despite the fact that the above-mentioned diagnoses have already been verified.

Affective Disorders

Social and cultural conditions can lead to syndrome changes in the sense of an increasing tendency to somatization. This is exemplarily illustrated by so-called "masked depression." The tendency toward somatization, i.e., the predominance of physical complaints, is not an infrequent occurrence among pilots suffering from depressive disorders, especially because aviators typically have a special relationship to their physical and mental well-being. Accurate diagnosis is difficult in such cases because patients typically "mask" or underplay affective symptoms and emphasize physical discomforts when they describe their problems.[3,4,6,10,11] For this reason, this disorder is also known as "*depressio sine depressione*." The ICD-10 categorizes these disorders under F32 ("depressive episode") or F33 ("recurrent depressive disorders"), each of which appears together "with somatic symptoms." Physical complaints, i.e., "presenting symptoms," are in the foreground, where they occupy the patients' attention — and frequently also the physicians' attention — for too long. It behooves a psychiatrist who is active as an AME to speak bluntly about this problem.

As early as 1973, field studies of 1000 physicians practicing in Germany, Austria, Switzerland, and France discovered that more than 10% of their patients suffered from depressive disorders, although these patients primarily complained about somatic symptoms.[10] In one Swiss study, patients of general practitioners and practitioners of internal medicine were subsequently subjected to psychiatric reevaluation. Approximately 15% of these patients were found to be suffering from depressive syndromes that were not initially diagnosed as such because somatic complaints had predominated. In individual cases, the specific type of somatoform disorder is often biographically explicable and is frequently related to symptoms the patient had already experienced in the past. The most common foci of somatic complaints are: the spinal column (i.e., the body's axial organ, which is essential for postural and expressive functions), the gastrointestinal tract, the cardiovascular system, and the head.[3,10]

Other factors contributing to masked depression are the widespread belief that only physical diseases are acceptable and the associated fear of the stigmatization a person might encounter if it became known that he was suffering from a psychiatric problem.[3–5] Somatic complaints, however, can only be properly treated after the underlying depressive disorder has been recognized and diagnosed. This is why the exploratory interview, which can be conducted either with or without structured components, constitutes such an important part of a psychiatric examination. This conversation, particularly during the first examination, is often psychotherapeutic and therefore requires an appropriate setting, sufficient patience, and adequate time.

Depressive disorders are used in Fig. 2 to serve as exemplary psychiatric disorders, illustrating the diagnostic procedure and eliminating the need for the presentation of numerous case studies. In the course of an interview with a patient, the general practitioner or AME seeks to isolate, from a potentially large number of varied symptoms, precisely those complaints that can be attributed to the depressive syndromes mentioned in the previous example. Syndrome-oriented therapy can be initiated if the symptoms are sufficiently severe, especially if there is reason to believe that the patient is contemplating or planning suicide. Phenomenological orientation should be followed by etiological clarification. Causal therapeutic treatment should be undertaken if the fundamental illness is cerebro-organic (CO) or if the brain participates in the underlying disease (SB). Nosological classification, which is often quite time-consuming, is not a primary therapeutic precondition. The therapy initially targets only the underlying depressive symptoms. Antidepressant treatment should predominate if there is reason to suspect the presence of recurrent affective disorders (ICD-10: F33, F31.3 to F31.5), formerly usually described as "endogenous." Psychotherapeutic measures, especially behavioral and cognitive therapies, are likewise helpful. Patients suffering from clearly defined depressive syndromes tend to be

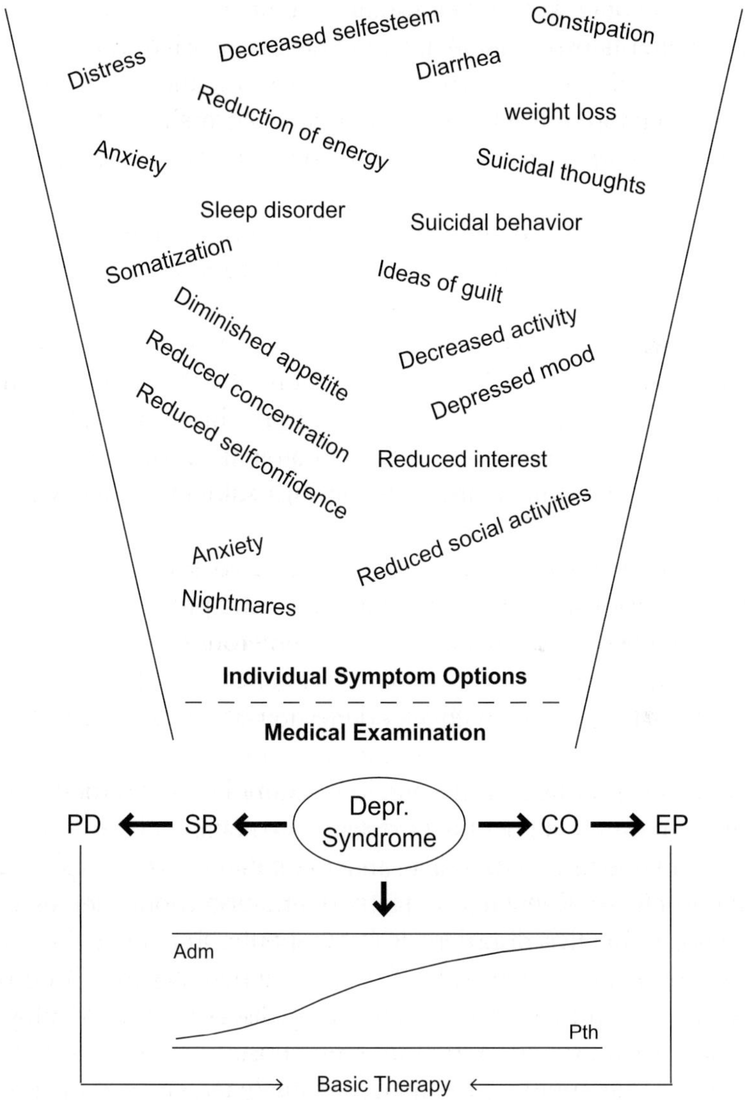

Figure 2. The medical/psychiatric examination reveals individual depressive symptoms leading to depressive syndromes. These may be characterized by agitation or inhibition. Phenomenological orientation should be followed by etiological clarification for causal therapy. CO: cerebro-organic; EP: encephalopathy; SB: secondary brain involvement; PD: primary diagnosis; Adm: antidepressant medication; Pth: psychotherapy.

uncommunicative at first, but usually become more communicative after psychopharmaceutical therapy begins to take effect. As the figure illustrates, this is why psychotherapeutic support gradually becomes increasingly important over time. In most cases, both the pharmacotherapy and the psychotherapy should be continued for a considerable time.

To select a suitable antidepressant, it is important to determine if a depressive syndrome is primarily characterized by agitation or inhibition. Previously widely disseminated schemata for antidepressive psychopharmacotherapy have become obsolete, primarily because new classes of substances have been synthesized. In every case, a finely tuned regimen of psychopharmaceutical therapy should be developed and supervised by a competent physician. Anyone, including a pilot with many years of professional experience, can potentially react to psychosocial stressors by developing a depression, which may result in suicidal symptoms and require hospitalization. The effect of the therapy and the specific category of the depressive disorder are both highly relevant for the aeromedical assessment.

Depressive episodes with a tendency to suffer relapses, especially when these episodes are associated with psychotic symptoms (e.g., delusions of guilt or poverty and accusatory or defamatory voices) entail unfitness for all classes of medical certification. This is also the case for chronically depressive and moderate-severe mood disturbances such as dysthymia (ICD-10: F34.1, "neurotic depression") and bipolar affective disorders (ICD-10: F31) with depressive (F31.1, F31.4, F31.5) and manic (F31.0, F31.1, F31.2) phases. Monopolar progression with manic or hypomanic episodes (without depressive episodes, F30) is very rare but particularly relevant in aviation medicine. Hypomania and mania differ only in the degree of psychopathologically conspicuous behavior. People suffering from manic and hypomanic disorders may exhibit, without obvious triggers, unmistakably euphoric moods, feelings of bliss and good fortune, enhanced motivation and psychomotor activity, increased physical and mental capabilities, heightened sociability, talkativeness with loosened associations and logorrhea, clumsy and unsolicited attempts at intimacy, increased libido with disregard for social norms, massive overconfidence to the point of megalomania, and heightened irritability with aggressive outbreaks. Despite their hyperactivity, patients feel scarcely any need for sleep and show no symptoms of sleep deprivation. The aforementioned symptoms typically lead to severe familial and occupational problems: non-sensical expenditures are not uncommon; bank directors may act irrationally, causing massive losses of money; and otherwise harmless citizens may find themselves pursued by the police in high-speed car chases.[3,4] Pilots have been known to ignore their flight plans and perform aerobatic flight maneuvers without regard for safety. We cite one final case study to round off our survey of affective disorders.

Case 6: At the prompting of the air traffic controller, a 50-year-old private pilot (PPL-A/PVT) with nearly 2000 hours of flight experience was escorted by the police to a psychiatric hospital, where he was hospitalized against his will. At the airfield, he had first planned to take off with an open canopy. He had then interfered with an aircraft taxiing toward its take-off position because he did not approve of the pilot's clothes. He ran barefoot back and forth on top of the aircraft's wing and obdurately ignored everyone shouting at him to come down. Upon admission to the psychiatric hospital, he failed to preserve conventional social distance and spoke with loose associations. He behaved erratically, first with exhilarated foolishness and then threateningly. He was convinced that his admission to the psychiatric hospital was being filmed by a hidden camera for subsequent broadcast on television as an episode of "Candid Camera." Holding a device that resembled a mobile phone, but which was later identified as a large cigarette lighter, he pretended to chat with important celebrities, alternately identifying himself as a military general or the owner of an international business. He repeatedly explained that he could simultaneously sing in soprano, tenor, and bass voices. He was wholly unaware of his own disorder. Interviews with his acquaintances revealed that he had purchased several costly automobiles a few days before his admission to the psychiatric clinic, that he had spent his money nonsensically, and that he had had behaved in a sexually importunate and uncharacteristic manner toward a female acquaintance. Days before, he had flown at altitudes between 4000 and 5000 meters (13 100 and 16 400 feet) without supplemental oxygen. The AME did not know that this patient had suffered a depressive phase at age 30, nor was the physician aware that the pilot had been hospitalized for treatment of a hypomanic phase at age 37. He did not submit to psychiatric evaluation of his flight fitness until after he had contested the revocation of his private pilot's licence. He was diagnosed as suffering from "bipolar affective disorder, most recently manic episodes with psychotic symptoms, currently in remission" (ICD-10: F31.2, F31.7). After successful treatment, his driver's licence was restored, limited to a two-year period. Furthermore, he had to regularly submit psychiatric reports, He was never recertified as a pilot.

In this case, we also encounter the problem posed by an "inconspicuous" medical history. This example likewise reaffirms that even a lengthy symptom-free interval cannot entirely rule out the possibility of relapses. If a relapse should occur, neither relevant experience nor comprehensive medical information (even if it also includes data furnished by the patent's personal contacts) can guarantee that the patient will be treated in time. Many other cases are known in which pilots have undergone comprehensive psychiatric examinations followed by certification to fly, despite the fact that they had previously suffered recurrent phases of affective disorders. Apparently unaware of the guidelines and requirements for aeromedical certification, the certifying physicians justified their affirmative decisions by citing their patients' good compliance, their own experience with similar cases, and the relatively few side effects associated with ingestion of well-tolerated prophylactic medications. Lithium or antiepileptics are the most commonly prescribed pharmaceuticals in such cases. But many patients, pilots included, opt to cease taking their medication when they feel better, so there remains a significant tendency to suffer relapses. We would strongly advise against the use of lithium or valproate prophylactics by pilots in the cockpit. International aeromedical consensus insists on permanent disqualification for flight duties in cases involving delusional and many affective disorders, especially manic episodes, bipolar affective disorders, severe depressive episodes with or without psychotic symptoms, and recurrent depressive disorders (formerly "endogenous" depressions).

Finally, it should be noted that screening for cocaine, amphetamines, barbiturates, and cannabinols as possible specific causes of the pilot's bizarre behavior all yielded negative results. From a phenomenological point of view, psychoses following intoxication with psychoactive drugs can exhibit psychopathological symptoms very similar to those associated with schizophrenic or affective psychoses (see Case 1).

PERSONALITY DISORDERS AND "NEUROSIS"

Several disorders are assigned to the largest group (see Fig. 1) under the heading of "personality disorders" ("neuroses"). These include: depressive reaction (ICD-10: F43.2); anxiety, compulsive, and somatoform disorders (ICD-10: F4); and personality and behavioral disorders (ICD-10: F6). This categorization seems reasonable from an aeromedical perspective: because the differential typology is so difficult, the specific disorder often cannot be diagnosed with the necessary degree of certainty within the framework of a psychiatric examination of flight fitness. 37% of all psychiatric diagnoses fall within one of these diagnostic groups. As mentioned above, the ICD-10 prioritizes an etiologically neutral and phenomenologically oriented classificatory system, and therefore, avoids using the noun "neurosis," although it repeatedly uses the adjectival form of the word. The concept of "neurosis" will be cited occasionally in the following paragraphs because personality disorders and the distinction between "psychosis" and "neurosis" remain highly significant regarding the differential diagnosis in the aeromedical context. This terminology still remains important in JAR-FCL 3.

Personality Disorders

Personality disorders primarily appear in adolescence and young adulthood. Estimated to affect more than 5% of the population, these disorders are characterized by obvious, long-lasting, and relatively unchanging behavioral patterns with deviations from usual social norms. If the deviations are sufficiently severe, they can cause problems for the affected individuals and for the people in their social surroundings. Persons suffering from personality disorders exhibit obvious, sustained, and non-episodic exaggerations of human character traits. Imbalances predominate in affect, motivation, impulse control, perception, thought and social relationships; reduced occupational and social competence may result from behavioral patterns that are inappropriate in many everyday situations. Therapeutic measures often fail to achieve long-lasting success. Unlike the situation in psychotic disorders, continuity of perception and contact with reality are maintained. It is sometimes difficult to distinguish personality disorders from anxiety, obsessive, and somatoform disorders ("neuroses"); lengthy observations of a patient's progress may often be required before such distinctions can be reliably drawn.

Anxiety, Obsessive, and Somatoform Disorders

Although patients suffering from psychiatric disorders classified in this group do not lose contact with objective reality, they often find it difficult to process their experiences, i.e., their patterns of response and behavior are disturbed. The associated subsequent psychopathological and somatic symptoms can be variously interpreted: from the perspective of learning theory, they can be interpreted as resulting from pathological behavioral models; from the point of view of depth psychology, they can be understood as expressions of intrapsychic conflicts. However, recent research has assigned progressively greater importance to the influence of genetically and neurobiologically determinable factors in these disorders. Regardless of the etiological model, symptoms associated with anxiety and obsessive-compulsive disorders can be activated under stressful circumstances and against the background of specific biological and/or psychological vulnerabilities in which early traumatic experiences can play an important role. Social conflicts can likewise cause problems that may overwhelm an individual's problem-solving strategies. Seriously insulting and frightening actions by third parties in childhood and adolescence may contribute to the formation of pathological behavioral patterns. If the affected person subsequently encounters circumstances which he perceives as similar to these early traumata (e.g. during interactions with flight instructors or captains), reactivation can ensue, accompanied by massive tensions that may be difficult for outsiders to understand. People suffering from such problematic constellations are repeatedly subjected to psychiatric examinations for evaluation of their fitness. Psychotherapeutic intervention frequently succeeds in solving their problems, thus enabling the patients to keep their medical certificate and remain competent for flight duties.

The foreground in psychiatric aviation medicine is occupied by anxiety disorders with acute symptom exacerbations, e.g., agoraphobia with panic disorder (ICD-10: F40.01), often mixed with depressive disorders. Simple agoraphobias without panic disorder (ICD-10: F40.00), claustrophobia, animal phobias, and social phobias play almost no role in aviation medicine. Fear of flying as an isolated phobia (ICD-10: F40.2) is not unknown among airborne personnel; flight attendants are its most common sufferers, although it also occasionally afflicts captains and first officers. Anxiety disorders are seldom a problem for anxious recreational aviators because these pilots tend either to avoid anxiety-provoking situations or to fly together with experienced pilots.

Case 7: An airline pilot with more than 4500 hours of flight experience and in line for promotion from first officer to captain was neurologically treated and psychologically tested on three occasions following an accident. As pilot flying (PF) of a B767 with 162 passengers aboard, he encountered poor visibility shortly after takeoff, collided with a radio tower, and was compelled to prepare for an emergency landing. After an emergency fuel dump, a safe emergency landing with no injuries to passengers or crew members ensued, thanks to good cooperation in the cockpit and the correct performance of all checklist procedures. During investigations into the accident, the behavior of an authority figure triggered an underlying authority conflict that exacerbated the pilot's reaction to stress and resulted in temporary free-floating anxieties in the form of panic attacks. Compulsive thoughts and impulsivity appeared briefly, also in the pilot's familial environment, but were well compensated. A flight phobia became progressively more problematic. The intensity of his anticipatory fears increased in direct proportion to the imminence of upcoming flight duty. Driving to work, he experienced cardiac palpitations, trepidation, trembling, and perspiration. In the cockpit, especially during nighttime transatlantic flights, he became increasingly prone to attacks of extreme trepidation and anxiety, accompanied by severe tachycardia, perspiration, problems with concentration, sensations of dizziness and globus, the fear of making major errors, the urge to leave his seat and "run away," worsening to experiences of derealization. These symptoms quickly dissipated after each flight, thus confirming the suspicion of a situation-related phobia with panic attacks. The first psychiatric referral resulted in disqualification for Class I according to JAR-FCL-3 and for Classes I and II according to FAA criteria, but his PPL was not revoked. The recommended inpatient behavioral therapy was discontinued because it focused on the agoraphobic problems in general rather than on this pilot's specific symptomatology. However, this encounter with behavioral therapy was sufficiently intensive to enable him to teach himself how to use its techniques, including systematic desensitization and flooding. This, in turn, gradually led to a reduction in the severity of his phobia. He initially copiloted and later piloted private aircraft, also on nighttime and international flights, and he again flew aerobatics. Eager for permission to improve his flying on a freelance basis, he applied for a CPL/IFR rating and received a favorable decision from his AME. After two subsequent years of flight experience had elapsed without complications (including problem-free long-haul flights to Africa and over the Atlantic), his AME recommended certification for ATPL. Following this, he re-attained his prior skill level, fully overcoming a disturbance that had been diagnosed as "panic disorder, isolated flight phobia" (ICD-10: F41.0, F40.2), and resumed his airline position with much contentment and success.

Similar successes were achieved in several other cases through the combination of initial inpatient treatment and subsequent outpatient therapy, along with intermittent support from medication. One such case involved a private pilot who developed aviophobia after witnessing a friend's fatal aircraft accident. Patients in other cases experienced adequate relief by refraining from flight duties (thus avoiding the specific stressors); they were therefore unable to develop sufficiently strong motivation to begin the relevant and sometimes stressful therapeutic regimen, and were consequently obliged to abandon their airborne duties.

Some first officers with many years of flight experience who switch to the left seat with the full responsibilities of a captain may develop serious constellations of problems associated with anxiety disorders, sometimes mixed with equally serious depressive symptoms (ICD-10: F41.2). Having switched from the right to the left seat, they may find themselves overwhelmed by the responsibilities of being a captain. Biographically explicable references can often be identified. Anxiety-sensitive primary personality characteristics (ICD-10: F60.8) are not infrequent in individuals who make contraphobic career choices. But career-related compensation can destabilize if corresponding professional responsibilities are perceived as overwhelming. Psychotherapy may have varying degrees of success, especially when somatic and conversion syndromes are present. In one case, a slight ankle injury was followed by therapy-resistant, neurologically and orthopedically inexplicable "paresis" ("nothing progresses anymore"). In another case, a mild concussion was followed by severe therapy-resistant headaches combined with deficiencies of concentration — doubtlessly the manifestations of an underlying anxiety disorder.

Possible diagnoses of the following case not only include panic disorder (F41.0) and aviophobia (F40.2), but perhaps also post-traumatic stress disorder (ICD-10: F43.1).

Case 8: A flight attendant suffered bruises and abrasions during severe turbulence. When she was checking out, the purser explained that their aircraft had entered the exhaust air stream of a "Galaxy" and that this could have created an extremely dangerous situation. Shortly thereafter, she heard the news about the crash of a neighboring country's airliner and the fate of its flight attendants. She subsequently developed increasingly severe aviophobic symptoms, for which she could compensate only with tremendous effort. Deplaning was delayed after landing at an Asian airport due to a shooting incident during which the airport manager was killed. She developed panic symptoms for the first time at her hotel during the ensuing curfew. Sometime later, after seeing a sunken B747 while landing in Hong Kong, she was just able to cope with the homeward flight, but never boarded an aircraft again. She experienced panicky anxiety with accompanying vegetative symptoms, especially tachycardia and perspiration, a feeling of pressure in the stomach, temporary disorientation, difficulty falling asleep due to the fear of nightmares, interrupted intervals of sleep, and symptoms of fatigue-induced depression. Despite therapy, she was unable to regain fitness for flight duties.

A delayed but diagnostically unmistakable reaction in the sense of a post-traumatic stress disorder (ICD-10: F43.1) was confirmed in one of two passengers who survived the crash of a Thai airliner. Reporters were so eager to interview the two survivors that the pair and others needed police protection during their emergency treatment at a hospital where they were taken after the crash. The survivors, as well as other patients who could scarcely walk under their own power, were lured to the telephone by reporters purporting to be their close relatives. The joy of having survived predominated initially, and the patients' misgivings were further allayed by the speedy healing of their physical injuries, but one of the survivors gradually began suffering from nightmares, later began to relive the traumatic crash in daytime flashbacks, and ultimately exhibited partial autistic withdrawal alternating with acute anxiety, aggressiveness, feelings of guilt, and a fundamentally depressive mood. Anhedonia, bleakness of outlook, and suicidal ideation increased after refusal to accept medication and after initial refusal to undergo psychotherapeutic treatment. This survivor experienced the hospital ward and its staff as continual reminders of the trauma. Improvement did not ensue until after the patient was transferred to another institution, where problem-focused psychotherapy was provided.

Subtypes of Behavioral and Personality Disorders

Now that we have described anxiety disorders and stress disorders, we turn our attention to personality disorders, which are generally regarded as resistant to therapeutic influence. Because symptoms of personality disorders are not easily distinguished from behavioral patterns associated with other psychiatric disturbances, the diagnosis of a personality disorder is difficult and is frequently possible only after repeated examinations and lengthy observation. Personality can be empirically defined as the sum of all behaviorally relevant attributes that combine to endow a person with his or her characteristic and unmistakable individuality.[3,4] Personality encompasses the entire spectrum of human behavior.

Personality disorders comprise a diagnostic group that is by no means as clearly describable as, for example, acute paranoid-hallucinatory schizophrenia. It is sometimes impossible to distinguish between a personality disorder, on the one hand, and behavior that is still "normal" and socially acceptable, on the other hand. The many-faceted diversity of personality structures is nearly impossible to categorize exhaustively. The widely accepted subtypes described in the ICD-10 are oriented toward specific and clearly defined forms, but these individual aspects may appear in diverse combinations. They become particularly obvious when they manifest as disturbances in interpersonal communication and interaction, e.g., in an aircraft's cockpit. Such disorders usually involve extreme variants of certain personality traits (e.g., mistrustfulness, lack of self-confidence, domineering behavior, and exaggerated precision to the point of perfectionism) or deviations of persistent character traits and the resultant behaviors. Personality disorders are only to a small degree susceptible to therapeutic influence: in most cases, the disorder itself interferes with the patient's ability to make lasting behavioral changes.

Indicatory criteria include obviously imbalanced attitudes and behavior in various functional domains such as motivation, affect, impulse control, perception, thought, self-criticism, and relationships with others. Standardized personality tests and structured interviews are useful diagnostic tools. Diagnostic criteria require that the abnormal behavioral patterns have developed in adolescence or young adulthood and have led to long-lasting reductions in occupational and social capabilities as well as subjective suffering, and/or have had severe negative impacts on the patient's surroundings.[1,2]

In the practice of aviation psychiatry, one encounters primarily schizoid, histrionic, obsessive-compulsive and paranoid personalities, and/or combinations of these subtypes. Borderline disorders occur in individual cases among members of cabin crews and/or applicants for crew positions. A greater number of options for avoidance and compensation, higher tolerance limits, and flexibility to reduce problems exist in the PPL realm. The experience of AMEs confirms that recreational pilots can compensate fairly well for many personality disorders. The risk of escalation is greater in the professional pilots' milieu with its predetermined schedules, obligatory teamwork, and frequent changes of personnel in both cockpit and cabin.

Case 9: In compliance with a court order, an aeromedical examination was undertaken of an air traffic controller who repeatedly deviated from predefined regulations and whose reduced ability to cooperate expressed itself through his failure to convey important information. Despite numerous warnings, and although he was thoroughly familiar with the regulations, the controller repeatedly erred in the guidance of aircraft and persisted in his arbitrary and idiosyncratic interpretations of the regulations. His case history described him as self-willed, eccentric with disturbed social behavior, mistrustful, and clumsily invasive to other people's personal space on several occasions. Inpatient therapy was discontinued because he failed to comply with the house rules. He insisted that well-founded criticisms of his behavior, which jeopardized flight safety, were exaggerated. Afterwards he believed himself to be unjustly under observation and a victim of "mobbing." A preliminary psychological examination characterized him as having paranoid, histrionic, and compulsive personality traits, as tending to overcompensate through a high degree of egocentricity, and as exhibiting exaggeratedly elevated self-assurance combined with latent aggressiveness and weak social contacts. Distortions of reality resulted from the paranoid orientation of his personality. He felt that nearly everything was directed solely against him; he became increasingly more idiosyncratic, argumentative, and undiscerning; and he found fault exclusively with others, never with himself. Unable to change his behavior and thus posing a risk to flight safety, he was assessed as mentally unfit for further air traffic control duties.

Abrogated self-criticism combined with exaggeratedly lofty self-esteem, extreme readiness to take offense at perceived insults, quarrelsome mistrustfulness, a tendency to misinterpret well-warranted criticism as evidence of deliberate hostility toward him, and situationally inappropriate insistence on the correctness of his own behavior combined to substantiate the diagnosis of a paranoid personality disorder (ICD-10: F60.0). Though aircraft captains' personality disorders frequently elude full detection by aptitude and practical tests, such disturbances repeatedly lead them to strongly criticize and reject the Crew Coordination Concept and Crew Resource Management (CCC/CRM — cf. "Operational and Clinical Aviation Psychology"). Such guidelines, the affected captains insist, are important and applicable only to others.

Case 10: An experienced, strongly self-assertive and highly intelligent airline captain had flown reliably and competently for many years. However, he repeatedly became involved in severe disruptions of collaboration in the cockpit. These disturbances became so massive that many FOs refused to fly with him. He was characterized as being stonily rigid, pedantic, exaggeratedly self-righteous, and emotionally unstable. His colleagues described him as lecturing, pontificating and cross-examining everyone, whereas he himself defended his behavior as "only intended to help the airline train the finest pilots." He combined offensive and demeaning behavior toward his FOs with an exaggerated tendency to feel that others had deliberately insulted him. He could be very meticulous and could become irritated about incidental matters, while simultaneously neglecting situationally important items such as checklists. He would justify his overlooking of items on the checklist by claiming to be "behind schedule" but he was adamantly unwilling to forgive FOs for what he perceived as errors, regardless of how slight or insignificant these mistakes actually were. An argument over an inconsequential bagatelle escalated toward the conclusion of a flight; the captain as pilot flying landed the aircraft with a forceful impact and subsequently blamed the FO for the hard landing. After check-out, the captain was jovial, conciliatory, and willing to compromise, but the slightest criticism triggered a return to his ingrained and undiscerning behavioral patterns. He usually did the FOs' preflight work himself, often beginning these tasks before the commencement of official duty time, because he insisted that "you people cannot be trusted." During one of his own preparations, he overlooked a NOTAM, under-calculated the amount of fuel, and later landed "below minimum." Line checks had never discovered noteworthy or conspicuous problems. His impaired ability to maintain social contacts also led to various private problems, including divorce from his wife. Massive abuse of alcohol ensued in a misguided attempt to solve the problems or seek relief from them, followed by an alcohol-related automobile accident with property damage — and revocation of his licence. He then immediately and permanently ceased his abuse of alcohol and also successfully gave up smoking. However, his interpersonal behavior remained unchanged because he failed to recognize and deal with its underlying causes. The psychiatric diagnosis infers the existence of a combined personality disorder with histrionic and obsessive traits, a tendency toward sensitive-paranoid reactions in stressful situations (ICD-10: F61.0), and abuse of alcohol. He was assessed as permanently unfit for all classes of medical certification.

This example illustrates a typical situation for an individual with an obvious personality disorder who suffers increasingly severe problems in his private and professional life, yet finds it nearly impossible to make the necessary profound and permanent behavioral changes. The patient's traumatic experience, which also led to alcohol abuse, is particularly obvious in this case. In other cases, the patient may be unaware of the emotional toll he inflicts upon the people in his surroundings.

Interdisciplinary comorbidities are often difficult to determine when they interact with personality disorders.

Case 11: A PPL-holder with over 2000 hours of flight experience hired a lawyer to assist him in waging many years of "paper-warfare," whereby the question repeatedly arose whether the dispute genuinely involved medical certification or was in fact merely a self-perpetuating case of self-righteous cantankerousness. The problems began after an aeromedical examiner had disqualified the pilot.

A psychiatric examination was carried out in response to a court order after the pilot had undertaken copious correspondence with the responsible authorities and the aeromedical certification committee. He had active parenchymal liver disease and immune deficiency in the wake of hepatitis A and B. Though his gamma-GT levels were chronically slightly elevated, he had nonetheless repeatedly been recertified as fit for flight duty. A new aeromedical examiner palpated the pilot's abdomen and subsequently ordered a sonogram, which confirmed the suspicion of an enlarged fatty liver (steatosis hepatis). The patient's gamma-GT levels were now significantly higher than the values measured after his hepatitis. Alcohol abuse was diagnosed for the first time and his medical certificate was revoked. He agreed to undergo examination as an inpatient, but failed to appear for his appointment. After having consumed inordinately large amounts of alcohol, he repeatedly became involved in conflicts at work and frequently failed to appear for scheduled shifts. Medical history revealed that alcoholism had been the cause for the revocation of his driver's licence on one occasion in the past. He refused to accept the aeromedical committee's revocation of his medical certificate and responded to the decision by leveling groundless accusations at the committee's members. This was followed by a series of seemingly histrionic scenarios, during which he attempted to pit one AME against another by presenting them "modified" medical histories. Some AMEs argued for temporary disqualification from flight duty because the patient's gamma-GT levels were between 161 and 314 i.u./L. (The upper normal level is 40 i.u./L.) His MCV values were marginally acceptable and only occasionally elevated. 12 separate tests conducted during intervals of abstinence from alcohol measured gamma-GT levels between 35 and 54 i.u./L, i.e., values that could be interpreted as indicative of a post-hepatitis condition. He underwent eight aeromedical examinations in rapid succession, each time presenting incomplete medical histories and exhibiting only slightly elevated gamma-GT levels, so that he could quickly collect eight positive aeromedical examinations, which he then presented to the authorities as the reports of "thorough medical examinations". He dismissed the results of other aeromedical examinations as "arbitrary and medically unprofessional procedures and erroneous conclusions based on ungrounded assumptions." He responded to a complaint by his supervisors with a counter-complaint and accused some of his physicians of personal misconduct and professional incompetence. His reputation, honor, and human dignity had been insulted by what he characterized as "a shocking falsification of the facts." Of his own accord, he arranged to have the head physician of an internal medicine department prepare a report recommending that he be declared fit for flight duty. The court based its rejection of his application on a previous examination by the aeromedical certification committee; after many delaying tactics, he grudgingly accepted this decision. He agreed to an appointment for another examination, but again failed to appear for the examination and likewise ignored the court's decision, obtaining instead, on the same day, another aeromedical evaluation confirming his flight fitness. A review of the records indicates that another negative medical examination was subsequently submitted, which the recalcitrant pilot reinterpreted and repeatedly criticized. At the ensuing court hearing, he no longer made the impression of being alcohol dependent, but seemed instead to be suffering from an extreme lack of self-criticism. He was cantankerous, blameful of others, and exhibited a distinct propensity to take offense and feel insulted, while simultaneously rebuking others with strongly derogatory language, which he subjectively regarded as "factually correct and fully justified." His histrionic declamations even strayed into the realm of pseudo-logic, i.e. his disorder caused him to misrepresent facts. His self-centeredness and lack of consideration for the opinions of others, his histrionic dramatizations, clearly exaggerated propensity to take offense at the slightest perceived insult, and ongoing manipulative behaviors to satisfy his own needs are all indicative of a histrionic personality disorder (ICD-10: F60.4), although other symptoms, e.g., paranoid accusations, could also be indicative of other disorders.

DISORDERS CAUSED BY PSYCHOTROPIC SUBSTANCES

The ICD-10 assigns disorders caused by psychotropic substances to the main groups F10 through F19. Decimal positions are used to codify the clinically observable phenomena of physical damage and psychopathologic disorders, epileptic episodes or delirium, as well as the estimation of the severity of the impairment. The ICD-10 thus differentiates between harmful use (abuse) and dependency (addiction). Dependency can be psychological and/or physical: psychological dependency is defined as an irresistible and overwhelming urge to ingest a particular substance, whereas physical addiction is characterized by the development of tolerance, i.e., the need for progressively stronger doses of the substance and the appearance of withdrawal symptoms when regular consumption is interrupted. Use and abuse of psychoactive substances is of particular importance within the aviation workplace. In Annex 1 — *Personnel Licensing*, ICAO uses the term 'problematic use of substances' and gives the following aeromedical definitions:

Problematic use of substances. The use of one or more psychoactive substances by aviation personnel in a way that:

a) constitutes a direct hazard to the user or endangers the lives, health or welfare of others; and/or
b) causes or worsens an occupational, social, mental or physical problem or disorder.

Psychoactive substances. Alcohol, opioids, cannabinoids, sedatives and hypnotics, cocaine, other psychostimulants, hallucinogens, and volatile solvents, whereas coffee and tobacco are excluded.

Guidance on suitable methods of identification of individuals who use psychoactive substances (which may include biochemical testing on such occasions as pre-employment, upon reasonable suspicion, after accidents/incidents, at intervals, and at random) and on other prevention topics is contained in the *Manual on Prevention of Problematic Use of Substances in the Aviation Workplace* (ICAO Doc 9654).

Readers interested in the problem of polytoxicomania are referred to Case No. 1. The combination of tranquilizers and alcohol is a principal cause of acute problems.

Benzodiazepines

The benzodiazepines deserve primary attention in the context of the misuse of pharmaceuticals, especially because physicians often prescribe these medications to members of cabin crews and to recreational pilots without the knowledge of the AMEs. Aeromedical examiners seem to be sufficiently familiar with the importance of not underestimating the potential for dependency, usually in cases of low-dosage misuse. Problems can arise in individual cases if patients consult various specialists, each of whom prescribes his own regimen of medication. Even if individual dosages remain unchanged, accumulation of active metabolites with long half-lives may lead to unintended pharmacological effects.

Figure 3 demonstrates this by showing several examples and listing the duration of various half-lives. A medication's half-life may be longer for a person of more advanced age. Especially when examining members of cabin crews assigned to long-haul flights, AMEs should specifically inquire about the use and possible abuse of tranquilizers.

Case 12: In good weather conditions and with clear visibility, an experienced private pilot landed a Cessna in a field near the airport. The fully fueled aircraft sustained no substantial damage during the landing and a technical inspection revealed no mechanical problems. The pilot had amnesia lasting several hours. The reconstruction of his medical history revealed that he had been taking benzodiazepines,

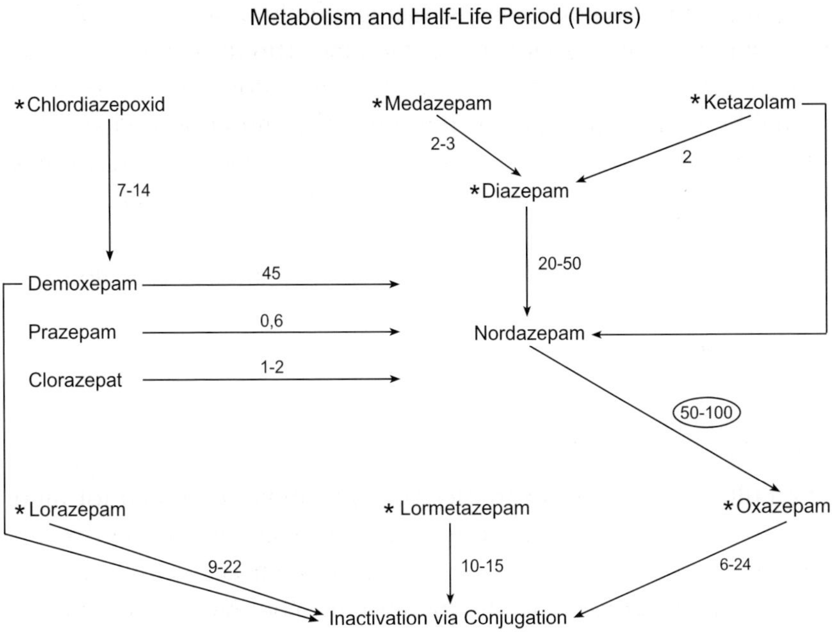

Figure 3. Benzodiazepine-tranquilizer with the risk of accumulation of pharmaceutical effects via metabolization of active metabolites. Some of these metabolites are individually prescribable benzodiazepines with long half-lives. Thus the same dosage may mask accumulative pharmaceutical effects (low dose dependency). The numbers represent half-lives in hours.

which have been known to trigger episodes of amnesia. No other plausible explanation for the emergency landing was found during two comprehensive inpatient examinations.

Nicotine

Legal drugs are particularly significant in the aeromedical context. Some nicotine addicts exhibit grossly aggressive behavioral abnormalities, especially on long-haul flights and when under the influence of alcohol. This problem has even prompted discussions about the potential merits of loosening restrictions against onboard smoking, but nonsmoking passengers and crew members should not be exposed to the risks of passive smoking merely to satisfy the cravings of people who are dependent on nicotine. The risks of secondhand smoke have been drastically underestimated for too long. Despite the available information about the health-related consequences of smoking, some young pilots (like their older colleagues) have been lured into using tobacco, thus suggesting that the potentials for smoking and dependency, as well as the harm tobacco causes to the health of those who smoke it, have been trivialized and denied.

Alcohol

Alcohol remains the principal problem, as is clearly shown in the 19%-bar in Fig. 1. Western societies embody a so-called "permissive culture" with regard to alcohol, but social tolerance for alcohol users decreases rapidly when its abuse causes severe health-related, private, or occupational problems. No clearly defined boundaries separate traditional enjoyment, harmful use, and dependency (addiction). Patterns and amounts of drinking are individual and highly variable. All social groups are affected. Factory workers are more likely to drink beer, whereas business executives may opt for champagne or cognac, but regardless of which type of inebriating beverage is consumed, the fact remains that alcohol is a dependency-inducing psychotropic substance. The volume of alcohol consumed by the populace has stabilized at a high level in Europe and USA. This correlates with high rates of alcohol-related morbidity and mortality. Among other reasons, the significantly reduced life expectancy of the average alcoholic is due to the fact that the suicide rate among people who are dependent upon alcohol can be as much as 20 times higher than the corresponding rate among the general public. Particularly tragic is the massive increase in alcohol-induced embryopathy as the most common cause of fetal damage.[3,4,12]

It would exceed the scope of this paper to provide an extensive discussion about alcoholism. Such a discussion would necessarily include the many-faceted causes of the substance's harmful use, dependency upon it, the various phases of the illness, and their fluent transitions. Comprehensive information about this topic is available in numerous textbooks and specialized literature. The medical provisions of ICAO stipulate that a mental or behavioral disorder due to use of psychoactive substances, including dependence syndrome induced by alcohol, entails unfitness for all classes of medical certification. The aeromedical examiner must investigate "if indicated," i.e., if he suspects the possibility of alcoholism. In our opinion, such suspicion renders him duty-bound to pursue further investigation. Regardless of their fields of specialization, all physicians should devote greater attention to alcoholism, and not solely as it relates to examinations of fitness for driving and flying. The widespread occupational and socio-medical consequences are more than obvious. Alcoholism ranks among the most frequent psychiatric causes of early retirement. More than 5% of all employed persons in the Western industrialized nations are estimated to be dependent on alcohol. The percentage of alcohol-dependent commercial and private pilots is believed to be substantially lower, but alcohol's hazards are uniquely grave for members of these occupational groups. Alcohol is a frequent cause of illness-related occupational absenteeism, as well as workplace and traffic accidents, some of which result in death.

The consequences of drinking even relatively small amounts of alcohol are often underestimated.[13] Experiments in driving and flying simulators have repeatedly shown that a blood alcohol concentration of as little as 0.3 g/L can cause drivers and pilots to misestimate distances and velocities, react more slowly, and be more likely to attempt risky maneuvers. Flight-simulator studies have shown that experienced airline pilots, flying familiar routes but with concentrations of 0.3 and 0.5 g/L alcohol in their bloodstreams, repeatedly deviate from their flight path and make other errors, some of which can be quite dangerous. This is an important fact that proves it is foolhardy to ignore even assumedly negligible amounts of residual alcohol, e.g., from drinks consumed the night before a takeoff.

Newspaper reports have time after time announced that airlines have suspended pilots because of alcohol problems. The media regularly reports about aviation accidents caused by alcohol-impaired pilots. Some of these mishaps are due to gross negligence at take-off, e.g., departure without preflight checks. In most reports, the journalists do not indicate whether the alcohol-related accident was the consequence of isolated misuse or chronic dependency (alcoholism). Thorough examinations are usually needed to distinguish between the two. An aeromedical examiner should therefore always bear in mind the possibility of alcohol abuse whenever he encounters a case of peculiar and atypical behavior in a pilot.

Case 13: A 42-year-old commercial pilot with over 6000 hours of flight experience, predominantly on short-haul and medium-haul turboprop cargo flights, experienced recurrent low back pains and lumbosciatic pain for many years. He suffered an acute and dramatic worsening of his condition, combined with the sudden appearance of a left-sided paresis of the quadriceps muscle, but therapy was delayed due to continued flight duties. Emergency surgical repair of a herniated disc (L3/L4) and subsequent lengthy rehabilitation resulted in near total regression of the paresis. Acute lumbosciatic pain recurred two years later, this time with progressively severe left-sided foot drop. A regularly scheduled aeromedical examination discovered that the pilot habitually adopted a pain-relieving posture and that he had developed lumbar paravertebral muscle hardening and near paralysis of the dorsal flexors of the foot and toes. The AME referred the patient to a neurologist, who immediately referred him to a neurosurgical department, where emergency surgery was performed on his spinal disc at the level of L4/L5. Despite intensive rehabilitation measures, no significant regression of the paresis occurred. The permanent insertion of a peroneal splint seemed unavoidable, but the pilot could still have retained his medical certificate pursuant to issuance of a special waiver. A subsequent medical examination, however, discovered conspicuous facial telangectasia ("spider veins"), untreated dental problems, and a blood-alcohol concentration of 0.3 g/L. Further information revealed that the patient's driver's licence had been revoked once in the past when he was found to have more than 1 g/L alcohol in his bloodstream while driving to an airport to check-in for a night flight. That same evening, before driving to the airport, he had consumed three bottles of beer and had taken diclofenac. The seriousness of the patient's drinking problem was further confirmed by the Munich alcoholism test (MALT 4, 12) and by spinal ataxia due to polyneuropathy (falling when the eyes are closed). As is typical among people suffering from alcohol-related problems, he rationalized and denied the severity of his alcohol consumption. An AME should surely investigate further whenever a patient fails to learn from prior experience and persists in his behavior despite repeated warnings from physicians. Self-inflicted injuries, sometimes to the point of protracted suicide, are typical among people who abuse alcohol or are alcohol dependent. The authors refer the reader to the extensive literature about alcohol-associated organ damage, e.g., injury to the liver, pancreas, gastrointestinal tract, immune system, endocrine system, cardiovascular system, musculature, and peripheral and central nervous systems.[10] Studies repeatedly confirm that patients suffering from alcohol-induced damage comprise *circa* 15% of the patients treated in internal medicine wards. In some cases, the affected organs are repeatedly treated, but the underlying problem either eludes recognition or is identified too late.

Regardless of the cultural milieu, alcohol abuse and dependency lead to relatively typical behavioral patterns, especially the creation of façades. Reduced capacity for self-criticism and projection of problems outward onto elements in the patient's environment are symptomatic of brain damage resulting from chronic intoxication. Such behaviors rarely involve mere lying in the conventional sense of the word, but are in fact genuine psychopathological symptoms. It is surprising, but nonetheless true, that even the closest friends and associates of a secretive drinker often fail to recognize the severity of his substance abuse, despite fluctuations and declines in the alcoholic's performance and despite his increasingly severe private and occupational deficiencies. The patient's façade of rationalization and denial is often so "successful" that even his physician may fail to see through it, despite obvious evidence of physical and psychological dependency. Failure to detect an alcohol problem is likely when obvious clues are overlooked.

Alcohol dependent patients in the so-called "tolerance phase" may remain astonishingly capable of appropriate action and reaction despite high levels of alcohol in their bloodstream. This paradoxical juxtaposition of seemingly unimpaired performance and a high level of alcohol in the blood is symptomatic of chronic alcoholism. As the following case study illustrates, this combination occurs when the enzymatic breakdown of alcohol via alcohol dehydrogenase is augmented by activation of the microsomal ethanol oxidizing system (MEOS), leading to a temporary "tolerance" for large volumes of alcoholic beverages.

Case 14: An AME discovered on several occasions that a glider pilot had steatosis (i.e., a fatty liver) and an elevated gamma-GT with levels between 95 and 385 i.u./L, although average corpuscular erythrocyte volumes (MCV) were only minimally elevated. The patient deliberately kept his physician uninformed about three previous grand-mal seizures, one of which occurred at the airport, and during which he had bitten his tongue, experienced urinary incontinence, exhibited tonic-clonic activity, lost consciousness for several minutes, and afterwards only gradually recovered his orientation. Despite inconspicuous levels of glucose in the patient's bloodstream, the AME noted a short-lived "hypoglycemic shock" on the examination form. Due to the suspicion of syncope and absolute arrhythmia resulting from atrial fibrillation, the pilot was admitted as an inpatient to an internal-medical ward for further examination.

Because atrial fibrillation with normal sinus node function cannot trigger a syncope, a consultant neurologist diagnosed alcoholism with alcohol-withdrawal seizures of grand-mal type. The senior physician, himself a private pilot, explained to the patient the consequences this diagnosis would have for his driver's and pilot's licences. Upon hearing this news, he left the hospital against the advice of his physicians. The next day, he caused a car accident while driving under the influence of alcohol. His blood-alcohol level was measured at 3.14 g/L immediately after the accident. Despite this high level of alcohol in his bloodstream, police found him capable of walking and answering questions with only mildly slurred speech.

His ability to function with near normality despite the high level of alcohol in his blood is clearly symptomatic of alcoholism in the "tolerance" phase. As only an insufficient ambulant treatment regimen had been undertaken, the following aeromedical examination ultimately disqualified him from further flying.

As the preceding case study shows, even experienced psychiatrists occasionally fail to diagnose longstanding alcohol abuse with clear dependency. Please note the "liver gap" in Fig. 1 (the aeromedical homunculus) in the neurology chapter. Pilots with drinking problems may deliberately keep their AME uninformed about grave incidents, e.g., grand-mal seizures. The relevant literature amply describes the difficulties of recognizing alcohol abuse and dependency. Bearing this in mind, it is particularly important for an aeromedical examiner to be alert for symptoms such as steatosis and elevated gamma-GT, and MCV. The reader is explicitly reminded of the significance of liver tests and in-flight grand-mal seizures in the overall context of a general aeromedical examination (see Case 4 in the chapter on neurology).

Not every instance of elevated gamma-GT is necessarily caused by chronic alcohol intoxication. However, if hepatobiliary and other potential causes can be ruled out, then high levels of gamma-GT strengthen the suspicion of alcoholism and obligate the physician to investigate in greater depth. Gamma-GT is a sensitive but relatively nonspecific marker. Elevated levels can ensue after an isolated bout of abnormally heavy drinking, but they may also be associated with a chronic alcohol-related problem. The MCV is a slowly reacting parameter, but elevation of MCV together with an elevated gamma-GT level is not uncommonly symptomatic of chronic and harmful misuse of alcohol. In this case, the physician should check whether the patient's normal levels of gamma-GT are likewise elevated. Teetotalers and people who drink little alcohol have considerably lower levels. Even regular consumption of low volumes of alcohol can have deleterious consequences.[13] The CDT (carbohydrate-deficient transferrin) level is a highly specific but less sensitive parameter, which, in our opinion, is utilized far too infrequently in aeromedical contexts.

The Exceptional Position of Dependency and the Therapeutic Goal

The human organism has three interactive systems for regulation and coordination: the neural, the endocrine (or neuro-endocrine), and the immune system. These systems are particularly susceptible to damage by toxins, which may lead to the problems and disorders described above. As is also the case in some other psychiatric disorders (e.g., psychoses), one characteristic of substance dependency is that the potential for corrective self-motivation becomes increasingly limited and is ultimately lost altogether as the dependency progresses. The dependency comes to dominate the entire personality, successfully asserting itself against all social bonds, long-range life goals, and financial common-sense. The path toward renewed competence in the activities of daily life cannot be trodden without insight into the disease process, motivation to undergo therapy, and willingness to accept professional help.

Aviation personnel, especially those who work in aircraft cockpits, typically have a high degree of occupational motivation, and this enthusiasm can also be used therapeutically. Several major airlines have successfully introduced occupationally specific programs of monitoring and therapy. These require continuously updated company-wide information, the abandonment of prejudices, and empathic understanding. Treatment of pilots who are suffering from alcohol-related problems always involves a combination of assistance and supervision. Essential components are group therapies, outpatient and inpatient treatment, integration of the patient's friends and loved ones, as well as appropriate and often long-term aftercare. The patient must also agree to submit to blood tests of biological markers at irregular intervals. In case of dependency, complete abstinence is the therapeutic goal. A diagnosis of alcoholism remains relevant throughout the patient's life. Therapies for nonprofessional pilots are frequently often less standardized and less carefully monitored than therapies for their professional colleagues, which helps explain why non-professional pilots with substance-dependency are less likely to regain their medical certificate. Prevention, early detection, and therapy are the logical steps. The traditional and socially sanctioned enjoyment of alcohol presupposes that this psychoactive and dependency-inducing drug be used in reasonable and moderate dosages.

SUICIDALITY

In many countries, the number of deaths due to suicide far exceeds the number of fatalities caused by traffic accidents. This chapter has already repeatedly referred to suicidality, including the use of airplanes as tools for so-called "hard suicide." The highest-risk groups are composed of people whose medical histories include alcoholism, dependency on medications and/or drugs, and depressive episodes, as well as elderly people and individuals who have threatened or attempted to commit suicide in the past. The intention to take one's own life is announced in advance in approximately 75% of all suicidal cases[3,4,6,11]; 25% of these suicidal individuals contact their family physicians a few days prior to their suicides, often expressing indirect innuendos and complaining of somatic symptoms. During the final decisive phase, and relatively independent of the etiology, the existent danger is often difficult to recognize, not only for people in the potential suicide's milieu, but also for specialists. When working with people in certain diagnostic groups, an aeromedical professional is therefore advised to proactively and systematically raise the subject of suicidal tendencies.

Suicide and the many methods used to commit it are multifaceted subjects, so the dominant factors can only be approached statistically. One should avoid hasty conclusions on the basis of individual and isolated cases. "Hard" methods (e.g., shooting, hanging, or jumping from great heights) are more common among alcoholics and psychotics; so-called "soft" methods (e.g., deliberate drug overdose) predominate among female suicides. The suicide rate is significantly higher among men than women. There is also a positive correlation with increasing age. The ratio between actual and attempted suicide is estimated to be about one to 10 among males, but comprehensive and decades-long analyses have found higher values, especially among younger men.

Although the individual intentions for attempting to take one's life are difficult to predict and categorize, non-fatal auto-aggressive behaviors can be subdivided into non-lethal failed attempts and parasuicidal behaviors (suicidal gestures). The reasons, the prior planning, and the physical means used in failed suicide attempts all reveal a very clear intention to end one's life. Survival (e.g., after jumping from the third floor of a building) is usually serendipitous. Suicide and failed attempted suicide are nearly identical from a psychopathological perspective. The desire to distance oneself from life's problems occupies the foreground in parasuicidal behaviors and the so-called "suicidal pause." Nonetheless, these behaviors should not be trivialized or underestimated, especially because of the indistinct boundary between parasuicide and failed attempted suicide. Chronic or current conflict constellations may overwhelm an individual's coping mechanisms and precipitate a suicide attempt, especially while the individual is under the influence of alcohol or benzodiazepines. Every suicidal gesture must be taken seriously: it requires understanding and it demands appropriate clarification and assistance. Underestimating the seriousness of the problem and simply remaining aloof from it are unacceptable. The relevant criterion that demands evaluation is the individual's sphere of subjective experience, not the objective severity of a triggering situation or the specific behavior undertaken.

After informing himself about the calculated risk of his act, a high-school graduate swallowed 10 tablets of a benzodiazepine and placed three empty vials on his nightstand. He knew when his family members would be returning home. The "objective situation" seemed so threatening that he was admitted to an intensive-care unit for two days. As is also true in the next example, this case with its histrionic background likewise demands unprejudiced clarification and help. A mildly retarded military draftee, who had been taken from his previously sheltered psychosocial situation, felt unable to cope with his new situation. He swallowed five "very large and very poisonous" antibiotic capsules. Although there was no "objective danger," the patient was firmly convinced that he had indeed swallowed a lethal dose.

Medical requirements pertaining to suicidality are clearly and restrictively formulated. If suicidal ideations are discovered in a patient's medical history, it behooves the aeromedical professional to undertake an appropriate examination, although this is very time consuming and requires psychopathometric clarification. The decision should be based on the specific characteristics of each individual case and should consider the determinative cause, the circumstances that might contribute toward the formation of a suicidal propensity, and the triggering factors. A psychosis can be one such determinative cause. In such cases, the aeromedical decision is clear. Chronic private and occupational stressors often increase the risk of suicide. The specific triggers can be seemingly trivial. People in the suicide's milieu may misidentify a petty quarrel or a misunderstanding as the determinative cause, and this can cause them to suffer long-lasting guilt feelings. The accessibility and availability "at arm's length" of the suicidal tool is another crucial factor: gun owners often turn their own weapons against themselves; pilots occasionally use their airplanes as the means to commit suicide.[7–9] Timely identification of the risk is often difficult, even for doctors, specialists, and psychologists, but constant vigilance remains indispensable. In the sense of "psychological autopsy" after a suicide or attempted suicide, many facts can be seen in a pilot's medical appraisal, which were either not known or only partially known by the AME. Nevertheless, the effort should be intensified to devote more attention and greater sensitivity to psychiatric disorders.

Antidepressant Treatment

As shown above, suicidal behavior is a main risk of depressive syndromes. Therefore, treatment in time by antidepressant medication and psychotherapy is necessary in order to prevent suicidal attempts. However, the ICAO, FAA, and JAA policies do not (yet) allow pilots to fly while taking antidepressant medication. This seems to be one of the major reasons why pilots and cabin attendants conceal even the indicated use of psychopharmacologic medication.[15] Many of them continue to fly while under such treatment, sometimes for years, without informing their AMEs. Current and ongoing studies show that flying personnel suffering from depressive syndromes under antidepressant treatment, especially with SSRIs, do not exhibit an increased number of incidents or accidents.[16]

Evidence for adverse safety outcomes arising from permitting individuals to operate as commercial or private aircrew while using antidepressants has not been found. Furthermore, the psychiatric follow-ups revealed more complete and reliable medical histories.

These findings strongly support changes of current policy. Based on our experience with treatment of depressive syndromes, we suggest that the aviation regulatory bodies should approve the therapeutic use of SSRIs for flying personal under psychiatric and aeromedical supervision.[16]

CONCLUSIONS

Even today, psychiatry and people suffering from psychiatric disorders still encounter prejudices and derogatory psychosocial labeling. Such prejudices and stigmatizations dissuade people, especially pilots, from seeking psychiatric help. Social pressure is often so strong that it influences peoples' descriptions of their complaints, frequently prompting patients to present somatic syndromes that even physicians may find difficult to diagnose.

A human being's sense of personal responsibility is the precondition for all legal systems, and these systems require people to accept social norms. Some mental disorders can drastically impair and, temporarily or permanently, interfere with personal self-determination, good judgment, and reasonable discrimination, so those affected may commit criminal and/or civil offenses. Along with the lack of insight that frequently accompanies disorders such as psychoses and substance dependency, this may contribute toward the stigmatization of mental disorders. Seminars and continuing education for aeromedical professionals should encourage unprejudiced openmindedness and greater attention to the psychiatric aspects of medical histories.

The following recapitulations are intentional. The phenomenological orientation of the contemporary psychiatric diagnostic system corresponds to syndrome-oriented therapeutic measures, but the clarification of somatic causes in the narrower sense should not be neglected. The dualistic model of "somatic versus psychogenic/psychological" is obsolete. The phenomenological similarity between organic and psychoreactive syndromes should not be overlooked. All psychopathological syndromes are ultimately nonspecific, i.e., until they have been thoroughly elucidated, they cannot serve as the basis for drawing conclusions about potential somatic or psychological causes.[3,4,14] No purely phenomenological, undoubtedly appraisable, and etiologically specific nosological entities exist within the specialized field of psychiatry. The ephemeral appearance of mental disorders, particularly those with lengthy symptom-free intervals, the often inconspicuous medical histories associated with such disorders, and the avoidance techniques practiced by patients suffering from such disorders, all combine to further exacerbate the difficulties confronted by aeromedical examiners.

Reasonable suspicion that a psychiatric problem may exist is sufficient to justify the implementation of all necessary diagnostic measures. An AME can use a pilot's desire to preserve or re-acquire his medical certificate as an effective motivational instrument for therapeutic intervention on behalf of the affected pilot. Most pilots are highly occupationally motivated, and this can be very helpful when they face lengthy and burdensome therapy. Every monitored therapeutic success enhances flight safety. Psychiatry overlaps extensively with other medical specialties and psychology. In the aeromedical and aeropsychological context, a distinction should be drawn between aptitude and application tests (which essentially select within normal psychological performance fields) on the one hand, and psychopathological and/or psychiatric clarification on the other hand. Pathological syndromes need special clinical training and experience (including inpatient care), and sometimes also require syndrome-oriented batteries of tests. The following chapters on psychology and neuropsychology should help the reader to recognize the differences and to order the additional expert examinations.

REFERENCES

1. Diagnostic and Statistical Manual of Mental Disorders. (2000) *DSM-IV-TR. 4th ed,* text revision. American Psychiatric Association, Washington.
2. *The ICD-10 Classification of Mental and Behavioral Disorders.* Diagnostic Criteria for Research. (1993) World Health Organization, Geneva.
3. Sadock BJ, Sadock VA. (2005) *Kaplan & Sadock's Comprehensive Textbook of Psychiatry.* Lippincott, Williams & Wilkins, Philadelphia.
4. Möller H-J, Laux G, Kapfhammer H-P. (2003) *Psychiatrie und Psychotherapie, 2nd ed.* Springer, Berlin, Heidelberg.
5. Kennedy SH, Lam RW, Nutt DJ. (2004) *Treating Depression Effectively. Applying Clinical Guidelines.* Dunitz, London, New York.
6. Heeringen K van. (2005) *Understanding Suicidal Behavior. The Suicidal Process Approach to Research, Treatment and Prevention.* Chichester Wiley.
7. Jones DR. (1977) Suicide by Aircraft. *Aviat Space Env Med* **48**: 454–459.
8. Siegel R. (2006) *NPR: My Final Landing: Suicide by Airplane.* Microsoft Internet Explorer.
9. National Transportation Safety Board. (10/02/2000) *Factual Report Aviation Occurrence.*
10. Pöldinger W. (1974) Die Behandlung der Depression in der täglichen Praxis. In: P Kielholz (ed), *Die Depression in der Praxis.* Huber Verlag, Bern.
11. Arolt V, Rothermundt M. (2004) Depression in Medical Patients. *Advances Psychosomatic Med* **26**: 98–117.
12. World Health Organization. (2004) *Global Status Report: Alcohol Policy.* Department of Mental Health and Substance Abuse, Geneva.
13. Aschoff JC, Knaps A. (1990) "Normal" Alcohol Consumption and Well-Being. In: L Deecke, JC Ecles, VB Mountcastle (eds), *From Neuron to Action,* pp. 531–537, Springer Verlag.
14. Kriebel J, Kriebel F. (2002) Psychiatrie für den Fliegerarzt. In: J Draeger, J Kriebel (eds), *Praktische Flugmedizin,* pp. 423–450. Ecomed Verlag, Landsberg.

15. Sen A, Akin A, Canfield DV, Charturvedi AK. (2007) Medical histories of 61 aviation accident pilots with postmortem SSRI antidepressant residues. *Aviat Space Env Med* **78**: 1055–1059.
16. Ross J, Griffith K, Dear K, *et al.* (2007) Antidepressant use and safety in civil aviation: A case-control study of 10 years of Australian data. *Aviat Space Environ Med* **78**: 749–755.

Part 6

PSYCHOLOGY

Chapter 21

Operational and Clinical Aviation Psychology

Konrad Steininger and Dirk Stelling*,[a]

INTRODUCTION

Fields of Application

As a branch of applied psychology, aviation psychology originated in response to the practical needs of the aviation and space industry. In Germany, there are two institutions for aviation psychology. One is located at the German Aerospace Center (DLR) in Cologne, the other at the German Air Force Base in Fürstenfeldbruck (FFB). The primary task of these institutions is the development, application, and scientific evaluation of diagnostic methods and selection procedures for the specific requirements of aviation and space flight personnel. In the area of civil aviation, a close cooperation with Lufthansa and other airlines has been established. Within Lufthansa, an additional demand for aviation psychology has arisen in the fields of leadership and management, caring for flight crews, flight safety programs, and aircrew training. Furthermore, there is

* Corresponding author.
Aviation and Space Psychology, Sportallee 54a, D-22335 German Aerospace Center (DLR e.V.), Hamburg, Germany.
[a] For their helpful comments and support, we wish to thank our colleagues: G. Fahnenbruck, K.-M. Goeters, H. Hansen, R. Kemmler, D. Manzey, M. A. Schuemann-Sen and B. Willkomm.

a long-term contract with the German Air Traffic Control (DFS) for the selection of controllers. All these experiences have contributed to the selection and training of German and other European astronauts for manned space flight.

In this chapter we use the term "operator" for all jobs of importance for safety in the aviation system, such as pilots, flight engineers, flight attendants, air traffic controllers, dispatchers, maintenance personnel, and space crews.

Aptitude versus Fitness

Mental and physical fitness does not automatically include the aptitude and suitability necessary for carrying out the different mental tasks and meeting the demands of piloting an aircraft. In German aviation law, the term aptitude has been avoided in favor of the term reliability. Reliability, however, is only one aspect of aptitude. In the aviation regulations, factors that make an applicant unreliable may be alcoholism, legal incapability, severe legal infractions, and traffic offences. The European regulations for flight crew licencing[1] also describe aptitude operationally: A psychological evaluation should be considered "... when the authority receives verifiable information from an identifiable source, which evokes doubt concerning the mental fitness or personality of a particular individual. Sources for this information can be accidents or incidents, problems in training or proficiency checks, delinquency or knowledge relevant to the safe exercise of the privileges of the applicable licences."

Fitness and aptitude are different categories and should be examined with different methods. Besides reliability, aptitude is comprised of the applicant's or pilot's cognitive and operational performance, behavior and personality. For example, the effects of alcohol abuse on a person's fitness to fly will rarely be determined by liver function tests alone, without checking for effects on performance and changes in the personality. The German and European reservations concerning aptitude refer to the applicant's entire personality. This chapter will outline how this is dealt with in Germany and what experiences have been made.

Aptitude implies the consideration of the entire personality with regard to specific requirements. The regulations describe many factors that may impair fitness to fly. Many of these are indisputable, being measurable and self-explanatory while certain other aspects of aptitude are less so. This is especially relevant to psychological aptitude testing where the partly subjective assessment process, based on numerous more or less objective data, requires the examiner to have extensive experience of both investigation techniques and aviation.

Clinical Psychology in Aviation

The term "clinical" refers to all kinds of behavioral problems that may cause people to seek help from a psychologist. Even professional selection, training, and leadership cannot prevent individuals, working in highly sensitive safety-relevant positions, from exceeding their limitations of performance and emotional stability in situations of high personal or job-related stress. The ensuing behavioral problems will directly affect work procedures and cooperation, and may cause depression, anxiety disorders, risk of suicide, and abuse of medicines, alcohol and drugs, as well as problems in social and sexual relations, and psychosomatic or physical disorders.

In order to maintain or regain their health, job performance level, and personal well-being, these individuals need competent counselling and treatment from a clinically trained psychologist. A qualified psychologist is trained in the application of diagnostic tests; he or she applies scientifically certified tests and knows how to interpret the results, using the classification of disorders according to DSM-IV or ICD-10. A psychologist who mainly works in clinical intervention deals with diagnostics and modification or prevention of maladaptation. An aviation psychologist is also able to recognize and assess specific problem areas within the aviation workplace due to his special knowledge of aviation.

Apart from pilot selection for different weapon systems and missions, the psychological care for crews under extreme operational conditions is a very important field of application in military aviation psychology. Clinical aviation psychology has been able to contribute substantially to accident investigations and to the rehabilitation and recovery of fitness after missions with high or extreme physical and psychological stress.[2,3] The accumulated knowledge and experience of psychological diagnostics and intervention has proven to be of higher value and effectiveness in maintaining or recovering operators' mental and physical fitness than psychiatric therapy.

Clinical psychological methods have gained significance for space flight as well. In the early years of manned space flight, only specially selected and experienced military pilots were recruited as astronauts, while today the number of scientist astronauts without much operational experiences has substantially increased. In addition to psychological selection, an efficient preparation of the mental and physical coping mechanisms needed in space flight has become important. The increasing duration of space missions (the world record, held by the Russian cosmonaut Valerie Polyakov, is 438 days) and the operation of the International Space Station have raised further questions concerning the psychological care of the crews during their stay in space. Among the procedures discussed in this context are the psychological and behavior-oriented methods of selection and assessment, (preventive) training — mainly in the areas of communication, conflict management, and stress management — and psychological as well as behavioral intervention methods in case of a crisis during a mission.[4,5]

OPERATIONAL AVIATION PSYCHOLOGY

Examination of Aviation Personnel

In civil aviation, the airlines determine how selection of aviation personnel is carried out. The procedures and methods applied vary. Psychological examination of applicants is being used by an increasing number of airlines. Aptitude testing of pilot applicants is also common practice. The job requirements define the level of required aptitude. The German Helicopter Rescue Service, for example, consults psychologists to evaluate applicants' capacities to cope with the specific requirements encountered in flight rescue operations. There are no legal regulations for the application of aptitude testing. Private companies make their own decisions about the methods and quality of their personnel selection. Consequently, aviation-psychological examinations are subject to the company's culture and personnel policies.

Psychological aptitude testing is an efficient way to minimize training risk and optimize economical personnel planning. The so-called negative selection, where only those applicants who are obviously unsuitable are rejected, is not sufficient. The mutual interest in a high quality psychological aptitude testing is to identify those applicants with the highest potential and most promising career prospects in aviation. The competent and consistent application of aviation-psychological aptitude testing has led to three results: first, unsuitable applicants are not accepted; second, the job-related failure rate is relatively low; and third, the number of problem cases is held at a tolerable level.

German Aerospace Center (DLR) support German Air Traffic Control (DFS) through the development and application of specific procedures for the selection of control personnel.[6] Supported by DLR, EUROCONTROL has given out recommendations and guidelines for planning and selecting personnel to other national flight safety organizations.[7]

Regarding the selection of applicants as astronauts for space flight missions, DLR has developed psychological procedures that are being applied in all participating European countries according to request from the European Space Agency (ESA).

Within the area of civil aviation, according to the current need, thousands of applicants are tested every year by DLR regarding their aptitude for different operational jobs in aviation.

In the military field, the demand is controlled by internal personnel structures. Every applicant for a career in the airforce is subjected to aviation-psychological aptitude testing. Prior to the beginning of the flight training, a medical examination of fitness is conducted. This may also include a thorough special clinical psychological or aviation psychological examination, according to specific regulations.

Legal requirements for the application of aviation-psychological aptitude testing only exist in national regulations and in JAR-FCL/Part 3 Appendix 17. Pursuant to these, a psychological evaluation is only required in case of verifiable doubt about an applicant's mental fitness and personality.[8]

Human Factors Training

Dealing with the issue of stress in aviation is always accompanied by the (unspoken) question, how to keep its effects as small as possible. Every measure and every technical solution to reduce the workload on the pilot can be foiled by "human error." An example is the "automation induced complacency," caused by the reduced workload that increasing automation on the flight deck has carried with it. The following sections on human factors explain the necessity for behavior modification of crews. Only continuous behavioral training, oriented towards the demands of contemporary aviation, can reduce the frequency of human errors and minimize their effect. The objective cannot be the elimination of human error, but the prevention of catastrophic outcomes.

A pilot's career is accompanied from the beginning by educational efforts toward safety-aware behavior. "Good airmanship" summarizes this behavior, comprised mainly of disciplined behavior, responsibility, risk awareness, adherence to "standard operating procedures" (SOP), critical self-assessment, etc. This type of airmanship does not evolve by itself or through technical training. Safety-relevant attitudes have to be positively reinforced continually and should be closely linked to the technical training; ideally, it should be an integral part of any training throughout the pilot's career.

Organizations and companies try to utilize the human resources optimally by means of personnel development measures. Consultants support them with tools such as counselling, supervision, mediation, and coaching. These methods have their roots in clinical psychology. International aviation has developed similar leadership concepts under the names of "Leadership Competence," "Crew Coordination Concept," and "Crew Resource Management" as efficient instruments for crew behavioral training. Despite efficient human factors training being acknowledged as necessary for front line operators, occasionally managers themselves do not practice such principles, which is unfortunate as they are in a position to set examples for their employees ("organizational safety and culture").

Human performance and limitations (HPL)

Technical skills, i.e., mastery of the functional skills and specific knowledge of procedures, are obvious prerequisites for obtaining an aviation licence. Professional flying schools are perfectly capable of teaching these technical skills. It is, however, known world-wide that certain behavioral skills are necessary for safe flying: discipline, self-control, critical self-awareness, decision-making ability, proficiency in team-oriented decision management, sense of responsibility, a good understanding of risk management, and social as well as communicative skills. For a long time it was expected that these non-technical skills would evolve by themselves as a side-product of a rigid technical training, according to strict training requirements. In reality, the desired non-technical behavior was coincidental, depending on the quality of the selection and various uncontrolled influences from the training personnel. These non-technical skills should be trained from the beginning in order to modify the behavior in the desired direction as early as possible.[9] HPL-Training has been integrated into basic training. The objective is to teach basic knowledge about human factors and to sensitize student pilots to different aspects of human factors in their aviation career. HPL-training is made up of two parts. "Basic physiology" deals with the physical environmental influences on flight performance. "Basic psychology" deals with personality, motivation, and the individual's and the team's performance, as well as information processing, decision-making, mental workload and stress management. The self-concept, i.e., critical self-awareness, and communication concepts are crucial to this training.

Multicrew coordination concept (MCC)

The next step of human factors training takes part during the advanced pilot training, as "crew (or multicrew) coordination concept" (CCC/MCC), according to JAR-FCL 1, Subpart F. This part of the training deals with the practical application of theoretical knowledge about responsibility, cooperation, roles, mutual acknowledgement of competencies, conflict management, communication, and allocation of tasks.

Significant improvement of flight safety occurred when a whole generation of senior flight captains began acknowledging that other crew members have competencies and should be treated as partners. This led to a new definition of the responsibilities on board: the pilot-in-command is in charge; the other crew members are responsible for their respective tasks, but every crew member is responsible also for the actions of the entire crew; thus every crew member has to keep an eye on the others and must react to any observed deviations from standard procedures, whether intentional or not.

In order to avoid or resolve conflicts in essential decision processes in the cockpit, specific rules have to be obeyed. Simultaneously, the communication style influences teamwork by building or removing barriers. The team's training objective is to acquire the skills for successful conflict management. For the resolution of interpersonal conflicts, it is important to keep in mind that there are three sides to every story: the crew member's own point of view, the other crew member's point of view, and the truth.

According to the technical set-up of cockpit and procedures, the formal allocation of responsibilities in the cockpit is precisely defined. It is explicitly designed for equal distribution of the workload among the crew members.

Crew resource management (CRM)

Accident investigation shows that even experienced crew members with comprehensive knowledge and highly trained functional abilities occasionally make wrong or dangerous decisions, either because of wrong assessment of a situation or because of misjudgment of their own skills. Human beings often cause critical situations, for instance by over-estimating their own abilities. An absolute necessity for successful CRM-training is an understanding of the human sources of error and the different causes for human error behavior, as already taught in HPL-training. The focus of CRM-training is on dealing practically with such behavior.

The training requirements are summarized in the following objectives:

- Self-awareness (introspection)
- Correct assessment of situations and problems (judgment)
- Correct problem solving strategy under conditions of uncertainty
- Timely decision-making
- Result control

Techniques belonging to these categories are meant to enable crews to cope with complex leadership tasks within the area of modern aviation. Among these are: planning ahead, disposition of resources, interpretation of data and information, assessment of facts, occurrences and appearances, decision between two alternatives, assessment by weighing the probability in uncertain situations, and integrating the other crew members into the decision process.

Finally, CRM requires the ability of re-orientation, critical evaluation of information, and disposition of every available aid and information during flight. Strategies of behavior control and work organization are meant to secure the necessary redundancy. The optimization of a flight operation requires mastery of leadership. Qualified CRM courses provide theoretical knowledge and practical training in all of these. The above-described HFT programs contain sensitive topics from the "soft sciences," which means that they require a high level of self-awareness in the participants in order to be accepted. Therefore, the instructors need a special qualification based on broad psychological knowledge. The training of these instructors requires much attention and continuous support (moderation) from competent psychologists. Instructors and moderators experienced with these HFT topics can contribute substantially to behavior modification. The European Association of Aviation Psychologists (EAAP), together with the Joint Research Center (JRC) of the European Commission, offers courses in human factors training for aviation psychologists and instructors.[10] The British Civil Aviation

Authority (CAA) has published a manual for instructors, "Guide to Performance Standards for Instructors of Crew Resource Management Training in Commercial Aviation."

Applied Research in Aviation Psychology

Job-requirement oriented aptitude tests are constantly being developed, *inter alia* at the German Aerospace Center in Germany, tested, and applied in cooperation with airlines and other aviation and space institutions. The professional application of such selection strategies has significantly enhanced the efficiency and reliability of complex systems.

As the development of such selection systems demands substantial knowledge of the job requirements for the operators' employment fields, extensive job analyses are carried out at different intervals.[11,12] One result of this research is that personality-related dimensions, especially in the interactive and social area, have been shown to be of greater significance for airline pilots than for student pilots. Air Traffic Control also benefits from this research and development work.[6]

Applied research does not only help aptitude testing progress with regard to predictive quality, it also provides clinical aviation psychology with improved methods, resulting in better insights into personality structures. In addition, assessment systems for non-technical skills are being developed, and assessor training, selection and training evaluations are being carried out.

APPROACHING CLINICAL-THERAPEUTIC INTERVENTION

The Human Factor

In the history of aviation, there has never been as dramatic a growth as there is now. The civil air traffic is expected to double within a few years, the product range is expanded constantly, and pressure for requirements on aviation systems is rapidly increasing. There is more and harder competition ("more traffic at lower cost"), while at the same time the high safety level in aviation has to be kept up and even improved in order to meet public expectations. International air transport has the highest safety standard in the entire transportation industry with an average of less than two fatal accidents per million flights. In recent years there have been about 20 hull loss accidents per year with a few hundred fatalities. Regarding the expected doubling of air traffic, these figures might increase drastically unless all precautions are taken and all means to improve safety are put into action. The multidimensional human factor definitely plays a prominent role in this process. This chapter will reflect on those dimensions of human factors that directly or indirectly influence the behavior of operators in the aviation environment.

All operators working in aviation are constantly subjected to different physical, mental, and emotional stressors, and not everyone is able to cope appropriately. For flight safety reasons, aviation personnel must submit to aeromedical examinations as well as ongoing performance checks, both regulated by law. The individual's adaptation to the aviation requirements is a permanent process that begins with the selection and the first medical examination, and continues with the basic education, flight training, further education programs, adaptation to new requirements, and ongoing aeromedical examinations.

Individuals are expected to cope not only with these aeromedical and technical requirements. Tasks in aviation are factual tasks and basically require factual competence from everyone involved. While performing factual tasks, the operator carry out normal actions that are not directly related to his or her emotional life. It is still often questioned what such vague factors as emotions, moods, attitudes, and motives have to do with the factual requirements in aviation. But human beings do not have a built-in mechanism that enables them to handle worries, conflicts, and errors autonomously.[13]

Stress and Stress Management

Physical, psychological, or mental strains are factors that have an effect on the operator in complex man-machine-systems; they are, therefore, stressors. The way that individuals feel and cope with strain can be very different, independent of the magnitude and type of stress generated by the strain. Everybody moderates stressors in his or her own way. Stress reactions show both the degree of strain and the way the individual handles it. People need stress as a stimulus for action. As long as this stress enables a person to perform well, it is healthy and useful. If a person cannot cope with stress factors adequately, there will be physical, performance related, or emotional consequences ("distress"). Thus, stress resistance is a very important criterion in the assessment of personality factors.

Physical stress reactions are mainly nervousness, hectic pace, muscle spasms, and disorders of motor coordination. Mental stress reactions can be diminished perception and attention, weakened concentration, mental block, memory gaps, decision errors, general confusion, irritation, and loss of action concept. Emotionally, stress can be felt as panic, anxiety, resignation, anger, annoyance, frustration, and aggressiveness. Chronic stressors like constant overtaxing, repeated traumatic experiences, and continuous impairment of self-esteem, can cause severe physical dysregulation and long-term decline of performance and health. In almost 40% of cases, pilots who become unfit for flying show psychological factors in the diseases that lead to unfitness. In the German Air Force, 30% of pilots, dismissed early for unfitness, were dismissed for psychological reasons.[2]

Anxiety, self-doubts, annoyance, anger, and frustration are dangerous triggers for aggression, failure, and mistakes. Psychological stress can cause distortions of the cognitive processes, loss of social relations, divorce, loss of motivation, loss of respect and competence, restlessness, sleeping disorders, eating disorders, depression, flight into illness, danger of addiction, and more. These kinds of annoyances disturb the emotional balance and are infectious for the people around as well. They ruin mutual confidence, infect discipline, paralyze creativity, and divert mental and emotional energy. A modification in the reactions to stressors, supported by qualified clinical-therapeutic intervention, will help in such cases. It is essential to provide this support.

Strain and stress reactions are nonspecific, i.e., they are independent of the type of stressor. The reactions are usually autonomous and involuntary. They become accessible to control though, when the individual becomes conscious of the effects. Operators in aviation and space flight have to learn about the reactions to expect under conditions of stress, and about how these may endanger the operating system. This applies especially to aircrews in military missions, who need special attention.[3] Numerous crash scenarios have shown that stress reactions have more catastrophic consequences the less they are controlled. Therefore, pilots and other operators should learn how to avoid stress situations and how to control stress reactions when stress is unavoidable. Consequently they need training in order to modify their attitudes towards conscious control of stress situations and in order to learn error-prevention strategies. The entire flight training should have a philosophy of stress management and error prevention as a background.

This also applies to coping with acute stress conditions. Crews must learn to recognize stress situations on the basis of behavioral symptoms. They should accept these as stress symptoms, communicate this to the other team members, and organize appropriate measures of behavior control. On top of theoretical training, compulsory seminars and practical training, additional aid should be provided in order to modify behavior and develop coping strategies. In the military field, a special care concept has been developed, "Psychological Mission Training and Counselling," comprised of the following four phases:[3] "pre-mission training → mission training → post-mission training → additional measures."

The main elements of stress management are:

- Self-awareness regarding the subjective stress level
- Stress and error prevention strategies
- Stress-coping strategies in acute situations
- After-action stress debriefing
- Treatment of long-term effects (e.g., post-traumatic stress and anti-airsickness training programs).

The Interpersonal Climate within the Air Crew

The work climate within the air crew is crucial for successful performance. Causes of tension in a crew include strong psychological differences between superiors and subordinates, differing understandings between cockpit and cabin crew of their respective roles, inappropriate self-assessment and inappropriate ambitions of some crew members, a know-all manner, poor willingness to cooperate and poor willingness to communicate and assist others. The true magnitude of this human "climate factor" has recently been investigated by Lufthansa in a large research project on flight safety (see Kemmler).[14]

The Importance of the Social Environment

Problems in a person's private life often influences his or her behavior and performance at work. This applies to any job but especially to jobs with high stress factors such as time pressure and demands of constant vigilance and attention; above all it applies to jobs with a high degree of responsibility and with extreme safety requirements such as those typical for the aerospace industry.

It is easier to learn how to deal with factual tasks than with emotions and conflicts. There is always a risk of not coping successfully with psychological conflicts and crises in the social environment. The affected individual ties the emotional energy to the conflict without being able to resolve it alone. Affected operators in any highly sensitive system run the risk of being vulnerable to aggressive behavior that disturbs cooperation and endangers safety. They are equally vulnerable to dubious methods of self-treatment, placation, trivialization, and suppression. This is likely to exert a strain on their private relationships, and they may develop psychosomatic disorders.[13] In severe cases, an affected person acquires a series of vague diagnoses and often ends up helpless as a person with "a personality disorder."

The social environment is also substantially marked by the climate in the organization, for which superiors in the hierarchy are responsible. Unjustified pressure from "above" causes grudges, loss of self-confidence, internal opposition, frustration, and loss of motivation — all of which curb commitment to maintain safety at the workplace.

CLINICAL AVIATION PSYCHOLOGY

Psychological Problem Areas in Aviation

In the field of civil aviation, psychological aptitude testing has a special status within fitness assessment, especially in countries where licensing regulations only allow psychological testing in cases of substantiated doubt about an applicant's aptitude. Doubt can appear prior to the beginning of training, during the first medical examination, or be based on information made available to the licensing authority. The instructor pilot might also find a student pilot's behavior bizarre or just out of the ordinary, and finally also trained pilots and controllers may display behavior that gives reason to doubt their reliability or aptitude.

Case report (1)

An airline pilot was found guilty of drunken driving a few years prior to his regular retirement. This caused the authorities to demand evidence of his reliability by means of an aviation-psychological aptitude test. Liver function tests were normal and there were no physical signs of alcohol abuse, nor were there any abnormal behavior or signs of mental disturbance. After a long period of habitual drinking, the pilot realized he was sitting on a "time-bomb." With the assistance of a psychologist, he self-critically tackled his wrong behavior. In order to get back his driving licence he underwent a medico-psychological examination, which once again showed no performance reduction and no toxic damages due to alcohol abuse.

Nevertheless, the results of the aviation-psychological examination led to substantial doubts about his capability to cope with the demands of professional flying. His performance profile was below average, also when adjusted for age. The pilot himself accepted having a reduced mental processing speed. Because of his objective difficulties in dealing with complex system requirements, it was not easy to make a favorable decision. However, his many years of experience and a successful check flight in a simulator had to be taken into account. The partly positive result of this aptitude test was favorably considered by the licensing authority but made contingent on successful refresher training.

In this case, the authority had a substantiated doubt about the pilot's suitability to continue his aviation activities and requested clarification by means of an aviation-psychological examination. This doubt originated from official information about his drunken driving sentence.

Another avenue for requests of aviation-psychological examinations is via the aeromedical examiner, who may detect significant and deep-rooted behavioral problems during the medical examination.

Cases where the licencing authority may decide to request aviation-psychological examination frequently result from the following observations:

- Difficulties in training, with considerable disturbances of the training process
- Specific flight-related performance deficits
- Cognitive performance deficits of perception, attention, and memory
- Obvious cognitive or psychomotor ability flaws
- Delinquency
- Drunken driving
- Alcohol or drug addiction
- Aggressiveness, intolerable social behavior
- Emotional instability
- Insufficient stress resistance, low frustration tolerance
- Traffic accidents, flight accidents or incidents
- Injury proneness and many accidents in everyday life
- Extreme personality traits that disturb teamwork in aviation or make it impossible
- Psychological behavior problems
- Psycho-somatic disorders

In Germany only experienced and authorized institutions are entitled to perform aviation-psychological examinations. In such institutions, most examination candidates appear for reasons of drunken driving and road traffic offences, followed by problems in training and psychological problems.[15,16]

In the military area, special aviation-psychological or clinical-psychological examinations have been ordered by flight surgeons for the following reasons:

- After accidents or incidents involving aircraft and where psychological factors are presumed involved or if there are doubts about the pilot's ability to cope
- Considerable flying-related performance deficits (e.g., due to age)
- Fear of flying and loss of flying motivation
- Recurring symptoms of airsickness, psychosomatic problems, neurotic and personality disorders, burn-out syndrome, behavioral problems, specific social conflict situations (job-related and private)
- Post-head injuries
- In case the ability to operate specific aircraft is questioned
- Pilots who were dismissed early from training for psychological or aviation-related reasons and are scheduled to perform a different task in aviation
- Before the transition to a different type of aircraft (propeller or helicopter to jet)

Psychological Methodology

The regulations define the procedures and methods for the aviation-psychological examination of fitness and aptitude of aviation personnel that meet these main demands: Aptitude testing must consider the specific strains of the aviation tasks; applied methods and test results must be valid for the specific group of persons; and results of the examination that were not gained by tests must be based on verifiable facts.

The methods of aviation-psychological examinations have been published in the European Regulations JAR-FCL/Part 3. They include biographical evaluation and testing of performance and personality dimensions.

Certain standards and criteria apply to the use of psychological tests.[17] Basic test principles demand comparability (with a norm group), objectivity (standardized application and processing of the results without subjective influence from test personnel), reliability (the test always measures the same dimension without significant deviations or measurement errors), and validity (the precision with which a test measures the target dimension and enables conclusions).

Extensive validation studies have been performed into the predictive validity of the different tests for successful training (for pilots: Maschke/Hörmann,[18] for air traffic controllers: Lorenz *et al.*)[19] The selection of pilot applicants ("*ab-initio*") shows a predictive validity of 95% for successful outcome of flight training. For licensed pilots ("ready-entry"), the correlation between the assessment during selection and their job-performance was similarly significant.

The basic test principles also apply to the application of tests in clinical psychology. Of these principles, the construct-related validity is of special importance for clinical and personality tests. In case clinical tests are used to support the aeromedical disposition, the criterion-oriented evidence of validity must be considered.

Case report (2)

During training for a CPL, the applicant (37 years and holder of a PPL) passed the theoretical examination at the third attempt. However, he did not pass the practical examination even after three attempts. He also repeatedly failed a test for flight instructors. The licensing authority now requested an aviation-psychological examination in order to determine whether the applicant was suitable for continued training for CPL, ATPL, and an instructor's licence.

The psychological tests showed a considerable deficiency in planned and controlled performance of complex coordination tasks. The psychologist described a deficiency in task-oriented performance in moments of high cognitive and emotional stress. This was manifest in his numerous failures at examinations and was confirmed by his unclear concept of his further career. The test results also indicated that he was substantially misjudging his own abilities.

Cases 1 and 2 point to the basic independence of aviation-psychological aptitude testing from aeromedical assessment of fitness. Case 2 demonstrates the necessity to supplement medical, operative, and laboratory results with psychological performance test results and insights into the personality (also after a psychological intervention) and to take into account the quality of flying experience for the assessment. Case 1 still holds a risk, which has to be controlled by close surveillance of the deployed pilot.

Cases 1 and 2 also show the need to consider the complete list of dimensions in the aviation-psychological assessment of problem cases, i.e., the biographical life history as well as performance and personality factors. Aviation psychologists should make sure to apply only such tests that are relevant to the aviation job requirements.

JAR-FCL/Part 3 (Medical) Subpart A, B, C, Section 2 lists the following psychological dimensions that should be looked at:

(1) Biographical anamnesis:

- General life history
- Education
- Critical behavioral incidents
- Delinquency
- Family
- Socio-economic status
- Diseases and accidents

(2) Operational attitudes (standardized tests for cognitive performance dimensions and operational ability):

- Logical reasoning
- Memory function (visual and auditory)
- Perception
- Psychomotor function
- Mental arithmetic
- Attention
- Spatial comprehension
- Multi-task abilities

(3) Personality dimensions (standardized questionnaires, clinical behavior observation, structured interview):

- Motivation and work orientation (need for achievement, vitality, mobility, readiness to acquire new knowledge and skills, acceptance of responsibility)

- Decision-making (problem-solving behavior, choice of alternatives, decision in situations of uncertainty, decision after assessing available information)
- Social capability (extroversion-introversion, dominance/assertiveness, empathy, aggression)
- Stress coping (emotional stability, readiness to bear privations, flexibility, stress management)

Extreme distinctiveness in certain dimensions, behavioral disorders, and obvious psycho-pathological and psychosomatic symptoms require the psychologist's special attention.

Case 2 also shows that, in spite of otherwise normal cognitive abilities, a performance deficiency in complex coordination tasks and a deficiency in concentration and emotional stability can reduce an individual's ability to control an aircraft to the extent that not even additional training will improve his performance. Futile extra training is not only uneconomic, but also demotivating. In general, unsuccessful training leads to a further loss of self-confidence and endangers flight safety. These deficiencies were not only visible in the applicant's performance behavior in test situations, but could also be seen when he flew on his own.

Case report (3)

A student pilot (56 years old), who wanted to acquire a PPL-A, failed the final practical check three times. The licensing authority requested an aviation-psychological examination. Several psychomotor tests were applied for different aspects of relevant psychomotor tasks. All of the results revealed considerable performance deficiencies. The student pilot had no problems with understanding test instructions and task concepts, but there was a deficiency in information processing. This behavioral deficiency was basically caused by his pronounced emotional instability and poor stress resistance. He was described as a very reflective, schizothyme person, unsure about himself and his performance, whose stress resistance appeared to be reduced considerably. In addition, at his relatively high age, it is not easy to acquire new psychomotor skills for demanding motor coordination and multiple task handling. Under conditions of stress, this can lead to learning problems, time-consuming extra training periods, and regression into simple and inappropriate behavior. This student pilot would never become be able to pilot an aircraft safely because such grave deficiencies cannot be compensated by additional flight training.

Case 3 describes grave performance deficiencies, observed during practical training, by the instructors. Their report to the licencing authority led to an aviation-psychological examination. The psychological report was the basis for the final licencing decision.

Assessment and Results

Any expert's recommendation about a pilot's fitness and aptitude requires integrity, especially in difficult cases. The interests of an individual's existence must be weighed against the safety interests of the general public. In cases of doubt, safety must be given priority. In borderline cases, it becomes obvious that a strictly objective judgement has its limitations. A classical and basically always valid question for the expert is: "Would I fly with this pilot?" The psychological expert can only make a recommendation if the following applies:

- The examination has been completed according to the above-mentioned criteria
- All available data have been considered
- The examination has been carried out with the support of a second psychologist or a trained test instructor in order to compare and check the results

If, after an aviation-psychological examination, doubt persists, limitations or restrictions of the licence can sometimes be imposed, allowing the pilot to fly without posing a danger to flight safety.

At DLR, 39% of the examined problem cases were first-time applicants, 30% were holders of ATPL, 18% had PPL, and 13% had CPL/IFR.[15] At FFB, the cases without a licence and with PPL were balanced (41% and 42%), and 11% had ATPL.[16]

Recommendation categories are: Suitable/unsuitable/temporarily unsuitable/suitable under conditions. At DLR, positive and negative recommendations are quite balanced (45% and 43%), and at FFB, the majority of cases qualified as positive (71%). 12% (DLR) and 10% (FFB) of the applicants were obliged to accept certain conditions, such as:

- Flight related conditions (e.g., licence limitations/restrictions)
- Behavior control
- Medical control (e.g., blood testing)
- Successfully completed educational air traffic classes
- Successful alcohol or drug withdrawal treatment
- Successfully completed psychotherapy
- Follow-up examination/s

Within a period of eight years, 396 airforce pilots with problems were examined psychologically for the following reasons:

- Flight-related performance deficiencies (e.g., accidents, incidents, mistakes, deterioration of performance, problems with transfer to more complex aircraft): N = 215; 87% rehabilitated, 13% dismissed
- Psychological maladaptation (e.g., fear of flying, fear of failure, reactive depression, alcoholism, simulation): N = 73; 59% rehabilitated, 41% dismissed
- Psychosomatic disorders (e.g., motion sickness, organic neuroses, sensory malfunction, vegetative dysregulation): N = 108; 58% rehabilitated, 42% dismissed.

Clinical Therapeutic Intervention

In aviation, psychology not only plays an integral role for the selection of suitable applicants, but also contributes substantially to the education and training of operational personnel. Helpful interventions range from the care for personnel subjected to high stress, to rehabilitation, i.e., the re-establishment of psychophysical and mental capacities.

When the task-induced and psychological stress reaches a level beyond a pilot's ability to cope alone, the professional adaptation process does not have to be interrupted if the pilot is willing to modify his attitudes and change his lifestyle. In order to achieve this, different means of psychological counselling, behavioral interventions, or psychotherapy are available. Self-help programs for civil aircrews have been introduced (e.g., "relapse prevention" for alcohol and drug problems, "employee assistance program (EAP)," and The Mayday Foundation), and professional clinical psychology offers a variety of interventions. An interdisciplinary cooperation with flight surgeons, aeromedical examiners, and experts from the licensing authority is generally helpful. In the civil area, the psychologist or aeromedical examiner can only recommend an individual to seek help. The affected pilot or controller must be willing to accept external therapeutic support. In the military area, clinical-therapeutic interventions are arranged by the flight surgeon or the commander.

Psychological interventions require a diagnostic process. Unlike the standardized and quantified examination procedures used in clinical aviation psychology, which can supplement the methods commonly applied in psychiatry, interventions are not determined by specific procedures. The choice of applicable methods has to be individually tailored. The first interview is essential as the treatment modality and the indication for specific methods are decided here. With the diagnostic tools previously mentioned, the consulting psychologist gains important insights into the individual's potential and personality. This is the basis for a goal-oriented treatment and its prognosis. Clinical-psychological consultation and psychotherapeutic treatment follow a structured sequence[20,3]:

1. Explanation of the test results and their significance for the individual case.
2. Indication of the necessary clinical therapeutic interventions, explanation of the planned counselling (or therapy), and the prognosis.
3. A maximum of three to four counselling sessions to talk about consequences based on self-competence and self-management.

4. Recommendations for further psychological behavioral training and/or treatment.
5. Carrying out the recommended measures. A clinical-psychological or psychotherapeutic treatment can only be conducted by external specialists.
6. Report the results of the measures to the responsible persons.
7. Judgement and evaluation of the results in view of their consequences for the course of the case regarding further treatment, the candidate's future deployment, and aptitude.
8. Quality control of the measures by the consulting psychologist, in cooperation with the aviation company after the candidate has resumed his job.
9. Establishing and improving a permanent network of responsible internal persons and external experts.

Case report (4)

A professional pilot who had been caught abusing and selling illicit drugs, had his CPL/IFR revoked by the licensing authority. An aviation-psychological examination was requested. The aptitude testing showed an intact and well-balanced person with an average level of intelligence and fully functioning operational skills. The examination also revealed a problematic, neurotic personality, marked by strong influences from his up-bringing at home and education at boarding school. The pilot had developed fear of examinations, which resulted in an anxiety disorder. He tried to fight his anxiety with drugs and became addicted. This development was encouraged by his psychoneurotic disposition. A lack of support in the social sphere is characteristic for the typical drug biography. Owing to this personality structure, a continuous high risk of addiction was diagnosed. In order to get back his licence, the pilot was obliged to complete the following:

- Successful withdrawal treatment (to be documented)
- Successful psychotherapy for his anxiety disorder
- Integration into a supportive social sphere

Accidents or critical incidents in aviation often result in traumatic stress with sustained shock and disorganization of lifestyle. In such cases, a stress debriefing, starting immediately after the event, can prevent worse post-traumatic effects. In the section of clinical psychology at the air force's medical institute, approximately 100 problem cases are psychologically examined and treated every year.[3] 74% of the pilots undergoing treatment were able to rejoin their units after successful interventions. It appeared that, for example, the fear of flying and airsickness were easier to treat than alcoholism or chronic psychosomatic disorders and neuroses with strong constitutional components.

However, cost-intensive and time-consuming psychotherapies should not be considered if the intervention, including refresher training, is to exceed a period of three months. Another aspect to bear in mind is that external therapists are unfamiliar with the field of aviation and, in case of military pilots, may not be available for consultation due to security reasons. Psychotherapy is justified, if:

- The pilot's performance was above average before his problems started
- The motivation for flying is unbroken
- The pilot shows insight and a strong will to cooperate
- The disorder can be treated efficiently in the available time period

Clinical psychology offers support in a variety of different conflicts (e.g., family and educational counselling, rehabilitation, withdrawal therapies, relaxation therapies, educational air traffic classes, emergency psychology, etc.). Cognitive behavioral therapy comprises training for the modification of behavior and deals with affects, attitudes, motives, and biographical aspects of the disorder. There is an evident demand for this kind of psychological support. With regard to job satisfaction, a long career in aviation, and last but not least, flight safety, individuals should be encouraged to accept these offers. In addition, it is necessary to establish a network of competent external experts to which pilots can be referred for clinical consultation and treatment.

Emergency psychology has developed concepts to deal with acute crises, which are applicable after accidents or catastrophic events ("critical incidents"), e.g., accidents with many casualties, life-threatening events, and exposure to terrorists, hijacking, and captivity (Kemmler).[20] The objective of such concepts is to make psychologically trained persons available to counteract stress and shock by early intervention. The "International Critical Incident Stress Foundation" in Baltimore trains helpers (e.g., psychologists, pilots) in critical incident stress management (CISM). The German Airforce has successfully applied this concept.[22]

CONCLUSIONS

This chapter describes the contribution of aviation psychology to aviation personnel at different career stages. A series of psychological measures is available during all the stages: starting with the psychological selection of personnel, through training syllabi ("human factors," HPL) and the obligatory leadership and cooperation seminars and training (CCC/MCC, CRM, and Captain Advanced Training), to the different forms of clinical intervention ("Emotional Balance Management," etc.) and psychotherapy, if necessary, in order to restore psychological fitness and aptitude.

This chapter also illustrates the necessity for preventive measures in order to avoid critical situations or cope with them appropriately. Critical incidents can have grave effects on an individual's health, performance, and motivation if they are not coped with adequately. In general, the objective is to continually develop prevention and coping strategies for the effects of stress, conflicts, risk exposure, and critical incidents.

Finally, there is substantial demand for the availability of emergency and crisis psychology in order to offer psychological help and care in cases of chaos and trauma. Helpers are affected as "secondary victims" in emergencies. After overcoming the acute crisis, the trauma and post-traumatic disorders must be treated.

In order to tackle all these tasks of clinical aviation psychology, a network of internal and external experts for clinical-psychological consultation, care and therapy of affected aviation personnel should be made available.

REFERENCES

1. JAA — Joint Aviation Authorities. (1996/2003) Flight Crew Licensing, Part 3 (Medical), Colorado: Global Engineering Documents.
2. Gerathewohl S. (1987) *Leitfaden der militärischen Flugpsychologie*. Verlag für Wehrwissenschaften, München.
3. Roth W. (1998) Clinical psychology applications in military aviation. In: Goeters Kl-M, *Aviation Psychology: A Science and a Profession*. Ashgate, Aldershot.
4. Kanas N. (1991) Psychological support for cosmonauts. *Aviat Space Env Med* **62**: 353–355.
5. Manzey D, Schiewe A, Fassbender C. (1995) Psychological countermeasures for extended manned spaceflight. *Acta Astronautica* **35**: 339–361.
6. Eissfeld H. (1998) The Selection of air traffic controllers. In: Goeters Kl-M (ed), *Aviation Psychology: A Science and a Profession*. Ashgate, Aldershot.
7. EUROCONTROL. (1996) *Guidelines for Selection Procedures and Tests for Ab-Initio Trainee Controllers*. HUM.ET1.ST04.10000-GUI-01.
8. Stelling D. (2004) Psychological requirements and examination guidelines in JAR-FCL 2. In: Goeters K-M (ed), *Aviation Psychology: Practice and Research*. Ashgate, Aldershot.
9. Steininger K. (1991) *Leadership Competence Training*. DLR — DLH, Internal Report.
10. Goeters Kl-M (ed). (1998) *Aviation Psychology: A Science and a Profession*. Ashgate, Aldershot.
11. Maschke P, Goeters Kl-M. (1999) *Anforderungen an Flugschüler in der Ab-initio-Ausbildung im Vergleich zu aktiven Linienflugzeugführern*. DLR Forschungsbericht 1999-16, Hamburg.
12. Heintz A. (1998) *Anforderungsanalysen in der Flugverkehrskontrolle: Ein Vergleich verschiedener Arbeitspositionen*. DLR Forschungsbericht 98-18, Hamburg.
13. King RE. (1999) *Aerospace Clinical Psychology*. Ashgate, Aldershot.

14. Kemmler R. (2000) *Analyse von Flugsituationen und Entwicklung präventiver Maßnahmen.* DLH Forschungsprojekt Flugsicherheit, Berliner Streßtage, 15.04.2000.
15. Stelling D. (1997) Psychological evaluations of problem cases in aviation. *EAAP/JRC Courses on Human Factors in Aviation,* Ispra.
16. Hansen D. (1999) *Flugpsychologische Untersuchung von zivilem Luftfahrtpersonal.* Interner Bericht Fl. Med. Inst. LW, Fürstenfeldbruck.
17. Goeters Kl-M. (1998) General standards of selection: Validity and utility analysis. In: Goeters Kl-M (ed), *Aviation Psychology: A Science and a Profession.* Ashgate, Aldershot.
18. Maschke P, Hörmann H-J. (1988) Zur Bewährung psychologischer Auswahlverfahren für operationelle Berufe in der Luft- und Raumfahrt. *Zeitschrift für Flugwissenschaften und Weltraumforschung* **12**: 181–186.
19. Lorenz B, Pecena Y, Eissfeld H. (1999) *Selection of Ab Initio Air Traffic Control Applicants for EUROCONTROL, Validation of the DLR-Battery against Training Effectiveness.* DLR Forschungsbericht 99-05, Hamburg.
20. Kemmler R. (1998) Clinical-psychological diagnostics and consultation in commercial aviation. In: Goeters Kl-M (ed), *Aviation Psychology: A Science and Profession,* Proceedings of the EAAP-Conference 1996, Ashgate, Aldershot.
21. Everly JS Jr, Mitchell JT. (1999) *Critical Incident Stress Management: A New Era and Standard of Care in Crisis Intervention, 2nd Ed.* Hevron Publishing Corporation, Ellicot City.
22. Willkomm B. (1999) *Critical Incident Stress Management (CISM) (nach MITCHELL), Maßnahmen zur akuten Krisenintervention und zur Prävention posttraumatischer Belastungsstörungen.* Flugmed Inst der LW, Abt VI-Flugpsychologie, Fürstenfeldbruck.

Chapter 22

Neuropsychological Disorders After Brain Injury and their Assessment

Josef Zihl*,† and Herbert Jacobs

DEFINITION

Neuropsychological disorders are impairments of mental health that include cognition, i.e. attention, learning, memory, executive function, language/speech, and sensorimotor functions, as well as motivation and emotion. (Behavioral) neurology, neuropsychology, psychiatry, and clinical psychology are involved in assessing these functional deficits.

Neuropsychology has become a neuroscientific specialty and its interdisciplinary character requires collaboration with other disciplines such as internal medicine and endocrinology. Clinical neuropsychology is concerned with assessing the cognitive, emotional, and behavioral consequences of brain dysfunction and their treatment.[1,2] Psychopathological symptoms such as affective and personality disorders are assessed in collaboration with clinical psychology and psychiatry.

High mental fitness is an indispensable prerequisite for safe flying. This prerequisite is critically related to the functional capacities

* Corresponding author.
† Department of Psychology, Ludwig Maximilians University, Munich, Leopoldstrasse 13, 80802 München, Germany, and Max Planck Institute of Psychiatry, Kraepleinstrasse 10, 80802 München, Germany.

and capabilities of the central nervous system (CNS). Brain injury and its consequences are often not adequately assessed. When mental functioning and performance are evaluated, cognitive impairments and psychopathological symptoms are often neither diagnosed nor considered. The variability of functional disturbances with respect to their clinical significance possibly explains this shortcoming. Furthermore, small lesions with skull injuries in particular may not always be detected by brain imaging (CT, MRI). Significant functional impairments can therefore exist without detectable morphological brain defects. In addition, despite evidence of brain injury from brain imaging, functional disturbances can nevertheless be absent. A comprehensive assessment of mental functioning requires objective, valid, and reliable psychometric tests. The personal history is an important component of the neuropsychological assessment although often of limited value. Patients seldom notice the cognitive impairment itself; they rather experience its effects on cognitive functioning, e.g. attentional impairments are often experienced as disturbances of memory, perception, and thought. Moreover, detection of cognitive deficits is often prevented by the patient's loss of insight into these disturbances; this so-called anosognosia (from Greek, meaning "unawareness of illness") is caused by brain injury and is regarded as a distinct disorder (see Section on *Awareness, Trivializing, and Malingering in Neuropsychological Assessment*). In addition, individuals with "mild" functional impairments often trivialize the consequences in order to protect their occupational activities or social status.

In summary, an objective, valid, and reliable assessment of the quality (type) and quantity (degree) of cognitive impairments is of high importance in aviation medicine and requires specific evaluation processes. A comprehensive assessment involves identifying not only the affected but also the preserved mental functions, i.e. a negative and positive performance profile. Determining whether functional deficits are primary or secondary deficits is crucial in this regard. Disorders of visual perception can lead to secondary impairments of memory, executive function, language/speech, and sensorimotor activities. As attention is the essential prerequisite for all mental functions, attentional impairment, depending on severity, can affect all mental areas. This also applies to disorders of motivation. Affective disorders such as depression influence a variety of cognitive functions,[3] which it is important to consider in neuropsychological assessments.

Brain injury can have transient or chronic effects on its functional capacities (for a review, see Ref. 1). Despite high variability of etiology, the resulting mental syndromes and cognitive symptoms are usually not unequivocally related to the etiology of brain injury or disease. Disorders of cognition and personality can appear in isolation or in combination, which should be considered in the diagnostic evaluation. In the International Classification of Diseases (ICD-10), they are classified as "organic mental disorders" (F0). ICD-10 offers only very few differentiation categories for mental and/or cognitive syndromes or symptoms (i.e. F00-F06, particularly F02.8, but also F07.2). Personality changes (in part included under cognitive symptoms such as F07.2) are classified as follows:

F07	Personality and behavioral disorders due to brain disease, damage, or dysfunction
F07.0	Organic personality disorder
F07.1	Post encephalitic syndrome
F07.2	Post concussional syndrome

DOMAINS OF COGNITION AND THEIR ASSESSMENT

Neuropsychological disorders vary with regard to their frequency of occurrence. Visual perception, attention, memory, and executive function are the most frequently affected cognitive domains. The resulting functional impairments are presented in detail in the following sections; disorders of language/speech, sensorimotor functions, and calculation are only briefly discussed. A comprehensive account of the various neuropsychological disorders and their assessment can be found in Lezak *et al.*[2]

Visual Perception

Our knowledge of the physical and social environment, as well as of our body, relies on information processing in our sensory systems; processed information is then stored in the subcortical and cortical structures of which these systems are comprised. Perception is the most important prerequisite for recognition, experience and action. The visual system plays a special role as it processes the majority of information about the far and near environment. The mental representation of the external world is predominantly visual in nature. Visual information is therefore indispensable for spatial orientation and enables exploration, navigation, and grasping.

The most common visual disorder caused by brain injury is a defect in the visual field (anopia), which affects the corresponding left or right hemifield (unilateral left- or right-sided homonymous hemianopia). The majority of patients with homonymous visual field defects have a relatively small residual visual field; in about 70% of cases the remaining visual field does not exceed five degrees. Typical functional consequences of homonymous visual field defects are the loss of overview, an impairment of visual scanning and visual search, and difficulties with reading (so-called hemianopic dyslexia).

Visual acuity is, as a rule, not affected after unilateral postchiasmatic injury. After bilateral injury, visual acuity may be unaffected yet it can also be impaired in such a way that visual acuity remains sufficient only for finger counting. Spatial contrast sensitivity (contrast vision), on the contrary, can be reduced after unilateral injury. Patients with this disorder report "blurred vision." Impairments of visual acuity or contrast vision primarily affect depth perception, visual recognition (particularly face identification), and reading. These impairments cannot be alleviated by optical correction.

Impairments of color vision manifest themselves as reduced foveal color discrimination (cerebral dyschromatopsia) or as a complete loss of color vision in corresponding (homonymous hemichromatopsia) or both hemifields (bilateral homonymous achromatopsia).

Disorders of visual space perception primarily affect the exact localization of objects, which leads to secondary impairments of, for example, visually-guided grasping and visual constructive skills; in some cases, reading and writing are also affected. The subjective visual straight-ahead direction may be shifted contralateral to the side of brain injury, which is frequently associated with homonymous visual field defects. Disorders of depth perception typically cause under- or overestimation of distances and impairments of stereoscopic (3D) vision. In cases with loss of stereoscopic vision, however, possible reductions in visual acuity or contrast vision and disorders of oculomotor functions (vergence, fusion, accommodation), which are known to interfere with depth perception, should be taken into account.

The (rare) impairment of visual recognition is also referred to as visual agnosia, i.e. the inability to visually recognize objects. Patients with visual agnosia misinterpret, for example, objects on the basis of identical or similar global (such as size, form) and/or local features (such as details of form, colors). Visual agnosia can be category specific and it can be differentiated between visual agnosia for objects (object agnosia), faces (prosopagnosia), localities and areas (topographagnosia, environmental agnosia), and letters and words (pure alexia).

Attention

Attention is an essential prerequisite for all activities in various functional realms, especially for all non-routine activities and processes that require (intentional) attentiveness, i.e. concentration. Attention has two broad dimensions, i.e. intensity and selectivity, according to which disorders of attention can be classified.

Disorders of the intensity dimension of attention primarily affect attention activation (alertness), information processing speed, cognitive performance speed, and the maintenance of attentiveness over time (sustained attention). Patients with a reduced cognitive processing speed ("cognitive slowing") require much more time for all cognitive tasks. Impaired sustained attention can manifest itself either as a reduction of the global level of attention or as a pathological fluctuation of attention when demanding tasks are performed.

Disorders of the selectivity dimension of attention include impaired focused or selective attention (concentration), divided attention, and spatial attention for one or both hemifields. Impaired divided attention can affect cognition and action in various ways as parallel multi-tasking is no longer possible and task components have to be executed serially (see also Section on *Executive Function*). For differential diagnosis, it is important to consider that selective attention crucially depends on the intensity aspect of attention. A reduction in attention intensity typically leads to secondary impairments of selective attention components. Disturbances of spatial attention include the unilateral (visual neglect syndrome) or bilateral restriction of the field of attention (Balint's syndrome). Both syndromes are rather rare but represent severe impairments for practically all activities of daily living, including visual spatial navigation, visuomotor guidance, reading, and writing. Another attentional deficit concerns the (rapid) shift of attention between stimuli in space, which occurs typically after frontal brain injury.

Memory

Temporary or long-term storage of information is one of the main requirements for transforming information into action. Furthermore, it guarantees — by means of learning processes — the acquisition of cognitive routines and habits as well as storing experience. Processing and transient storage of information in working memory plays a particularly important role in spatial navigation. A disturbance of working memory is a very frequent memory deficit, which can occur in every sensory modality (e.g. visual, auditory), and for each category of information (e.g. forms, colors, objects, faces, places, signs, words, auditory signals, language). Other memory disorders are the loss of semantic memory (verbal, visual knowledge), episodic memory (memory for episodes and events), and autobiographical memory (personal experiences). Loss of remote memory (acquired semantic and episodic knowledge before brain injury) is labeled retrograde amnesia while the loss of storing new information (acquisition of knowledge by learning, storing of new experiences, episodes and events after brain injury) is known as anterograde amnesia. The terms "global amnesia" or "amnesic syndrome" refer to the combination of antero- and retrograde amnesia.

Executive Function

The concept of "executive function" includes higher cognitive processes and activities, i.e. planning and problem solving, supervision of one's own activities (monitoring), flexible adaptation to a changing environment and tasks, error detection, management and correction, as well as the evaluation of actions, also with respect to intentions and desired actions. Executive dysfunction (dysexecutive syndrome) causes an impairment or loss of these functions and capacities, affects the allocation of attentional resources (intensity, selectivity) as well as motivation and reward perception. These patients have difficulties in performing tasks that require multi-tasking. In addition, planning and problem solving cannot be flexibly adapted to changing task conditions anymore, which affects optimizing action strategies. Motor or action control may also be affected, and difficulties with response inhibition emerge, i.e. responses are made to stimuli or changes in the environment, which should be ignored. The guidance of behavior lacks cognitive control. As a consequence, considering changing task conditions for decision making is no longer possible, and rigid behavior emerges. The loss of cognitive flexibility also manifests itself as perseverative responses, i.e. the patient is unable to change his or her behavior although the task requires a different response. Lack of response inhibition can also affect social behavior. Social signals immediately "trigger" (inappropriate) behavior, characterized by impulsivity. Another symptom of the dysexecutive syndrome is the supramodal impairment of working memory (see Section on *Memory*).

Language

Disorders of language and speech after acquired brain injury (i.e. any brain injury that happens after birth) are called "aphasia."

Aphasias are supramodal disorders that affect understanding and producing spoken and written language (reading and writing). Commonly, aphasia occurs after injury to the language-dominant (usually left) cerebral hemisphere. Aphasias are classified according to speech production (fluent versus non-fluent aphasias), or according to the main pathological symptoms with regard to semantic memory (amnesic aphasia), speech production (Broca's aphasia), and understanding of speech (Wernicke's aphasia). The combination of Broca's and Wernicke's aphasia is referred to as global aphasia. These aphasic syndromes typically occur after focal strokes in the language-dominant hemisphere. Traumatic brain injuries can cause a combination of divergent aphasic symptoms, which cannot be classified as one of the four syndromes mentioned. Reading and writing can be affected selectively (so-called pure alexia and pure agraphia).

Calculation

Disturbances of calculation abilities are frequently associated with an aphasic syndrome, yet selective calculation deficits do occur. Typical symptoms are loss of operational knowledge (addition, subtraction, division, multiplication) or of meaning of the spatial digit-positions within a number, or an impairment of estimating the order of sizes.

Sensorimotor Functions

Sensorimotor functions include sensorimotor coordination with respect to hand and finger movements and visually guided oculomotor activities. In ocular apraxia, the intentional spatio-temporal guidance of the scan path, and therefore visual scanning and exploration, is impaired. This impairment can be identified best by recording eye movements. The registration of eye movements is also a valuable tool for diagnosing disorders of visual scanning and visual exploration associated with homonymous visual field loss, visual spatial disorientation, and visual neglect.

Important Factors Influencing Neuropsychological Assessment

A variety of factors have to be taken into consideration when planning and performing a neuropsychological examination in order to prevent false positive or negative assessment outcomes:

- Peripheral sensory disorders (e.g. visual, auditory) can, depending on their severity, interfere with the correct application of neuropsychological tests.
- Cerebral visual disorders as well as oculomotor disorders (accommodation or vergence) have a negative impact on assessing cognitive functions as most tests require adequate visual functions and capacities (especially overview, visual acuity, and contrast vision).
- Disorders of hand function reduce the applicability of many test procedures, as nearly all tests require either a motor response or finger movement skills (e.g. paper-pencil tests).
- Speech and language disorders prevent an adequate comprehension of task instructions, and may distort the assessment of verbal memory.
- Sedating and stimulating medication can alter the examination results as they affect attentional functions, which can cause secondary impairments of memory and executive deficits.

Interpretation of Neuropsychological Test Results

Assessing cognitive impairments after acquired brain injury requires an estimate of the individual premorbid intellectual level; otherwise, poor cognitive performance might be incorrectly interpreted as deficit.

For estimation of the premorbid intellectual level, the following strategy can be used. According to the two-factor theory of intelligence proposed by Cattell,[4] human intelligence consists of "fluid" and "crystallized" intelligence. Fluid intelligence is understood as cognitive-intellectual potential, which is largely independent of culture and education. Basic cognitive functions, e.g. the information processing, cognitive speed, storage of information, and the ability to create logical connections for non-verbal, numerical, and culture-free material are components of fluid intelligence. Crystallized intelligence develops by learning (practice) and optimizing cognitive abilities, which result in successful and flexible routines and skills. Crystallized intelligence therefore depends crucially on education and cultural background.

Since crystallized intelligence is less vulnerable than fluid intelligence, it is a useful measure for individual premorbid intelligence. A standardized measure for the assessment of crystallized intelligence is, for example, vocabulary (recognition conditions). Vocabulary strongly depends on the level of education and is highly correlated with the overall intelligence of the individual. The case history (anamnesis) and information about education/occupation as well as strengths/weaknesses in cognitively demanding activities provide additional information. This information is also valuable for estimating individual differences regarding the overall intelligence level due to particular skills or special training, and builds the framework for a more valid interpretation of the individual test results in terms of "normal" or "impaired." The assessed cognitive performance level of an individual can then be compared with the respective expected level. In addition, standardized norm data are used for interpreting specific test results.

For valid and reliable neuropsychological test results, it also has to be considered that reduced cognitive performance might also be caused by normal mental aging processes, increased distress experienced in the testing situation, and uncertainty about one's own performance capabilities. Expectations of the subject, difficulties in comprehending task instructions, concerns regarding one's own occupational and/or private future, increased (internal) distractibility, and symptoms of depression and anxiety may also affect cognitive performance during neuropsychological assessment. Furthermore, the outcome of neuropsychological tests can also be influenced by functional substitution or compensation of the deficit. For example, a visual field loss may be compensated by systematic gaze shifts so that more time is required to perform a task; this may incorrectly be interpreted as cognitive slowing. A subject with memory difficulties may use written notes or special time organizers to cope with this impairment in daily life. Reduced perceptual and cognitive capacities may thus become evident in conditions where the subject cannot adequately compensate for his functional impairments.

Diagnostic classification relies on the results of the neuropsychological assessment. Significant deviations from standardized norm data indicate a reduction, i.e. impairment, of the assessed cognitive function. Yet, the variety of factors that can distort test results and their interpretation has to be taken into account. These influential factors should be considered when assessing cognitive performance and interpreting the outcome in the various cognitive tests.

Awareness, Trivializing, and Malingering in Neuropsychological Assessment

It is generally understood as "normal" that brain-injured subjects have sufficient awareness of and insight into their functional disabilities (handicaps); this is, however, only partly true for subjects with acquired brain injury. This also raises the question: what kind of behavioral reaction to acquired cognitive impairments can be classified as "normal" or "adequate" in this undoubtedly pathological condition?

Individual personality traits and life experiences certainly play an important role in gaining insight into functional impairments after brain injury. Factors of "pathological" nature that hinder the subject to detect, analyze, and interpret correctly his or her functional deficits can only be adequately assessed by means of a valid clinical psychological and psychiatric interview and assessment with standardized tests. It sometimes remains unclear whether and to what extent subjects are able to detect their functional deficits and interpret them adequately. For example, 20–30% of patients with hemiplegia and about 30% of patients with homonymous hemianopia are not aware of and have no (full) insight into their disorders. Often, disorders are attributed to external factors, i.e. patients are convinced that they are perfectly healthy and it is the external world that has changed. This loss of awareness and insight into one's own functional deficits is called anosognosia and is understood as a genuine disorder after acquired brain injury, which cannot be explained by (premorbid) personality traits or by global cognitive deterioration.[5] Yet, reduced awareness and "insight" can also be caused by other factors. Subjects may implicitly make use of compensatory strategies so that the impairment is not (fully) "noticeable" for him or her in daily life. Some subjects report cognitive difficulties without being able to classify them correctly according to the primary affected cognitive domain (e.g. attention or memory).

Functional impairments and their consequences may also be experienced as embarrassing and are therefore often trivialized or not at all reported by the patient. This may also apply to the patient's relatives when they are asked for the patient's difficulties in everyday life activities. Trivializing the resulting consequences may also be used in order to protect occupational activities or social status. The severity of functional deficits can also be intentionally exaggerated, often motivated by wish of secondary gain such as early retirement and various kinds of compensation or insurance claims. Detecting such tendencies requires different observational methods, and malingering is likely when ...

- the patient has an incentive to exaggerate or simulate symptoms
- subjective complaints are inconsistent with the neurological, psychopathological, or neuropsychological condition
- premorbid personality disorders exist
- reasonable doubts exist concerning the patient's efforts during the examination
- results from neuropsychological tests are contradictory and invalid as is the case if, for example, results from tests with low cognitive demands are worse than those from tests with higher demands.

PERSONALITY DISORDERS OF ORGANIC ORIGIN

Symptomatology

Personality changes and disorders are often associated with cognitive disorders and can occur as consequences of acquired brain injury. An accentuation of premorbid personality traits are referred to as (quantitative) personality changes, whereas an altered affect and lowered impulse control is referred to as a (qualitative) personality disorder. Relatives or colleagues often regard such behavior as strange when compared to premorbid personality characteristics. Personality changes and disorders manifest themselves as motivational disorders (e.g. reduced motivation), behavioral disinhibition (increased distractibility, logorrhea, aggressive behavior), and affect lability. These symptoms typically occur after frontal lobe injury, are commonly associated with executive disorders (dysexecutive syndrome; see Section on *Executive Function*), and are part of the "frontal lobe syndrome". Affect lability and response disinhibition are sometimes also associated with a deficient adequate evaluation of one's own capabilities and performance. These symptoms pose severe limitations, and are therefore particularly disabling for patients with professions that require highly demanding cognitive capacities, a high level of social competence, and superior responsibilities.

Diagnostic Problems

Personality changes caused by acquired brain injury are often not reliably detectable with standardized tests. Psychological personality inventories are not suitable because they do not allow identification of personality changes or disorders. Furthermore, it should be noted that the predictive value of personality questionnaires critically depends on the ability and willingness of the subject to provide reliable information. Many items address (actual) behavior and experiences, and attitudes, which are rather stable over time.

Personality changes after brain injury are often not experienced by the subject or the relatives, because accentuations of personal traits are often hardly noticeable. Patients with significant behavioral deviations often attribute the effects of these deviations to other people. The required diagnostic information can therefore only be obtained by carefully establishing case histories and collecting information from relatives and colleagues.

Case histories and information from others may not be sufficiently reliable to provide an adequate basis for a diagnostic statement regarding personality changes or disorders. Changes have to persist for a certain period of time to be noticed and experienced by the patient who then becomes aware of possible consequences in a given social context. Associated cognitive, language, and speech disorders usually have to diminish or become at least stable before personality changes become unequivocally evident. Yet, not all personality changes are caused by the brain lesion itself but rather emerge as a consequence of the functional limitations after brain injury. Functional limitations can lead to changes in personal interests and attitudes, biased interpretation of situations and the behavior of others, "unusual" affective responses, and sometimes, radical changes in habits. Thus, personality "changes" may represent inappropriate or appropriate coping strategies. Personality changes and disorders after acquired brain injury have to persist for a substantial period of time before a definitive diagnosis can be made.

AN ILLUSTRATIVE CASE

Mr. H, a military helicopter pilot, was involved, together with his wife, in a motor vehicle accident. A vehicle from the oncoming traffic came into his lane and collided with his vehicle. His wife was only slightly injured, but since then suffered from nightmares related to the accident. Mr. H was seriously injured, suffered severe head injury, and remained in a comatose state for six days. Brain imaging showed a cerebral contusion. After discharge from the hospital, he was referred to a rehabilitation center. A few months later, he underwent a neuropsychological assessment; at that time, he seemed to have almost totally recovered. He showed full orientation concerning person, place, and time. His verbal IQ was 118. Considering his educational and professional status (completion of professional technical school, helicopter training, and officer in the German Air Force), this IQ result was regarded as being similar to his premorbid intelligence level and therefore as being equal to the expected intellectual/cognitive level. Cognitive speed and verbal memory performance were significantly lower than the expected (or pre-morbid) values. Visual retention performance was significantly below average. Analytic-synthetic and spatial-cognitive abilities were normal. Sustained attention was below the range of average.

After this initial neuropsychological assessment, Mr. H was examined every six months. During each examination he expressed the hope to be able to fly again soon, which, in his view, he had not been allowed to do "because of the doctors." Personality changes were not observed. He had no memories of the accident, which he experienced as an "uncomfortable void," yet at the same time he was happy that he was not haunted by nightmares like his wife.

Two years later, there was no longer any evidence of morphological brain injury from brain imaging. Only minimal deficits in visual memory and a slight reduction of cognitive speed were identified in neuropsychological assessment. However, in his daily life he noticed pronounced concentration deficits, particularly over longer periods of time. He returned to work but could not cope despite low task demand and reduced workload (he worked only for a few hours daily). At this point, he began to understand that flying a helicopter would exceed his concentration and memory capacities as well as his ability to process information quickly and accurately. He experienced a change in affective reactivity and noticed a reduction of his cognitive flexibility. Furthermore, he reported that in the first year after the accident, for reasons unknown to him, he was often quite aggressive and even hit his wife. He regarded his behavior as totally strange, inadequate, and as being inconsistent with his personality. This was extremely embarrassing for him and he felt very sorry for it. Fortunately, these aggressive outbursts disappeared later on and his self-control returned to normal. His impression was that he was now much more stable, was able to accept his situation, and had learned how to cope with his impairments and their consequences for his professional and private life.

SUMMARY AND FINAL REMARKS

Neuropsychological and clinical psychological diagnoses require an adequate and comprehensive assessment of impaired and intact cognitive functions, level of adaptation to the deficits in terms of coping strategies, psychopathological symptoms, and premorbid personality traits. It also requires subjective reports from the patient, family members and colleagues about the various functional consequences. Behavioral observations during assessment can also provide additional information; it is important to observe how patients deal with the demands of particularly challenging tasks as well as take notice of characteristic error types, the motivation to cooperate and make every effort, and fluctuations of the performance level over a testing period of about two hours (i.e. the average duration of a neuropsychological examination). From a methodological viewpoint, standardized tests fulfilling the criteria objectivity, reliability, and validity should be preferred. Experimental procedures may be useful if standardized procedures are not available to assess the functional impairment of interest. Adequate norm data that correct for age, sex, and education are required for ensuring a valid diagnosis. Finally, it should also be noted that non-neurological diseases can cause cognitive disorders if the CNS is indirectly affected, e.g. in diabetes, hormonal disorders, heavy metal or organic solvent intoxication, and drug abuse.

Personality indices or symptom lists should not be used to validate or exclude cognitive or other functional disturbances. This also applies to intelligence tests as the resulting total or partial scores do not provide evidence for reliable conclusions regarding underlying functional disturbances. For example, disorders of (visual) information processing systems or attention cannot be detected by using a subset of such tests because of their insufficient validity.

Considering the requirements for piloting an aircraft, (visual) information processing, attention, and executive abilities (e.g. problem-solving, monitoring of activities) are of great importance. These cognitive domains also represent the determining factors of the so-called multi-tasking performance and therefore should be particularly considered in assessing and diagnosing neuropsychological disorders in aviation medicine.

Considering the complex cognitive and psychomotor requirements in aviators, even minimal evidence of reduced performance and/or personality changes due to acquired brain injury require immediate assessment and should be taken seriously. Of course, assessing the relevant cognitive and psychomotor functions requires tests with high ecological validity, computerized flight simulation tests, and possibly even real flights check.

GLOSSARY

Brain dysfunction

Any kind of consequence of pathological alterations of brain function due to structural, biochemical, or other causes, including diabetes, intoxication, metabolic disorders, etc.

Cognition

All forms of knowing and awareness, including perception, attention, learning and memory, and executive functions (planning, problem solving, monitoring, etc.). Cognitive abilities are skills of, or aptitudes for cognition.

Intelligence

Ability to select information, learn from experience, adapt to the environment, interpret and correctly utilize problem solving and planning.

Multi-tasking

Carrying out several tasks in parallel or in succession, which requires monitoring, task switching, and maintaining future goals while current goals are being dealt with.

Personality

The configuration of characteristics and behavior that comprises an individual's adaptation to life, including drivers, interests, abilities, major traits, values, self-concept, and emotional/affective patterns. The complex integration of this configuration includes among others hereditary and constitutional components, individual cognitive and social experiences, and culturally conditioned values and rules.

REFERENCES

1. Heilman KM, Valenstein E (eds). (2003) *Clinical Neuropsychology*. Oxford University Press, Oxford.
2. Lezak MD, Howieson DB, Loring DW. (2004) *Neuropsychological Assessment*. Oxford University Press, Oxford.
3. Austin MP, Mitchell P, Goodwin GM. (2001) Cognitive deficits in depression. *British J Psych* **178**: 200–206.
4. Cattel RB. (1971) *Abilities, Their Structure, Growth, and Action*. Houghton Mifflin, New York.
5. Adair JC, Schwartz RL, Barrett AM. (2003) Anosognosia. In: Heilman KM and Valenstein E (eds), *Clinical Neuropsychology*, pp. 185–214. Oxford University Press, Oxford.

Chapter 23

The Man-Man Interface in the Man-Machine System of Commercial Aviation Aircraft

Reiner W. Kemmler*

INTRODUCTION

Flight safety standards in commercial aviation are remarkably high compared to other transportation systems. IATA-statistics for recent years show 15–25 hull loss accidents per year of commercial aircraft (over 20 tons gross weight) among IATA members.

Due to the small statistical sample size, these events cannot be used as an empirical basis for analysis of the pilot's impact on flight safety. An optimum alternative approach is to interrogate a large number of professional airline pilots regarding their experience with safety-relevant in-flight situations, how they were involved in these events, and how they recovered from them. This concept was designed and carried out for all Lufthansa flight operations: Passenger Airline, CityLine, Cargo and Condor.[1,2] The IATA-accident category system was the basis of this "Cockpit Safety Survey" and consisted of four causal factors: Technical, Environmental, Organizational, and Human.

Based on the assumption that human factors not only consist of failures and errors, but also of social interaction deficits, these latter were included as aggravating factors. For statistical analysis, the IATA-category environmental and organizational factors were put

---

* Praxis für Luftfahrt psychologie und Krisenmanagement, Schillerstr. 27, D64546 Mörfelden-Walldorf, Germany.

together into one, pilot-independent factor, called operational. Human factors were differentiated into two: pilot failures/errors and social interaction deficits.

The expectation was to obtain more valid information regarding dangerous flight safety components, especially the influence of human factors in various combinations.

Determinants of Safety-Relevant Flight Situations

An anonymous questionnaire was distributed to 4400 pilots of all four Lufthansa flight operations. 2070 (47.2%) pilots responded, and only 73 (3.5%) of them reported no events. How pilots experience the event-determining factors was one of the central questions. Are there mainly single causes responsible for events or are combinations of several factors more frequent?

Interestingly (see Table 1), social interaction deficits do not play a significant role as a single cause. Technical factors rank highest at 7.7%, significantly higher than human failure.

Table 1. Frequency Distribution by Event-Configurations

Single Factors (14.5%)	
Technical	7.7%
Human failure/error	4.9%
Social interaction deficits	0.7%
Operational	1.2%

Table 2. Frequency Distribution by Event-Configurations

Combination of Two Factors (30.8%)	
Human failure/error + social interaction deficits	13.7%
Operational + human failure/error	8.3%
Technical + Operational	4.1%
Technical + social interaction deficits	2.6%
Operational + social interaction deficits	1.2%
Technical + human failure/error	0.9%

Table 3. Frequency Distribution by Event-Configurations

Combination of Three Factors	
Operational + Human failure/error + Social interaction deficits	37.8%
Technical + Operational + Social interaction deficits	4.1%
Technical + Operational + Human failure/error	2.5%
Technical + Human failure/error + Social interaction deficits	1.9%

The largest number of two-factor combinations (see Table 2) comes from human failure/error and social interaction problems. The common perception that a combination of human failure and technical factors is the most dangerous combination for flight safety is not supported by these results. On the contrary, it is the least important combination.

Most of the safety-relevant events are created by a combination of three factors. Two of them are human factors and one is operational. Operational factors in our survey represent pilot-independent characteristics, e.g., weather conditions, airport features, or organizational conditions (see Table 3).

These results focus on the importance of social skills and competence. We like to name this dimension "turbo-factor," because its effect boosts the combination of human failure and operational factors by a factor of nearly five.

In the history of flight safety, the most catastrophic accident in commercial aviation happened in March 1977 at the airport of Tenerife. It was the consequence of three such factors. Under extreme weather conditions two B-747 jumbos collided on the ground. In addition to the operational (airport) conditions — low visibility due to heavy fog — human errors and interpersonal deficits played a major role in the cockpit of one of the aircraft. The collision resulted in 583 fatalities.

This accident is also remarkable for giving rise to the concept of crew resource management.[3] Since that time much effort has been given to crew resource management training and emphasis has been placed on the improvement of social skills in cockpit crews.

Table 4. Frequency Distribution by Event-Configuration

Combination of Four Factors	
Technical + Operational + Human failure/error + Interpersonal deficits	9.1%

All four factors are present only in 9.1% (see Table 4) of all events. It seems that technical factors when combined with other factors have a reducing effect on the number of events, possibly due to the use of checklists indicating suitable procedures. Checklists may have a controlling effect on human factors and thus improve the situation.

Further studies and discussions are necessary to determine whether checklists and detailed procedures to specifically control human factors would be helpful and should be established. In the basic flight training program there are currently some commonly required training lessons called Human Performance and Limitations,[4] Crew Resource Management,[5] Line Oriented Flight Training (LOFT) and/or Threat and Error Management[6] for line pilots.

Social Interaction Deficits

All behavior items in the questionnaire that indicated social interaction deficits underwent a statistical factor analysis. The most plausible result was a four-factor structure with the following interaction deficit dimensions:

1. Information management between persons
2. Quality of communication
3. Impaired fitness for duty
4. Social climate

These four dimensions reflect the cockpit crew's problems when handling social interactions.

The most prominent is the transfer of information among crewmembers in the cockpit and between the cockpit and cabin crew, ATC, and other people in the air or on the ground. The second is the quality of communication, which is surprising as there is already a highly standardized phraseology in use in aviation.

The third dimension indicates the importance of the cockpit crew's situational (psycho-physiological) state, which significantly influences the social interaction. Social climate stands for spontaneous situational parameters of open-mindedness and sympathy versus ignorance and aversion.

All four behavior characteristics describe the broad spectrum of social interrelations.

In detail, the dimensions consist of a variety of specific behavior markers:

Information management

This dimension focuses on information transfer among persons, not only between persons and electronic systems. It is the most important behavior category. It refers to problems with information exchange among cockpit crew members, with cabin crew members and ATCO's or other people in the air or on the ground.

Behavior markers of this dimension are: Relevant messages not transferred, important statements disregarded, doubts not expressed, and distractions due to inadequate communication, all defined as transfer of information.

Quality of communication

This dimension generally focuses on the so-called "authority gradient." There is either a steep gradient due to a very dominant person, usually the captain, or a flat or even reverse gradient.

The behavior markers are: Solo attempt, lack of crew coordination because of distraction, authoritarian behavior, and too close relationships between crew members so that discipline is reduced.

Impaired fitness for duty

The third dimension indicates the importance of the cockpit crew's situational state, which significantly influences social interaction.

The behavior markers are: Physical and/or psychological strain. Physical strain is mostly related to fatigue caused by change of biorhythm due to time zone shift or flight schedule.

Psychological strain is linked predominantly to emotional states (anger, frustration) and interpersonal conflicts. An interpretation of this could be that these markers oppose each other with regard to arousal on a psycho-physiological dimension.

Social climate

Social climate stands for situational parameters of open-mindedness and sympathy versus ignorance and aversion.

The behavior markers are: Disorganized and irritating behavior, lack of self-assertion, and unnerving, intimidating behavior.

These markers describe strange behaviors of people working closely together in a team. It seems as if this is an effect of team members' cognitive and emotional incongruence, which can only be resolved if immediately addressed.

Safety-Relevant Determinants and Risk

In order to assess how dangerous the safety-related events had been, pilots were asked to estimate the degree to which they had lost control over the situation they were describing in the survey. They could respond on a scale from 1: "there was a risk, but no impairment of safety," up to 6: "the situation was completely out of control." The distribution of the mean risk (see Table 5) for all four event analysis categories in the survey indicates how detrimental the effects of social interaction deficits were.

Technical problems produce the least risk, social factors the highest. What is noteworthy is that operational factors in combination

Table 5. Risk Scale

Event-analysis Category	Mean
Technical factors	3.28
Human failure/error	3.46
Operational factors	3.47
Social interaction deficits	3.49

with social factors lead to the highest risk (3.62). The combination of operational problems with social factors and human failure/error result in a risk level of 3.56. All four factors combined create a risk level of 3.52. It is important to note that a risk level of over 3.5 indicates partial loss of control over the situation.

Conclusion and Consequences

For a long time most flight safety experts have concentrated on human failure and error. Since the end of the 1970s, there has been an increased focus on human factors in flight safety.

In the beginning it was unclear what specific aspects of social interaction, besides behavior markers of specific authority and communication, would influence performance and flight safety, and in which way.

Now we can state that not only human failure and error but also specific human interaction skills play a decisive role in the cockpit of commercial aviation aircraft. The most prominent and most dangerous combination of factors is that of human factors (human failure/error plus social interaction deficits) with pilot-independent, operational factors. The consequences are always, to some degree, loss of control over the situation.

In addition, global statistical analyses, such as the Annual Safety Reports from IATA, do not encompass research about combinations of different causative factors and their inherent risk levels. It seems a great step forward now to know much more about human factors on the basis of this large and representative research study.[1,2]

Since the beginning of specific human factor training activities, several generations of Crew Resource Management-Training have been developed. It is obvious that these countermeasures in combination with permanently optimized pilot selection are still not sufficient.

This could be the result of a didactic problem of training, an effect of financial restrictions, or a consequence of being unable to differentiate clearly between a variety of social interaction factors and their effects. Social factors belong to a very complex culture-dependant field of human behavior parameters, which are not easy to identify in a closed workplace like the cockpit of a commercial aircraft. Furthermore, trustful cooperation between pilots, human factor experts and research institutions is necessary if significant progress in this complex area is to be achieved. For the sake of flight safety, such cooperation is urgently needed.

REFERENCES

1. Braun P, Kemmler R, Eckerle T, Neb H, Lee I. (1999) Lufthansa Flight Safety Study: "Analysis of In-flight Situations and Development of Preventive Measurements," Part I: Frequency of event-configurations and problem aspects, Part II: Risk Analysis, Internal Report.
2. Baberg T, Kemmler R. (2001) *The Impact of Human Factors on the Development and Risk of Safety-Relevant Factors*, pp. 133–149. Flight Safety Foundation, EASS-Proc, Amsterdam, Netherlands.
3. Hawkins FH. (1987) *Human Factors in Flight.* Gower Technical Press.
4. Campbell RD, Bagshaw M. (eds) (2002) *Human Performance and Limitations in Aviation*. Blackwell Service, Oxford.
5. Wiener E, Kanki B, Helmreich RL. (eds) (1993) *Cockpit Resource Management.* Academic Press, San Diego.
6. Helmreich RL, Merrit AC. (1999) *Error and Error Management.* Technical Report. Austin, TX.

Part 7

PASSENGERS

Chapter 24

Passenger Health

Petra A. Illig*

INTRODUCTION

Aviation medicine has historically focused on the health of cockpit crew members with an occasional nod to the cabin and ground crew. In the last few years, attention has begun to be paid to the health of passengers as well, especially those whose medical problems could be exacerbated by the physical stressors of flying.

More than one billion (10^9) people travel by air every year throughout the world. Despite the financial struggles of the airline industry, airline travel is currently growing, and is estimated to double over the next 20 years.[1,2] The advent of super jumbo aircraft such as the Airbus A380, which carries more passengers for longer times over greater distances, combined with an aging flying population, makes the incidence of on-board medical emergencies likely to increase.[3]

Airline companies are increasingly challenged to provide reasonable medical assistance to ill passengers. For example, since April 2004, automated external defibrillators (AED) and enhanced emergency medical kits (EEMK) have been required by the Federal Aviation Administration (FAA) to be on board all US passenger airliners with a minimum payload capacity of 7500 pounds and serviced by at least one flight attendant. Passengers who are physicians often find themselves volunteering to assist in medical emergency

* Aviation Medical Services, 5011 Spenard Road 102, Anchorage, AL 99517, USA.

situations and can find themselves outside their clinical comfort zones. Unnecessary diversions based on medical incidents are costly to the airline industry and very disruptive to the passengers. In today's legal atmosphere, airlines are less likely to allow flight attendants to give even simple advice for commonly encountered in-flight medical problems, such as ear pain caused by cabin pressure changes.

In response to consumer pressure and media sensationalism, passenger health has become an issue visible enough to be addressed by the US Federal Air Surgeon.[4,5] Some articles and studies have been published in general medical literature,[7,18,19,24] and most recently, passenger health has its own chapter in a reputable textbook of aerospace medicine.[8] Several medical specialty societies have chimed in as well.[6,13]

Reports on passenger health by industry groups, such as the International Air Transport Association (IATA),[9] government (FAA),[11,12] as well as international professional groups, especially the World Health Organization (WHO),[27] the International Civil Aviation Organization (ICAO) and European Civil Aviation Conference (ECAC), have also been published.[16]

Airline companies are increasingly publishing basic passenger health advice on their websites. Even the House of Lords in the British Parliament has taken an interest in passenger health issues, primarily in the area of cabin air quality and traveler's thrombosis.[17]

Through their knowledge of aviation physiology, aerospace medicine practitioners usually have a greater awareness of the challenges facing passengers with chronic and acute medical conditions than their terrestrially oriented colleagues. There are numerous factors that primary care physicians and their passenger-patients might not recognize as being potentially problematic, especially on long flights. It is quite common for patients to be discharged from hospitals and sent home via commercial airlines rather than air ambulances, often with little consideration given to possible deterioration en route. Patients who normally use supplemental oxygen at home will at times decide not to arrange for in-flight supplemental oxygen due to the expense, not understanding that cabin pressure is kept to a much higher altitude than that to which they are accustomed. Terminally ill individuals will often try to fly great distances to die at home, and sometimes may not survive to reach their destination.

Traditional travel medicine will not be covered in this chapter, as the focus here is primarily on in-flight passenger health issues. Immunizations and prophylactic medications are well-defined in other publications, and are also easily available through the websites of the World Health Organization (WHO) (http://www.who.int/ith/en/) and the Center for Disease Control and Prevention (CDC) (http://www.cdc.gov/). Air ambulance issues will also not be covered in this chapter, as these are outside the realm of this subject matter and can be found in numerous other publications.

INCIDENCE OF IN-FLIGHT AND POST-FLIGHT MEDICAL EVENTS

It is difficult to accurately determine the incidence of passenger medical emergencies on-board commercial aircraft, as there are no regulatory requirements within the aviation industry to keep track of such events. The few studies that have been done indicate that in-flight illness is a rather uncommon event and is usually minor in nature, although serious conditions do occur.[18]

It has been estimated that about one in 10 000 to 40 000 passengers has a medical incident during air transport.[18,20] Of these, approximately one in 150 000 requires use of in-flight medical equipment or drugs. From a variety of studies, deaths have been estimated at 0.04 to one per million passengers. However, in one review of eight years' data by IATA, derived from international carriers, a death rate of 0.3 per million passengers was found, with about two-thirds of these deaths having been caused by cardiac problems.[19]

One can extrapolate from these data that a few hundred deaths may be occurring annually worldwide on board commercial aircraft at current air travel rates.

According to Dr. Jon Jordan (Federal Air Surgeon 1969–2005), during a mandatory reporting year (July 1998–June 1999) in the United States, the FAA received airline reports of "188 deaths or threat-of-death incidents resulting in a total of 108 deaths, 43 of which occurred inflight."[5] It is estimated that 600 million passengers flew on US domestic carriers during that study year.

In a study of the medical events of a major US carrier,[20] there were over 2000 reported events during one year, at a rate of about two medical complaints per 100 flights. There were seven in-flight deaths. An automated external defibrillator (AED) was used 32 times (most often as a monitoring unit rather than for providing shocks), and emergency medical kits were used nearly 1200 times.

According to one in-flight medical advisory company, MedAire, their 2002 statistics[21] revealed that "flight crews of 40 airlines called on the ground-based physicians more than 8400 times for assistance in dealing with in-flight medical incidents and emergencies — the most common of which was people fainting." More than 65% of all in-flight medical emergencies fell under one of just five different types of events:

1) Vasovagal (i.e., syncope) — 21.5%
2) Gastrointestinal — 15.4%
3) Respiratory — 10.2%
4) Cardiac — 9.6%
5) Neurological — 8.7%

It is reassuring that with the availability of trained flight attendants, on-board medical kits and AED's, ground-based medical consultants (when available), and in-flight volunteer medical assistance, medical care is almost always available during long haul flights. It should be noted that use of emergency equipment such as an AED is only effective if there is a medically appropriate diversion site available within a short period of time. Successful resuscitations cannot be expected in flights where there are no such diversions possible, such as over oceans or polar routes. However, it is clear that pre-flight evaluation of patients with medical conditions is the key to avoiding many such on-board medical emergencies. Only with more research will it be possible to intelligently develop more focused prevention strategies. On-board medical emergencies increase risk not only to other passengers, but can also affect the safety of the flight itself, not to mention the financial burden associated with diversions. If little is known about in-flight medical events, even less is known about post-flight medical incidents that could be related to air travel. A common concern is deep venous thrombosis (DVT), also known as traveler's thrombosis, and the potentially deadly sequel of pulmonary emboli (PE). Current research appears to support that there is no greater risk from flying than from other forms of transportation requiring long periods of immobility.[22,26]

Other potential post-flight problems, such as communicable diseases, have also not been quantified, even though perceived by the traveling public as being problematic. They are often incorrectly assumed to be caused by recirculated cabin air. In today's environment, concerns associated with potential new pandemics such as SARS and H5N1 avian influenza, as well as old communicable diseases such as tuberculosis and measles, make it even more important to understand the factors involved in the transmissibility of infectious illnesses of public health concern. Additional issues on the horizon are hypoxia and possible acute mountain sickness,[14] bioterrorism, cosmic radiation, and health risks associated with disinsection.

IS THERE A DOCTOR ON BOARD?

The majority of commercial flights in the US seem to have a physician or other health care provider on-board.[23] Whether or not they identify themselves as such at the time of an on-board medical event is dependent on a number of factors. These could include the country in which the doctor is registered to practice, his or her clinical specialty, concerns about liability, prior ingestion of alcohol, personal desires not to become involved, and other medical consultants available to the flight attendant. This was illustrated by a study of one airline where doctors offered to help in nearly a third of the incidents, nurses about 10% of the time, and others, such as paramedics, helped in another 10% of the cases.[20] This means that in half of the incidents, the flight attendant received help from an on-board health care professional.

In 1998 in the US, the Aviation Medical Assistance Act (Public Law 105-170, 49 USC 44701) created a federal Good Samaritan Law that limits liability for individuals and airlines providing a medical response to in-flight medical emergencies. Although not always understood by responding voluntary physicians, it seems obvious that such a Good Samaritan Act makes it inappropriate for a physician then to bill the airline for professional services provided during the flight. This act therefore not only indemnifies the responding voluntary physician (or other health care volunteer) provided he or she acts in a reasonable and professional manner, but also allows the volunteer to offer medical assistance in the airspace over a state where he or she does not have a license to practice medicine. Physicians who submit a bill for payment would lose their protection under this act and become fully liable for the treatment and outcomes.

As stated in the introduction, the Aviation Medical Assistance Act has also required that domestic US carriers carry AED's and EEMK's on all passenger aircraft weighing over 7500 pounds and having at least one flight attendant. The European Joint Aviation Authorities have mandated similar requirements. The availability of such equipment and medications provides an increased capability for treating unexpected cardiac arrest and arrhythmias as well as other medical emergencies. It should go without saying that this equipment is intended for emergency use only and is never to be utilized as primary or back-up equipment for a passenger with a known medical instability. British Airways, in a previous website for passenger medical clearance, summed it up well by stating, "The passenger cabin of a commercial airliner is designed to carry the maximum number of passengers in comfort and safety, within the constraints of cost effectiveness. It is incompatible with providing the facilities of an ambulance, an emergency room, an intensive care unit, a delivery suite, or a mortuary."

Furthermore, it is important to define the role of the flight attendant in a medical emergency. Commercial carriers around the world train their flight attendants to recognize common symptoms of distress and to respond to medical emergencies with first aid and basic resuscitation techniques. They are also trained in the use of medical oxygen, and more recently, often in the proper use of the AED. In some countries they are trained and allowed to give parenteral medications, although that is not the case in the US (unless they also have an additional medical degree that allows such treatment). It is important to recognize that at least in the US, flight attendants are given initial and recurrent training in these basic skills, but they do not necessarily carry any formal medical certification.

If a passenger requires emergency medical oxygen, this is usually provided by bottled oxygen by the cabin crew. The drop-down emergency oxygen masks are not intended for this purpose, as they need to be available for emergency decompression events.

Due to safety concerns, passengers are not allowed to bring their own bottled oxygen tanks on board, and must make arrangements with the airline prior to flight if this form of supplemental oxygen is required en route. The passenger's physician must submit a written request for the necessary flow rates, and the number of bottles per flight leg are then ordered. This can be expensive and logistically challenging, especially if long flights and aircraft changes are involved, or if there are any flight delays or cancellations. Fortunately, since August 2005, the FAA has implemented a new rule governing the use of portable oxygen concentrators, allowing this form of personal oxygen supplementation on-board. It should be pointed out that this rule *allows*, but does not *require*, airlines to let patients use approved portable oxygen concentrators on-board their airplanes. Currently, the portable oxygen concentrators approved by the FAA for in-flight use are:

- Inogen One Portable Oxygen Concentrator
- SeQual Eclipse Portable Oxygen Concentrator
- AirSep Lifestyle
- AirSep Freestyle
- Respironics EverGo

Supplemental oxygen is discussed in greater detail in the next section on medical conditions affected by flight.

An informal review by the author of passenger medical incident reports for three years (1998–2001) at a major US carrier identified several recurrent complaints from medical incident responders. The concerns demonstrate the difficulty of supplying equipment that is both familiar to the individuals, yet economical and useful for equipping all aircraft. One of the most frequent complaints concerned the perceived poor quality of the inexpensive stethoscopes, which were thought by some physicians to be inadequate for accurately assessing heart and lung sounds. It is doubtful that more expensive stethoscopes would be more helpful, as the in-flight noise and vibration make it nearly impossible to perform a detailed heart and lung evaluation anyway. During in-flight medical emergencies it is often a matter of determining whether heart and breath sounds exist or are absent, rather than identifying subtle auscultatory qualities. Other physicians have complained about the digital sphygmomanometers, as they were often unfamiliar with their use. Again, the noise of the aircraft makes it very difficult to auscultate blood pressure, making the digital semi-automatic devices more appropriate in the setting of an airplane cabin. Additionally, these digital devices are easier to use for non-medical personnel, such as flight attendants.

There were also physicians who complained about the lack of their favorite emergency drugs in the EEMK, yet there were others who praised the equipment and were pleasantly surprised by the variety of medications and tools available to them (Fig. 1). A listing of the currently required medications and equipment in the EEMK can be found in the Appendix. It is important to note that it is usually not possible to provide continuous suction on standard commercial aircraft, making difficult intubation procedures or events requiring gastric emptying problematic.

The volunteer physician also needs to be prepared to make decisions pertaining to possible diversions. The task of determining whether or not a flight needs to be diverted for a medical reason is made by the captain who bases his or her decision on the recommendation of a volunteer health care provider, a trained ground-based physician, or an unassisted flight attendant. This decision should be biased toward safety but the choice between making diversion decisions

CONTENTS	QUANTITY
Sphygmomanometer	1
Stethoscope	1
Airways, oropharyngeal (3 sizes): 1 pediatric, 1 small adult, 1 large adult or equivalent	3
Self-inflating manual resuscitation device with 3 masks (1 pediatric, 1 small adult, 1 large adult or equivalent)	1:3 masks
CPR mask (3 sizes) 1 pediatric, 1 small adult, 1 large adult or equivalent	3
IV Admin Set, Tubing w/2 Y connectors	1
Alcohol sponges	2
Adhesive tape, 1-inch standard roll adhesive	1
Tape scissors	1 pair
Tourniquet	1
Saline solution , 500 cc	1
Protective nonpermeable gloves or equivalent	1 pair*
Needles (2-18 ga., 2-20 ga., 2-22 ga., or sizes necessary to administer required medications)	6
Syringes (1-5 cc, 2-10 cc, or sizes necessary to administer required medications)	4
Analgesic, non-narcotic, tablets, 325 mg	4
Antihistamine tablets, 25 mg	4
Antihistamine injectable, 50 mg (single dose ampuleor equivalent)	2
Atropine, 0.5 mg, 5 cc (single dose ampule or equivalent)	2
Aspirin tablets, 325 mg	4
Bronchodilator, inhaled (metered dose inhaler or equivalent)	1
Dextrose, 50%/50 cc injectable (single dose ampule or equivalent)	1
Epinephrine 1:1000, 1 cc, injectable (single dose ampule or equivalent)	2
Epinephrine 1:10,000, 2 cc, injectable (single dose ampule or equivalent)	2
Lidocaine, 5 cc, 20 mg/ml, injectable (single dose ampule or equivalent)	2
Nitroglycerine tablets, 0.4 mg	10
Basic instructions for use of the drugs in the kit	1

* Although the FAA requires only one pair of protective gloves, it recommends that operators keep additional pairs accessible on the aircraft. This would allow crewmembers to access a pair of gloves without having to locate and open an EEMK.

Figure 1. Enhanced emergency medical kit contents.

that may prove to be unnecessary versus the desire to continue on to the scheduled destination is never easy. There have been no studies to indicate how volunteer physicians make these recommendations. It has been shown, however, that when physicians participate in the decision to divert, either as on-board volunteers or a ground-based medical consultants, more appropriate divert decisions are likely to be made.[20]

Many airlines have highly trained ground-based physicians available either by satellite phone or by cockpit radio-phone patch to support the medical volunteer or flight attendant in any medical or diversion decisions that need to be made. Information pertaining to the facilities available on the ground should impact the decision of where to land. It is often more reasonable to fly a little longer in order to land at an airport near a hospital where appropriate medical care is available, rather than to divert to the nearest airport, which might not have the necessary medical facility close by.

MEDICAL CONDITIONS AFFECTED BY FLIGHT

Fortunately for the vast majority of airline passengers, no noticeable adverse health effects occur that can be directly attributable to the flight.[6] The cabin altitude up to 8000 feet at routine cruise flight levels is generally well tolerated by healthy people, and most passengers seem to have no ill effects. The physical discomforts endured by the passengers do not seem to be significantly hazardous, although there is a general dissatisfaction with such issues as seat pitch and leg room, food service (or lack thereof), and cabin air quality.

Certain individuals might be at greater risk for acute exacerbations of their underlying medical problems. While all the mechanisms of action have not been clearly delineated, exacerbations are most often related to barometric pressure changes, especially lower ambient oxygen partial pressure at cruising altitude[14] and orthostatic events. Other relevant factors include low cabin humidity, restricted mobility, seating constraints, vibration and noise, number of time zones crossed, and the length of flight. In this post September 11 world, additional stressors related to passenger screening are frequently encountered. The altitude of the destination airport should also be considered. As a general rule, an individual with an unstable medical condition should not fly.

The greatest of these stressors is hypoxia. At sea level, the barometric pressure is about 760 mmHg, with a corresponding PaO_2 of 95 mmHg and an SaO_2 of about 96–98% in healthy individuals. At a maximum cabin altitude of 8000 feet (2438 m), barometric pressure drops to 565 mmHg, and in the healthy individual the PaO_2 drops to 60 mmHg with a corresponding SaO_2 of about 90%. Although most healthy passengers can easily compensate for this

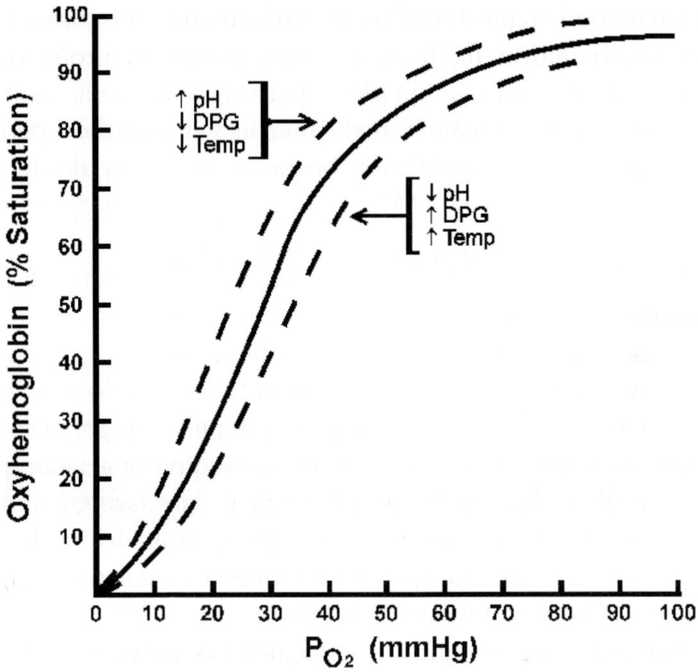

Figure 2. Oxyhemoglobin desaturation curve.

amount of hypoxemia, those with cardiac, pulmonary, cerebrovascular, and anemic conditions might not fare as well. By starting out at a lower PaO_2, these individuals are at a much steeper part of the oxygen desaturation curve prior to flight (Fig. 2).

Lowered ambient pressure can also be problematic in body areas where gas expansion could be hazardous. This can be critical for individuals who have had recent surgery with trapped air inside closed spaces. People who have problems associated with equilibration of gas trapped in areas such as the sinuses, ears, lungs, or GI tract, can also be adversely affected. Decompression illness can occur in persons who have been diving and inhaling compressed air prior to flight.

Preflight assessment of fitness to fly is very important, and the personal physician as well as the medical department of the airline, if available, should be involved in the clearance process early on.

Patients with both acute and chronic medical problems that could be exacerbated by airline flight often underestimate the problems they might encounter. Things as simple as packing vital medications into checked luggage can create a medical crisis within a short period of time if that particular medication becomes necessary during flight (and is not available in the EEMK) or if the critical baggage does not arrive at the destination.

The ability to monitor passengers is usually quite limited: a stethoscope, a sphygmomanometer, and the visual monitor on an AED, although some airlines are beginning to utilize telemetric equipment.

It is obvious that in order to avoid in-flight medical emergencies, the passenger should consult with his or her personal physician, and the physician needs to have a good understanding of aviation physiology as well as the constraints of medical care offered on-board commercial aircraft. The following section offers advice to the medical practitioner who faces a patient desiring to fly. It should be noted that some medical problems can be dealt with as long as there is a competent medical assistant caring for the passenger; however, this needs to be thoroughly evaluated in case of unanticipated worsening of the medical condition.

The Role of the Airline Medical Department

Whether or not an airline has a medical department depends on many factors, primarily the economic health of the particular airline and the laws applying to its operations. Certain airlines are required by their governments to support their employees with occupational health care and facilities. Some of these airlines extend their medical services to passengers as well. In the post September 11 world, however, airlines are being severely economically stretched. Many of the major US carriers have reduced or eliminated their medical departments, especially with respect to passenger medical assistance.

According to convention, airline medical departments are responsible for ensuring, as far as possible, that passenger health does not deteriorate during the journey, and to assure that there are adequate measures in place to deal with common, yet unforeseen medical emergencies.[9] In reality, airlines have no real means of ensuring that all passengers are fit to begin their journey. Additional issues, such as the Americans with Disabilities Act (ADA), make it difficult to provide standardized medical clearances on a worldwide basis.

Major international airlines have traditionally offered medical clearance assistance and rely on forms such as the Frequent Traveler's Medical Card (FREMEC) and the Medical Information Sheet (MEDIF) provided by their airlines (Fig. 3). In the past, "medical clearance" documentation from personal physicians was required for those passengers with particular medical needs that could be problematic during flight. However, practical experience has shown that physicians who do not have a thorough understanding of air transportation may not be fully familiar with all the particular medical challenges involved. These clearance certificates should then be taken into account by the airline medical department, and assessed individually as to whether or not, and under what conditions, the passenger is acceptable for flight.

The following section on medical clearance guidelines indicates when medical clearance might be required by the airline's medical department. At a minimum, consideration should be given if the passenger:

a) suffers from any disease that is believed to be actively contagious and communicable;
b) has any physical or behavioral condition that is likely to be a hazard or may cause discomfort to other passengers;
c) is considered to be a potential hazard to the safety or punctuality of the flight, including the possibility of diversion of the flight or an unscheduled landing;
d) is incapable of caring for him or herself and requires special assistance, particularly in the event of an emergency; or
e) has a medical condition that may be adversely affected by the flight environment.[9]

Hopefully, as the industry recovers and the need for solid passenger health advice is increasingly recognized, these medical departments

MEDICAL INFORMATION SHEET
Resolution 700 (MEDIF) Attachment B

*This form is intended to provide **confidential** information to enable the airlines **medical** departments to assess the fitness of the passenger to travel. If the passenger is acceptable, this information will permit the issuance of necessary directives designed to provide for the passenger's welfare and comfort.*
*The physician attending the incapacitated passenger is requested to **answer all questions (1)**. Enter a cross (x) in the appropriate 'yes' or 'no' boxes, and/or give precise concise answers.*

Confidential
To be completed by attending physician
The form must be returned to the Airline Medical Clearance Department

Airlines ref. code		
MEDA01	**Patient's name**	______ Initials__☐ M☐ F__☐ Date of birth______
MEDA02	**Attending physician** Name Address Telephone	______ ______ Business ______ Home ______
MEDA03	Medical data Diagnosis in details *(including vital signs)*	______ Date of first symptoms ______ ______ Date of diagnosis ______ ______ Date of operation ______
MEDA04	Prognosis for the flight(s)	______
MEDA05	Contagious and communicable disease	☐ no ☐ yes, specify ______
MEDA06	Would physical/mental condition patient likely cause distress/discomfort to other passenger(s)	☐ no ☐ yes, specify ______
NEDA07	Can patient use normal aircraft seat with seatback placed in the **upright** position	☐ no ☐ yes
MEDA08	Can patient take care of his own needs on board **unassisted (2)** (including meals, visit to toilet, etc.)	☐ no ☐ yes If not, type of help needed ______
MEDA09	If to be **escorted**, is the arrangement satisfactory for you	☐ no ☐ yes type of escort ______ If not, proposed by you ______

Figure 3. Medical information sheet (MEDIF).

MEDA10	Does patient need **oxygen (3)** equipment in flight ☐no	☐yes, Liters per minute ______ L. Continuous	☐ no	☐ yes
MEDA11	Does patient need only **Medication (2)** other than self administered, and/or the use of special apparatus such as respirator, incubator, etc.	a. **on the ground** while at the airport(s)	☐ no	☐ yes
		if yes, specify ______		
MEDA12		b. **on board of the aircraft**	☐ no	☐ yes
		if yes, specify ______		
MEDA13	Does patient need **hospitalization** *(if yes, indicate arrangements made, or if none were made, indicate 'no action taken')*	during long layover or nightstop a. **at connection points** en route	☐ no	☐ yes
		if yes, action ______		
EDA14		b. **upon arrival at destination**	☐no	☐yes
		If yes, action ______		
MEDA15	Other remarks or information in the interest of your patient's smooth and comfortable transportation	☐none ☐yes, specify **(2)** ______		
MEDA16	Other arrangements made by the attending physician	______		

Important notes:

1 Fees, if any, relevant to the provision of this information are to be paid by the passenger concerned.

2 Cabin attendants are **not** authorized to give special assistance to particular passengers (e.g. lifting). Additionally, they are trained only in **first aid** and are **not permitted** to administer any injection, or to give medication.

3 Fees for carrier-provided special equipment are to be paid by the passenger concerned.

Date ______

Place ______

Physician Signature ______

Passenger's declaration

I hereby authorize (doctor's name) ______
to provide the airlines with the information required by those airlines medical departments for the purpose of determining my fitness for carriage by air and in consideration thereof I hereby relieve that physician of his/her professional duty of confidentiality in respect of such information, and agree to meet such physician's fees in connection therewith. I take note that, if accepted for carriage, my journey will be subject to the general conditions of carriage/tariffs of the carrier concerned and that the carrier does not assume any special liability exceeding those conditions/tariffs. I agree to reimburse the carrier upon demand for any special expenditures or costs in connection with my carriage.
(Where needed, to be read by/to the passenger, dated and signed by him/her or on his/her behalf).

Date ______

Passenger Signature ______

Figure 3. *(Continued).*

may rise from the ashes and become prominent again in assisting passengers with special medical needs and providing advice to their physicians.

MEDICAL CLEARANCE GUIDELINES

The objective of medical clearance is to provide safe and healthy travel, and to prevent delays and diversions to the flight as a result of deterioration of a passenger's medical situation. It is often up to individual physicians to provide this information, since not all airlines have medical departments that are able to give guidance in this area. There are excellent recent guidelines developed by the Aerospace Medical Association (AsMA)[1,2] WHO[27] and IATA,[9] and will only be briefly described in this chapter. Other professional organizations, such as the Canadian Cardiovascular Society and the British Medical Association, have also made recommendations.[13,24]

IATA has published a Medical Information Form (MEDIF) (Fig. 3), which has a passenger and a physician section. Many airlines require this to be completed well in advance of flight so that proper arrangements can be made for passengers with additional needs. Although there is some variation in opinions among the experts pertaining to medical clearance issues, the following recommendations are based on the Medical Guidelines for Airline Travel (second edition) compiled by AsMA in 2003.[1] These recommendations are intended for flight, but additional consideration should be used in evaluating a patient's ability to navigate a crowded airport.

Cardiovascular disease should be carefully evaluated prior to each flight unless it is very stable, with co-morbid conditions taken into consideration.

1. *Angina*: As long as the stress of air travel is not likely to precipitate symptoms, most stable patients can fly. They must be cautious to carry their medications with them on-board. Unstable angina is a clear contraindication to flight.
2. *Myocardial infarction* (MI): For the uncomplicated MI, patients should not fly for at least two to three weeks and until they have

resumed normal activities. Patients with complicated MI, especially those with limited mobility, should wait longer until they are stabilized medically. Symptom-limited stress testing can be very helpful in estimating ability to fly.

3. *Congestive heart failure* (CH): Severe decompensated heart failure is a contraindication to flight. Individuals with stable CHF with NYHA Class III–IV or with baseline PaO_2 of 70 mmHg or less should be advised to arrange for supplemental oxygen.
4. *Coronary artery bypass graft*: If surgery is uncomplicated, fully recovered CABG patients should wait 10–14 days post surgery to allow for surgically introduced intrathoracic air to be absorbed.
5. *Percutaneous coronary artery interventions*: Uncomplicated angioplasty or stent operations usually carry a low risk, provided the patient is medically stable and has returned to his or her normal activities.
6. *Symptomatic valvular heart disease*: This is a relative contraindication to flight, so these patients should be carefully assessed. Fitness to fly is determined by severity of symptoms, functional status, left ventricular ejection fraction, and whether or not pulmonary hypertension and baseline hypoxia exist.
7. *Hypertension*: As long as the hypertension is under reasonable control, there is no contraindication to flight.
8. *Pacemakers and implantable cardiac defibrillators* (ICD): These devices are low risk for commercial airline travel, once the patient is medically stable after having the device implanted. The commonly used bipolar devices are very unlikely to have electromagnetic interferences with airline or security devices, and even the older unifocal devices are unlikely to cause interference problems. [Note that any equipment carried on-board an aircraft must meet the radio frequency interference requirements of the regulatory authority (e.g., FAA or EASA).] Passengers with these devices should carry copies of their electrocardiogram (ECG) (both with and without magnets) as well as copies of their pacemaker or ICD cards. The reason for this is that it might not be possible to transmit electronic telephone checks of pacemaker function via international satellite telephone systems.

General Risk Factors

- Impairment of blood clotting mechanisms, such as clotting factor abnormality
- Estrogen hormone therapy, including oral contraception
- Extremes of height
- Fight greater than four hours' duration
- Cardiovascular disease
- Current or history of malignancy
- Recent major surgery
- Recent trauma to lower limbs or abdomen
- Personal family history of DVT
- Pregnancy
- Age above 40 years
- Prior prolonged immobilization
- Depletion of body fluids causing increased blood viscosity (Note that this is not dehydration as a result of dry cabin air.)

Suggested DVT Prophylaxis
(with kind permission for reproduction from 2003 AsMA Medical Guidelines Task Force)

	Risk Categories	Prophylaxis
Low risk	Age over 40; obesity; active inflammation; recent minor surgery (within last 3 days)	Advice about mobilization and hydration, +/- support tights/ non-elasticized long socks
Moderate risk	Varicose veins; heart failure (uncontrolled); recent myocardial infarction (within 6 weeks); hormone therapy (including oral contraception); polycythemia; pregnancy/ postnatal; lower limb paralysis; recent lower limb trauma (within 6 weeks)	Passenger advised to consult own medical practitioner who may recommend the above + aspirin (if not contraindicated) +/- graduated compression stockings
High risk	Previous VTE; known thrombophilia; recent Major surgery (within 6 weeks); previous CVA; malignancy; family history of VTE	As above, but passenger's medical practitioner may recommend low molecular weight heparin instead of aspirin

Figure 4. DVT risk factors and prophylaxis for flight.

9. *Deep venous thrombosis*: DVT *per se* is not a dangerous condition, but the sequel of pulmonary embolism (PE) can be life threatening. Provided the condition is stable and the passenger is on appropriate anti-coagulation with resolution of the clot, there is no contraindication to flying. Passengers with risk factors (Fig. 4) for DVT should be counseled about preventive activities such as walking in the cabin aisles during flight, in-seat stretching

exercises, and adequate hydration. Depending on the severity of their risk factors, they might consult with their physician about medical preventive therapy (Fig. 4). All passengers should be educated about the signs and symptoms of DVT, with instructions given as to how to seek medical assistance at their destination, as DVT and PE can develop hours or days afterwards.[7]

10. *Miscellaneous contraindicated cardiovascular medical conditions*: This includes cardiovascular accidents within two weeks of flight, uncontrolled ventricular or supraventricular tachycardia, and Eisenmenger's syndrome. Of course, all cardiac patients should be reminded to carry a list of their medications with them, and make certain that they have more than sufficient quantities of medications to last them through their entire trip.

Consideration must be made to accommodate for limited physical reserve by reducing long airport walks and heavy baggage. It goes without saying that if there are special needs, such as wheelchairs, special seats or meal requirements, arrangements need to be made with the carrier well in advance. Even though special meals are ordered, they are not always available. Thus, those with special meal requirements should carry emergency foodstuffs.

Pulmonary diseases require attention to the possible need for supplemental oxygen and rescue medications in case of exacerbations. The physician should consider the type, reversibility, and functional severity of the pulmonary disorder, evaluate altitude tolerance, and determine the anticipated altitude and duration of the flight. Pulmonary function tests and arterial blood gas determinations can be very helpful in this evaluation. As stated in the cardiac section, the baseline PaO_2 is the most useful indicator of altitude tolerance. A more sophisticated test is the hypoxia altitude simulation test (HAST), which determines the patient's PaO_2 while breathing mixed gases simulating the aircraft cabin environment at altitude. A PaO_2 of less than 55 mmHg saturation at simulated cabin altitude requires supplemental oxygen during flight. Individuals with PaO_2 less than 70 mmHg may also warrant supplemental oxygen.

1. *Asthma*: Air travel is contraindicated for patients with severe, labile disease that requires frequent hospitalization. For stable individuals, it is important to remind them that they must hand-carry their medications, particularly their inhalers. A course of oral steroids might be indicated for all but the mildest asthmatics.
2. *Bronchiectasis and cystic fibrosis*: These patients should be carefully evaluated, with measures taken to effectively loosen and clear secretions. Infections should be treated and stabilized prior to flight, and in-flight oxygen therapy might be essential. Aerosolized enzyme deoxyribonuclease should be considered prior to, and possibly also during flight.
3. *Interstitial lung disease*: Most of these patients can generally tolerate air travel, although supplemental oxygen therapy might be necessary.
4. *Malignancies*: Lung cancer is not contraindicated for flight, provided the passenger is otherwise medically stable. Medications during flight might be needed to relieve pain, and supplemental oxygen might be necessary.
5. *Neuromuscular disease*: Patients who have neurological or skeletal disorders that affect breathing can require manual and/or mechanical assistance, which can be problematic for long flights. Often they require an assistant to accompany them. The low humidity in the aircraft can exacerbate excessive dryness of the respiratory mucosa. These cases should be thoroughly discussed with the air carrier in advance of flight.
6. *Pulmonary infections*: Those with actively contagious infections are unsuitable for air travel until documented control of the infection can be obtained. To avoid spread of the virus to nearby passengers and cabin crew, individuals with even "mild" viral infections should not be allowed on-board
7. *Pneumothorax*: The presence of pneumothorax or pneumomediastinum is a contraindication as these conditions can progress to a tension pneumothorax by gas expansion during flight. Treated patients can usually travel within two to three weeks of successful drainage. Patients with recurrent spontaneous pneumothorax

should be individually counseled; end-expiratory chest radiographs can be helpful in identification of suspicious cases.

8. *Pleural effusions*: Large collections require drainage prior to flight, with at least 14 days recovery for both diagnostic and therapeutic reasons. A chest radiograph might be needed prior to flight to rule out reaccumulation or induced pneumothorax.
9. *Pulmonary vascular disease*: Patients with preexisting PE or pulmonary hypertension are at risk for hypoxia-induced pulmonary vasoconstriction with an ultimate reduction in cardiac output. These patients necessitate careful preflight evaluation, as they might need a combination of anticoagulation, medical oxygen, restricted exertion, compression stockings, and in-seat isometric exercises.
10. *Sleep apnea*: Passenger who use CPAP devices often take them along on long-haul flights. They must pass TSA inspection, so the passenger should call the airline in advance for information regarding bringing these devices on-board.
11. *Special conditions*: These patients require close coordination between the physician and the air carrier if unusual or special medical equipment is required on-board.

Recent surgery should be evaluated individually. With the increase of ambulatory surgery, patients frequently fly home after an outpatient procedure. General anesthesia *per se* is not a contraindication for flight, as the gases used do not predispose one to decompression illness. However, it should be kept in mind that post-operative patients have increased oxygen consumption due to the trauma of surgery, and oxygen delivery might be impaired. Post-operative anemia must be assessed. Patients with recent thoracic surgery are especially sensitive to intrathoracic pressure changes, as gas expands 25–30% at cabin altitude. Neurosurgical patients must be shown to have no trapped intracranial air, and patients with any cerebrospinal leak should avoid flying because of the possibility of backflow and bacterial contamination during pressure changes. This gas expansion also puts post-abdominal surgery patients at risk, therefore air travel should be discouraged for at least one to two weeks for individuals who have had an intestinal lumen opened. Even after a simple colonoscopy with polypectomy procedure, flight should be delayed for at least 24 hours. Laparoscopic procedures are less likely to cause problems because of the rapid diffusion of the residual CO_2. Travelers with colostomy bags are not at increased risk during air travel, but might need larger bags due to the increased fecal output produced by intestinal distention and gas expansion.

Consideration should also be given to wound care requirements, pressure-sensitive tubing, IV fluids, and medications, along with ambulatory and positional requirements.

Pregnancy in general is compatible with airline flight. Because of the properties of fetal hemoglobin, fetal PaO_2 changes very little, despite a potential substantial drop in maternal PaO_2 at altitude. However, the physical changes associated with pregnancy can make flight more challenging, in that motion sickness might be aggravated, intra-abdominal gas expansion might be worse than in the non-pregnant female, and orthostatic changes can be accentuated. High risk pregnancies at risk for preterm labor should be discouraged from prolonged flight. First trimester travelers should not fly if they have either bleeding or pain associated with their pregnancy. Most airlines require medical certification from the obstetrician to allow flight after the 36th gestational week (32nd in the case of a multiple pregnancy) in order to avoid the onset of labor during flight.

Travel with children has few caveats. Infants should be at least seven days old in order to assure lack of serious congenital defects or respiratory distress. Risk of Eustachian tube dysfunction can be decreased by having the babies suck on a bottle, breast or pacifier, and older children can drink from a cup during decent. Just as with adults, children with respiratory congestion can benefit from decongestion medications given orally 30 minutes before descent. Otitis media is not contraindicated, provided appropriate antibiotics are being used for 36 hours and the Eustachian tube is patent. Diarrheal illnesses should be remedied with appropriate electrolyte solutions.

TRAVELING WEST

Usual Regimen	Day of Departure/Travel (West Bound)	First Day at Destination
Multiple injection regimen with pre-meal soluble insulin and overnight intermediate insulin.	Usual pre-meal soluble insulin. Additional soluble insulin injection with additional meal or snack. Modest reduction (1/3) in overnight intermediate insulin to avoid nocturnal hypoglycemia.	Return to usual insulin regimen. Additional soluble insulin (1/3 of usual morning dose) should be considered if fasting blood glucose >14mmol/L (250 mg/dl).

Usual Regimen	Day of Departure	18 Hour After Morning Dose	First Morning at Destination
Two-dose schedule	Usual morning and evening doses	1/3 usual dose followed by meal or snack if blood glucose > 14 mmol/L (250 mg/dl)	Usual two doses
Single dose schedule	Usual dose	1/3 usual dose followed by meal or snack	Usual dose

TRAVELING EAST

Usual Regimen	Day of Departure/Travel (East Bound)	First Day at Destination
Multiple injection regimen with pre-meal soluble insulin and overnight intermediate insulin.	Usual pre-meal soluble insulin. If less than 4 hours between meals this requires a slightly reduced dose of the third soluble injection (by 1/3) and additional carbohydrate (i.e. extra large evening snack if one meal is missed) and a reduction (1/3) in overnight intermediate insulin to avoid nocturnal hypoglycemia.	Return to usual insulin regimen if you have overcompensated with the reduction of the evening intermediate insulin. Additional soluble insulin (1/3 of usual morning dose) should be considered if fasting blood glucose >14 mmol/L (250 mg/dl).

Usual Regimen	Day of Departure	First Morning at Destination	10 hr after Morning Dose	Second day at Destination
Two-dose schedule	Usual morning and evening doses	2/3 usual morning dose	Usual evening dose plus remaining 1/3 of morning dose if blood sugar > 250 mg/dl	Usual two doses
Single-dose schedule			Remaining 1/3 of morning dose if blood sugar > 250 mg/dl	Usual dose

Figure 5. Insulin adjustments when traveling across multiple time zones (five or more time zones) (with kind permission for reproduction from 2003 AsMA Medical Guidelines Task Force).

Cerebrovascular disease patients, if otherwise stable, should be able to travel within a few days of having a cerebral vascular accident (CVA). For those with cerebral artery insufficiency, the relative hypoxia in the aircraft might necessitate supplemental oxygen. Some airlines require medical clearance if traveling within 10 days of a stroke.

Ear, nose and throat (ENT) disturbances that affect an individual's ability to equilibrate pressure through the Eustachian tubes or sinuses might cause barotrauma. Any condition that is associated with vertigo or motion sickness is likely to be worsened in flight. ENT surgeries in general should preclude flight for 10–14 days, except for ear tube placements or myringotomy (which ventilate the middle ear). Patients with tracheo-laryngeal surgeries may need extra moisturization and possibly removal of thickened secretions caused by the low humidity of the cabin air. Facial plastic surgery patients can generally fly once drains are removed. Penetrating eye injuries should not fly within six days of the injury or surgery due to the danger of gas expansion inside the globe. Passengers whose jaws are wired shut should only fly with an escort with appropriate wire cutters, or have self-quick-release wiring in case of vomiting or aspiration.

Diabetes is not a contraindication to flight, provided passengers can administer their own medications and understand the problems associated with time zone and nutritional changes. For insulin dependent diabetics, insulin vials, syringes, and monitoring supplies should be carried by the passenger on-board and not in checked baggage. A prescription or letter from the treating physician will expedite security clearance. The cabin altitude should not affect the accuracy of most glucose meters. Journeys across several time zones may shorten or lengthen the 24-hour day, and adjustments need to be made to compensate for this. (See Fig. 5 for insulin adjustment schedules.) It is, of course, important to have snacks available as countermeasure against hypoglycemia, especially if meal service is delayed. Passengers should alert cabin crew to their medical condition and wear medical alert ID tags.

The Transport Security Administration (TSA) in the US requires specific medical documentation of the need to carry insulin syringes on-board when going through security checkpoints at the airport. Only the necessary number of syringes for the length of flight is acceptable, with any additional syringes packed into the checked luggage. Insulin dependent diabetics should be reminded not to dispose of their syringes in areas of the aircraft that might likely injure others, such as seat back pockets and lavatory waste baskets. Cabin cleaning crews and fight attendants are often injured by these syringes; it can cause the worker considerable anxiety if punctured by one. An alternative is the insulin pen, which is a compact, portable device that serves exactly the same function as a needle and syringe, but is handier and more convenient to use. These come preloaded with the proper amount of soluble insulin, and are very convenient for frequent travelers.

Non-insulin dependent diabetics do not have the same issues with medical management. Additional tablets are not usually required to cover an extended day, and a normal dose might be omitted in the case of a significantly shortened day. Most important is careful planning and consultation with their diabetic specialist.

Communicable diseases can be a concern on airplanes, but they are probably no more likely to be transmitted in aircraft than in other public areas where people are in close proximity, despite public opinion to the contrary.[24]

Communicable diseases need to be investigated if a significant public health risk exists, such as infectious tuberculosis. Because of the potential serious consequences in compromised individuals, certain common childhood diseases in their infectious states should not be allowed onto aircraft, such as chickenpox, measles, mumps, rubella, scarlet fever, and pertussis. Similarly, those with other common highly contagious illnesses, such as influenza, should not be on-board because of the potential serious sequelae in at-risk people and the possibility of airborne transmission. Passengers with less serious infectious illnesses, e.g., the common cold (URI), frequently fly, because these illnesses are very common. Fortunately, they pose little risk as a public health hazard. Long haul flights, primarily international, are of particular concern, as these do increase the likelihood of even low virulence diseases, such as tuberculosis, to infect other passengers. Acute food poisoning on an airplane is particularly problematic, and potentially dangerous if it affects the flight crew. Although airlines are not allowed to knowingly board passengers with actively contagious diseases, passengers are often unwilling to admit their illnesses because of their motivation to travel. They might also perceive themselves as being well enough to fly, and ignore the potential of passing the disease on to others.

Difficulties arise in that many infectious diseases are contagious during a prodromal stage before symptoms actually develop, and even influenza may be entirely asymptomatic. Other challenges occur when dealing with emotionally charged conditions, for example tuberculosis or certain blood-borne pathogens. The SARS epidemic in 2003 highlighted the potential for an airborne illness to rapidly travel around the world.

Terminal illness are not necessarily disqualifying for flight, provided the illness is stable enough to allow the patient to withstand the flight. Patients are often discharged from hospitals with terminal illnesses and then fly home, while others wish to return to their native countries to die after being diagnosed with a terminal disease.

Orthopedic fractures can be a challenging situation for accommodation on passenger airlines. Most domestic US carriers do not allow stretcher cases, and require that a passenger must be able to sit in a regular seat. Some international carriers that are accustomed to repatriating sick passengers are able to accommodate stretcher configurations, and with adequate preparation, may even be able to provide accompanying medical personnel. It must be kept in mind that just because a passenger can fit into an airline seat with a short leg cast does not mean that he or she will tolerate it for several hours. Following application of a plaster cast, flights under two hours duration should be avoided for 24 hours, and longer flights for 48 hours.

If the cast is bivalved, these restrictions can be liberalized, although elevation is still a critical factor. Passengers with air casts should be advised to bring the air pump in their carry-on baggage, as the air in the bladders will expand at altitude requiring the removal of some of the air. Upon descent, as the air contracts, additional air will need to be placed in the bladders to stabilize the fracture.

Prescription medications with international travel require the original prescription bottles with labels on them, if traveling to certain countries. Some countries even require a prescription for pseudoephedrine hydrochloride, which is a common non-prescription decongestant in other countries. It is always a good idea to take copies of prescriptions along, in case of loss of the original medications.

Unattended minors with medical problems or prescription medications require careful coordination with the airlines. Children with medical problems, especially those requiring medications en route, must be discussed with the airline's medical department in order to avoid medication incidents. Such children, if below an appropriate developmental age to take their own medications, should not travel alone. Each airline has its own regulations concerning unaccompanied minors, and should be investigated before flight plans are made.

Blood disorders with reduced tolerance to hypoxia also require special consideration. Patients with hemoglobin levels below 7.5 g/dL should be provided supplemental oxygen, especially if the anemia has been acute in onset. Sometimes the cause of the anemia is enough to preclude stability for flight. Sickle cell trait patients should in general be able to travel without supplemental oxygen, but those with sickle cell disease should have supplemental oxygen in flight, and certainly not fly within 10 days of suffering a crisis.

Psychiatric illness, whether acute or chronic, should be stable and unlikely to deteriorate during flight. In some circumstances, medical escorts might be required.

Substance abuse cannot be tolerated on-board aircraft. Anyone who seems impaired or intoxicated should not be allowed on-board.

Personal medical devices need to be cleared in advance of flight, as not only do the airlines have rules regarding certain devices, but the security screening agencies may prohibit some being brought on-board. It is therefore important to discuss this with the airline well in advance of the flight.

TRANSPORTING ILL PASSENGERS

If a person is seriously ill, too unstable, or unable to sit in a normal airline seat, arrangements should be made for transportation on a stretcher, in a patient transport compartment, or via air ambulance. There are many aviation companies that provide transportation for patients locally, regionally, or internationally with specialized aircraft (ambulance aircraft or air ambulances).

Most US domestic carriers require that a passenger be able to sit in a normal seat. Some carriers, particularly those that fly internationally, are accustomed to providing room for stable stretcher cases by removing several seats. The innovative Patient Transport Compartment (PTC) system has been developed by Lufthansa German Airlines, which is a portable intensive care unit that can be quickly installed in a B-747 or A340-300. Lufthansa does not provide the accompanying physician, but will provide the additional specialty training for the medical personnel required to care for the patient en route.

Chronically ill passengers needing minor medical or personal assistance can often travel with an appropriate assistant. If unusual medications or medical devices will need to be utilized during flight, the customer service department of the airline must be notified in advance for guidance. There may be safety or regulatory limitations pertaining to many of these devices. In addition, depending on local laws, airlines may require a medical certificate. Failure to provide any requested information could result in denied boarding until the matter is resolved.

MISCELLANEOUS TOPICS

Airline passengers often have a variety of common complaints, some of which have more to do with comfort than with health issues. Concerns vary with the stability of the airline industry, as well as natural causes outside of human control. Bioterrorism and security are topics with political ramifications, and topics like "economy class syndrome" have achieved media notoriety. Issues such as air rage have lessened somewhat, while others like cabin air quality seem never to go away.

It is beyond the scope of this chapter to go into extensive detail on these topics, but at least a brief comment on a few of them is warranted. The author hopes these comments are representative of the opinions of the aeromedical community, but certainly future research will shed more light on the nature of medical problems associated with commercial airline flight.

Health Hazards versus Discomfort Issues

What is perceived by the traveling public to be a health hazard is often only a discomfort issue. Because of the low moisture in cabin air, symptoms such as a dry cough and sore throat are often misconstrued by the passenger as being caused by a contagious exposure during flight. It is a common misconception that respiratory infections spread quickly throughout the cabin. Viral infections travel in airplanes the same way as in other public facilities, primarily by contaminated hands and droplets, and usually not by airborne spread.

Passenger exposures to ground exhaust fumes reinforce this belief that the air is unhealthy. Contrary to popular belief, cramped seating in coach class does not appear to increase one's risk of DVT over that of sitting in first class.

Cabin Air Quality

Nearly all commercial airliners built after the late 1980's recirculate 10–50% of the cabin air, and utilize high-efficiency particle air

(HEPA) filters, which are the same as used in hospital operating rooms. These filters remove over 99.9% of particles over the size of 0.3 micrometers. It is of interest to note that the size of the *Mycobacterium tuberculosis* organism is 0.5–1 micrometers in diameter. Nonetheless, the topic of cabin air quality has remained one of the most contentious areas of passenger health. After many years of being a highly politicized and maligned issue, serious attempts to study the air quality in the aircraft cabin have been undertaken. The CabinAir project is a European funded consortium, bringing together 15 organizations from seven nations to investigate the issues surrounding cabin air quality. As part of this project, key air quality parameters have been monitored on 14 flights from "flag carrier" fleets made up of the BAe 146 (ventilation mode selected to provide 100% outside air to the cabin) and Boeing 737-300 (supply into the cabin is a mixture of outside and recirculated air). Overall, levels of measured air pollutants were always below any recommended health limits. Other agencies, such as the CDC and FAA, are currently working with industry partners to better assess cabin air quality.

Many questions still remain unanswered, however. More research is needed in order to understand whether there are health hazards associated with the levels of ozone, carbon dioxide, volatile organic compounds (VOC's), and bioaerosols, such as endotoxins, found in aircraft cabin air.

Hand Washing

Antiseptic hand cleaners have become popular for use in aircraft that do not have hand washing facilities readily available. These cleaners kill a variety of viruses and bacteria found on hands, but only washing with soap and water actually removes them.

DVT

Clotting of blood in deep veins, usually occurring in the lower legs, is known as deep venous thrombosis. Sensationalized in the press as "economy class syndrome," this term is misleading, because the risk of DVT seems to have no relationship to the amount of leg room available to the passenger. Individuals seated in cars, buses, and trains may all be at similar risk, and the term "traveler's thrombosis" is much more accurate. In order to understand this phenomenon, a large-scale study, the WRIGHT (WHO Research Into Global Hazards of Travel) project, has been undertaken by the World Health Organization. Set up in June 2001, it is a comprehensive project consisting "of a series of research studies to fill the key information gaps in available knowledge on the suspected link between air travel and DVT. The studies, which cover epidemiological, clinical, and physiological areas, will provide key information on the frequency of venous thrombosis, the magnitude of its association with air travel, and the caused mechanisms to possible prevention strategies for air travelers."[26] Phase I of this project, recently published, has demonstrated that the risk of DVT approximately doubles after a lengthy flight (defined as over four hours), but also with other forms of travel that involve prolonged seated immobility. Longer travel durations and multiple flights within a short period of time further increases the risk, as do the following risk factors: extremes of height, use of oral contraception, and the presence of prothrombotic hematological abnormalities. The absolute risk of DVT in these flights over four hours in a cohort of healthy individuals was found to be 1:6000. There are more studies to be conducted under Phase II related to the effects of preventive interventions.

For additional information, please also see the section on DVT in the cardiology section of this book.

Cosmic Radiation

The International Commission on Radiological Protection (ICRP) recommends a maximum annual occupational exposure of 20 millisievert (mSv) per year averaged over a period of five years. On average, dose rates received by passengers on long haul aircraft are on the order of 5 microsievert (μSv) per hour, and on short haul aircraft,

1–3 μSv per hour, depending on the altitude flown. The effects of ionizing radiation on airline passengers or pregnancies appears to be negligible, even for frequent fliers. Please also see the section on cosmic radiation for further details.

Disinsection

Control of disease-causing insect vectors is important not only in order to reduce the likelihood of spread of unwanted insects to other countries, but also to reduce the risk of passengers being bitten. One case of "runway malaria" has been attributed to mosquito entry into the cabin during a night layover with the aircraft doors open.

There are generally four WHO approved methods of disinsection, all of which use pyrethrin. The most common methods are to spray the cabin for approximately 10 minutes with passengers inside either at push back, top of descent, or on arrival. In theory, the mosquitoes will be shaken out of their hiding places and into contact with the aerosol. The fourth is to treat the surface of the cabin interior with a residual pyrethroid while passengers are absent. Disinsection has been regulated by the World Health Organization (WHO) since 1949. A 1995 study undertaken by the WHO showed no adverse health effects from properly performed disinsection, although some passengers and crew members might experience transient discomfort.

Currently a few countries require routine disinsection prior to arrival, although most reserve the right to do so in selected situations. Travelers who may be adversely affected by these aerosols sprays should be advised to contact their airline well in advance to obtain specific information regarding possible disinsection procedures and chemical exposures during a particular flight.

Public Health Issues

As stated in the Medical Clearance section of this chapter, communicable diseases are a controversial subject within the airline industry. Although they currently do not generally pose a significant public health hazard, airline passengers could potentially disseminate serious communicable diseases and, if conditions are right, do so on a global scale. Particularly worrisome are organisms that are highly contagious and for which there is little human immunity. Serious worldwide public health concerns could be unleashed if such an organism had an incubation period long enough for travelers to go long distances while they were infectious, but before they develop symptoms. SARS in 2003 certainly exposed this vulnerability. Under the right circumstances, catastrophic epidemics could be caused by naturally occurring viruses (e.g. hemorrhagic viral illnesses), genetic mutations that cause human-to-human transmission (avian flu), or novel strains of pandemic influenza.

A newly revised International Health Regulations (2005) was rolled out on June 15, 2007, with the technical support of WHO. This document enhances national, regional, and international public health security against acute public health risks that can spread internationally and have a devastating impact on human health.

Quarantine

With the eradication of naturally occurring smallpox, most United States quarantine stations were closed in the late 1960's. However, in the post-SARS world, the US Congress began to allocate funds in order to increase the number of quarantine stations. It should be noted that US federal regulations, Title 42, Part 71.21(b), requires that "the commander of an aircraft destined for a US airport shall report immediately to the quarantine station at or nearest the airport at which the aircraft will arrive, the occurrence, on board, of any death or ill person among passengers or crew." Currently this is interpreted as:

- severe diarrhea
- fever >2 days
- fever and:
  - — rash
  - — swollen lymph nodes

— jaundice
— difficulty breathing
— persistent cough
— headache and stiff neck
— decreased level of consciousness
— unexplained bleeding

Currently, the quarantinable diseases by law are:

- infectious tuberculosis
- diphtheria
- smallpox
- yellow fever
- viral hemorrhagic fever(s)
- cholera
- plague
- SARS
- novel strain of influenza

Much work is being done by the CDC in the area of disease transmissibility on commercial aircraft. It is worthy to note that infectious tuberculosis is only considered a concern to other passengers if the flight is greater than eight hours in duration.[28]

Passenger Medical Clearance at the Boarding Gate

Occasionally a passenger becomes ill prior to a flight and appears at the boarding gate with worrisome symptoms. Gate agents should not summon emergency medical personnel unless a real or perceived medical emergency exists. To request a "medical clearance" evaluation is not an appropriate utilization of emergency ambulance personnel. Such problems should be handled with the airlines' medical department, or if none exists, the passenger should be requested to seek an evaluation from a medical clinic.

Air Rage

Reasons for extreme misbehavior by unruly passengers include excessive alcohol consumption, smoking bans, crowding, long flights, psychological problems with authority figures, and mental illness. In addition to placing other passengers and crew members at risk, air rage passengers have accidentally been killed during attempts by other passengers to subdue them. The incidence of air rage seems to have lessened since September 11 due to heightened security and passenger awareness.

Additional Medical Equipment

Occasionally a passenger will need to bring on-board additional medical equipment. Although many of these items are approved, there might be problems bringing them on-board if gate agents or cabin crew are unfamiliar with them. It is important for the passenger to obtain approval through the airline well in advance before the flight in order to avoid such last minute complications.

Fear of Flying

This is a complex psychological issue, one that has been made more difficult by the security concerns of the last few years. Some self-help programs exist to alleviate symptoms. Physicians can also assist with judicious use of anti-anxiety medication in appropriate circumstances.

Fatigue and Jet Lag

Travelers rapidly crossing three or more time zones will experience some form of circadian desynchronization. It is exacerbated by stress, over-eating, dehydration, increasing age, traveling east, sleep deprivation, and alcohol consumption. It can be minimized by taking short flights, taking transit breaks, and appropriately timed exposure to sunlight on arrival. There is some evidence that judicious use of melatonin may be of help in some individuals. Depending on the individual, it can take a full day for each hour of time zone change above three hours to fully recover from jet lag. Besides fatigue and general discomfort, there are potential problems associated with dosage adjustments of such medications as insulin, narcoleptics, anticonvulsants, and anticoagulants.

Elderly Passengers

Even without medical problems, elderly passengers are subjected to greater stress with air travel due to their physical limitations. In addition to needing more time and assistance with baggage and negotiating the airport environment, in-flight considerations should be made, like providing seats near washrooms on long flights.

Telemedicine

Transmission of medical data from patients to remote site physicians has long been in use, and this technology is continuously improving. Although still prohibitively expensive for routine commercial airline use, telemedicine will probably be increasingly utilized as jetliners carry more passengers, especially over routes where diversion landing sites are not always possible.

Airport Medical Clinics

Many large airports, especially international airports, have medical clinics on the premises. Some of these facilities are free-standing, others are part of their government's medical services. In general, they serve airport personnel and passengers in transit, but are usually not receiving units for passengers who become ill during flight.

Handling of On-Board Deaths

As stated earlier in this chapter, it has been estimated that the incidence of in-flight deaths from medical conditions is 0.3–1 per million passengers. With the large numbers of passengers flying every day, it is not surprising that there will occasionally be on-board deaths, especially on long haul flights. The cabin attendants have the primary responsibility of attending to the situation. Only a medical doctor can formally pronounce a person dead. In addition, many airlines will not acknowledge a "do not resuscitate" (DNR) order due to jurisdiction issues. Close cooperation between the airline and the involved governmental agencies needs to be established and carefully followed.

Post Airline Accident Tragedy Care

The difference between the public perceptions concerning the handling of the two tragedies, TWA Flight 800 (1996) and Swiss Air 111 (1998), demonstrate the importance of a well organized airline tragedy response team. Following the crash and the ensuing public relations difficulties of TWA Flight 800, all airlines flying in the United States are required by federal law to have a family assistance plan in place that must be activated following a fatal air accident. The National Transportation and Safety Board has been tasked with the mission of being the federal coordinator for services to the families of the victims of aviation disasters, in order to ensure that family members are treated well and given access to crash sites, personal effects, and the remains of their loved ones.

THE FUTURE OF MEDICAL CLEARANCE: THE SPACE TOURIST

Commercial space tourism had its start with Dennis Tito (age 60-USA) on Soyuz TM-32 in April 2001. There have been five others as of this writing. These candidates had to undergo intense medical and physiological evaluation before selection, then continue with rigorous cosmonaut training in Star City, Russia. This, and a payment of over US$20 million, provides space tourists a stay of several days in the International Space Station.

With the successful flights in 2004 of SpaceShipOne, suborbital flight has been opened for much less rigorous and expensive commercial space tourism. It is likely that by the end of this decade space tourists will be regularly attaining altitudes of 100 km (62 miles, or 328 000 feet). These flights will be relatively short (under an hour) with only a few minutes of weightlessness.

Positive G-loads are expected to be between two and 4.5. These passengers will not be required to perform any missions, requiring much less physiological training, and allowing for medical conditions that would currently be disqualifying. Medical guidelines for commercial space tourists are already being discussed for suborbital trips[25] as well as orbital.[29] The focus is not on the kinds of medical problems the passenger might bring to the flight, but rather the passengers' fitness to survive the flight. Even terminally ill individuals could safely experience suborbital flight, as long as they are otherwise healthy enough to endure the physiological stressors.

In February 2005, the Federal Aviation Administration's (FAA) Commercial Space Transportation announced that the agency does not plan to certify the health of space tourists, and leaves that decision up to a physician "trained in the concepts of aerospace medicine". And, until an accident or close call occurs, the Department of Transportation (DOT) and the FAA will apparently not step in and issue regulations to govern the design and operation of private space-launch vehicles, according to a provision in the Commercial Space Launch Amendments Act of 2004.

SUMMARY

The vast majority of airline passengers travel safely, without noticeable impact on their health. Historically, regulatory agencies have been concerned with the safety aspects of the flight *per se*, and have shown little interest in passenger health issues. A combination of media sensationalism, inadequate research, and perceived disregard by the airlines have resulted in a variety of passenger health topics that are poorly understood by the traveling public and their health care providers.

Although complaints about health risks abound in the form of criticism by passengers and sensationalism by the lay media, not enough research has been performed to investigate the true incidence of passenger illness on commercial flights. It could be stated that more is known about the health effects of space flight on astronauts than is known about the health risks of routine commercial flights on normal people. Perhaps syncope and anxiety, which are common in-flight medical events, are an expression of underlying mild hypoxia. Perhaps passengers with relatively unstable diseases are now more willing to fly, falsely believing that the medical kits on board would be able to manage any unanticipated medical events. Perhaps passengers with risk factors for DVT should be encouraged to get up and walk the aisles; such measures should be weighed against the possibility of injuries from turbulence.

The paucity of research into the area of passenger health stems primarily from the hesitancy of the airlines to expose their medical events to public scrutiny. In times of shrinking airline budgets, medical departments are hit especially hard. The aerospace medical community should pool its collective experience and address topics that have the greatest relevance to passenger health. Some topics are begging for research and are quite appropriate areas for airline companies to assist in data collection. The airline industry should recognize that the promotion of passenger health issues will again increase their customers' support, loyalty, and trust, without necessarily exposing themselves to increased liabilities.

Passengers and their physicians should be well informed and proactive in cases where medical conditions exist that could be adversely affected by flight. The aerospace medical community should continue to provide recommendations to these passengers, based on empirical evidence, which unfortunately remains profoundly inadequate. Despite the fact that passenger health is highly fertile ground for further study, a number of roadblocks has prevented meaningful research into this field. One can understand the reluctance of airlines to make information on passenger medical events available; however, this could be done anonymously through a central scientific organization such as AsMA or a non-biased governmental agency such as ICAO. This research would help aerospace medicine physicians develop a much better basis from which to make recommendations on in-flight passenger health issues.

The author hopes this chapter, as an introduction to the topic of airline passenger health, will motivate those readers, who are in aerospace medicine research, to conduct some meaningful studies in this area, and that those readers from the airline industry are equally convinced that such research is worthwhile to support. It is neither obtrusive to the passengers nor is it a negative marketing factor. In contrast, it will be viewed by the customers as an indicator that the airlines are finally appreciating their physical needs. If the airlines respond to the outcomes, the passengers will thank them for it.

REFERENCES

1. Aerospace Medical Association Task Force. (2003) Medical guidelines for airline travel, 2nd ed. *Aviat Space Env Med* **74**(5).
2. *Medical Guidelines for Airline Passengers.* (2002) Aerospace Medical Association.
3. Rayman RB. (1997) Passenger safety, health, and comfort: A review. *Aviat Space Env Med* **68**: 432–440.
4. Jordan Jon L. (2000) Medical risks associated with air travel, editorial, *The Federal Air Surgeon's Bulletin,* Winter ed.
5. *Statement of Dr Jon L Jordan.* (2000) Federal Air Surgeon, Federal Aviation Administration, before the committee on Transportation and Infrastructure, Subcommittee on Aviation, US House of Representatives, concerning implementation of the Aviation Medical Assistance Act of 1998.
6. British Geriatrics Society. (2002) Air travel in older people. *Age and Aging* **31**: 17–22.
7. Bettes Thomas, McKenas David K. (1999) Medical advice for commercial air travelers. *American Family Physician, American Academy of Family Practice Physicians,* Vol 60.

8. Rayman RB, Williams Kenneth A. (2002) The passenger and the patient in-flight, in: RH DeHart & JR Davis (eds), *Fundamentals of Aerospace Medicine*, 3rd ed.
9. *Medical Manual.* (2004) International Air Transport Association, 1st ed.
10. *Useful Tips for Airline Travel.* (2001) Aerospace Medical Association.
11. Wolbrink Alex. Deep vein thrombosis and travel. *FAA Publication* **AAM-400-03/2**.
12. Lomangino Nicholas. (2001) Thromboembolic disease: Risk for passengers and aircrew? *The Federal Air Surgeon's Medical Bulletin,* Spring ed.
13. Canadian Cardiovascular Society Consensus Conference. (2003) *Assessment of the Cardiac Patient for Fitness to Drive and Fly.*
14. Muhm JM, Rock PB. (2007) Effect of aircraft-cabin altitude on passenger discomfort. *NEJM* **357**: 18–27.
15. www.who.int/csr/ihr/en/
16. http://www.icao.int/icaolen/assembl/a35/wp/wp122-en.pdf
17. House of Lords, Science and Technology. (2005) Fifth Report, Nov. 15.
18. Gendreau MA, DeJohn C. (2002) Responding to medical events during commercial airline flights. *N Engl J Med* **346**: 1067–1073.
19. Cummins RO, *et al.* (1988) In-flight deaths during commercial air travel. How big is the problem? *JAMA* **259**: 1983–1988.
20. DeLaune EF, Lucas RH Illig P. (2003) In-flight medical events and aircraft diversions: One airline's experience. *Aviat Space Env Med* **74**: 62–68.
21. http://www.medaire.com/2002_stat_nr.html
22. Bagshaw M, Air Transport Medicine Committee of the Aerospace Medical Association. (2001) Traveler's thrombosis: A review of deep vein thrombosis associated with travel. *Aviat Space Env Med* **72**: 848–851.
23. Hordinsky JR, George MH. (1991) Utilization of emergency kits by air. *DOT/FAA report* **AM-91/2**.
24. *The Impact of Flying on Passenger Health, A Guide for Healthcare Professionals.* (2004) British Medical Association.
25. Aerospace Medical Association Task Force on Space Travel (2001 & 2002) Medical guidelines for space passengers. *Aviat Space Env Med* **72(10)**: 948–950 & Part II **73(11)**: 1132–1134.

26. http://www.who.int/cardiovascular_diseases/wright_project/en/
27. International Travel and Health. (2008) World Health Organization (www.int/ith/en).
28. Tuberculosis and Air Travel: Guidelines for prevention and control. 2nd edition (2005) World Health Organization.
29. Antunano M, Gerzer R. (2008) *Medical Safety Consideration for Passengers on Short-Duration Commercial Orbital Space Flights.* International Academy of Astronautics Study Group.

Appendix I

International Standards and Recommended Practices

Chapter 1. Definitions and General Rules Concerning Licenses

1.1 DEFINITIONS

When the following terms are used in the Standards and Recommended Practices for Personnel Licensing, they have the following meanings:

Accredited medical conclusion. The conclusion reached by one or more medical experts acceptable to the Licensing Authority for the purposes of the case concerned, in consultation with flight operations or other experts as necessary.

Aeroplane. A power-driven heavier-than-air aircraft, deriving its lift in flight chiefly from aerodynamic reactions on surfaces which remain fixed under given conditions of flight.

Aircraft. Any machine that can derive support in the atmosphere from the reactions of the air other than the reactions of the air against the earth's surface.

Aircraft avionics. A term designating any electronic device — including its electrical part — for use in an aircraft, including radio, automatic flight control and instrument systems.

Aircraft — category. Classification of aircraft according to specified basic characteristics, e.g. aeroplane, helicopter, glider, free balloon.

Aircraft certificated for single-pilot operation. A type of aircraft which the State of Registry has determined, during the certification process, can be operated safely with a minimum crew of one pilot.

Aircraft required to be operated with a co-pilot. *A* type of aircraft that is required to be operated with a co-pilot, as specified in the flight manual or by the air operator certificate.

Aircraft — type of. All aircraft of the same basic design including all modifications thereto except those modifications which result in a change in handling or flight characteristics.

Airmanship. The consistent use of good judgement and well-developed knowledge, skills and attitudes to accomplish flight objectives.

Airship. A power-driven lighter-than-air aircraft.

Approved maintenance organization. An organization approved by a Contracting State, in accordance with the requirements of Annex 6, Part I, Chapter 8 — Aeroplane Maintenance, to perform maintenance of aircraft or parts thereof and operating under supervision approved by that State.

Note. — Nothing in this definition is intended to preclude that the organization and its supervision be approved by more than one State.

Approved training. Training conducted under special curricula and supervision approved by a Contracting State that, in the case of flight crew members, is conducted within an approved training organization.

Approved training organization. An organization approved by a Contracting State in accordance with the requirements of Annex 1, 1.2.8.2 and Appendix 2 to perform flight crew training and operating under the supervision of that State.

Balloon. A non-power-driven lighter-than-air aircraft.

Note. — For the purposes of this Annex, this definition applies to free balloons.

Certify as airworthy (to). To certify that an aircraft or parts thereof comply with current airworthiness requirements after maintenance has been performed on the aircraft or parts thereof.

Commercial air transport operation. An aircraft operation involving the transport of passengers, cargo or mail for remuneration or hire.

Competency. A combination of skills, knowledge and attitudes required to perform a task to the prescribed standard.

Competency element. An action that constitutes a task that has a triggering event and a terminating event that clearly defines its limits, and an observable outcome.

Competency unit. A discrete function consisting of a number of competency elements.

Co-pilot. A licensed pilot serving in any piloting capacity other than as pilot-in-command but excluding a pilot who is on board the aircraft for the sole purpose of receiving flight instruction.

Credit. Recognition of alternative means or prior qualifications.

Cross-country. A flight between a point of departure and a point of arrival following a pre-planned route using standard navigation procedures.

Dual instruction time. Flight time during which a person is receiving flight instruction from a properly authorized pilot on board the aircraft.

Error. An action or inaction by the flight crew that leads to deviations from organizational or flight crew intentions or expectations.

Error management. The process of detecting and responding to errors with countermeasures that reduce or eliminate the consequences of errors and mitigate the probability of further errors or undesired aircraft states.

Note. — See Attachment C to Chapter 3 of the Procedures for Air Navigation Services — Training *(PANS-TRG, Doc 9868) for a description of undesired aircraft states.*

Flight crew member. A licensed crew member charged with duties essential to the operation of an aircraft during a flight duty period.

Flight plan. Specified information provided to air traffic services units, relative to an intended flight or portion of a flight of an aircraft.

Flight procedures trainer. *See* Flight simulation training device.

Flight simulation training device. Any one of the following three types of apparatus in which flight conditions are simulated on the ground:

A flight simulator, which provides an accurate representation of the flight deck of a particular aircraft type to the extent that the mechanical, electrical, electronic, etc. aircraft systems control functions, the normal environment of flight crew members, and the performance and flight characteristics of that type of aircraft are realistically simulated;

A flight procedures trainer, which provides a realistic flight deck environment, and which simulates instrument responses, simple control functions of mechanical, electrical, electronic, etc. aircraft systems, and the performance and flight characteristics of aircraft of a particular class;

A basic instrument flight trainer, which is equipped with appropriate instruments, and which simulates the flight deck environment of an aircraft in flight in instrument flight conditions.

Flight simulator. *See* Flight simulation training device.

Flight time — aeroplanes. The total time from the moment an aeroplane first moves for the purpose of taking off until the moment it finally comes to rest at the end of the flight.

Note. — Flight time as here defined is synonymous with the term "block to block" time or "chock to chock" time in general usage which is measured from the time an aeroplane first moves for the purpose of taking off until it finally stops at the end of the flight.

Flight time — helicopters. The total time from the moment a helicopter's rotor blades start turning until the moment the helicopter finally comes to rest at the end of the flight, and the rotor blades are stopped.

Glider. A non-power-driven heavier-than-air aircraft, deriving its lift in flight chiefly from aerodynamic reactions on surfaces which remain fixed under given conditions of flight.

Glider flight time. The total time occupied in flight, whether being towed or not, from the moment the glider first moves for the purpose of taking off until the moment it comes to rest at the end of the flight.

Helicopter. A heavier-than-air aircraft supported in flight chiefly by the reactions of the air on one or more power-driven rotors on substantially vertical axes.

Human performance. Human capabilities and limitations which have an impact on the safety and efficiency of aeronautical operations.

Instrument flight time. Time during which a pilot is piloting an aircraft solely by reference to instruments and without external reference points.

Instrument ground time. Time during which a pilot is practising, on the ground, simulated instrument flight in a flight simulation training device approved by the Licensing Authority.

Instrument time. Instrument flight time or instrument ground time.

Licensing Authority. The Authority designated by a Contracting State as responsible for the licensing of personnel.

Note. — *In the provisions of this Annex, the Licensing Authority is deemed to have been given the following responsibilities by the Contracting State:*

a) *assessment of an applicant's qualifications to hold a license or rating;*
b) *issue and endorsement of licenses and ratings;*
c) *designation and authorization of approved persons;*
d) *approval of training courses;*

e) *approval of the use of flight simulation training devices and authorization for their use in gaining the experience or in demonstrating the skill required for the issue of a license or rating; and*
f) *validation of licenses issued by other Contracting States.*

Likely. In the context of the medical provisions in Chapter 6, ***likely*** means with a probability of occurring that is unacceptable to the medical assessor.

Maintenance. The performance of tasks required to ensure the continuing airworthiness of an aircraft, including any one or combination of overhaul, inspection, replacement, defect rectification, and the embodiment of a modification or repair.

Medical Assessment. The evidence issued by a Contracting State that the license holder meets specific requirements of medical fitness.

Medical assessor. A physician qualified and experienced in the practice of aviation medicine who evaluates medical reports submitted to the Licensing Authority by medical examiners.

Medical examiner. A physician with training in aviation medicine and practical knowledge and experience of the aviation environment, who is designated by the Licensing Authority to conduct medical examinations of fitness of applicants for licenses or ratings for which medical requirements are prescribed.

Night. The hours between the end of evening civil twilight and the beginning of morning civil twilight or such other period between sunset and sunrise, as may be prescribed by the appropriate authority.

Note. — Civil twilight ends in the evening when the centre of the sun's disc is 6 degrees below the horizon and begins in the morning when the centre of the sun's disc is 6 degrees below the horizon.

Performance criteria. Simple, evaluative statements on the required outcome of the competency element and a description of the criteria used to judge whether the required level of performance has been achieved.

Pilot (to). To manipulate the flight controls of an aircraft during flight time.

Pilot-in-command. The pilot designated by the operator, or in the case of general aviation, the owner, as being in command and charged with the safe conduct of a flight.

Pilot-in-command under supervision. Co-pilot performing, under the supervision of the pilot-in-command, the duties and functions of a pilot-in-command, in accordance with a method of supervision acceptable to the Licensing Authority.

Powered-lift. A heavier-than-air aircraft capable of vertical take-off, vertical landing, and low-speed flight, which depends principally on engine-driven lift devices or engine thrust for the lift during these flight regimes and on non-rotating aerofoil(s) for lift during horizontal flight.

Problematic use of substances. The use of one or more psychoactive substances by aviation personnel in a way that:

a) constitutes a direct hazard to the user or endangers the lives, health or welfare of others; and/or
b) causes or worsens an occupational, social, mental or physical problem or disorder.

Psychoactive substances. Alcohol, opioids, cannabinoids, sedatives and hypnotics, cocaine, other psychostimulants, hallucinogens, and volatile solvents, whereas coffee and tobacco are excluded.

Quality system. Documented organizational procedures and policies; internal audit of those policies and procedures; management review and recommendation for quality improvement.

Rated air traffic controller. An air traffic controller holding a license and valid ratings appropriate to the privileges to be exercised.

Rating. An authorization entered on or associated with a license and forming part thereof, stating special conditions, privileges or limitations pertaining to such license.

Rendering (a license) valid. The action taken by a Contracting State, as an alternative to issuing its own license, in accepting a license issued by any other Contracting State as the equivalent of its own license.

Sign a maintenance release (to). To certify that maintenance work has been completed satisfactorily in accordance with the applicable Standards of airworthiness, by issuing the maintenance release referred to in Annex 6.

Significant. In the context of the medical provisions in Chapter 6, ***significant*** means to a degree or of a nature that is likely to jeopardize flight safety.

Solo flight time. Flight time during which a student pilot is the sole occupant of an aircraft.

Threat. Events or errors that occur beyond the influence of the flight crew, increase operational complexity and must be managed to maintain the margin of safety.

Threat management. The process of detecting and responding to threats with countermeasures that reduce or eliminate the consequences of threats and mitigate the probability of errors or undesired aircraft states.

Note. — See Attachment C to Chapter 3 of the Procedures for Air Navigation Services — Training *(PANS-TRG, Doc 9868) for a description of undesired aircraft states.*

1.2 GENERAL RULES CONCERNING LICENSES

Note 1. — Although the Convention on International Civil Aviation allocates to the State of Registry certain functions which that State is entitled to discharge, or obligated to discharge, as the case may be, the Assembly recognized, in Resolution A23–13, that the State of Registry may be unable to fulfil its responsibilities adequately in instances where aircraft are leased, chartered or interchanged — in particular without crew — by an operator of another State and that the

Convention may not adequately specify the rights and obligations of the State of an operator in such instances until such time as Article 83 bis *of the Convention enters into force. Accordingly, the Council urged that if, in the above-mentioned instances, the State of Registry finds itself unable to discharge adequately the functions allocated to it by the Convention, it delegate to the State of the Operator, subject to acceptance by the latter State, those functions of the State of Registry that can more adequately be discharged by the State of the Operator. While Article 83* bis *of the Convention entered into force on 20 June 1997 in respect of Contracting States which have ratified the related Protocol (Doc 9318), the foregoing action will remain particularly relevant for those Contracting States which do not have treaty relations under Article 83* bis. *It was understood that pending entry into force of Article 83* bis *of the Convention, the foregoing action would only be a matter of practical convenience and would not affect either the provisions of the Chicago Convention prescribing the duties of the State of Registry or any third State. However, as Article 83* bis *of the Convention entered into force on 20 June 1997, such transfer agreements will have effect in respect of Contracting States which have ratified the related Protocol (Doc 9318) upon fulfilment of the conditions established in Article 83* bis.

Note 2. — International Standards and Recommended Practices are established for licensing the following personnel:

a) Flight crew
- *— private pilot — aeroplane, airship, helicopter or powered-lift;*
- *— commercial pilot — aeroplane, airship, helicopter or powered-lift;*
- *— multi-crew pilot — aeroplane;*
- *— airline transport pilot — aeroplane, helicopter or powered-lift*
- *— glider pilot;*
- *— free balloon pilot;*
- *— flight navigator;*
- *— flight engineer.*

b) Other personnel
- *— aircraft maintenance (technician/engineer/mechanic);*

— *air traffic controller;*
— *flight operations officer/flight dispatcher;*
— *aeronautical station operator.*

1.2.1 Authority to Act as a Flight Crew Member

A person shall not act as a flight crew member of an aircraft unless a valid license is held showing compliance with the specifications of this Annex and appropriate to the duties to be performed by that person. The license shall have been issued by the State of Registry of that aircraft or by any other Contracting State and rendered valid by the State of Registry of that aircraft.

Note. — Article 29 of the Convention on International Civil Aviation requires that the flight crew members carry their appropriate licenses on board every aircraft engaged in international air navigation.

1.2.2 Method of Rendering a License Valid

1.2.2.1 When a Contracting State renders valid a license issued by another Contracting State, as an alternative to the issuance of its own license, it shall establish validity by suitable authorization to be carried with the former license accepting it as the equivalent of the latter. When a State limits the authorization to specific privileges, the authorization shall specify the privileges of the license which are to be accepted as its equivalent. The validity of the authorization shall not extend beyond the period of validity of the license. The authorization ceases to be valid if the license upon which it was issued is revoked or suspended.

Note. — This provision is not intended to preclude the State that issued the license from extending, by a suitable notification, the period of validity of the license without necessarily requiring either the physical return of the license or the appearance of the license holder before the Authorities of that State.

1.2.2.2 When an authorization under 1.2.2.1 is issued for use in commercial air transport operations, the Licensing Authority shall confirm the validity of the other Contracting State's license before issuing the authorization.

1.2.1.3 **Recommendation.** — *A pilot license issued by a Contracting State should be rendered valid by other Contracting States for use in private flights.*

Note. — Contracting States which, without formality, render valid a license issued by another Contracting State for use in private flights are encouraged to notify this facility in their Aeronautical Information Publications.

1.2.3 Privileges of the Holder of a License

A Contracting State shall not permit the holder of a license to exercise privileges other than those granted by that license.

1.2.4 Medical Fitness

Note 1. — Guidance material is published in the Manual of Civil Aviation Medicine *(Doc 8984).*

Note 2. — To satisfy the licensing requirements of medical fitness for the issue of various types of licenses, the applicant must meet certain appropriate medical requirements which are specified as three classes of Medical Assessment. Details are given in 6.2, 6.3, 6.4 and 6.5. To provide the necessary evidence to satisfy the requirements of 1.2.4.1, the Licensing Authority issues the license holder with the appropriate Medical Assessment, Class 1, Class 2 or Class 3. This can be done in several ways such as a suitably titled separate certificate, a statement on the license, a national regulation stipulating that the Medical Assessment is an integral part of the license, etc.

1.2.4.1 An applicant for a license shall, when applicable, hold a Medical Assessment issued in accordance with the provisions of Chapter 6.

1.2.4.2 The period of validity of a Medical Assessment shall begin on the day the medical examination is performed. The duration of the period of validity shall be in accordance with the provisions of 1.2.5.2.

1.2.4.2.1 The period of validity of a Medical Assessment may be extended, at the discretion of the Licensing Authority, up to 45 days.

Note. — It is advisable to let the calendar day on which the Medical Assessment expires remain constant year after year by allowing the expiry date of the current Medical Assessment to be the beginning of the new validity period under the proviso that the medical examination takes place during the period of validity of the current Medical Assessment but no more than 45 days before it expires.

1.2.4.3 Except as provided in 1.2.5.2.4, flight crew members or air traffic controllers shall not exercise the privileges of their license unless they hold a current Medical Assessment appropriate to the license.

1.2.4.4 Contracting States shall designate medical examiners, qualified and licensed in the practice of medicine, to conduct medical examinations of fitness of applicants for the issue or renewal of the licenses or ratings specified in Chapters 2 and 3, and of the appropriate licenses specified in Chapter 4.

1.2.4.4.1 Medical examiners shall have received training in aviation medicine and shall receive refresher training at regular intervals. Before designation, medical examiners shall demonstrate adequate competency in aviation medicine.

1.2.4.4.2 Medical examiners shall have practical knowledge and experience of the conditions in which the holders of licenses and ratings carry out their duties.

Note. — Examples of practical knowledge and experience are flight experience, simulator experience, on-site observation or any other hands-on experience deemed by the Licensing Authority to meet this requirement.

1.2.4.5 Applicants for licenses or ratings for which medical fitness is prescribed shall sign and furnish to the medical examiner a declaration stating whether they have previously undergone such an examination and, if so, the date, place and result of the last examination. They shall indicate to the examiner whether a Medical Assessment has previously been refused, revoked or suspended and, if so, the reason for such refusal, revocation or suspension.

1.2.4.5.1 Any false declaration to a medical examiner made by an applicant for a license or rating shall be reported to the Licensing Authority of the issuing State for such action as may be considered appropriate.

1.2.4.6 Having completed the medical examination of the applicant in accordance with Chapter 6, the medical examiner shall coordinate the results of the examination and submit a signed report, or equivalent, to the Licensing Authority, in accordance with its requirements, detailing the results of the examination and evaluating the findings with regard to medical fitness.

1.2.4.6.1 If the medical report is submitted to the Licensing Authority in electronic format, adequate identification of the examiner shall be established.

1.2.4.6.2 If the medical examination is carried out by two or more medical examiners, Contracting States shall appoint one of these to be responsible for coordinating the results of the examination, evaluating the findings with regard to medical fitness, and signing the report.

1.2.4.7 Contracting States shall use the services of medical assessors to evaluate reports submitted to the Licensing Authorities by medical examiners.

1.2.4.7.1 The medical examiner shall be required to submit sufficient medical information to the Licensing Authority to enable the Authority to audit Medical Assessments.

Note. — The purpose of such auditing is to ensure that medical examiners meet applicable standards for good practice.

1.2.4.8 If the medical Standards prescribed in Chapter 6 for a particular license are not met, the appropriate Medical Assessment shall not be issued or renewed unless the following conditions are fulfilled:

a) accredited medical conclusion indicates that in special circumstances the applicant's failure to meet any requirement, whether numerical or otherwise, is such that exercise of the privileges of the license applied for is not likely to jeopardize flight safety;
b) relevant ability, skill and experience of the applicant and operational conditions have been given due consideration; and
c) the license is endorsed with any special limitation or limitations when the safe performance of the license holder's duties is dependent on compliance with such limitation or limitations.

1.2.4.9 Medical confidentiality shall be respected at all times.

1.2.4.9.1 All medical reports and records shall be securely held with accessibility restricted to authorized personnel.

1.2.4.9.2 When justified by operational considerations, the medical assessor shall determine to what extent pertinent medical information is presented to relevant officials of the Licensing Authority.

1.2.5 Validity of Licenses

1.2.5.1 A Contracting State, having issued a license, shall ensure that the privileges granted by that license, or by related ratings, are not exercised unless the holder maintains competency and meets the requirements for recent experience established by that State.

1.2.5.1.1 **Recommendation.** — *A Contracting State should establish maintenance of competency and recent experience requirements for pilot licenses and ratings based on a systematic approach to accident prevention and should include a risk assessment process and analysis of current operations, including accident and incident data appropriate to that State.*

1.2.5.1.2 A Contracting State, having issued a license, shall ensure that other Contracting States are enabled to be satisfied as to the validity of the license.

Note 1. — The maintenance of competency of flight crew members, engaged in commercial air transport operations, may be satisfactorily established by demonstration of skill during proficiency flight checks completed in accordance with Annex 6.

Note 2. — Maintenance of competency may be satisfactorily recorded in the operator's records, or in the flight crew member's personal log book or license.

Note 3. — Flight crew members may, to the extent deemed feasible by the State of Registry, demonstrate their continuing competency in flight simulation training devices approved by that State.

Note 4. — See the Manual of Criteria for the Qualification of Flight Simulators *(Doc 9625).*

Note 5. — See the Manual of Procedures for Establishment and Management of a State's Personnel Licensing System *(Doc 9379) for guidance material on the development of a risk assessment process.*

1.2.5.2 Except as provided in 1.2.5.2.1, 1.2.5.2.2, 1.2.5.2.3, 1.2.5.2.4, 1.2.5.2.5 and 1.2.5.2.6, a Medical Assessment issued in accordance with 1.2.4.5 and 1.2.4.6 shall be valid from the date of the medical examination for a period not greater than:

60 months for the private pilot license — aeroplane, airship, helicopter and powered-lift;
12 months for the commercial pilot license — aeroplane, airship, helicopter and powered-lift;
12 months for the multi-crew pilot license — aeroplane;
12 months for the airline transport pilot license — aeroplane, helicopter and powered-lift;
60 months for the glider pilot license;
60 months for the free balloon pilot license;
12 months for the flight navigator license;
12 months for the flight engineer license;
48 months for the air traffic controller license.

Note 1. — The periods of validity listed above may be extended by up to 45 days in accordance with 1.2.4.2.1.

Note 2. — When calculated in accordance with 1.2.5.2 and its subparagraphs, the period of validity will, for the last month counted, include the day that has the same calendar number as the date of the medical examination or, if that month has no day with that number, the last day of that month.

1.2.5.2.1 The period of validity of a Medical Assessment may be reduced when clinically indicated.

1.2.5.2.2 When the holders of airline transport pilot licenses — aeroplane, helicopter and powered-lift, and commercial pilot licenses — aeroplane, airship, helicopter and powered-lift, who are engaged in single-crew commercial air transport operations carrying passengers, have passed their 40th birthday, the period of validity specified in 1.2.5.2 shall be reduced to six months.

1.2.5.2.3 When the holders of airline transport pilot licenses — aeroplane, helicopter and powered-lift, commercial pilot licenses — aeroplane, airship, helicopter and powered-lift, and multi-crew pilot licenses — aeroplane, who are engaged in commercial air transport operations, have passed their 60th birthday, the period of validity specified in 1.2.5.2 shall be reduced to six months.

1.2.5.2.4 When the holders of private pilot licenses — aeroplane, airship, helicopter and powered-lift, free balloon pilot licenses, glider pilot licenses and air traffic controller licenses have passed their 40th birthday, the period of validity specified in 1.2.5.2 shall be reduced to 24 months.

1.2.5.2.5 **Recommendation.** — *When the holders of private pilot licenses — aeroplane, airship, helicopter and powered-lift, free balloon pilot licenses, glider pilot licenses and air traffic controller licenses have passed their 50th birthday, the period of validity specified in 1.2.5.2 should be further reduced to 12 months.*

Note. — The periods of validity listed above are based on the age of the applicant at the time of undergoing the medical examination.

1.2.5.2.6 *Circumstances in which a medical examination may be deferred.* The prescribed re-examination of a license holder operating in an area distant from designated medical examination facilities may be deferred at the discretion of the Licensing Authority, provided that such deferment shall only be made as an exception and shall not exceed:

a) a single period of six months in the case of a flight crew member of an aircraft engaged in non-commercial operations;
b) two consecutive periods each of three months in the case of a flight crew member of an aircraft engaged in commercial operations provided that in each case a favorable medical report is obtained after examination by a designated medical examiner of the area concerned, or, in cases where such a designated medical examiner is not available, by a physician legally qualified to practise medicine in that area. A report of the medical examination shall be sent to the Licensing Authority where the license was issued;
c) in the case of a private pilot, a single period not exceeding 24 months where the medical examination is carried out by an examiner designated under 1.2.4.4 by the Contracting State in which the applicant is temporarily located. A report of the medical examination shall be sent to the Licensing Authority where the license was issued.

1.2.6 Decrease in Medical Fitness

1.2.6.1 Holders of licenses provided for in this Annex shall not exercise the privileges of their licenses and related ratings at any time when they are aware of any decrease in their medical fitness which might render them unable to safely and properly exercise these privileges.

1.2.6.1.1 **Recommendation.** — *License holders should inform the Licensing Authority of confirmed pregnancy or any decrease in medical fitness of a duration of more than 20 days or which requires continued treatment with prescribed medication or which has required hospital treatment.*

1.2.6.1.2 **Recommendation.** — *Each Contracting State should, as far as practicable, ensure that license holders do not exercise the privileges of their licenses and related ratings during any period in which their medical fitness has, from any cause, decreased to an extent that would have prevented the issue or renewal of their Medical Assessment.*

1.2.7 Use of Psychoactive Substances

1.2.7.1 Holders of licenses provided for in this Annex shall not exercise the privileges of their licenses and related ratings while under the influence of any psychoactive substance which might render them unable to safely and properly exercise these privileges.

1.2.7.2 Holders of licenses provided for in this Annex shall not engage in any problematic use of substances.

1.2.7.3 **Recommendation.** — *Contracting States should ensure, as far as practicable, that all license holders who engage in any kind of problematic use of substances are identified and removed from their safety-critical functions. Return to the safety-critical functions may be considered after successful treatment or, in cases where no treatment is necessary, after cessation of the problematic use of substances and upon determination that the person's continued performance of the function is unlikely to jeopardize safety.*

Note. — Guidance on suitable methods of identification (which may include biochemical testing on such occasions as pre-employment, upon reasonable suspicion, after accidents/incidents, at intervals, and at random) and on other prevention topics is contained in the Manual on Prevention of Problematic Use of Substances in the Aviation Workplace *(Doc 9654).*

1.2.8 Approved Training and Approved Training Organization

Note. — The qualifications required for the issue of personnel licenses can be more readily and speedily acquired by applicants who undergo closely supervised, systematic and continuous courses of training, conforming to a planned syllabus or curriculum. Provision has accordingly been made for some reduction in the experience requirements for the issue of certain licenses and ratings prescribed in these Standards and Recommended Practices, in respect of an applicant who has satisfactorily completed a course of approved training.

1.2.8.1 Approved training shall provide a level of competency at least equal to that provided by the minimum experience requirement for personnel not receiving such approved training.

1.2.8.2 The approval of a training organization by a State shall be dependent upon the applicant demonstrating compliance with the requirements of Appendix 2.

Note. — Guidance on approval of a flight crew training organization can be found in the Manual on the Approval of Flight Crew Training Organizations *(Doc 9841).*

1.2.9 Language Proficiency

1.2.9.1 Aeroplane, airship, helicopter and powered-lift pilots and those flight navigators who are required to use the radio telephone aboard an aircraft shall demonstrate the ability to speak and understand the language used for radiotelephony communications.

Note. — Pursuant to Article 42 of the Convention on International Civil Aviation, paragraph 1.2.9.1 does not apply to personnel whose licenses are originally issued prior to 5 March 2004 but, in any case, does apply to personnel whose licenses remain valid after 5 March 2008.

1.2.9.2 Air traffic controllers and aeronautical station operators shall demonstrate the ability to speak and understand the language used for radiotelephony communications.

1.2.9.3 **Recommendation.** — *Flight engineers, and glider and free balloon pilots should have the ability to speak and understand the language used for radiotelephony communications.*

1.2.9.4 As of 5 March 2008, aeroplane, airship, helicopter and powered-lift pilots, air traffic controllers and aeronautical station operators shall demonstrate the ability to speak and understand the language used for radiotelephony communications to the level specified in the language proficiency requirements in Appendix 1.

1.2.9.5 **Recommendation.** — *Aeroplane, airship, helicopter and powered-lift pilots, flight navigators required to use the radiotelephone aboard an aircraft, air traffic controllers and aeronautical station operators should demonstrate the ability to speak and understand the language used for radiotelephony communications to the level specified in the language proficiency requirements in Appendix 1.*

1.2.9.6 As of 5 March 2008, the language proficiency of aeroplane, airship, helicopter and powered-lift pilots, air traffic controllers and aeronautical station operators who demonstrate proficiency below the Expert Level (Level 6) shall be formally evaluated at intervals in accordance with an individual's demonstrated proficiency level.

1.2.9.7 **Recommendation.** — *The language proficiency of aeroplane, airship, helicopter and powered-lift pilots, flight navigators required to use the radiotelephone aboard an aircraft, air traffic controllers and aeronautical station operators who demonstrate proficiency below the Expert Level (Level 6) should be formally evaluated at intervals in accordance with an individual's demonstrated proficiency level, as follows:*

a) those demonstrating language proficiency at the Operational Level (Level 4) should be evaluated at least once every three years; and
b) those demonstrating language proficiency at the Extended Level (Level 5) should be evaluated at least once every six years.

Note 1. — Formal evaluation is not required for applicants who demonstrate expert language proficiency, e.g. native and very proficient non-native speakers with a dialect or accent intelligible to the international aeronautical community.

Note 2. — The provisions of 1.2.9 refer to Annex 10, Volume II, Chapter 5, whereby the language used for radiotelephony communications may be the language normally used by the station on the ground or English. In practice, therefore, there will be situations whereby flight crew members will only need to speak the language normally used by the station on the ground.

Chapter 6. Medical Provisions for Licensing

Note 1. — The Standards and Recommended Practices established in this chapter cannot, on their own, be sufficiently detailed to cover all possible individual situations. Of necessity, many decisions relating to the evaluation of medical fitness must be left to the judgement of the individual medical examiner. The evaluation must, therefore, be based on a medical examination conducted throughout in accordance with the highest standards of medical practice.

Note 2. — Predisposing factors for disease, such as obesity and smoking, may be important for determining whether further evaluation or investigation is necessary in an individual case.

Note 3. — In cases where the applicant does not fully meet the medical requirements and in complicated and unusual cases, the evaluation may have to be deferred and the case submitted to the medical assessor of the Licensing Authority for final evaluation. In such cases due regard must be given to the privileges granted by the license applied for or held by the applicant for the Medical Assessment, and the conditions under which the license holder is going to exercise those privileges in carrying out assigned duties.

Note 4. — Attention is called to the administrative clause in 1.2.4.8 dealing with accredited medical conclusion.

Note 5. — Guidance material to assist Licensing Authorities and medical examiners is published separately in the Manual of Civil Aviation Medicine *(Doc 8984). This guidance material also contains a discussion of the terms "likely" and "significant" as used in the context of the medical provisions in Chapter 6.*

6.1 MEDICAL ASSESSMENTS — GENERAL

6.1.1 Classes of Medical Assessment

Three classes of Medical Assessment shall be established as follows:

a) Class 1 Medical Assessment;
applies to applicants for, and holders of:
— commercial pilot licenses — aeroplane, airship, helicopter and powered-lift
— multi-crew pilot licenses — aeroplane
— airline transport pilot licenses — aeroplane, helicopter and powered-lift

b) Class 2 Medical Assessment;
applies to applicants for, and holders of:
— flight navigator licenses
— flight engineer licenses
— private pilot licenses — aeroplane, airship, helicopter and powered-lift
— glider pilot licenses
— free balloon pilot licenses

c) Class 3 Medical Assessment;
applies to applicants for, and holders of:
— air traffic controller licenses.

6.1.2 The applicant for a Medical Assessment shall provide the medical examiner with a personally certified statement of medical facts concerning personal, familial and hereditary history. The applicant shall be made aware of the necessity for giving a statement that is as complete and accurate as the applicant's knowledge permits, and any false statement shall be dealt with in accordance with 1.2.4.5.1.

6.1.3 The medical examiner shall report to the Licensing Authority any individual case where, in the examiner's judgement, an applicant's failure to meet any requirement, whether numerical or otherwise, is such that exercise of the privileges of the license being applied for, or held, is not likely to jeopardize flight safety (1.2.4.8).

6.1.4 The requirements to be met for the renewal of a Medical Assessment are the same as those for the initial assessment except where otherwise specifically stated.

Note. — The intervals between routine medical examinations for the purpose of renewing Medical Assessments are specified in 1.2.5.2.

6.2 REQUIREMENTS FOR MEDICAL ASSESSMENTS

6.2.1 General

An applicant for a Medical Assessment issued in accordance with the terms of 1.2.4.1 shall undergo a medical examination based on the following requirements:

a) physical and mental;
b) visual and colour perception; and
c) hearing.

6.2.2 Physical and Mental Requirements

An applicant for any class of Medical Assessment shall be required to be free from:

a) any abnormality, congenital or acquired; or
b) any active, latent, acute or chronic disability; or
c) any wound, injury or sequelae from operation; or
d) any effect or side-effect of any prescribed or non-prescribed therapeutic, diagnostic or preventive medication taken;

such as would entail a degree of functional incapacity which is likely to interfere with the safe operation of an aircraft or with the safe performance of duties.

Note. — Use of herbal medication and alternative treatment modalities requires particular attention to possible side-effects.

6.2.3 Visual Acuity Test Requirements

6.2.3.1 The methods in use for the measurement of visual acuity are likely to lead to differing evaluations. To achieve uniformity, therefore, Contracting States shall ensure that equivalence in the methods of evaluation be obtained.

6.2.3.2 **Recommendation.**— *The following should be adopted for tests of visual acuity:*

a) Visual acuity tests should be conducted in an environment with a level of illumination that corresponds to ordinary office illumination (30–60 cd/m^2).
b) Visual acuity should be measured by means of a series of Landolt rings or similar optotypes, placed at a distance from the applicant appropriate to the method of testing adopted.

6.2.4 Colour Perception Requirements

6.2.4.1 Contracting States shall use such methods of examination as will guarantee reliable testing of colour perception.

6.2.4.2 The applicant shall be required to demonstrate the ability to perceive readily those colours the perception of which is necessary for the safe performance of duties.

6.2.4.3 The applicant shall be tested for the ability to correctly identify a series of pseudoisochromatic plates in daylight or in artificial light of the same colour temperature such as that provided by CIE standard illuminants C or D_{65} as specified by the International Commission on Illumination (CIE).

6.2.4.4 An applicant obtaining a satisfactory result as prescribed by the Licensing Authority shall be assessed as fit. An applicant failing to obtain a satisfactory result in such a test shall be assessed as unfit unless able to readily distinguish the colours used in air navigation and correctly identify aviation coloured lights. Applicants who fail to meet these criteria shall be assessed as unfit except for Class 2 assessment with the following restriction: valid daytime only.

Note. — Guidance on suitable methods of assessing colour vision is contained in the Manual of Civil Aviation Medicine *(Doc 8984).*

6.2.4.4.1 **Recommendation.** — *Sunglasses worn during the exercise of the privileges of the license or rating held should be non-polarizing and of a neutral grey tint.*

6.2.5 Hearing Test Requirements

6.2.5.1 Contracting States shall use such methods of examination as will guarantee reliable testing of hearing.

6.2.5.2 Applicants shall be required to demonstrate a hearing performance sufficient for the safe exercise of their license and rating privileges.

6.2.5.3 Applicants for Class 1 Medical Assessments shall be tested by pure-tone audiometry at first issue of the Assessment, not less than once every five years up to the age of 40 years, and thereafter not less than once every two years.

6.2.5.3.1 Alternatively, other methods providing equivalent results may be used.

6.2.5.4 Applicants for Class 3 Medical Assessments shall be tested by pure-tone audiometry at first issue of the Assessment, not less than once every four years up to the age of 40 years, and thereafter not less than once every two years.

6.2.5.4.1 Alternatively, other methods providing equivalent results may be used.

6.2.5.5 **Recommendation.** — *Applicants for Class 2 Medical Assessment should be tested by pure-tone audiometry at first issue of the Assessment and, after the age of 50 years, not less than once every two years.*

6.2.5.6 At medical examinations, other than those mentioned in 6.2.5.3, 6.2.5.4 and 6.2.5.5, where audiometry is not performed, applicants shall be tested in a quiet room by whispered and spoken voice tests.

Note 1. — The reference zero for calibration of pure-tone audiometers is that of the pertinent Standards of the current edition of the Audiometric Test Methods, published by the International Organization for Standardization (ISO).

Note 2. — For the purpose of testing hearing in accordance with the requirements, a quiet room is a room in which the intensity of the background noise is less than 35 dB(A).

Note 3. — For the purpose of testing hearing in accordance with the requirements, the sound level of an average conversational voice at 1 m from the point of output (lower lip of the speaker) is c. 60 dB(A) and that of a whispered voice c. 45dB(A). At 2 m from the speaker, the sound level is 6 dB(A) lower.

Note 4. — Guidance on assessment of applicants who use hearing aids is contained in the Manual of Civil Aviation Medicine *(Doc 8984).*

Note 5. — Attention is called to 2.7.1.3.1 on requirements for the issue of instrument rating to applicants who hold a private pilot license.

6.3 CLASS 1 MEDICAL ASSESSMENT

6.3.1 Assessment Issue and Renewal

6.3.1.1 An applicant for a commercial pilot license —aeroplane, airship, helicopter or powered-lift, a multi-crew pilot license — aeroplane, or an airline transport pilot license — aeroplane, helicopter or powered-lift shall undergo an initial medical examination for the issue of a Class 1 Medical Assessment.

6.3.1.2 Except where otherwise stated in this section, holders of commercial pilot licenses — aeroplane, airship, helicopter or powered-lift, multi-crew pilot licenses — aeroplane, or airline transport pilot licenses — aeroplane, helicopter or powered-lift shall have their Class 1 Medical Assessments renewed at intervals not exceeding those specified in 1.2.5.2.

6.3.1.3 When the Licensing Authority is satisfied that the requirements of this section and the general provisions of 6.1 and 6.2 have been met, a Class 1 Medical Assessment shall be issued to the applicant.

6.3.2 Physical and Mental Requirements

6.3.2.1 The applicant shall not suffer from any disease or disability which could render that applicant likely to become suddenly unable either to operate an aircraft safely or to perform assigned duties safely.

6.3.2.2 The applicant shall have no established medical history or clinical diagnosis of:

a) an organic mental disorder;
b) a mental or behavioural disorder due to use of psychoactive substances; this includes dependence syndrome induced by alcohol or other psychoactive substances;
c) schizophrenia or a schizotypal or delusional disorder;
d) a mood (affective) disorder;
e) a neurotic, stress-related or somatoform disorder;
f) a behavioural syndrome associated with physiological disturbances or physical factors;
g) a disorder of adult personality or behaviour, particularly if manifested by repeated overt acts;
h) mental retardation;
i) a disorder of psychological development;
j) a behavioural or emotional disorder, with onset in childhood or adolescence; or
k) a mental disorder not otherwise specified;

such as might render the applicant unable to safely exercise the privileges of the license applied for or held.

Note. — Mental and behavioural disorders are defined in accordance with the clinical descriptions and diagnostic guidelines of the World Health Organization as given in the International Statistical Classification of Diseases and Related Health Problems, 10th Edition — Classification of Mental and Behavioural Disorders, *WHO 1992. This document contains detailed descriptions of the diagnostic requirements, which may be useful for their application to medical assessment.*

6.3.2.3 The applicant shall have no established medical history or clinical diagnosis of any of the following:

a) a progressive or non-progressive disease of the nervous system, the effects of which are likely to interfere with the safe exercise of the applicant's license and rating privileges;
b) epilepsy; or
c) any disturbance of consciousness without satisfactory medical explanation of cause.

6.3.2.4 The applicant shall not have suffered any head injury, the effects of which are likely to interfere with the safe exercise of the applicant's license and rating privileges.

6.3.2.5 The applicant shall not possess any abnormality of the heart, congenital or acquired, which is likely to interfere with the safe exercise of the applicant's license and rating privileges.

6.3.2.5.1 An applicant who has undergone coronary bypass grafting or angioplasty (with or without stenting) or other cardiac intervention or who has a history of myocardial infarction or who suffers from any other potentially incapacitating cardiac condition shall be assessed as unfit unless the applicant's cardiac condition has been investigated and evaluated in accordance with best medical practice and is assessed not likely to interfere with the safe exercise of the applicant's license or rating privileges.

6.3.2.5.2 An applicant with an abnormal cardiac rhythm shall be assessed as unfit unless the cardiac arrhythmia has been investigated and evaluated in accordance with best medical practice and is assessed not likely to interfere with the safe exercise of the applicant's license or rating privileges.

Note. — Guidance on cardiovascular evaluation is contained in the Manual of Civil Aviation Medicine *(Doc 8984).*

6.3.2.6 Electrocardiography shall form part of the heart examination for the first issue of a Medical Assessment.

6.3.2.6.1 Electrocardiography shall be included in re-examinations of applicants over the age of 50 no less frequently than annually.

6.3.2.6.2 **Recommendation.** — *Electrocardiography should be included in re-examinations of applicants between the ages of 30 and 50 no less frequently than every two years.*

Note 1. — The purpose of routine electrocardiography is case finding. It does not provide sufficient evidence to justify disqualification without further thorough cardiovascular investigation.

Note 2. — Guidance on resting and exercise electrocardiography is contained in the Manual of Civil Aviation Medicine *(Doc 8984).*

6.3.2.7 The systolic and diastolic blood pressures shall be within normal limits.

6.3.2.7.1 The use of drugs for control of high blood pressure shall be disqualifying except for those drugs, the use of which is compatible with the safe exercise of the applicant's license and rating privileges.

Note. — Guidance on the subject is contained in the Manual of Civil Aviation Medicine *(Doc 8984).*

6.3.2.8 There shall be no significant functional nor structural abnormality of the circulatory system.

6.3.2.9 There shall be no acute disability of the lungs nor any active disease of the structures of the lungs, mediastinum or pleurae likely to result in incapacitating symptoms during normal or emergency operations.

6.3.2.9.1 **Recommendation.** — *Chest radiography should form part of the initial examination.*

Note. — Periodic chest radiography is usually not necessary but may be a necessity in situations where asymptomatic pulmonary disease can be expected.

6.3.2.10 Applicants with chronic obstructive pulmonary disease shall be assessed as unfit unless the applicant's condition has been investigated and evaluated in accordance with best medical practice and is assessed not likely to interfere with the safe exercise of the applicant's license or rating privileges.

6.3.2.11 Applicants with asthma causing significant symptoms or likely to cause incapacitating symptoms during normal or emergency operations shall be assessed as unfit.

6.3.2.11.1 The use of drugs for control of asthma shall be disqualifying except for those drugs, the use of which is compatible with the safe exercise of the applicant's license and rating privileges.

Note. — Guidance on hazards of medication and drugs is contained in the Manual of Civil Aviation Medicine *(Doc 8984).*

6.3.2.12 Applicants with active pulmonary tuberculosis shall be assessed as unfit.

6.3.2.12.1 Applicants with quiescent or healed lesions which are known to be tuberculous, or are presumably tuberculous in origin, may be assessed as fit.

Note 1. — Guidance on assessment of respiratory diseases is contained in the Manual of Civil Aviation Medicine *(Doc 8984).*

Note 2. — Guidance on hazards of medications and drugs is contained in the Manual of Civil Aviation Medicine *(Doc 8984).*

6.3.2.13 Applicants with significant impairment of function of the gastrointestinal tract or its adnexa shall be assessed as unfit.

6.3.2.13.1 Applicants shall be completely free from those hernias that might give rise to incapacitating symptoms.

6.3.2.14 Applicants with sequelae of disease of, or surgical intervention on, any part of the digestive tract or its adnexa, likely to cause incapacitation in flight, in particular any obstruction due to stricture or compression, shall be assessed as unfit.

6.3.2.14.1 **Recommendation.** — *An applicant who has undergone a major surgical operation on the biliary passages or the digestive tract or its adnexa with a total or partial excision or a diversion of any of these organs should be assessed as unfit until such time as the medical assessor, having access to the details of the operation concerned, considers that the effects of the operation are not likely to cause incapacitation in flight.*

6.3.2.15 Applicants with metabolic, nutritional or endocrine disorders that are likely to interfere with the safe exercise of their license and rating privileges shall be assessed as unfit.

6.3.2.16 Applicants with insulin-treated diabetes mellitus shall be assessed as unfit.

6.3.2.16.1 Applicants with non-insulin-treated diabetes mellitus shall be assessed as unfit unless the condition is shown to be satisfactorily controlled by diet alone or by diet combined with oral antidiabetic medication, the use of which is compatible with the safe exercise of the applicant's license and rating privileges.

Note. — Guidance on assessment of diabetic applicants is contained in the Manual of Civil Aviation Medicine *(Doc 8984).*

6.3.2.17 Applicants with diseases of the blood and/or the lymphatic system shall be assessed as unfit unless adequately investigated and their condition found unlikely to interfere with the safe exercise of their license and rating privileges.

Note. — Sickle cell trait or other haemoglobinopathic traits are usually compatible with a fit assessment.

6.3.2.18 Applicants with renal or genito-urinary disease shall be assessed as unfit, unless adequately investigated and their condition found unlikely to interfere with the safe exercise of their license and rating privileges.

6.3.2.18.1 Urine examination shall form part of the medical examination and abnormalities shall be adequately investigated.

Note. — Guidance on urine examination and evaluation of abnormalities is contained in the Manual of Civil Aviation Medicine *(Doc 8984).*

6.3.2.19 Applicants with sequelae of disease of or surgical procedures on the kidneys or the genito-urinary tract, in particular obstructions due to stricture or compression, shall be assessed as unfit unless the applicant's condition has been investigated and evaluated in accordance with best medical practice and is assessed not likely to interfere with the safe exercise of the applicant's license or rating privileges.

6.3.2.19.1 Applicants who have undergone nephrectomy shall be assessed as unfit unless the condition is well compensated.

6.3.2.20 Applicants with acquired immunodeficiency syndrome (AIDS) shall be assessed as unfit.

6.3.2.20.1 Applicants who are seropositive for human immunodeficiency virus (HIV) shall be assessed as unfit unless full investigation provides no evidence of clinical disease.

Note 1. — Evaluation of applicants who are seropositive for human immunodeficiency virus (HIV) requires particular attention to their mental state, including the psychological effects of the diagnosis.

Note 2. — Guidance on the assessment of applicants who are seropositive for human immunodeficiency virus (HIV) is contained in the Manual of Civil Aviation Medicine *(Doc 8984).*

6.3.2.21 Applicants with gynaecological disorders that are likely to interfere with the safe exercise of their license and rating privileges shall be assessed as unfit.

6.3.2.22 Applicants who are pregnant shall be assessed as unfit unless obstetrical evaluation and continued medical supervision indicate a low-risk uncomplicated pregnancy.

6.3.2.22.1 **Recommendation.** — *For applicants with a low-risk uncomplicated pregnancy, evaluated and supervised in accordance with 6.3.2.22, the fit assessment should be limited to the period* *from the end of the 12th week until the end of the 26th week of gestation.*

6.3.2.23 Following confinement or termination of pregnancy, the applicant shall not be permitted to exercise the privileges of her license until she has undergone re-evaluation in accordance with best medical practice and it has been determined that she is able to safely exercise the privileges of her license and ratings.

6.3.2.24 The applicant shall not possess any abnormality of the bones, joints, muscles, tendons or related structures which is likely to interfere with the safe exercise of the applicant's license and rating privileges.

Note. — *Any sequelae after lesions affecting the bones, joints, muscles or tendons, and certain anatomical defects will normally require functional assessment to determine fitness.*

6.3.2.25 The applicant shall not possess any abnormality or disease of the ear or related structures which is likely to interfere with the safe exercise of the applicant's license and rating privileges.

6.3.2.26 There shall be:

a) no disturbance of vestibular function;
b) no significant dysfunction of the Eustachian tubes; and
c) no unhealed perforation of the tympanic membranes.

6.3.2.26.1 A single dry perforation of the tympanic membrane need not render the applicant unfit.

Note. — *Guidance on testing of the vestibular function is contained in* Manual of Civil Aviation Medicine *(Doc 8984).*

6.3.2.27 There shall be:

a) no nasal obstruction; and
b) no malformation nor any disease of the buccal cavity or upper respiratory tract

which is likely to interfere with the safe exercise of the applicant's license and rating privileges.

6.3.2.28 Applicants with stuttering or other speech defects sufficiently severe to cause impairment of speech communication shall be assessed as unfit.

6.3.3 Visual Requirements

The medical examination shall be based on the following requirements.

6.3.3.1 The function of the eyes and their adnexa shall be normal. There shall be no active pathological condition, acute or chronic, nor any sequelae of surgery or trauma of the eyes or their adnexa likely to reduce proper visual function to an extent that would interfere with the safe exercise of the applicant's license and rating privileges.

6.3.3.2 Distant visual acuity with or without correction shall be 6/9 or better in each eye separately, and binocular visual acuity shall be 6/6 or better. No limits apply to uncorrected visual acuity. Where this standard of visual acuity can be obtained only with correcting lenses, the applicant may be assessed as fit provided that:

a) such correcting lenses are worn during the exercise of the privileges of the license or rating applied for or held; and
b) in addition, a pair of suitable correcting spectacles is kept readily available during the exercise of the privileges of the applicant's license.

Note 1. — 6.3.3.2 b) is the subject of Standards in Annex 6, Part I.

Note 2. — An applicant accepted as meeting these provisions is deemed to continue to do so unless there is reason to suspect otherwise, in which case an ophthalmic report is required at the discretion of the Licensing Authority. Both uncorrected and corrected visual acuity are normally measured and recorded at each re-examination. Conditions which indicate a need to obtain an ophthalmic report include: a substantial decrease in the uncorrected visual acuity, any decrease in best corrected visual acuity, and the occurrence of eye disease, eye injury or eye surgery.

6.3.3.2.1 Applicants may use contact lenses to meet this requirement provided that:

a) the lenses are monofocal and non-tinted;
b) the lenses are well tolerated; and
c) a pair of suitable correcting spectacles is kept readily available during the exercise of the license privileges.

Note. — Applicants who use contact lenses may not need to have their uncorrected visual acuity measured at each re-examination provided the history of their contact lens prescription is known.

6.3.3.2.2 Applicants with a large refractive error shall use contact lenses or high-index spectacle lenses.

Note. — If spectacles are used, high-index lenses are needed to minimize peripheral field distortion.

6.3.3.2.3 Applicants whose uncorrected distant visual acuity in either eye is worse than 6/60 shall be required to provide a full ophthalmic report prior to initial Medical Assessment and every five years thereafter.

Note 1. — The purpose of the required ophthalmic examination is (1) to ascertain normal visual performance, and (2) to identify any significant pathology.

Note 2. — Guidance on the assessment of monocular applicants under the provisions of 1.2.4.8 is contained in the Manual of Civil Aviation Medicine *(Doc 8984).*

6.3.3.3 Applicants who have undergone surgery affecting the refractive status of the eye shall be assessed as unfit unless they are free from those sequelae which are likely to interfere with the safe exercise of their license and rating privileges.

6.3.3.4 The applicant shall have the ability to read, while wearing the correcting lenses, if any, required by 6.3.3.2, the N5 chart or its equivalent at a distance selected by that applicant in the range of 30 to 50 cm and the ability to read the N14 chart or its equivalent at a distance of 100 cm. If this requirement is met only by the use of near correction, the applicant may be assessed as fit provided that this near correction is added to the spectacle correction already prescribed in accordance with 6.3.3.2; if no such correction is prescribed, a pair of spectacles for near use shall be kept readily available during the exercise of the privileges of the license. When near correction is required, the applicant shall demonstrate that one pair of spectacles is sufficient to meet both distant and near visual requirements.

Note 1. — N5 and N14 refer to the size of typeface used. For further details, see the Manual of Civil Aviation Medicine *(Doc 8984).*

Note 2. — An applicant who needs near correction to meet this requirement will require "look-over", bifocal or perhaps multifocal lenses in order to read the instruments and a chart or manual held in the hand, and also to make use of distant vision, through the windscreen, without removing the lenses. Single-vision near correction (full lenses of one power only, appropriate for reading) significantly reduces distant visual acuity and is therefore not acceptable.

Note 3. — Whenever there is a requirement to obtain or renew correcting lenses, an applicant is expected to advise the refractionist of reading distances for the visual flight deck tasks relevant to the types of aircraft in which the applicant is likely to function.

6.3.3.4.1 When near correction is required in accordance with this paragraph, a second pair of near-correction spectacles shall be kept available for immediate use.

6.3.3.5 The applicant shall be required to have normal fields of vision.

6.3.3.6 The applicant shall be required to have normal binocular function.

6.3.3.6.1 Reduced stereopsis, abnormal convergence not interfering with near vision, and ocular misalignment where the fusional reserves are sufficient to prevent asthenopia and diplopia need not be disqualifying.

6.3.4 Hearing Requirements

6.3.4.1 The applicant, when tested on a pure-tone audiometer, shall not have a hearing loss, in either ear separately, of more than 35 dB at any of the frequencies 500, 1000 or 2000 Hz, or more than 50 dB at 3000 Hz.

6.3.4.1.1 An applicant with a hearing loss greater than the above may be declared fit provided that the applicant has normal hearing performance against a background noise that reproduces or simulates the masking properties of flight deck noise upon speech and beacon signals.

Note 1. — It is important that the background noise be representative of the noise in the cockpit of the type of aircraft for which the applicant's license and ratings are valid.

Note 2. — In the speech material for discrimination testing, both aviation-relevant phrases and phonetically balanced words are normally used.

6.3.4.1.2 Alternatively, a practical hearing test conducted in flight in the cockpit of an aircraft of the type for which the applicant's license and ratings are valid may be used.

6.4 CLASS 2 MEDICAL ASSESSMENT

6.4.1 Assessment Issue and Renewal

6.4.1.1 An applicant for a private pilot license — aeroplane, airship, helicopter or powered-lift, a glider pilot license, a free balloon pilot license, a flight engineer license or a flight navigator license shall undergo an initial medical examination for the issue of a Class 2 Medical Assessment.

6.4.1.2 Except where otherwise stated in this section, holders of private pilot licenses — aeroplane, airship, helicopter or powered-lift, glider pilot licenses, free balloon pilot licenses, flight engineer licenses or flight navigator licenses shall have their Class 2 Medical Assessments renewed at intervals not exceeding those specified in 1.2.5.2.

6.4.1.3 When the Licensing Authority is satisfied that the requirements of this section and the general provisions of 6.1 and 6.2 have been met, a Class 2 Medical Assessment shall be issued to the applicant.

6.4.2 Physical and Mental Requirements

The medical examination shall be based on the following requirements.

6.4.2.1 The applicant shall not suffer from any disease or disability which could render that applicant likely to become suddenly unable either to operate an aircraft safely or to perform assigned duties safely.

6.4.2.2 The applicant shall have no established medical history or clinical diagnosis of:

a) an organic mental disorder;
b) a mental or behavioural disorder due to psychoactive substance use; this includes dependence syndrome induced by alcohol or other psychoactive substances;
c) schizophrenia or a schizotypal or delusional disorder;
d) a mood (affective) disorder;
e) a neurotic, stress-related or somatoform disorder;
f) a behavioural syndrome associated with physiological disturbances or physical factors;
g) a disorder of adult personality or behaviour, particularly if manifested by repeated overt acts;
h) mental retardation;
i) a disorder of psychological development;
j) a behavioural or emotional disorder, with onset in childhood or adolescence; or
k) a mental disorder not otherwise specified;

such as might render the applicant unable to safely exercise the privileges of the license applied for or held.

Note. — Mental and behavioural disorders are defined in accordance with the clinical descriptions and diagnostic guidelines of the World Health Organization as given in the International Statistical Classification of Diseases and Related Health Problems, 10th Edition — Classification of Mental and Behavioural Disorders, *WHO 1992. This document contains detailed descriptions of the diagnostic requirements, which may be useful for their application to medical assessment.*

6.4.2.3 The applicant shall have no established medical history or clinical diagnosis of any of the following:

a) a progressive or non-progressive disease of the nervous system, the effects of which are likely to interfere with the safe exercise of the applicant's license and rating privileges;
b) epilepsy;
c) any disturbance of consciousness without satisfactory medical explanation of cause.

6.4.2.4 The applicant shall not have suffered any head injury, the effects of which are likely to interfere with the safe exercise of the applicant's license and rating privileges.

6.4.2.5 The applicant shall not possess any abnormality of the heart, congenital or acquired, which is likely to interfere with the safe exercise of the applicant's license and rating privileges.

6.4.2.5.1 An applicant who has undergone coronary by-pass grafting or angioplasty (with or without stenting) or other cardiac intervention or who has a history of myocardial infarction or who suffers from any other potentially incapacitating cardiac condition shall be assessed as unfit unless the applicant's cardiac condition has been investigated and evaluated in accordance with best medical practice and is assessed not likely to interfere with the safe exercise of the applicant's license or rating privileges.

6.4.2.5.2 An applicant with an abnormal cardiac rhythm shall be assessed as unfit unless the cardiac arrhythmia has been investigated and evaluated in accordance with best medical practice and is assessed not likely to interfere with the safe exercise of the applicant's license or rating privileges.

Note. — Guidance on cardiovascular evaluation is contained in the Manual of Civil Aviation Medicine *(Doc 8984).*

6.4.2.6 Electrocardiography shall form part of the heart examination for the first issue of a Medical Assessment after the age of 40.

6.4.2.6.1 Electrocardiography shall be included in re-examinations of applicants after the age of 50 no less than every two years.

6.4.2.6.2 **Recommendation.** — *Electrocardiography should form part of the heart examination for the first issue of a Medical Assessment.*

Note 1. — The purpose of routine electrocardiography is case finding. It does not provide sufficient evidence to justify disqualification without further thorough cardiovascular investigation.

Note 2. — Guidance on resting and exercise electrocardiography is contained in the Manual of Civil Aviation Medicine *(Doc 8984).*

6.4.2.7 The systolic and diastolic blood pressures shall be within normal limits.

6.4.2.7.1 The use of drugs for control of high blood pressure shall be disqualifying except for those drugs, the use of which is compatible with the safe exercise of the applicant's license and rating privileges.

Note. — Guidance on the subject is contained in the Manual of Civil Aviation Medicine *(Doc 8984).*

6.4.2.8 There shall be no significant functional nor structural abnormality of the circulatory system.

6.4.2.9 There shall be no disability of the lungs nor any active disease of the structures of the lungs, mediastinum or pleura likely to result in incapacitating symptoms during normal or emergency operations.

6.4.2.9.1 **Recommendation.** — *Chest radiography should form part of the initial and periodic examinations in cases where asymptomatic pulmonary disease can be expected.*

6.4.2.10 Applicants with chronic obstructive pulmonary disease shall be assessed as unfit unless the applicant's condition has been investigated and evaluated in accordance with best medical practice and is assessed not likely to interfere with the safe exercise of the applicant's license or rating privileges.

6.4.2.11 Applicants with asthma causing significant symptoms or likely to cause incapacitating symptoms during normal or emergency operations shall be assessed as unfit.

6.4.2.11.1 The use of drugs for control of asthma shall be disqualifying except for those drugs, the use of which is compatible with the safe exercise of the applicant's license and rating privileges.

Note. — Guidance on hazards of medication and drugs is contained in the Manual of Civil Aviation Medicine *(Doc 8984).*

6.4.2.12 Applicants with active pulmonary tuberculosis shall be assessed as unfit.

6.4.2.12.1 Applicants with quiescent or healed lesions, known to be tuberculous or presumably tuberculous in origin, may be assessed as fit.

Note 1. — Guidance on assessment of respiratory diseases is contained in the Manual of Civil Aviation Medicine *(Doc 8984).*

Note 2. — Guidance on hazards of medication and drugs is contained in the Manual of Civil Aviation Medicine *(Doc 8984).*

6.4.2.13 Applicants shall be completely free from those hernias that might give rise to incapacitating symptoms.

6.4.2.13.1 Applicants with significant impairment of the function of the gastrointestinal tract or its adnexa shall be assessed as unfit.

6.4.2.14 Applicants with sequelae of disease of or surgical intervention on any part of the digestive tract or its adnexa, likely to cause incapacitation in flight, in particular any obstruction due to stricture or compression, shall be assessed as unfit.

6.4.2.14.1 **Recommendation.** — *An applicant who has undergone a major surgical operation on the biliary passages or the digestive tract or its adnexa with a total or partial excision or a diversion of any of these organs should be assessed as unfit until such time as the medical assessor, having access to the details of the operation concerned, considers that the effects of the operation are not likely to cause incapacitation in flight.*

6.4.2.15 Applicants with metabolic, nutritional or endocrine disorders that are likely to interfere with the safe exercise of their license and rating privileges shall be assessed as unfit.

6.4.2.16 Applicants with insulin-treated diabetes mellitus shall be assessed as unfit.

6.4.2.16.1 Applicants with non-insulin-treated diabetes mellitus shall be assessed as unfit unless the condition is shown to be satisfactorily controlled by diet alone or by diet combined with oral anti-diabetic medication, the use of which is compatible with the safe exercise of the applicant's license and rating privileges.

Note. — Guidance on assessment of diabetic applicants is contained in the Manual of Civil Aviation Medicine *(Doc 8984).*

6.4.2.17 Applicants with diseases of the blood and/or the lymphatic system shall be assessed as unfit unless adequately investigated and their condition found unlikely to interfere with the safe exercise of their license and rating privileges.

Note. — Sickle cell trait and other haemoglobinopathic traits are usually compatible with fit assessment.

6.4.2.18 Applicants with renal or genito-urinary disease shall be assessed as unfit unless adequately investigated and their condition found unlikely to interfere with the safe exercise of their license and rating privileges.

6.4.2.18.1 Urine examination shall form part of the medical examination and abnormalities shall be adequately investigated.

Note. — Guidance on urine examination and evaluation of abnormalities is contained in the Manual of Civil Aviation Medicine *(Doc 8984).*

6.4.2.19 Applicants with sequelae of disease of, or surgical procedures on, the kidneys or the genito-urinary tract, in particular obstructions due to stricture or compression, shall be assessed as unfit unless the applicant's condition has been investigated and evaluated in accordance with best medical practice and is assessed not likely to interfere with the safe exercise of the applicant's license or rating privileges.

6.4.2.19.1 Applicants who have undergone nephrectomy shall be assessed as unfit unless the condition is well compensated.

6.4.2.20 Applicants with acquired immunodeficiency syndrome (AIDS) shall be assessed as unfit.

6.4.2.20.1 Applicants who are seropositive for human immunodeficiency virus (HIV) shall be assessed as unfit unless full investigation provides no evidence of clinical disease.

Note 1. — Evaluation of applicants who are seropositive for human immunodeficiency virus (HIV) requires particular attention to their mental state, including the psychological effects of the diagnosis.

Note 2. — Guidance on the assessment of applicants who are seropositive for human immunodeficiency virus (HIV) is contained in the Manual of Civil Aviation Medicine *(Doc 8984).*

6.4.2.21 Applicants with gynaecological disorders that are likely to interfere with the safe exercise of their license and rating privileges shall be assessed as unfit.

6.4.2.22 Applicants who are pregnant shall be assessed as unfit unless obstetrical evaluation and continued medical supervision indicate a low-risk uncomplicated pregnancy.

6.4.2.22.1 **Recommendation.** — *For applicants with a low-risk uncomplicated pregnancy, evaluated and supervised in accordance with 6.4.2.22, the fit assessment should be limited to the period from the end of the 12th week until the end of the 26th week of gestation.*

6.4.2.23 Following confinement or termination of pregnancy, the applicant shall not be permitted to exercise the privileges of her license until she has undergone re-evaluation in accordance with best medical practice and it has been determined that she is able to safely exercise the privileges of her license and ratings.

6.4.2.24 The applicant shall not possess any abnormality of the bones, joints, muscles, tendons or related structures which is likely to interfere with the safe exercise of the applicant's license and rating privileges.

Note. — Any sequelae after lesions affecting the bones, joints, muscles or tendons, and certain anatomical defects will normally require functional assessment to determine fitness.

6.4.2.25 The applicant shall not possess any abnormality or disease of the ear or related structures which is likely to interfere with the safe exercise of the applicant's license and rating privileges.

6.4.2.26 There shall be:

a) no disturbance of the vestibular function;
b) no significant dysfunction of the Eustachian tubes; and
c) no unhealed perforation of the tympanic membranes.

6.4.2.26.1 A single dry perforation of the tympanic membrane need not render the applicant unfit.

Note. — Guidance on testing of the vestibular function is contained in the Manual of Civil Aviation Medicine *(Doc 8984).*

6.4.2.27 There shall be:

a) no nasal obstruction; and
b) no malformation nor any disease of the buccal cavity or upper respiratory tract;

which is likely to interfere with the safe exercise of the applicant's license and rating privileges.

6.4.2.28 Applicants with stuttering and other speech defects sufficiently severe to cause impairment of speech communication shall be assessed as unfit.

6.4.3 Visual Requirements

The medical examination shall be based on the following requirements.

6.4.3.1 The function of the eyes and their adnexa shall be normal. There shall be no active pathological condition, acute or chronic, nor any sequelae of surgery or trauma of the eyes or their adnexa likely to reduce proper visual function to an extent that would interfere with the safe exercise of the applicant's license and rating privileges.

6.4.3.2 Distant visual acuity with or without correction shall be 6/12 or better in each eye separately, and binocular visual acuity shall be 6/9 or better. No limits apply to uncorrected visual acuity. Where this standard of visual acuity can be obtained only with correcting lenses, the applicant may be assessed as fit provided that:

a) such correcting lenses are worn during the exercise of the privileges of the license or rating applied for or held; and
b) in addition, a pair of suitable correcting spectacles is kept readily available during the exercise of the privileges of the applicant's license.

Note. — An applicant accepted as meeting these provisions is deemed to continue to do so unless there is reason to suspect otherwise, in which case an ophthalmic report is required at the discretion of the Licensing Authority. Both uncorrected and corrected visual acuity are normally measured and recorded at each re-examination. Conditions which indicate a need to obtain an ophthalmic report include: a substantial decrease in the uncorrected visual acuity, any decrease in best corrected visual acuity, and the occurrence of eye disease, eye injury or eye surgery.

6.4.3.2.1 Applicants may use contact lenses to meet this requirement provided that:

a) the lenses are monofocal and non-tinted;
b) the lenses are well tolerated; and
c) a pair of suitable correcting spectacles is kept readily available during the exercise of the license privileges.

Note. — Applicants who use contact lenses may not need to have their uncorrected visual acuity measured at each re-examination provided the history of their contact lens prescription is known.

6.4.3.2.2 Applicants with a large refractive error shall use contact lenses or high-index spectacle lenses.

Note. — If spectacles are used, high-index lenses are needed to minimize peripheral field distortion.

6.4.3.2.3 **Recommendation.** — *Applicants whose uncorrected distant visual acuity in either eye is worse than 6/60 should be required to provide a full ophthalmic report prior to initial Medical Assessment and every five years thereafter.*

Note 1. — The purpose of the required ophthalmic examination is (1) to ascertain normal visual performance, and (2) to identify any significant pathology.

Note 2. — Guidance on the assessment of monocular applicants under the provisions of 1.2.4.8 is contained in the Manual of Civil Aviation Medicine *(Doc 8984).*

6.4.3.3 Applicants who have undergone surgery affecting the refractive status of the eye shall be assessed as unfit unless they are free from those sequelae which are likely to interfere with the safe exercise of their license and rating privileges.

6.4.3.4 The applicant shall have the ability to read, while wearing the correcting lenses, if any, required by 6.4.3.2, the N5 chart or its equivalent at a distance selected by that applicant in the range of 30 to 50 cm. If this requirement is met only by the use of near correction, the applicant may be assessed as fit provided that this near correction is added to the spectacle correction already prescribed in accordance with 6.4.3.2; if no such correction is prescribed, a pair of spectacles for near use shall be kept readily available during the exercise of the privileges of the license. When near correction is required, the applicant shall demonstrate that one pair of spectacles is sufficient to meet both distant and near visual requirements.

Note 1. — N5 refers to the size of typeface used. For further details, see the Manual of Civil Aviation Medicine *(Doc 8984).*

Note 2. — An applicant who needs near correction to meet the requirement will require "look-over", bifocal or perhaps multifocal lenses in order to read the instruments and a chart or manual held in the hand, and also to make use of distant vision, through the windscreen, without removing the lenses. Single-vision near correction (full lenses of one power only, appropriate for reading) significantly reduces distant visual acuity and is therefore not acceptable.

Note 3. — Whenever there is a requirement to obtain or renew correcting lenses, an applicant is expected to advise the refractionist of the reading distances for the visual flight deck tasks relevant to the types of aircraft in which the applicant is likely to function.

6.4.3.4.1 When near correction is required in accordance with this paragraph, a second pair of near-correction spectacles shall be kept available for immediate use.

6.4.3.5 The applicant shall be required to have normal fields of vision.

6.4.3.6 The applicant shall be required to have normal binocular function.

6.4.3.6.1 Reduced stereopsis, abnormal convergence not interfering with near vision, and ocular misalignment where the fusional reserves are sufficient to prevent asthenopia and diplopia need not be disqualifying.

6.4.4 Hearing Requirements

Note. — Attention is called to 2.7.1.3.1[a] *on requirements for the issue of instrument rating to applicants who hold a private pilot license.*

6.4.4.1 Applicants who are unable to hear an average conversational voice in a quiet room, using both ears, at a distance of 2 m from the examiner and with the back turned to the examiner, shall be assessed as unfit.

6.4.4.2 When tested by pure-tone audiometry, an applicant with a hearing loss, in either ear separately, of more than 35 dB at any of the frequencies 500, 1000 or 2000 Hz, or more than 50 dB at 3000 Hz, shall be assessed as unfit.

6.4.4.3 **Recommendation.** — *An applicant who does not meet the requirements in 6.4.4.1 or 6.4.4.2 should undergo further testing in accordance with 6.3.4.1.1.*

6.5 CLASS 3 MEDICAL ASSESSMENT

6.5.1 Assessment Issue and Renewal

6.5.1.1 An applicant for an air traffic controller license shall undergo an initial medical examination for the issue of a Class 3 Medical Assessment.

6.5.1.2 Except where otherwise stated in this section, holders of air traffic controller licenses shall have their Class 3 Medical Assessments renewed at intervals not exceeding those specified in 1.2.5.2.

---

[a]2.7.1.3 *Medical fitness.*

2.7.1.3.1 Applicants who hold a private pilot licence shall have established their hearing acuity on the basis of compliance with the hearing requirements for the issue of a Class 1 Medical Assessment.

2.7.1.3.2 **Recommendation.** — *Contracting States should consider requiring the holder of a private pilot licence to comply with the physical and mental, and visual requirements for the issue of a Class 1 Medical Assessment.*

6.5.1.3 When the Licensing Authority is satisfied that the requirements of this section and the general provisions of 6.1 and 6.2 have been met, a Class 3 Medical Assessment shall be issued to the applicant.

6.5.2 Physical and Mental Requirements

6.5.2.1 The applicant shall not suffer from any disease or disability which could render that applicant likely to become suddenly unable to perform duties safely.

6.5.2.2 The applicant shall have no established medical history or clinical diagnosis of:

a) an organic mental disorder;
b) a mental or behavioural disorder due to psychoactive substance use; this includes dependence syndrome induced by alcohol or other psychoactive substances;
c) schizophrenia or a schizotypal or delusional disorder;
d) a mood (affective) disorder;
e) a neurotic, stress-related or somatoform disorder;
f) a behavioural syndrome associated with physiological disturbances or physical factors;
g) a disorder of adult personality or behaviour, particularly if manifested by repeated overt acts;
h) mental retardation;
i) a disorder of psychological development;
j) a behavioural or emotional disorder, with onset in childhood or adolescence; or
k) a mental disorder not otherwise specified;

such as might render the applicant unable to safely exercise the privileges of the license applied for or held.

Note. — Mental and behavioural disorders are defined in accordance with the clinical descriptions and diagnostic guidelines of the World Health Organization as given in the International Statistical Classification of Diseases and Related Health Problems,

10th Edition — Classification of Mental and Behavioural Disorders, *WHO 1992. This document contains detailed descriptions of the diagnostic requirements which may be useful for their application to medical assessment.*

6.5.2.3 The applicant shall have no established medical history or clinical diagnosis of any of the following:

a) a progressive or non-progressive disease of the nervous system, the effects of which are likely to interfere with the safe exercise of the applicant's license and rating privileges;
b) epilepsy; or
c) any disturbance of consciousness without satisfactory medical explanation of cause.

6.5.2.4 The applicant shall not have suffered any head injury, the effects of which are likely to interfere with the safe exercise of the applicant's license and rating privileges.

6.5.2.5 The applicant shall not possess any abnormality of the heart, congenital or acquired, which is likely to interfere with the safe exercise of the applicant's license and rating privileges.

6.5.2.1 An applicant who has undergone coronary bypass grafting or angioplasty (with or without stenting) or other cardiac intervention or who has a history of myocardial infarction or who suffers from any other potentially incapacitating cardiac condition shall be assessed as unfit unless the applicant's cardiac condition has been investigated and evaluated in accordance with best medical practice and is assessed not likely to interfere with the safe exercise of the applicant's license and rating privileges.

6.5.2.2 An applicant with an abnormal cardiac rhythm shall be assessed as unfit unless the cardiac arrhythmia has been investigated and evaluated in accordance with best medical practice and is assessed not likely to interfere with the safe exercise of the applicant's license and rating privileges.

Note. — Guidance on cardiovascular evaluation is contained in the Manual of Civil Aviation Medicine *(Doc 8984).*

6.5.2.6 Electrocardiography shall form part of the heart examination for the first issue of a Medical Assessment.

6.5.2.6.1 Electrocardiography shall be included in re-examinations of applicants after the age of 50 no less frequently than every two years.

Note 1. — The purpose of routine electrocardiography is case finding. It does not provide sufficient evidence to justify disqualification without further thorough cardiovascular investigation.

Note 2. — Guidance on resting and exercise electrocardiography is contained in the Manual of Civil Aviation Medicine *(Doc 8984).*

6.5.2.7 The systolic and diastolic blood pressures shall be within normal limits.

6.5.2.7.1 The use of drugs for control of high blood pressure is disqualifying except for those drugs, the use of which is compatible with the safe exercise of the applicant's license privileges.

Note. — Guidance on this subject is contained in the Manual of Civil Aviation Medicine *(Doc 8984).*

6.5.2.8 There shall be no significant functional nor structural abnormality of the circulatory system.

6.5.2.9 There shall be no disability of the lungs nor any active disease of the structures of the lungs, mediastinum or pleurae likely to result in incapacitating symptoms.

Note. — Chest radiography is usually not necessary but may be indicated in cases where asymptomatic pulmonary disease can be expected.

6.5.2.10 Applicants with chronic obstructive pulmonary disease shall be assessed as unfit unless the applicant's condition has been investigated and evaluated in accordance with best medical practice and is assessed not likely to interfere with the safe exercise of the applicant's license or rating privileges.

6.5.2.11 Applicants with asthma causing significant symptoms or likely to cause incapacitating symptoms shall be assessed as unfit.

6.5.2.11.1 The use of drugs for control of asthma shall be disqualifying except for those drugs, the use of which is compatible with the safe exercise of the applicant's license and rating privileges.

Note. — Guidance on hazards of medications is contained in the Manual of Civil Aviation Medicine *(Doc 8984).*

6.5.2.12 Applicants with active pulmonary tuberculosis shall be assessed as unfit.

6.5.2.12.1 Applicants with quiescent or healed lesions, known to be tuberculous or presumably tuberculous in origin, may be assessed as fit.

Note 1. — Guidance on assessment of respiratory diseases is contained in the Manual of Civil Aviation Medicine *(Doc 8984).*

Note 2. — Guidance on hazards of medication and drugs is contained in the Manual of Civil Aviation Medicine *(Doc 8984).*

6.5.2.13 Applicants with significant impairment of the function of the gastrointestinal tract or its adnexae shall be assessed as unfit.

6.5.2.14 Applicants with sequelae of disease of or surgical intervention on any part of the digestive tract or its adnexa, likely to cause incapacitation, in particular any obstructions due to stricture or compression, shall be assessed as unfit.

6.5.2.14.1 **Recommendation.** — *An applicant who has undergone a major surgical operation on the biliary passages or the digestive tract or its adnexa, with a total or partial excision or a diversion of any of these organs should be assessed as unfit until such time as the medical assessor, having access to the details of the operation concerned, considers that the effects of the operation are not likely to cause incapacitation.*

6.5.2.15 Applicants with metabolic, nutritional or endocrine disorders that are likely to interfere with the safe exercise of their license and rating privileges shall be assessed as unfit.

6.5.2.16 Applicants with insulin-treated diabetes mellitus shall be assessed as unfit.

6.5.2.16.1 Applicants with non-insulin-treated diabetes shall be assessed as unfit unless the condition is shown to be satisfactorily controlled by diet alone or by diet combined with oral anti-diabetic medication, the use of which is compatible with the safe exercise of the applicant's license and rating privileges.

Note. — Guidance on assessment of diabetic applicants is contained in the Manual of Civil Aviation Medicine *(Doc 8984).*

6.5.2.17 Applicants with diseases of the blood and/or the lymphatic system shall be assessed as unfit, unless adequately investigated and their condition found unlikely to interfere with the safe exercise of their license and rating privileges.

6.5.2.18 Applicants with renal or genito-urinary disease shall be assessed as unfit unless adequately investigated and their condition found unlikely to interfere with the safe exercise of their license and rating privileges.

6.5.2.18.1 Urine examination shall form part of the medical examination and abnormalities shall be adequately investigated.

Note. — Guidance on urine examination and evaluation of abnormalities is contained in the Manual of Civil Aviation Medicine *(Doc 8984).*

6.5.2.19 Applicants with sequelae of disease of, or surgical procedures on the kidneys or the genito-urinary tract, in particular obstructions due to stricture or compression, shall be assessed as unfit unless the applicant's condition has been investigated and evaluated in accordance with best medical practice and is assessed not likely to interfere with the safe exercise of the applicant's license or rating privileges.

6.5.2.19.1 Applicants who have undergone nephrectomy shall be assessed as unfit unless the condition is well compensated.

6.5.2.20 Applicants with acquired immunodeficiency syndrome (AIDS) shall be assessed as unfit.

6.5.2.20.1 Applicants who are seropositive for human immunodeficiency virus (HIV) shall be assessed as unfit unless full investigation provides no evidence of clinical disease.

Note 1. — Evaluation of applicants who are seropositive for human immunodeficiency virus (HIV) requires particular attention to their mental state, including the psychological effects of the diagnosis.

Note 2. — Guidance on the assessment of applicants who are seropositive for human immunodeficiency virus (HIV) is contained in the Manual of Civil Aviation Medicine *(Doc 8984).*

6.5.2.21 Applicants with gynaecological disorders that are likely to interfere with the safe exercise of their license and rating privileges shall be assessed as unfit.

6.5.2.22 Applicants who are pregnant shall be assessed as unfit unless obstetrical evaluation and continued medical supervision indicate a low-risk uncomplicated pregnancy.

6.5.2.22.1 **Recommendation.** — *During the gestational period, precautions should be taken for the timely relief of an air traffic controller in the event of early onset of labour or other complications.*

6.5.2.22.2 **Recommendation.** — *For applicants with a low-risk uncomplicated pregnancy, evaluated and supervised in accordance with 6.5.2.22, the fit assessment should be limited to the period until the end of the 34th week of gestation.*

6.5.2.23 Following confinement or termination of pregnancy the applicant shall not be permitted to exercise the privileges of her license until she has undergone re-evaluation in accordance with best medical practice and it has been determined that she is able to safely exercise the privileges of her license and ratings.

6.5.2.24 The applicant shall not possess any abnormality of the bones, joints, muscles, tendons or related structures which is likely to interfere with the safe exercise of the applicant's license and rating privileges.

Note. — Any sequelae after lesions affecting the bones, joints, muscles or tendons, and certain anatomical defects will normally require functional assessment to determine fitness.

6.5.2.25 The applicant shall not possess any abnormality or disease of the ear or related structures which is likely to interfere with the safe exercise of the applicant's license and rating privileges.

6.5.2.26 There shall be no malformation nor any disease of the nose, buccal cavity or upper respiratory tract which is likely to interfere with the safe exercise of the applicant's license and rating privileges.

6.5.2.27 Applicants with stuttering or other speech defects sufficiently severe to cause impairment of speech communication shall be assessed as unfit.

6.5.3 Visual Requirements

The medical examination shall be based on the following requirements.

6.5.3.1 The function of the eyes and their adnexa shall be normal. There shall be no active pathological condition, acute or chronic, nor any sequelae of surgery or trauma of the eyes or their adnexa likely to reduce proper visual function to an extent that would interfere with the safe exercise of the applicant's license and rating privileges.

6.5.3.2 Distant visual acuity with or without correction shall be 6/9 or better in each eye separately, and binocular visual acuity shall be 6/6 or better. No limits apply to uncorrected visual acuity. Where this standard of visual acuity can be obtained only with correcting lenses, the applicant may be assessed as fit provided that:

a) such correcting lenses are worn during the exercise of the privileges of the license or rating applied for or held; and

b) in addition, a pair of suitable correcting spectacles is kept readily available during the exercise of the privileges of the applicant's license.

Note. — *An applicant accepted as meeting these provisions is deemed to continue to do so unless there is reason to suspect otherwise, in which case an ophthalmic report is required at the discretion of the Licensing Authority. Both uncorrected and corrected visual acuity are normally measured and recorded at each re-examination. Conditions which indicate a need to obtain an ophthalmic report include: a substantial decrease in the uncorrected visual acuity, any decrease in best corrected visual acuity, and the occurrence of eye disease, eye injury or eye surgery.*

6.5.3.2.1 Applicants may use contact lenses to meet this requirement provided that:

a) the lenses are monofocal and non-tinted;
b) the lenses are well tolerated; and
c) a pair of suitable correcting spectacles is kept readily available during the exercise of the license privileges.

Note. — *Applicants who use contact lenses may not need to have their uncorrected visual acuity measured at each re-examination provided the history of their contact lens prescription is known.*

6.5.3.2.2 Applicants with a large refractive error shall use contact lenses or high-index spectacle lenses.

Note. — *If spectacles are used, high-index lenses are needed to minimize peripheral field distortion.*

6.5.3.2.3 Applicants whose uncorrected distant visual acuity in either eye is worse than 6/60 shall be required to provide a full ophthalmic report prior to initial Medical Assessment and every five years thereafter.

Note 1. — *The purpose of the required ophthalmic examination is (1) to ascertain normal vision performance, and (2) to identify any significant pathology.*

Note 2. — Guidance on the assessment of monocular applicants under the provisions of 1.2.4.8 is contained in the Manual of Civil Aviation Medicine *(Doc 8984).*

6.5.3.3 Applicants who have undergone surgery affecting the refractive status of the eye shall be assessed as unfit unless they are free from those sequelae which are likely to interfere with the safe exercise of their license and rating privileges.

6.5.3.4 The applicant shall have the ability to read, while wearing the correcting lenses, if any, required by 6.5.3.2, the N5 chart or its equivalent at a distance selected by that applicant in the range of 30 to 50 cm and the ability to read the N14 chart or its equivalent at a distance of 100 cm. If this requirement is met only by the use of near correction, the applicant may be assessed as fit provided that this near correction is added to the spectacle correction already prescribed in accordance with 6.5.3.2; if no such correction is prescribed, a pair of spectacles for near use shall be kept readily available during the exercise of the privileges of the license. When near correction is required, the applicant shall demonstrate that one pair of spectacles is sufficient to meet both distant and near visual requirements.

Note 1. — N5 and N14 refer to the size of typeface used. For further details, see the Manual of Civil Aviation Medicine *(Doc 8984).*

Note 2. — An applicant who needs near correction to meet the requirement will require "look-over", bifocal or perhaps multi-focal lenses in order to read radar screens, visual displays and written or printed material and also to make use of distant vision, through the windows, without removing the lenses. Single-vision near correction (full lenses of one power only, appropriate for reading) may be acceptable for certain air traffic control duties. However, it should be realized that single-vision near correction significantly reduces distant visual acuity.

Note 3. — Whenever there is a requirement to obtain or renew correcting lenses, an applicant is expected to advise the refractionist of reading distances for the air traffic control duties the applicant is likely to perform.

6.5.3.4.1 When near correction is required in accordance with this paragraph, a second pair of near-correction spectacles shall be kept available for immediate use.

6.5.3.5 The applicant shall be required to have normal fields of vision.

6.5.3.6 The applicant shall be required to have normal binocular function.

6.5.3.6.1 Reduced stereopsis, abnormal convergence not interfering with near vision, and ocular misalignment where the fusional reserves are sufficient to prevent asthenopia and diplopia need not be disqualifying.

6.5.4 Hearing Requirements

6.5.4.1 The applicant, when tested on a pure-tone audiometer shall not have a hearing loss, in either ear — separately, of more than 35 dB at any of the frequencies 500, 1000 or 2000 Hz, or more than 50 dB at 3000 Hz.

6.5.4.1.1 An applicant with a hearing loss greater than the above may be declared fit provided that the applicant has normal hearing performance against a background noise that reproduces or simulates that experienced in a typical air traffic control working environment.

Note 1. — The frequency composition of the background noise is defined only to the extent that the frequency range 600 to 4800 Hz (speech frequency range) is adequately represented.

Note 2. — In the speech material for discrimination testing, both aviation-relevant phrases and phonetically balanced words are normally used.

6.5.4.1.2 Alternatively, a practical hearing test conducted in an air traffic control environment representative of the one for which the applicant's license and ratings are valid may be used.

Appendix 1. Requirements for Proficiency in Languages Used for Radiotelephony Communications

(Chapter 1, Section 1.2.9, refers)

1. GENERAL

Note. — The ICAO language proficiency requirements include the holistic descriptors at Section 2 and the ICAO Operational Level (Level 4) of the ICAO Language Proficiency Rating Scale in Attachment A. The language proficiency requirements are applicable to the use of both phraseologies and plain language.

To meet the language proficiency requirements contained in Chapter 1, Section 1.2.9, an applicant for a license or a license holder shall demonstrate, in a manner acceptable to the licensing authority, compliance with the holistic descriptors at Section 2 and with the ICAO Operational Level (Level 4) of the ICAO Language Proficiency Rating Scale in Attachment A.

2. HOLISTIC DESCRIPTORS

Proficient speakers shall:

a) communicate effectively in voice-only (telephone/radiotelephone) and in face-to-face situations;
b) communicate on common, concrete and work-related topics with accuracy and clarity;
c) use appropriate communicative strategies to exchange messages and to recognize and resolve misunderstandings (e.g. to check,

confirm, or clarify information) in a general or work-related context;

d) handle successfully and with relative ease the linguistic challenges presented by a complication or unexpected turn of events that occurs within the context of a routine work situation or communicative task with which they are otherwise familiar; and

e) use a dialect or accent which is intelligible to the aeronautical community.

Appendix 2. Approved Training Organization

(Chapter 1, 1.2.8.2 refers)

1. ISSUE OF APPROVAL

1.1 The issuance of an approval for a training organization and the continued validity of the approval shall depend upon the training organization being in compliance with the requirements of this Appendix.

1.2 The approval document shall contain at least the following:

a) organization's name and location;
b) date of issue and period of validity (where appropriate);
c) terms of approval.

2. TRAINING AND PROCEDURES MANUAL

2.1 The training organization shall provide a training and procedures manual for the use and guidance of personnel concerned. This manual may be issued in separate parts and shall contain at least the following information:

a) a general description of the scope of training authorized under the organization's terms of approval;
b) the content of the training programmes offered including the courseware and equipment to be used;
c) a description of the organization's quality assurance system in accordance with 4;
d) a description of the organization's facilities;

e) the name, duties and qualification of the person designated as responsible for compliance with the requirements of the approval in 6.1;
f) a description of the duties and qualification of the personnel designated as responsible for planning, performing and supervising the training in 6.2;
g) a description of the procedures used to establish and maintain the competence of instructional personnel as required by 6.3;
h) a description of the method used for the completion and retention of the training records required by 7;
i) a description, when applicable, of additional training needed to comply with an operator's procedures and requirements; and
j) when a State has authorized an approved training organization to conduct the testing required for the issuance of a license or rating in accordance with 9, a description of the selection, role and duties of the authorized personnel, as well as the applicable requirements established by the Licensing Authority.

2.2 The training organization shall ensure that the training and procedures manual is amended as necessary to keep the information contained therein up-to-date.

2.3 Copies of all amendments to the training and procedures manual shall be furnished promptly to all organizations or persons to whom the manual has been issued.

3. TRAINING PROGRAMMES

3.1 A Licensing Authority may approve a training programme for a private pilot license, commercial pilot license or instrument rating that allows an alternative means of compliance with the experience requirements established by Annex 1, provided that the approved training organization demonstrates to the satisfaction of the Licensing Authority that the training provides a level of competency at least equivalent to that provided by the minimum experience requirements for personnel not receiving such approved training.

3.2 When a Licensing Authority approves a training programme for a multi-crew pilot license, the approved training organization shall demonstrate to the satisfaction of the Licensing Authority that the training provides a level of competency in multi-crew operations at least equal to that met by holders of a commercial pilot license, instrument rating and type rating for an aeroplane certificated for operation with a minimum crew of at least two pilots.

Note. — Guidance on the approval of training programmes can be found in the Manual on the Approval of Flight Crew Training Organizations *(Doc 9841).*

4. QUALITY ASSURANCE SYSTEM

The training organization shall establish a quality assurance system, acceptable to the Licensing Authority granting the approval, which ensures that training and instructional practices comply with all relevant requirements.

5. FACILITIES

5.1 The facilities and working environment shall be appropriate for the task to be performed and be acceptable to the Licensing Authority.

5.2 The training organization shall have, or have access to, the necessary information, equipment, training devices and material to conduct the courses for which it is approved.

5.3 Synthetic training devices shall be qualified according to requirements established by the State and their use shall be approved by the Licensing Authority to ensure that they are appropriate to the task.

Note. — The Manual of Criteria for the Qualification of Flight Simulators *(Doc 9625) provides guidance on the approval of flight simulators.*

6. PERSONNEL

6.1 The training organization shall nominate a person responsible for ensuring that it is in compliance with the requirements for an approved organization.

6.2 The organization shall employ the necessary personnel to plan, perform and supervise the training to be conducted.

6.3 The competence of instructional personnel shall be in accordance with procedures and to a level acceptable to the Licensing Authority.

6.4 The training organization shall ensure that all instructional personnel receive initial and continuation training appropriate to their assigned tasks and responsibilities. The training programme established by the training organization shall include training in knowledge and skills related to human performance.

Note. — Guidance material to design training programmes to develop knowledge and skills in human performance can be found in the Human Factors Training Manual *(Doc 9683).*

7. RECORDS

7.1 The training organization shall retain detailed student records to show that all requirements of the training course have been met as agreed by the Licensing Authority.

7.2 The training organization shall maintain a system for recording the qualifications and training of instructional and examining staff, where appropriate.

7.3 The records required by 7.1 shall be kept for a minimum period of two years after completion of the training. The records required by 7.2 shall be retained for a minimum period of two years after the instructor or examiner ceases to perform a function for the training organization.

8. OVERSIGHT

Contracting States shall maintain an effective oversight programme of the approved training organization to ensure continuing compliance with the approval requirements.

9. EVALUATION AND CHECKING

When a State has authorized an approved training organization to conduct the testing required for the issuance of a license or rating, the testing shall be conducted by personnel authorized by the Licensing Authority or designated by the training organization in accordance with criteria approved by the Licensing Authority.

Appendix 3. Requirements for the Issue of the Multicrew Pilot License — Aeroplane

(Chapter 2, Section 2.5, refers)

1. TRAINING

1.1 In order to meet the requirements of the multi-crew pilot license in the aeroplane category, the applicant shall have completed an approved training course. The training shall be competency-based and conducted in a multi-crew operational environment.

1.2 During the training, the applicant shall have acquired the knowledge, skills and attitudes required as the underpinning attributes for performing as a co-pilot of a turbine-powered air transport aeroplane certificated for operation with a minimum crew of at least two pilots.

2. ASSESSMENT LEVEL

The applicant for the multi-crew pilot license in the aeroplane category shall have satisfactorily demonstrated performance in all the nine competency units specified in 3, at the advanced level of competency as defined in Attachment B.

Note. — The training scheme for the multi-crew pilot license in the aeroplane category, including the various levels of competency are contained in the Procedures for Air Navigation Services — Training *(PANS-TRG, Doc 9868).*

3. COMPETENCY UNITS

The nine competency units that an applicant has to demonstrate in accordance with Chapter 2, 2.5.1.3, are as follows:

1) apply threat and error management (TEM) principles;
2) perform aeroplane ground operations;
3) perform take-off;
4) perform climb;
5) perform cruise;
6) perform descent;
7) perform approach;
8) perform landing; and
9) perform after-landing and aeroplane post-flight operations.

Note 1. — Competency units are broken down into their constituent elements, for which specific performance criteria have been defined. Competency elements and performance criteria are contained in the Procedures for Air Navigation Services — Training *(PANSTRG, Doc 9868).*

Note 2. — The application of threat and error management principles is a specific competency unit that is to be integrated with each of the other competency units for training and testing purposes.

4. SIMULATED FLIGHT

4.1 The flight simulation training devices used to gain the experience specified in Chapter 2, 2.5.3.3, shall have been approved by the Licensing Authority.

4.2 Flight simulation training devices shall be categorized as follows:

a) *Type I.* E-training and part tasking devices approved by the Licensing Authority that have the following characteristics:
   — involve accessories beyond those normally associated with desktop computers, such as functional replicas of a throttle quadrant, a sidestick controller, or an FMS keypad; and

— involve psychomotor activity with appropriate application of force and timing of responses.

b) *Type II.* A flight simulation training device that represents a generic turbine-powered aeroplane.

Note. — This requirement can be met by a flight simulation training device equipped with a daylight visual system and otherwise meeting, at a minimum, the specifications equivalent to FAA FTD Level 5, or JAA FNPT II, MCC.

c) *Type III.* A flight simulation training device that represents a multi-engined turbine-powered aeroplane certificated for a crew of two pilots with enhanced daylight visual system and equipped with an autopilot.

Note. — This requirement can be met by a flight simulation training device equipped with a daylight visual system and otherwise meeting, at a minimum, the specifications equivalent to a Level B simulator as defined in JAR STD IA, as amended; and in FAA AC I20–40B, as amended, including Alternate Means of Compliance (AMOC), as permitted in AC 120–40B. (Some previously evaluated Level A full flight simulators that have been approved for training and checking required manoeuvres may be used.)

d) *Type IV.* Fully equivalent to a Level D flight simulator or to a Level C flight simulator with an enhanced daylight visual system.

Note. — This requirement can be met by a flight simulation training device meeting, at a minimum, the specifications equivalent to a Level C and Level D simulator as defined in JAR STD 1A, as amended; and in FAA AC 120–40B, as amended, including Alternate Means of Compliance (AMOC), as permitted in AC 120–40B.

ATTACHMENT A

ICAO LANGUAGE PROFICIENCY RATING SCALE

1.1 Expert, extended and operational levels

LEVEL	PRONUNCIATION Assumes a dialect and/or accent intelligible to the aeronautical community	STRUCTURE Relevant grammatical structures and sentence patterns are determined by language functions appropriate to the task	VOCABULARY	FLUENCY	COMPREHENSION	INTERACTIONS
Expert 6	Pronunciation, stress, rhythm, and intonation, though possibly influenced by the first language or regional variation, almost never interfere with ease of understanding.	Both basic and complex grammatical structures and sentence patterns are consistently well controlled. sometimes interfere	Vocabulary range and accuracy are sufficient to communicate effectively on a wide variety of familiar and unfamiliar topics. Vocabulary is idiomatic, nuanced, and sensitive to register.	Able to speak at length with a natural, effortless flow. Varies speech flow for stylistic effect, e.g. to emphasize a point. Uses appropriate discourse markers and connectors spontaneously.	Comprehension is consistently accurate in nearly all contexts and includes comprehension of linguistic and cultural subtleties.	Interacts with ease in nearly all situations. Is sensitive to verbal and non-verbal cues and responds to them appropriately.

(Continued)

(*Continued*)

LEVEL	**PRONUNCIATION** Assumes a dialect and/or accent intelligible to the aeronautical community	**STRUCTURE** Relevant grammatical structures and sentence patterns are determined by language functions appropriate to the task	VOCABULARY	FLUENCY	COMPREHENSION	INTERACTIONS
Extended 5	Pronunciation, stress, rhythm, and intonation, though influenced by the first language or regional variation, rarley interfere with ease of understanding.	Basic grammatical structures and sentence patterns are consistently well controlled. Complex structures are attempted but with errors which sometimes interfere with meaning.	Vocabulary range and accuracy are sufficient to communicate effectively on common, concrete, and work-related topics. Paraphrases consistently and successfully. Vocabulary is sometimes idiomatic.	Able to speak at length with relative ease on familiar topics but may not vary speech flow as a stylistic device. Can make use of appropriate discourse markers or connectors.	Comprehension is accurate on common, concrete, and work-related topics and mostly accurate when the speaker is confronted with a linguistic or situational complication or an unexpected turn of events. Is able to comprehend a range of speech varieties (dialect and/or accent) or registers.	Responses are immediate, appropriate, and informative. Manages the speaker/ listener relationship effectively.

(*Continued*)

(Continued)

LEVEL	PRONUNCIATION Assumes a dialect and/or accent intelligible to the aeronautical community	STRUCTURE Relevant grammatical structures and sentence patterns are determined by language functions appropriate to the task	VOCABULARY	FLUENCY	COMPREHENSION	INTERACTIONS
Operational 4	Pronunciation, stress, rhythm, and intonation are influenced by the first language or regional variation but only sometimes interfere with ease of understanding.	Basic grammatical structures and sentence patterns are used creatively and are usually well controlled. Errors may occur, particularly in unusual or unexpected circumstances, but rarely interfere with meaning.	Vocabulary range and accuracy are usually sufficient to communicate effectively on common, concrete, and work-related topics. Can often paraphrase successfully when lacking vocabulary in unusual or unexpected circumstances.	Produces stretches of language at an appropriate tempo. There may be occasional loss of fluency on transition from rehearsed or formulaic speech to spontaneous interaction, but this does not prevent effective communication. Can make	Comprehension is mostly accurate on common, concrete, and work-related topics when the accent or variety used is sufficiently intelligible for an international community of users. When the speaker is confronted with a linguistic or situational	Responses are usually immediate, appropriate, and informative. Initiates and maintains exchanges even when dealing with an unexpected turn of events. Deals adequately with apparent

(Continued)

(*Continued*)

LEVEL	PRONUNCIATION Assumes a dialect and/or accent intelligible to the aeronautical community	STRUCTURE Relevant grammatical structures and sentence patterns are determined by language functions appropriate to the task	VOCABULARY	FLUENCY	COMPREHENSION	INTERACTIONS
				limited use of discourse markers or connectors. Fillers are not distracting.	complication or an unexpected turn of events, comprehension may be slower or require clarification strategies.	misunder-standings by checking, confirming, or clarifying.

1.2 Pre-operational, elementary and pre-elementary levels

LEVEL	PRONUNCIATION Assumes a dialect and/or accent intelligible to the aeronautical community	STRUCTURE Relevant grammatical structures and sentence patterns are determined by language functions appropriate to the task	VOCABULARY	FLUENCY	COMPREHENSION	INTERACTIONS
Pre-operational 3	Pronunciation, stress, rhythm, and intonation are influenced by the first language or regional variation and frequently interfere with ease of understanding.	Basic grammatical structures and sentence patterns associated with predictable situations are not always well controlled. Errors frequently interfere with meaning.	Vocabulary range and accuracy are often sufficient to communicate on common, concrete, or work-related topics, but range is limited and the word choice often inappropriate. Is often unable to paraphrase successfully when lacking vocabulary.	Produces stretches of language, but phrasing and pausing are often inappropriate. Hesitations or slowness in language processing may prevent effective communication. Fillers are sometimes distracting.	Comprehension is often accurate on common, concrete, and work-related topics when the accent or variety used is sufficiently intelligible for an international community of users. May fail to understand a linguistic or situational complication or	Responses are sometimes immediate, appropriate, and informative. Can initiate and maintain exchanges with reasonable ease on familiar topics and in predictable situations. Generally inadequate

(Continued)

(**Continued**)

LEVEL	PRONUNCIATION Assumes a dialect and/or accent intelligible to the aeronautical community	STRUCTURE Relevant grammatical structures and sentence patterns are determined by language functions appropriate to the task	VOCABULARY	FLUENCY	COMPREHENSION	INTERACTIONS
					an unexpected turn of events.	when dealing with an unexpected turn of events.
Elementary 2	Pronunciation, stress, rhythm, and intonation are heavily influenced by the first language or regional variation and usually interfere	Shows only limited control of a few simple memorized grammatical structures and sentence patterns.	Limited vocabulary range consisting only of isolated words and memorized phrases.	Can produce very short, isolated, memorized utterances with frequent pausing and a distracting use of fillers to	Comprehension is limited to isolated, memorized phrases when they are carefully and	Response time is slow and often inappropriate. Interaction is limited to simple

(*Continued*)

(*Continued*)

LEVEL	PRONUNCIATION Assumes a dialect and/or accent intelligible to the aeronautical community	STRUCTURE Relevant grammatical structures and sentence patterns are determined by language functions appropriate to the task	VOCABULARY	FLUENCY	COMPREHENSION	INTERACTIONS
	with ease of understanding.			search for expressions and to articulate less familiar words.	slowly articulated.	routine exchanges.
Preelementary 1	Performs at a level below the Elementary level.	Performs at a level below the Elementary level.	Performs at a level below the Elementary level.	Performs at a level below the Elementary level.	Performs at a level below the Elementary level.	Performs at a level below the Elementary level.

Note. — The Operational Level (Level 4) is the minimum required proficiency level for radiotelephony communication. Levels 1 through 3 describe Pre-elementary, Elementary, and Pre-operational levels of language proficiency, respectively, all of which describe a level of proficiency below the ICAO language proficiency requirement. Levels 5 and 6 describe Extended and Expert levels, at levels of proficiency more advanced than the minimum required Standard. As a whole, the scale will serve as benchmarks for training and testing, and in assisting candidates to attain the ICAO Operational Level (Level 4).

Attachment B

Multi-crew Pilot License — Aeroplane Levels of Competency

1. CORE FLYING SKILLS

The level of competency at which the applicant shall have complied with the requirements for the private pilot license specified in Chapter 2, 2.3, including night flight requirements, and, in addition, have completed, smoothly and with accuracy, all procedures and manoeuvres related to upset training and flight with reference solely to instruments. From the outset, all training is conducted in an integrated multi-crew, competency-based and threat and error management (TEM) environment. Initial training and instructional input levels are high as core skills are being embedded in the *ab initio* application. Assessment at this level confirms that control of the aeroplane is maintained at all times in a manner such that the successful outcome of a procedure or a manoeuvre is assured.

2. LEVEL 1 (BASIC)

The level of competency at which assessment confirms that control of the aeroplane or situation is maintained at all times and in such a manner that if the successful outcome of a procedure or manoeuvre is in doubt, corrective action is taken. Performance in the generic cockpit environment does not yet consistently meet the Standards of knowledge, operational skills and level of achievement required in the core competencies. Continual training input is required to meet an acceptable initial operating standard. Specific performance improvement/personal development plans will be agreed and the details recorded. Applicants will be continuously assessed as to their suitability to progress to further training and assessment in successive phases.

3. LEVEL 2 (INTERMEDIATE)

The level of competency at which assessment confirms that control of the aeroplane or situation is maintained at all times and in such a manner that the successful outcome of a procedure or manoeuvre is assured. The training received at Level 2 shall be conducted under the instrument flight rules, but need not be specific to any one type of aeroplane. On completion of Level 2, the applicant shall demonstrate levels of knowledge and operational skills that are adequate in the environment and achieves the basic standard in the core capability. Training support may be required with a specific development plan to maintain or improve aircraft handling, behavioural performance in leadership or team management. Improvement and development to attain the Standard is the key performance objective. Any core competency assessed as less than satisfactory should include supporting evidence and a remedial plan.

4. LEVEL 3 (ADVANCED)

The level of competency required to operate and interact as a co-pilot in a turbine-powered aeroplane certificated for operation with a minimum crew of at least two pilots, under visual and instrument conditions. Assessment confirms that control of the aeroplane or situation is maintained at all times in such a manner that the successful outcome of a procedure or manoeuvre is assured. The applicant shall consistently demonstrate the knowledge, skills and attitudes required for the safe operation of an applicable aeroplane type as specified in the performance criteria.

Note. — Material on the development of performance criteria can be found in the Procedures for Air Navigation Services — Training *(PANS-TRG, Doc 9868).*

Appendix II

Electronic Code of Federal Regulations

e-CFR Data is current as of September 11, 2008

Title 14: Aeronautics and Space

PART 67 — MEDICAL STANDARDS AND CERTIFICATION

Section Contents

Subpart A — General

Subpart B — First-Class Airman Medical Certificate

Subpart C — Second-Class Airman Medical Certificate

§67.201 Eligibility.
§67.203 Eye.
§67.205 Ear, nose, throat, and equilibrium.
§67.207 Mental.
§67.209 Neurologic.
§67.211 Cardiovascular.
§67.213 General medical condition.
§67.215 Discretionary issuance.

Subpart D — Third-Class Airman Medical Certificate

§67.301 Eligibility.
§67.303 Eye.
§67.305 Ear, nose, throat, and equilibrium.
§67.307 Mental.
§67.309 Neurologic.
§67.311 Cardiovascular.
§67.313 General medical condition.
§67.315 Discretionary issuance.

Subpart E — Certification Procedures

§67.401 Special issuance of medical certificates.
§67.403 Applications, certificates, logbooks, reports, and records: Falsification, reproduction, or alteration; incorrect statements.
§67.405 Medical examinations: Who may perform?
§67.407 Delegation of authority.
§67.409 Denial of medical certificate.
§67.411 [Reserved]
§67.413 Medical records.
§67.415 Return of medical certificate after suspension or revocation.

Authority: 49 U.S.C. 106(g), 40113, 44701–44703, 44707, 44709–44711, 45102–45103, 45301–45303.

Source: Docket No. 27940, 61 FR 11256, Mar. 19, 1996, unless otherwise noted.

Subpart A — General

§67.1 Applicability.

This part prescribes the medical standards and certification procedures for issuing medical certificates for airmen and for remaining eligible for a medical certificate.

§67.3 Issue.

A person who meets the medical standards prescribed in this part, based on medical examination and evaluation of the person's history and condition, is entitled to an appropriate medical certificate.

[Doc. No. FAA–2007–27812, 73 FR 43065, July 24, 2008]

§67.4 Application.

An applicant for first-, second- and third-class medical certification must:

(a) Apply on a form and in a manner prescribed by the Administrator;
(b) Be examined by an aviation medical examiner designated in accordance with part 183 of this chapter. An applicant may obtain a list of aviation medical examiners from the FAA Office of Aerospace Medicine homepage on the FAA Web site, from any FAA Regional Flight Surgeon, or by contacting the Manager of the Aerospace Medical Education Division, P.O. Box 26200, Oklahoma City, Oklahoma 73125.
(c) Show proof of age and identity by presenting a government-issued photo identification (such as a valid U.S. driver's license, identification card issued by a driver's license authority, military identification, or passport). If an applicant does not have government-issued identification, he or she may use non-photo, government-issued identification (such as a birth certificate or voter registration card) in conjunction with photo identification (such as a work identification card or a student identification card).

[Doc. No. FAA–2007–27812, 73 FR 43065, July 24, 2008]

§67.7 Access to the National Driver Register.

At the time of application for a certificate issued under this part, each person who applies for a medical certificate shall execute an express consent form authorizing the Administrator to request the chief driver licensing official of any state designated by the Administrator to transmit information contained in the National Driver Register about the person to the Administrator. The Administrator shall make information received from the National Driver Register, if any, available on request to the person for review and written comment.

Subpart B — First-Class Airman Medical Certificate

§67.101 Eligibility.

To be eligible for a first-class airman medical certificate, and to remain eligible for a first-class airman medical certificate, a person must meet the requirements of this subpart.

§67.103 Eye.

Eye standards for a first-class airman medical certificate are:

(a) Distant visual acuity of 20/20 or better in each eye separately, with or without corrective lenses. If corrective lenses (spectacles or contact lenses) are necessary for 20/20 vision, the person may be eligible only on the condition that corrective lenses are worn while exercising the privileges of an airman certificate.
(b) Near vision of 20/40 or better, Snellen equivalent, at 16 inches in each eye separately, with or without corrective lenses. If age 50 or older, near vision of 20/40 or better, Snellen equivalent, at both 16 inches and 32 inches in each eye separately, with or without corrective lenses.
(c) Ability to perceive those colors necessary for the safe performance of airman duties.
(d) Normal fields of vision.
(e) No acute or chronic pathological condition of either eye or adnexa that interferes with the proper function of an eye, that

may reasonably be expected to progress to that degree, or that may reasonably be expected to be aggravated by flying.

(f) Bifoveal fixation and vergence-phoria relationship sufficient to prevent a break in fusion under conditions that may reasonably be expected to occur in performing airman duties. Tests for the factors named in this paragraph are not required except for persons found to have more than 1 prism diopter of hyperphoria, 6 prism diopters of esophoria, or 6 prism diopters of exophoria. If any of these values are exceeded, the Federal Air Surgeon may require the person to be examined by a qualified eye specialist to determine if there is bifoveal fixation and an adequate vergence-phoria relationship. However, if otherwise eligible, the person is issued a medical certificate pending the results of the examination.

§67.105 Ear, nose, throat, and equilibrium.

Ear, nose, throat, and equilibrium standards for a first-class airman medical certificate are:

(a) The person shall demonstrate acceptable hearing by at least one of the following tests:
    (1) Demonstrate an ability to hear an average conversational voice in a quiet room, using both ears, at a distance of 6 feet from the examiner, with the back turned to the examiner.
    (2) Demonstrate an acceptable understanding of speech as determined by audiometric speech discrimination testing to a score of at least 70 percent obtained in one ear or in a sound field environment.
    (3) Provide acceptable results of pure tone audiometric testing of unaided hearing acuity according to the following table of worst acceptable thresholds, using the calibration standards of the American National Standards Institute, 1969 (11 West 42d Street, New York, NY 10036):

Frequency (Hz)	500 Hz	1000 Hz	2000 Hz	3000 Hz
Better ear (Db)	35	30	30	40
Poorer ear (Db)	35	50	50	60

(b) No disease or condition of the middle or internal ear, nose, oral cavity, pharynx, or larynx that —
   (1) Interferes with, or is aggravated by, flying or may reasonably be expected to do so; or
   (2) Interferes with, or may reasonably be expected to interfere with, clear and effective speech communication.
(c) No disease or condition manifested by, or that may reasonably be expected to be manifested by, vertigo or a disturbance of equilibrium.

§67.107 Mental.

Mental standards for a first-class airman medical certificate are:

(a) No established medical history or clinical diagnosis of any of the following:
   (1) A personality disorder that is severe enough to have repeatedly manifested itself by overt acts.
   (2) A psychosis. As used in this section, "psychosis" refers to a mental disorder in which:
      (i) The individual has manifested delusions, hallucinations, grossly bizarre or disorganized behavior, or other commonly accepted symptoms of this condition; or
      (ii) The individual may reasonably be expected to manifest delusions, hallucinations, grossly bizarre or disorganized behavior, or other commonly accepted symptoms of this condition.
   (3) A bipolar disorder.
   (4) Substance dependence, except where there is established clinical evidence, satisfactory to the Federal Air Surgeon, of recovery, including sustained total abstinence from the substance(s) for not less than the preceding 2 years. As used in this section —
      (i) "Substance" includes: Alcohol; other sedatives and hypnotics; anxiolytics; opioids; central nervous system stimulants such as cocaine, amphetamines, and similarly acting sympathomimetics; hallucinogens; phencyclidine or similarly acting arylcyclohexylamines; cannabis; inhalants; and other psychoactive drugs and chemicals; and

(ii) "Substance dependence" means a condition in which a person is dependent on a substance, other than tobacco or ordinary xanthine-containing (e.g., caffeine) beverages, as evidenced by —

(A) Increased tolerance;

(B) Manifestation of withdrawal symptoms;

(C) Impaired control of use; or

(D) Continued use despite damage to physical health or impairment of social, personal, or occupational functioning.

(b) No substance abuse within the preceding 2 years defined as:

(1) Use of a substance in a situation in which that use was physically hazardous, if there has been at any other time an instance of the use of a substance also in a situation in which that use was physically hazardous;

(2) A verified positive drug test result, an alcohol test result of 0.04 or greater alcohol concentration, or a refusal to submit to a drug or alcohol test required by the U.S. Department of Transportation or an agency of the U.S. Department of Transportation; or

(3) Misuse of a substance that the Federal Air Surgeon, based on case history and appropriate, qualified medical judgment relating to the substance involved, finds —

(i) Makes the person unable to safely perform the duties or exercise the privileges of the airman certificate applied for or held; or

(ii) May reasonably be expected, for the maximum duration of the airman medical certificate applied for or held, to make the person unable to perform those duties or exercise those privileges.

(c) No other personality disorder, neurosis, or other mental condition that the Federal Air Surgeon, based on the case history and appropriate, qualified medical judgment relating to the condition involved, finds —

(1) Makes the person unable to safely perform the duties or exercise the privileges of the airman certificate applied for or held; or

(2) May reasonably be expected, for the maximum duration of the airman medical certificate applied for or held, to make the person unable to perform those duties or exercise those privileges.

[Doc. No. 27940, 61 FR 11256, Mar. 19, 1996, as amended by Amdt. 67–19, 71 FR 35764, June 21, 2006]

§67.109 Neurologic.

Neurologic standards for a first-class airman medical certificate are:

(a) No established medical history or clinical diagnosis of any of the following:
   (1) Epilepsy;
   (2) A disturbance of consciousness without satisfactory medical explanation of the cause; or
   (3) A transient loss of control of nervous system function(s) without satisfactory medical explanation of the cause.

(b) No other seizure disorder, disturbance of consciousness, or neurologic condition that the Federal Air Surgeon, based on the case history and appropriate, qualified medical judgment relating to the condition involved, finds —
   (1) Makes the person unable to safely perform the duties or exercise the privileges of the airman certificate applied for or held; or
   (2) May reasonably be expected, for the maximum duration of the airman medical certificate applied for or held, to make the person unable to perform those duties or exercise those privileges.

§67.111 Cardiovascular.

Cardiovascular standards for a first-class airman medical certificate are:

(a) No established medical history or clinical diagnosis of any of the following:
   (1) Myocardial infarction;
   (2) Angina pectoris;
   (3) Coronary heart disease that has required treatment or, if untreated, that has been symptomatic or clinically significant;
   (4) Cardiac valve replacement;
   (5) Permanent cardiac pacemaker implantation; or
   (6) Heart replacement;

(b) A person applying for first-class medical certification must demonstrate an absence of myocardial infarction and other clinically significant abnormality on electrocardiographic examination:
 (1) At the first application after reaching the 35th birthday; and
 (2) On an annual basis after reaching the 40th birthday.
(c) An electrocardiogram will satisfy a requirement of paragraph (b) of this section if it is dated no earlier than 60 days before the date of the application it is to accompany and was performed and transmitted according to acceptable standards and techniques.

§67.113 General medical condition.

The general medical standards for a first-class airman medical certificate are:

(a) No established medical history or clinical diagnosis of diabetes mellitus that requires insulin or any other hypoglycemic drug for control.
(b) No other organic, functional, or structural disease, defect, or limitation that the Federal Air Surgeon, based on the case history and appropriate, qualified medical judgment relating to the condition involved, finds —
 (1) Makes the person unable to safely perform the duties or exercise the privileges of the airman certificate applied for or held; or
 (2) May reasonably be expected, for the maximum duration of the airman medical certificate applied for or held, to make the person unable to perform those duties or exercise those privileges.
(c) No medication or other treatment that the Federal Air Surgeon, based on the case history and appropriate, qualified medical judgment relating to the medication or other treatment involved, finds —
 (1) Makes the person unable to safely perform the duties or exercise the privileges of the airman certificate applied for or held; or

(2) May reasonably be expected, for the maximum duration of the airman medical certificate applied for or held, to make the person unable to perform those duties or exercise those privileges.

§67.115 Discretionary issuance.

A person who does not meet the provisions of §§67.103 through 67.113 may apply for the discretionary issuance of a certificate under §67.401.

Subpart C — Second-Class Airman Medical Certificate

§67.201 Eligibility.

To be eligible for a second-class airman medical certificate, and to remain eligible for a second-class airman medical certificate, a person must meet the requirements of this subpart.

§67.203 Eye.

Eye standards for a second-class airman medical certificate are:

(a) Distant visual acuity of 20/20 or better in each eye separately, with or without corrective lenses. If corrective lenses (spectacles or contact lenses) are necessary for 20/20 vision, the person may be eligible only on the condition that corrective lenses are worn while exercising the privileges of an airman certificate.
(b) Near vision of 20/40 or better, Snellen equivalent, at 16 inches in each eye separately, with or without corrective lenses. If age 50 or older, near vision of 20/40 or better, Snellen equivalent, at both 16 inches and 32 inches in each eye separately, with or without corrective lenses.
(c) Ability to perceive those colors necessary for the safe performance of airman duties.
(d) Normal fields of vision.
(e) No acute or chronic pathological condition of either eye or adnexa that interferes with the proper function of an eye, that may reasonably be expected to progress to that degree, or that may reasonably be expected to be aggravated by flying.

(f) Bifoveal fixation and vergence-phoria relationship sufficient to prevent a break in fusion under conditions that may reasonably be expected to occur in performing airman duties. Tests for the factors named in this paragraph are not required except for persons found to have more than 1 prism diopter of hyperphoria, 6 prism diopters of esophoria, or 6 prism diopters of exophoria. If any of these values are exceeded, the Federal Air Surgeon may require the person to be examined by a qualified eye specialist to determine if there is bifoveal fixation and an adequate vergence-phoria relationship. However, if otherwise eligible, the person is issued a medical certificate pending the results of the examination.

§67.205 Ear, nose, throat, and equilibrium.

Ear, nose, throat, and equilibrium standards for a second-class airman medical certificate are:

(a) The person shall demonstrate acceptable hearing by at least one of the following tests:
  (1) Demonstrate an ability to hear an average conversational voice in a quiet room, using both ears, at a distance of 6 feet from the examiner, with the back turned to the examiner.
  (2) Demonstrate an acceptable understanding of speech as determined by audiometric speech discrimination testing to a score of at least 70 percent obtained in one ear or in a sound field environment.
  (3) Provide acceptable results of pure tone audiometric testing of unaided hearing acuity according to the following table of worst acceptable thresholds, using the calibration standards of the American National Standards Institute, 1969:

Frequency (Hz)	500 Hz	1000 Hz	2000 Hz	3000 Hz
Better ear (Db)	35	30	30	40
Poorer ear (Db)	35	50	50	60

(b) No disease or condition of the middle or internal ear, nose, oral cavity, pharynx, or larynx that —
   (1) Interferes with, or is aggravated by, flying or may reasonably be expected to do so; or
   (2) Interferes with, or may reasonably be expected to interfere with, clear and effective speech communication.
(c) No disease or condition manifested by, or that may reasonably be expected to be manifested by, vertigo or a disturbance of equilibrium.

§67.207 Mental.

Mental standards for a second-class airman medical certificate are:

(a) No established medical history or clinical diagnosis of any of the following:
   (1) A personality disorder that is severe enough to have repeatedly manifested itself by overt acts.
   (2) A psychosis. As used in this section, "psychosis" refers to a mental disorder in which:
      (i) The individual has manifested delusions, hallucinations, grossly bizarre or disorganized behavior, or other commonly accepted symptoms of this condition; or
      (ii) The individual may reasonably be expected to manifest delusions, hallucinations, grossly bizarre or disorganized behavior, or other commonly accepted symptoms of this condition.
   (3) A bipolar disorder.
   (4) Substance dependence, except where there is established clinical evidence, satisfactory to the Federal Air Surgeon, of recovery, including sustained total abstinence from the substance(s) for not less than the preceding 2 years. As used in this section —
      (i) "Substance" includes: Alcohol; other sedatives and hypnotics; anxiolytics; opioids; central nervous system stimulants such as cocaine, amphetamines, and similarly acting sympathomimetics; hallucinogens; phencyclidine or similarly acting arylcyclohexylamines; cannabis; inhalants; and other psychoactive drugs and chemicals; and
      (ii) "Substance dependence" means a condition in which a person is dependent on a substance, other than tobacco

or ordinary xanthine-containing (e.g., caffeine) beverages, as evidenced by —
(A) Increased tolerance;
(B) Manifestation of withdrawal symptoms;
(C) Impaired control of use; or
(D) Continued use despite damage to physical health or impairment of social, personal, or occupational functioning.

(b) No substance abuse within the preceding 2 years defined as:
(1) Use of a substance in a situation in which that use was physically hazardous, if there has been at any other time an instance of the use of a substance also in a situation in which that use was physically hazardous;
(2) A verified positive drug test result, an alcohol test result of 0.04 or greater alcohol concentration, or a refusal to submit to a drug or alcohol test required by the U.S. Department of Transportation or an agency of the U.S. Department of Transportation; or
(3) Misuse of a substance that the Federal Air Surgeon, based on case history and appropriate, qualified medical judgment relating to the substance involved, finds—
(i) Makes the person unable to safely perform the duties or exercise the privileges of the airman certificate applied for or held; or
(ii) May reasonably be expected, for the maximum duration of the airman medical certificate applied for or held, to make the person unable to perform those duties or exercise those privileges.

(c) No other personality disorder, neurosis, or other mental condition that the Federal Air Surgeon, based on the case history and appropriate, qualified medical judgment relating to the condition involved, finds —
(1) Makes the person unable to safely perform the duties or exercise the privileges of the airman certificate applied for or held; or
(2) May reasonably be expected, for the maximum duration of the airman medical certificate applied for or held, to make the person unable to perform those duties or exercise those privileges.

[Doc. No. 27940, 61 FR 11256, Mar. 19, 1996, as amended by Amdt. 67–19, 71 FR 35764, June 21, 2006]

§67.209 Neurologic.

Neurologic standards for a second-class airman medical certificate are:

(a) No established medical history or clinical diagnosis of any of the following:
   (1) Epilepsy;
   (2) A disturbance of consciousness without satisfactory medical explanation of the cause; or
   (3) A transient loss of control of nervous system function(s) without satisfactory medical explanation of the cause;
(b) No other seizure disorder, disturbance of consciousness, or neurologic condition that the Federal Air Surgeon, based on the case history and appropriate, qualified medical judgment relating to the condition involved, finds —
   (1) Makes the person unable to safely perform the duties or exercise the privileges of the airman certificate applied for or held; or
   (2) May reasonably be expected, for the maximum duration of the airman medical certificate applied for or held, to make the person unable to perform those duties or exercise those privileges.

§67.211 Cardiovascular.

Cardiovascular standards for a second-class medical certificate are no established medical history or clinical diagnosis of any of the following:

(a) Myocardial infarction;
(b) Angina pectoris;
(c) Coronary heart disease that has required treatment or, if untreated, that has been symptomatic or clinically significant;
(d) Cardiac valve replacement;

(e) Permanent cardiac pacemaker implantation; or
(f) Heart replacement.

§67.213 General medical condition.

The general medical standards for a second-class airman medical certificate are:

(a) No established medical history or clinical diagnosis of diabetes mellitus that requires insulin or any other hypoglycemic drug for control.
(b) No other organic, functional, or structural disease, defect, or limitation that the Federal Air Surgeon, based on the case history and appropriate, qualified medical judgment relating to the condition involved, finds —
    (1) Makes the person unable to safely perform the duties or exercise the privileges of the airman certificate applied for or held; or
    (2) May reasonably be expected, for the maximum duration of the airman medical certificate applied for or held, to make the person unable to perform those duties or exercise those privileges.
(c) No medication or other treatment that the Federal Air Surgeon, based on the case history and appropriate, qualified medical judgment relating to the medication or other treatment involved, finds —
    (1) Makes the person unable to safely perform the duties or exercise the privileges of the airman certificate applied for or held; or
    (2) May reasonably be expected, for the maximum duration of the airman medical certificate applied for or held, to make the person unable to perform those duties or exercise those privileges.

§67.215 Discretionary issuance.

A person who does not meet the provisions of §§67.203 through 67.213 may apply for the discretionary issuance of a certificate under §67.401.

Subpart D — Third-Class Airman Medical Certificate

§67.301 Eligibility.

To be eligible for a third-class airman medical certificate, or to remain eligible for a third-class airman medical certificate, a person must meet the requirements of this subpart.

§67.303 Eye.

Eye standards for a third-class airman medical certificate are:

(a) Distant visual acuity of 20/40 or better in each eye separately, with or without corrective lenses. If corrective lenses (spectacles or contact lenses) are necessary for 20/40 vision, the person may be eligible only on the condition that corrective lenses are worn while exercising the privileges of an airman certificate.
(b) Near vision of 20/40 or better, Snellen equivalent, at 16 inches in each eye separately, with or without corrective lenses.
(c) Ability to perceive those colors necessary for the safe performance of airman duties.
(d) No acute or chronic pathological condition of either eye or adnexa that interferes with the proper function of an eye, that may reasonably be expected to progress to that degree, or that may reasonably be expected to be aggravated by flying.

§67.305 Ear, nose, throat, and equilibrium.

Ear, nose, throat, and equilibrium standards for a third-class airman medical certificate are:

(a) The person shall demonstrate acceptable hearing by at least one of the following tests:
    (1) Demonstrate an ability to hear an average conversational voice in a quiet room, using both ears, at a distance of 6 feet from the examiner, with the back turned to the examiner.
    (2) Demonstrate an acceptable understanding of speech as determined by audiometric speech discrimination testing to a score

of at least 70 percent obtained in one ear or in a sound field environment.

(3) Provide acceptable results of pure tone audiometric testing of unaided hearing acuity according to the following table of worst acceptable thresholds, using the calibration standards of the American National Standards Institute, 1969:

Frequency (Hz)	500 Hz	1000 Hz	2000 Hz	3000 Hz
Better ear (Db)	35	30	30	40
Poorer ear (Db)	35	50	50	60

(b) No disease or condition of the middle or internal ear, nose, oral cavity, pharynx, or larynx that —
  (1) Interferes with, or is aggravated by, flying or may reasonably be expected to do so; or
  (2) Interferes with clear and effective speech communication.

(c) No disease or condition manifested by, or that may reasonably be expected to be manifested by, vertigo or a disturbance of equilibrium.

§67.307 Mental.

Mental standards for a third-class airman medical certificate are:

(a) No established medical history or clinical diagnosis of any of the following:
  (1) A personality disorder that is severe enough to have repeatedly manifested itself by overt acts.
  (2) A psychosis. As used in this section, "psychosis" refers to a mental disorder in which —
    (i) The individual has manifested delusions, hallucinations, grossly bizarre or disorganized behavior, or other commonly accepted symptoms of this condition; or
    (ii) The individual may reasonably be expected to manifest delusions, hallucinations, grossly bizarre or disorganized behavior, or other commonly accepted symptoms of this condition.
  (3) A bipolar disorder.

(4) Substance dependence, except where there is established clinical evidence, satisfactory to the Federal Air Surgeon, of recovery, including sustained total abstinence from the substance(s) for not less than the preceding 2 years. As used in this section —
   (i) "Substance" includes: alcohol; other sedatives and hypnotics; anxiolytics; opioids; central nervous system stimulants such as cocaine, amphetamines, and similarly acting sympathomimetics; hallucinogens; phencyclidine or similarly acting arylcyclohexylamines; cannabis; inhalants; and other psychoactive drugs and chemicals; and
   (ii) "Substance dependence" means a condition in which a person is dependent on a substance, other than tobacco or ordinary xanthine-containing (e.g., caffeine) beverages, as evidenced by —
      (A) Increased tolerance;
      (B) Manifestation of withdrawal symptoms;
      (C) Impaired control of use; or
      (D) Continued use despite damage to physical health or impairment of social, personal, or occupational functioning.

(b) No substance abuse within the preceding 2 years defined as:
   (1) Use of a substance in a situation in which that use was physically hazardous, if there has been at any other time an instance of the use of a substance also in a situation in which that use was physically hazardous;
   (2) A verified positive drug test result, an alcohol test result of 0.04 or greater alcohol concentration, or a refusal to submit to a drug or alcohol test required by the U.S. Department of Transportation or an agency of the U.S. Department of Transportation; or
   (3) Misuse of a substance that the Federal Air Surgeon, based on case history and appropriate, qualified medical judgment relating to the substance involved, finds—
      (i) Makes the person unable to safely perform the duties or exercise the privileges of the airman certificate applied for or held; or
      (ii) May reasonably be expected, for the maximum duration of the airman medical certificate applied for or held, to make

the person unable to perform those duties or exercise those privileges.

(c) No other personality disorder, neurosis, or other mental condition that the Federal Air Surgeon, based on the case history and appropriate, qualified medical judgment relating to the condition involved, finds —
   (1) Makes the person unable to safely perform the duties or exercise the privileges of the airman certificate applied for or held; or
   (2) May reasonably be expected, for the maximum duration of the airman medical certificate applied for or held, to make the person unable to perform those duties or exercise those privileges.

[Doc. No. 27940, 61 FR 11256, Mar. 19, 1996, as amended by Amdt. 67–19, 71 FR 35764, June 21, 2006]

§67.309 Neurologic.

Neurologic standards for a third-class airman medical certificate are:

(a) No established medical history or clinical diagnosis of any of the following:
   (1) Epilepsy;
   (2) A disturbance of consciousness without satisfactory medical explanation of the cause; or
   (3) A transient loss of control of nervous system function(s) without satisfactory medical explanation of the cause.

(b) No other seizure disorder, disturbance of consciousness, or neurologic condition that the Federal Air Surgeon, based on the case history and appropriate, qualified medical judgment relating to the condition involved, finds —
   (1) Makes the person unable to safely perform the duties or exercise the privileges of the airman certificate applied for or held; or
   (2) May reasonably be expected, for the maximum duration of the airman medical certificate applied for or held, to make the person unable to perform those duties or exercise those privileges.

§67.311 Cardiovascular.

Cardiovascular standards for a third-class airman medical certificate are no established medical history or clinical diagnosis of any of the following:

(a) Myocardial infarction;
(b) Angina pectoris;
(c) Coronary heart disease that has required treatment or, if untreated, that has been symptomatic or clinically significant;
(d) Cardiac valve replacement;
(e) Permanent cardiac pacemaker implantation; or
(f) Heart replacement.

§67.313 General medical condition.

The general medical standards for a third-class airman medical certificate are:

(a) No established medical history or clinical diagnosis of diabetes mellitus that requires insulin or any other hypoglycemic drug for control.
(b) No other organic, functional, or structural disease, defect, or limitation that the Federal Air Surgeon, based on the case history and appropriate, qualified medical judgment relating to the condition involved, finds —
    (1) Makes the person unable to safely perform the duties or exercise the privileges of the airman certificate applied for or held; or
    (2) May reasonably be expected, for the maximum duration of the airman medical certificate applied for or held, to make the person unable to perform those duties or exercise those privileges.
(c) No medication or other treatment that the Federal Air Surgeon, based on the case history and appropriate, qualified medical judgment relating to the medication or other treatment involved, finds —
    (1) Makes the person unable to safely perform the duties or exercise the privileges of the airman certificate applied for or held; or
    (2) May reasonably be expected, for the maximum duration of the airman medical certificate applied for or held, to make the person unable to perform those duties or exercise those privileges.

§67.315 Discretionary issuance.

A person who does not meet the provisions of §§67.303 through 67.313 may apply for the discretionary issuance of a certificate under §67.401.

Subpart E — Certification Procedures

§67.401 Special issuance of medical certificates.

(a) At the discretion of the Federal Air Surgeon, an Authorization for Special Issuance of a Medical Certificate (Authorization), valid for a specified period, may be granted to a person who does not meet the provisions of subparts B, C, or D of this part if the person shows to the satisfaction of the Federal Air Surgeon that the duties authorized by the class of medical certificate applied for can be performed without endangering public safety during the period in which the Authorization would be in force. The Federal Air Surgeon may authorize a special medical flight test, practical test, or medical evaluation for this purpose. A medical certificate of the appropriate class may be issued to a person who does not meet the provisions of subparts B, C, or D of this part if that person possesses a valid Authorization and is otherwise eligible. An airman medical certificate issued in accordance with this section shall expire no later than the end of the validity period or upon the withdrawal of the Authorization upon which it is based. At the end of its specified validity period, for grant of a new Authorization, the person must again show to the satisfaction of the Federal Air Surgeon that the duties authorized by the class of medical certificate applied for can be performed without endangering public safety during the period in which the Authorization would be in force.

(b) At the discretion of the Federal Air Surgeon, a Statement of Demonstrated Ability (SODA) may be granted, instead of an Authorization, to a person whose disqualifying condition is static or nonprogressive and who has been found capable of performing airman duties without endangering public safety. A SODA does not expire and authorizes a designated aviation medical examiner to issue a medical certificate of a specified class if the examiner finds that the condition described on its face has not adversely changed.

(c) In granting an Authorization or SODA, the Federal Air Surgeon may consider the person's operational experience and any medical facts that may affect the ability of the person to perform airman duties including —
 (1) The combined effect on the person of failure to meet more than one requirement of this part; and
 (2) The prognosis derived from professional consideration of all available information regarding the person.

(d) In granting an Authorization or SODA under this section, the Federal Air Surgeon specifies the class of medical certificate authorized to be issued and may do any or all of the following:
 (1) Limit the duration of an Authorization;
 (2) Condition the granting of a new Authorization on the results of subsequent medical tests, examinations, or evaluations;
 (3) State on the Authorization or SODA, and any medical certificate based upon it, any operational limitation needed for safety; or
 (4) Condition the continued effect of an Authorization or SODA, and any second- or third-class medical certificate based upon it, on compliance with a statement of functional limitations issued to the person in coordination with the Director of Flight Standards or the Director's designee.

(e) In determining whether an Authorization or SODA should be granted to an applicant for a third-class medical certificate, the Federal Air Surgeon considers the freedom of an airman, exercising the privileges of a private pilot certificate, to accept reasonable risks to his or her person and property that are not acceptable in the exercise of commercial or airline transport pilot privileges, and, at the same time, considers the need to protect the safety of persons and property in other aircraft and on the ground.

(f) An Authorization or SODA granted under the provisions of this section to a person who does not meet the applicable provisions of subparts B, C, or D of this part may be withdrawn, at the discretion of the Federal Air Surgeon, at any time if —

(1) There is adverse change in the holder's medical condition;
(2) The holder fails to comply with a statement of functional limitations or operational limitations issued as a condition of certification under this section;
(3) Public safety would be endangered by the holder's exercise of airman privileges;
(4) The holder fails to provide medical information reasonably needed by the Federal Air Surgeon for certification under this section; or
(5) The holder makes or causes to be made a statement or entry that is the basis for withdrawal of an Authorization or SODA under §67.403.

(g) A person who has been granted an Authorization or SODA under this section based on a special medical flight or practical test need not take the test again during later physical examinations unless the Federal Air Surgeon determines or has reason to believe that the physical deficiency has or may have degraded to a degree to require another special medical flight test or practical test.

(h) The authority of the Federal Air Surgeon under this section is also exercised by the Manager, Aeromedical Certification Division, and each Regional Flight Surgeon.

(i) If an Authorization or SODA is withdrawn under paragraph (f) of this section the following procedures apply:
(1) The holder of the Authorization or SODA will be served a letter of withdrawal, stating the reason for the action;
(2) By not later than 60 days after the service of the letter of withdrawal, the holder of the Authorization or SODA may request, in writing, that the Federal Air Surgeon provide for review of the decision to withdraw. The request for review may be accompanied by supporting medical evidence;
(3) Within 60 days of receipt of a request for review, a written final decision either affirming or reversing the decision to withdraw will be issued; and
(4) A medical certificate rendered invalid pursuant to a withdrawal, in accordance with paragraph (a) of this section, shall be surrendered to the Administrator upon request.

(j) An Authorization or SODA granted under the provisions of this section to a person who does not meet the applicable provisions of subparts B, C, or D of this part must be in that person's physical possession or readily accessible in the aircraft.

[Docket No. 27940, 61 FR 11256, Mar. 19, 1996, as amended by Amdt. 67–20, 73 FR 43066, July 24, 2008]

§67.403 Applications, certificates, logbooks, reports, and records: Falsification, reproduction, or alteration; incorrect statements.

(a) No person may make or cause to be made —
   (1) A fraudulent or intentionally false statement on any application for a medical certificate or on a request for any Authorization for Special Issuance of a Medical Certificate (Authorization) or Statement of Demonstrated Ability (SODA) under this part;
   (2) A fraudulent or intentionally false entry in any logbook, record, or report that is kept, made, or used, to show compliance with any requirement for any medical certificate or for any Authorization or SODA under this part;
   (3) A reproduction, for fraudulent purposes, of any medical certificate under this part; or
   (4) An alteration of any medical certificate under this part.
(b) The commission by any person of an act prohibited under paragraph (a) of this section is a basis for —
   (1) Suspending or revoking all airman, ground instructor, and medical certificates and ratings held by that person;
   (2) Withdrawing all Authorizations or SODA's held by that person; and
   (3) Denying all applications for medical certification and requests for Authorizations or SODA's.
(c) The following may serve as a basis for suspending or revoking a medical certificate; withdrawing an Authorization or SODA; or denying an application for a medical certificate or request for an authorization or SODA:

(1) An incorrect statement, upon which the FAA relied, made in support of an application for a medical certificate or request for an Authorization or SODA.
(2) An incorrect entry, upon which the FAA relied, made in any logbook, record, or report that is kept, made, or used to show compliance with any requirement for a medical certificate or an Authorization or SODA.

§67.405 Medical examinations: Who may perform?

(a) *First-class.* Any aviation medical examiner who is specifically designated for the purpose may perform examinations for the first-class medical certificate.
(b) *Second- and third-class.* Any aviation medical examiner may perform examinations for the second- or third-class medical certificate.

[Doc. No. FAA–2007–27812, 73 FR 43066, July 24, 2008]

§67.407 Delegation of authority.

(a) The authority of the Administrator under 49 U.S.C. 44703 to issue or deny medical certificates is delegated to the Federal Air Surgeon to the extent necessary to —
  (1) Examine applicants for and holders of medical certificates to determine whether they meet applicable medical standards; and
  (2) Issue, renew, and deny medical certificates, and issue, renew, deny, and withdraw Authorizations for Special Issuance of a Medical Certificate and Statements of Demonstrated Ability to a person based upon meeting or failing to meet applicable medical standards.
(b) Subject to limitations in this chapter, the delegated functions of the Federal Air Surgeon to examine applicants for and holders of medical certificates for compliance with applicable medical standards and to issue, renew, and deny medical certificates are also delegated to aviation medical examiners and to authorized representatives of the Federal Air Surgeon within the FAA.

(c) The authority of the Administrator under 49 U.S.C. 44702, to reconsider the action of an aviation medical examiner is delegated to the Federal Air Surgeon; the Manager, Aeromedical Certification Division; and each Regional Flight Surgeon. Where the person does not meet the standards of §§67.107(b)(3) and (c), 67.109(b), 67.113(b) and (c), 67.207(b)(3) and (c), 67.209(b), 67.213(b) and (c), 67.307(b)(3) and (c), 67.309(b), or 67.313(b) and (c), any action taken under this paragraph other than by the Federal Air Surgeon is subject to reconsideration by the Federal Air Surgeon. A certificate issued by an aviation medical examiner is considered to be affirmed as issued unless an FAA official named in this paragraph (authorized official) reverses that issuance within 60 days after the date of issuance. However, if within 60 days after the date of issuance an authorized official requests the certificate holder to submit additional medical information, an authorized official may reverse the issuance within 60 days after receipt of the requested information.

(d) The authority of the Administrator under 49 U.S.C. 44709 to re-examine any civil airman to the extent necessary to determine an airman's qualification to continue to hold an airman medical certificate, is delegated to the Federal Air Surgeon and his or her authorized representatives within the FAA.

§67.409 Denial of medical certificate.

(a) Any person who is denied a medical certificate by an aviation medical examiner may, within 30 days after the date of the denial, apply in writing and in duplicate to the Federal Air Surgeon, Attention: Manager, Aeromedical Certification Division, AAM–300, Federal Aviation Administration, P.O. Box 26080, Oklahoma City, Oklahoma 73126, for reconsideration of that denial. If the person does not ask for reconsideration during the 30-day period after the date of the denial, he or she is considered to have withdrawn the application for a medical certificate.

(b) The denial of a medical certificate —

(1) By an aviation medical examiner is not a denial by the Administrator under 49 U.S.C. 44703.
(2) By the Federal Air Surgeon is considered to be a denial by the Administrator under 49 U.S.C. 44703.
(3) By the Manager, Aeromedical Certification Division, or a Regional Flight Surgeon is considered to be a denial by the Administrator under 49 U.S.C. 44703 except where the person does not meet the standards of §§67.107(b)(3) and (c), 67.109(b), or 67.113(b) and (c); 67.207(b)(3) and (c), 67.209(b), or 67.213(b) and (c); or 67.307(b)(3) and (c), 67.309(b), or 67.313(b) and (c).

(c) Any action taken under §67.407(c) that wholly or partly reverses the issue of a medical certificate by an aviation medical examiner is the denial of a medical certificate under paragraph (b) of this section.

(d) If the issue of a medical certificate is wholly or partly reversed by the Federal Air Surgeon; the Manager, Aeromedical Certification Division; or a Regional Flight Surgeon, the person holding that certificate shall surrender it, upon request of the FAA.

§67.411 [Reserved]

§67.413 Medical records.

(a) Whenever the Administrator finds that additional medical information or history is necessary to determine whether you meet the medical standards required to hold a medical certificate, you must:
(1) Furnish that information to the FAA; or
(2) Authorize any clinic, hospital, physician, or other person to release to the FAA all available information or records concerning that history.

(b) If you fail to provide the requested medical information or history or to authorize its release, the FAA may suspend, modify, or revoke your medical certificate or, in the case of an applicant, deny the application for a medical certificate.

(c) If your medical certificate is suspended, modified, or revoked under paragraph (b) of this section, that suspension or modification remains in effect until you provide the requested information, history, or authorization to the FAA and until the FAA determines that you meet the medical standards set forth in this part.

[Doc. No. FAA–2007–27812, 73 FR 43066, July 24, 2008]

§67.415 Return of medical certificate after suspension or revocation.

The holder of any medical certificate issued under this part that is suspended or revoked shall, upon the Administrator's request, return it to the Administrator.

Index